Sectional Anatomy
by MRI and CT

Sectional Anatomy by MRI and CT

THIRD EDITION

Georges Y. El-Khoury, MD
Professor
Departments of Radiology and Orthopaedic Surgery
University of Iowa College of Medicine
Iowa City, Iowa

William J. Montgomery, MD
Associate Professor
Department of Radiology
University of Florida College of Medicine
Gainesville, Florida

Ronald A. Bergman, PhD
Professor Emeritus
Department of Anatomy
University of Iowa College of Medicine
Iowa City, Iowa

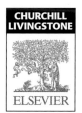

CHURCHILL
LIVINGSTONE

ELSEVIER

CHURCHILL LIVINGSTONE
ELSEVIER

1600 John F. Kennedy Blvd.
Ste 1800
Philadelphia, PA 19103-2899

SECTIONAL ANATOMY BY MRI AND CT ISBN: 978-0-443- 06666-5

Copyright © 2007, 1995, 1990 by Churchill Livingstone, an imprint of Elsevier Inc.

Notice

Neither the Publisher nor the Editors assume any responsibility for any loss or injury and/or damage to persons or property arising out of or related to any use of the material contained in this book. It is the responsibility of the treating practitioner, relying on independent expertise and knowledge of the patient, to determine the best treatment and method of application for the patient.

The Publisher

Library of Congress Cataloging-in-Publication Data
El-Khoury, Georges Y.
  Sectional anatomy by MRI and CT / Georges Y. El-Khoury, William J. Montgomery, Ronald A. Bergman.—3rd ed.
    p. ; cm.
  Rev. ed. of: Sectional anatomy by MRI / Georges Y. El-Khoury, Ronald A. Bergman, William J. Montgomery. 1995.
    ISBN-13: 978-0-443-06666-5   ISBN-10: 0-443-06666-3
    1. Human anatomy—Atlases. 2. Magnetic resonance imaging—Atlases. 3. Tomography—Atlases. I. Montgomery, William J. II. Bergman, Ronald A. (Ronald Arly). III. El-Khoury, Georges Y. Sectional anatomy by MRI. IV. Title.
    [DNLM: 1. Anatomy, Regional—Atlases. 2. Magnetic Resonance Imaging—Atlases. QS 17 E44s 2007]
  QM25.E38 2007
  611'.90222–dc22

                              2006030553

ISBN: 978-0-443-06666-5

Acquisitions Editor: Rebecca Gaertner
Developmental Editor: Kim Davis and Scott Scheidt
Publishing Services Manager: Tina Rebane
Project Manager: Amy Norwitz
Design Direction: Lou Forgione

Cover illustrations are by Leonardo da Vinci and were made available by The Royal Collection © 2006 Her Majesty Queen Elizabeth II.

Printed in the United States of America

Working together to grow libraries in developing countries

www.elsevier.com | www.bookaid.org | www.sabre.org

ELSEVIER   BOOK AID International   Sabre Foundation

Last digit is the print number: 9 8 7 6 5 4 3 2

To our wives, Salam, Phyllis, and Nancy.
Without their love and support, this work would not have been possible.

Associate Editors

Carol A. Boles, MD
Associate Professor
Department of Radiology
Wake-Forest University School of Medicine
Winston-Salem, North Carolina

Mark J. Kransdorf, MD
Professor
Department of Radiology
Mayo Clinic Jacksonville
Jacksonville, Florida

Brian F. Mullan, MD
Associate Professor
Department of Radiology
University of Iowa College of Medicine
Iowa City, Iowa

Alan H. Stolpen, MD, PhD
Associate Professor
Department of Radiology
University of Iowa College of Medicine
Iowa City, Iowa

Contributors

Timothy Averion-Mahloch, MD
Department of Radiology
Lexington Clinic
Lexington, Kentucky

Carol A. Boles, MD
Associate Professor
Department of Radiology
Wake-Forest University School of Medicine
Winston-Salem, North Carolina

Kousei Ishigami, MD
Staff Radiologist
Department of Radiology
Abdominal Imaging Group
Kyushu University Hospital
Fukuoka City, Fukuoka
Japan

Mark J. Kransdorf, MD
Professor
Department of Radiology
Mayo Clinic Jacksonville
Jacksonville, Florida

Thomas P. Martin, MD
X-Ray Associates of New Mexico
Albuquerque, New Mexico

William J. Montgomery, MD
Associate Professor
Department of Radiology
University of Florida College of Medicine
Gainesville, Florida

Brian F. Mullan, MD
Associate Professor
Department of Radiology
University of Iowa College of Medicine
Iowa City, Iowa

Akihiro Nishie, MD
Visiting Assistant Professor
Department of Radiology
University of Iowa College of Medicine
Iowa City, Iowa

Alan H. Stolpen, MD, PhD
Associate Professor
Department of Radiology
University of Iowa College of Medicine
Iowa City, Iowa

Preface

It has been 17 years since publication of the first edition of this atlas, and 12 years since the second edition. In the past 12 years, magnetic resonance imaging (MRI) improved and multi-detector row computed tomography (MDCT) came into being. This resulted in stunning advances in the imaging subspecialties as tiny structures and minimal abnormalities became easier to visualize. Three years ago, we started contacting experts from the different subspecialties to help us acquire and annotate high-quality images. Because of the advances in imaging, we have replaced all of the images from the previous two editions with state-of-the-art images.

We have made some organizational changes since the last edition. We have included complete sets of MR and MDCT images of the thorax and abdomen and have assigned them separate chapters. Because MRI studies of the shoulder focus on the shoulder joint and do not include muscles of the shoulder girdle, which originate from the chest wall, we added a new chapter, "MRI of the Pectoral Girdle and Chest Wall." In the past few years shoulder MR arthrography and hip MR arthrography have become common diagnostic procedures, so we dedicated specific chapters to these topics. For MRI studies of the ankle, we observed that thorough evaluation often requires images in more than the standard three planes (axial, sagittal, and coronal), and to rectify this we added an imaging sequence obtained in the oblique axial plane.

To maintain uniformity throughout the atlas, we implemented a few other changes. Imaging of all extremity parts was acquired from structures on the right side of the body. All axial series in this atlas start proximally (or cephalic) and progress distally (or caudad). Sagittal series start laterally and progress medially. Coronal sections start anteriorly (or ventrally) and progress posteriorly. We have used familiar abbreviations to save space and provide a key at the beginning of each chapter.

In the previous editions, we invested a significant amount of time and space on creating text to describe anatomic relations for each image. In response to users' feedback that the text was not essential in the typical daily practice of radiology, we have eliminated the text and have used the space for additional MR and CT images.

While anatomy is an enduring discipline in which little or no changes occur, it is obvious, when comparing images from the previous editions with the current ones, that the detail and spatial resolution have made a quantum leap.

We are excited about this edition, and we hope that for the next few years this atlas will continue to fulfill the needs of our colleagues in diagnostic radiology.

Georges Y. El-Khoury, MD
William J. Montgomery, MD
Ronald A. Bergman, PhD

Acknowledgments

We would like to acknowledge Paul Reimann for creating the line drawings that accompany the labeled images, and Phyllis S. Bergman for her assistance with editorial issues. We thank Dr. Joong Mo Ahn for his expertise and help with some of the anatomic details in the musculoskeletal system. We are also grateful to Mary McBride for secretarial assistance during the entire project. Ms. Kim Davis, Developmental Editor, gave us daily advice and guidance, and we are greatly appreciative of this help. Thanks also to Amy Norwitz, Senior Project Manager, for her expertise. We would also like to thank our Associate Editors and Contributors, who put numerous hours of work into this book.

Georges Y. El-Khoury, MD
William J. Montgomery, MD
Ronald A. Bergman, PhD

Contents

Upper Extremity

Chapter 1

MRI of the Pectoral Girdle and Chest Wall

AXIAL

Figure 1.1.1

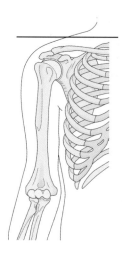

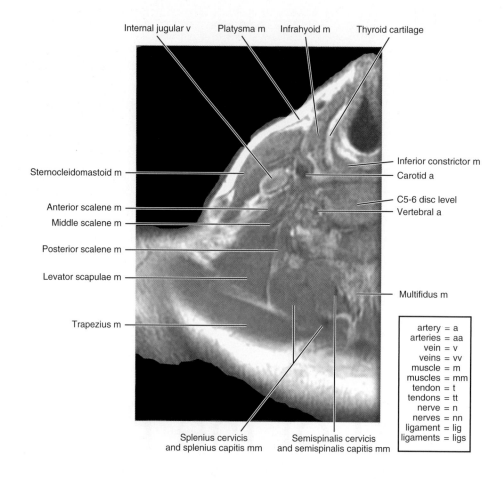

Internal jugular v   Platysma m   Infrahyoid m   Thyroid cartilage

Sternocleidomastoid m

Anterior scalene m

Middle scalene m

Posterior scalene m

Levator scapulae m

Trapezius m

Inferior constrictor m

Carotid a

C5-6 disc level

Vertebral a

Multifidus m

Splenius cervicis
and splenius capitis mm

Semispinalis cervicis
and semispinalis capitis mm

artery	= a
arteries	= aa
vein	= v
veins	= vv
muscle	= m
muscles	= mm
tendon	= t
tendons	= tt
nerve	= n
nerves	= nn
ligament	= lig
ligaments	= ligs

Figure 1.1.2

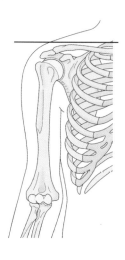

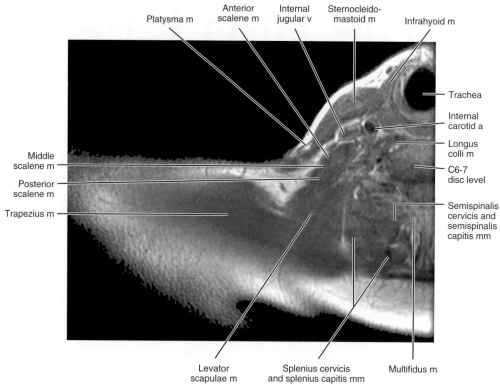

Platysma m   Anterior
scalene m   Internal
jugular v   Sternocleidomastoid m   Infrahyoid m

Middle
scalene m

Posterior
scalene m

Trapezius m

Trachea

Internal
carotid a

Longus
colli m

C6-7
disc level

Semispinalis
cervicis and
semispinalis
capitis mm

Levator
scapulae m

Splenius cervicis
and splenius capitis mm

Multifidus m

Figure 1.1.3

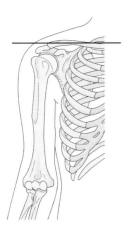

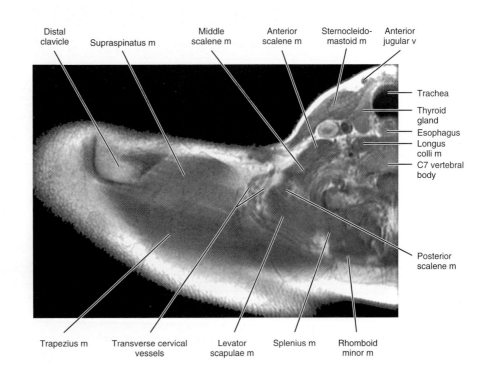

Distal clavicle — Supraspinatus m — Middle scalene m — Anterior scalene m — Sternocleido-mastoid m — Anterior jugular v

Trachea
Thyroid gland
Esophagus
Longus colli m
C7 vertebral body

Posterior scalene m

Trapezius m — Transverse cervical vessels — Levator scapulae m — Splenius m — Rhomboid minor m

Figure 1.1.4

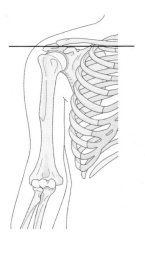

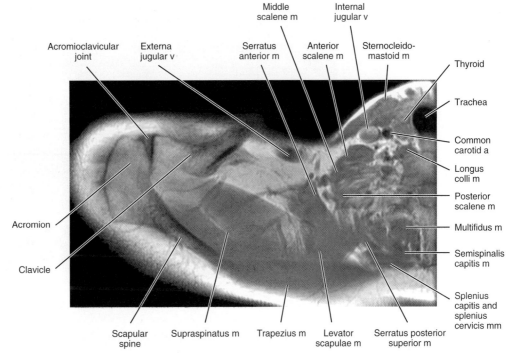

Acromioclavicular joint — Externa jugular v — Serratus anterior m — Middle scalene m — Anterior scalene m — Internal jugular v — Sternocleido-mastoid m

Thyroid
Trachea
Common carotid a
Longus colli m
Posterior scalene m
Multifidus m
Semispinalis capitis m
Splenius capitis and splenius cervicis mm

Acromion

Clavicle

Scapular spine — Supraspinatus m — Trapezius m — Levator scapulae m — Serratus posterior superior m

Figure 1.1.5

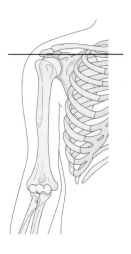

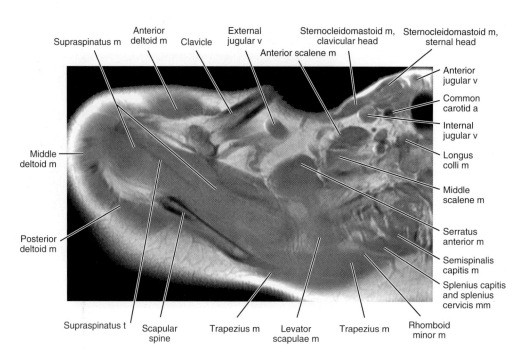

Supraspinatus m — Anterior deltoid m — Clavicle — External jugular v — Sternocleidomastoid m, clavicular head — Sternocleidomastoid m, sternal head — Anterior scalene m

Anterior jugular v
Common carotid a
Internal jugular v
Longus colli m
Middle scalene m
Serratus anterior m
Semispinalis capitis m
Splenius capitis and splenius cervicis mm

Middle deltoid m

Posterior deltoid m

Supraspinatus t — Scapular spine — Trapezius m — Levator scapulae m — Trapezius m — Rhomboid minor m

Figure 1.1.6

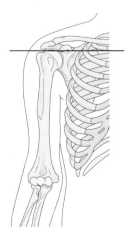

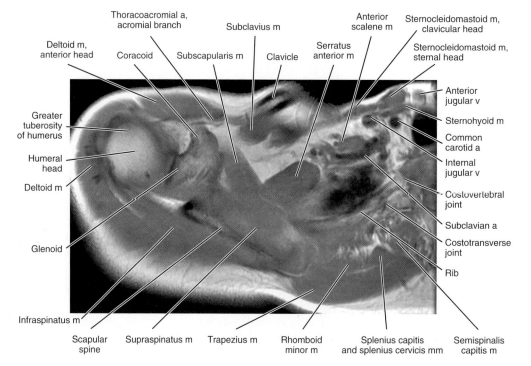

Thoracoacromial a, acromial branch — Subclavius m — Anterior scalene m — Sternocleidomastoid m, clavicular head

Deltoid m, anterior head — Coracoid — Subscapularis m — Clavicle — Serratus anterior m — Sternocleidomastoid m, sternal head

Greater tuberosity of humerus

Humeral head

Deltoid m

Glenoid

Anterior jugular v
Sternohyoid m
Common carotid a
Internal jugular v
Costovertebral joint
Subclavian a
Costotransverse joint
Rib

Infraspinatus m — Scapular spine — Supraspinatus m — Trapezius m — Rhomboid minor m — Splenius capitis and splenius cervicis mm — Semispinalis capitis m

Figure 1.1.7

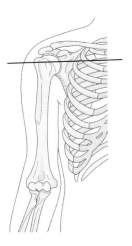

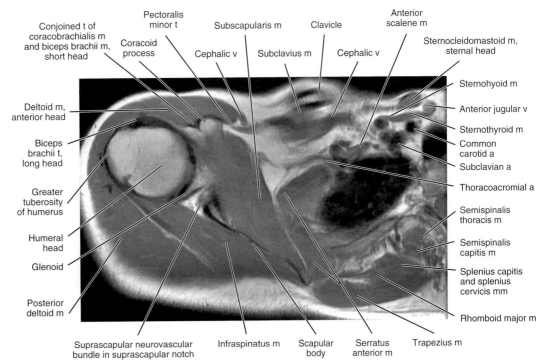

Conjoined t of coracobrachialis m and biceps brachii m, short head

Coracoid process

Pectoralis minor t

Cephalic v

Subscapularis m

Subclavius m

Clavicle

Cephalic v

Anterior scalene m

Sternocleidomastoid m, sternal head

Deltoid m, anterior head

Biceps brachii t, long head

Greater tuberosity of humerus

Humeral head

Glenoid

Posterior deltoid m

Sternohyoid m

Anterior jugular v

Sternothyroid m

Common carotid a

Subclavian a

Thoracoacromial a

Semispinalis thoracis m

Semispinalis capitis m

Splenius capitis and splenius cervicis mm

Rhomboid major m

Suprascapular neurovascular bundle in suprascapular notch

Infraspinatus m

Scapular body

Serratus anterior m

Trapezius m

Figure 1.1.8

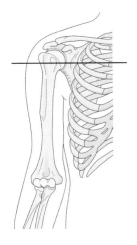

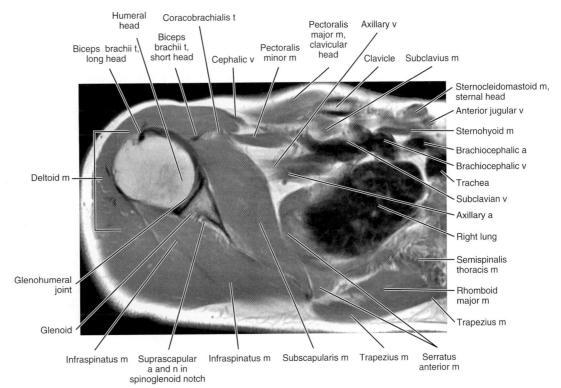

Humeral head

Coracobrachialis t

Biceps brachii t, long head

Biceps brachii t, short head

Cephalic v

Pectoralis minor m

Pectoralis major m, clavicular head

Axillary v

Clavicle

Subclavius m

Deltoid m

Glenohumeral joint

Glenoid

Sternocleidomastoid m, sternal head

Anterior jugular v

Sternohyoid m

Brachiocephalic a

Brachiocephalic v

Trachea

Subclavian v

Axillary a

Right lung

Semispinalis thoracis m

Rhomboid major m

Trapezius m

Infraspinatus m

Suprascapular a and n in spinoglenoid notch

Infraspinatus m

Subscapularis m

Trapezius m

Serratus anterior m

Figure 1.1.9

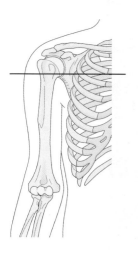

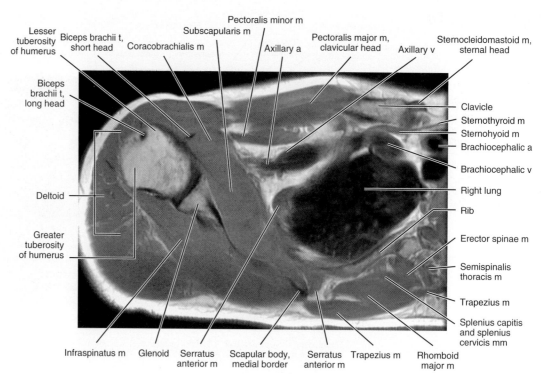

Lesser tuberosity of humerus
Biceps brachii t, short head
Coracobrachialis m
Pectoralis minor m
Subscapularis m
Axillary a
Pectoralis major m, clavicular head
Axillary v
Sternocleidomastoid m, sternal head

Biceps brachii t, long head

Deltoid

Greater tuberosity of humerus

Clavicle
Sternothyroid m
Sternohyoid m
Brachiocephalic a
Brachiocephalic v
Right lung
Rib
Erector spinae m
Semispinalis thoracis m
Trapezius m
Splenius capitis and splenius cervicis mm

Infraspinatus m
Glenoid
Serratus anterior m
Scapular body, medial border
Serratus anterior m
Trapezius m
Rhomboid major m

Figure 1.1.10

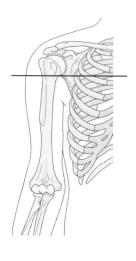

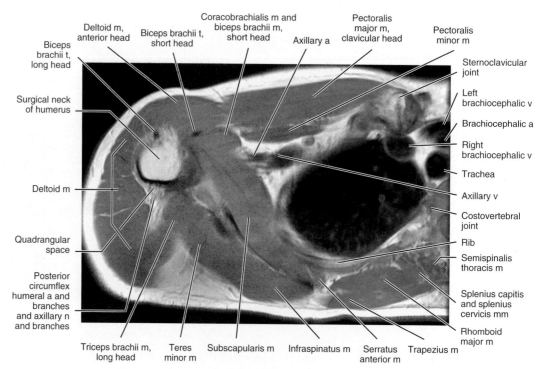

Deltoid m, anterior head
Biceps brachii t, short head
Coracobrachialis m and biceps brachii m, short head
Axillary a
Pectoralis major m, clavicular head
Pectoralis minor m

Biceps brachii t, long head

Surgical neck of humerus

Deltoid m

Quadrangular space

Posterior circumflex humeral a and branches and axillary n and branches

Sternoclavicular joint
Left brachiocephalic v
Brachiocephalic a
Right brachiocephalic v
Trachea
Axillary v
Costovertebral joint
Rib
Semispinalis thoracis m
Splenius capitis and splenius cervicis mm
Rhomboid major m

Triceps brachii m, long head
Teres minor m
Subscapularis m
Infraspinatus m
Serratus anterior m
Trapezius m

Figure 1.1.11

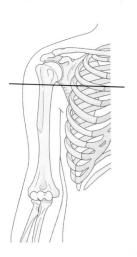

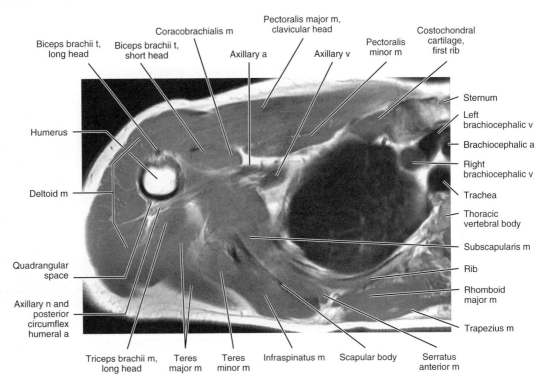

Biceps brachii t, long head
Biceps brachii t, short head
Coracobrachialis m
Axillary a
Pectoralis major m, clavicular head
Axillary v
Pectoralis minor m
Costochondral cartilage, first rib
Humerus
Sternum
Left brachiocephalic v
Brachiocephalic a
Right brachiocephalic v
Deltoid m
Trachea
Thoracic vertebral body
Subscapularis m
Quadrangular space
Rib
Rhomboid major m
Axillary n and posterior circumflex humeral a
Trapezius m
Triceps brachii m, long head
Teres major m
Teres minor m
Infraspinatus m
Scapular body
Serratus anterior m

Figure 1.1.12

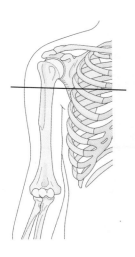

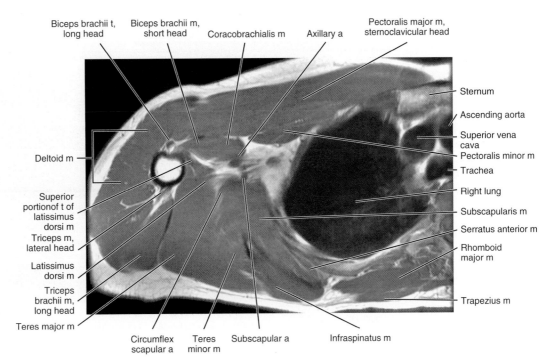

Biceps brachii t, long head
Biceps brachii m, short head
Coracobrachialis m
Axillary a
Pectoralis major m, sternoclavicular head
Deltoid m
Sternum
Ascending aorta
Superior vena cava
Pectoralis minor m
Superior portionof t of latissimus dorsi m
Trachea
Triceps m, lateral head
Right lung
Subscapularis m
Latissimus dorsi m
Serratus anterior m
Rhomboid major m
Triceps brachii m, long head
Teres major m
Trapezius m
Circumflex scapular a
Teres minor m
Subscapular a
Infraspinatus m

Figure 1.1.13

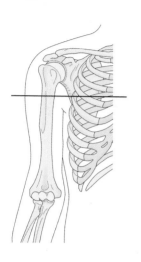

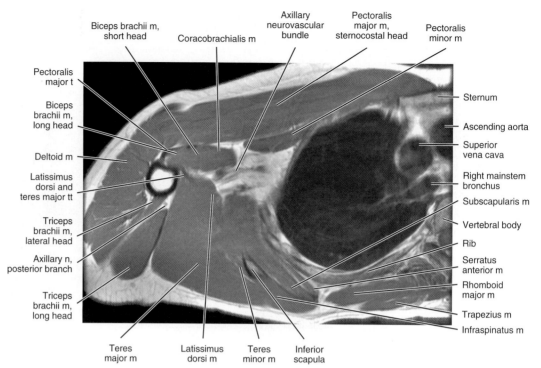

Biceps brachii m, short head

Coracobrachialis m

Axillary neurovascular bundle

Pectoralis major m, sternocostal head

Pectoralis minor m

Pectoralis major t

Biceps brachii m, long head

Deltoid m

Latissimus dorsi and teres major tt

Triceps brachii m, lateral head

Axillary n, posterior branch

Triceps brachii m, long head

Sternum

Ascending aorta

Superior vena cava

Right mainstem bronchus

Subscapularis m

Vertebral body

Rib

Serratus anterior m

Rhomboid major m

Trapezius m

Infraspinatus m

Teres major m

Latissimus dorsi m

Teres minor m

Inferior scapula

Figure 1.1.14

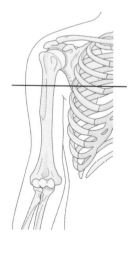

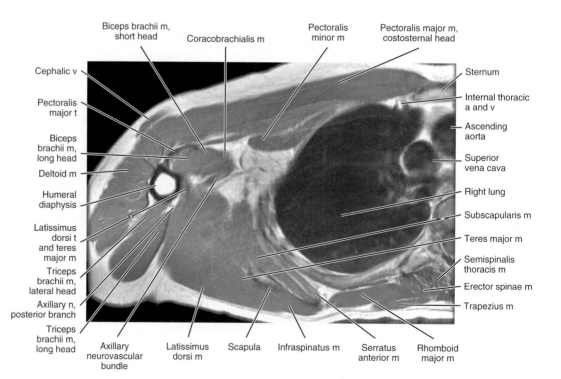

Biceps brachii m, short head

Coracobrachialis m

Pectoralis minor m

Pectoralis major m, costosternal head

Cephalic v

Pectoralis major t

Biceps brachii m, long head

Deltoid m

Humeral diaphysis

Latissimus dorsi t and teres major m

Triceps brachii m, lateral head

Axillary n, posterior branch

Triceps brachii m, long head

Axillary neurovascular bundle

Latissimus dorsi m

Scapula

Infraspinatus m

Serratus anterior m

Rhomboid major m

Sternum

Internal thoracic a and v

Ascending aorta

Superior vena cava

Right lung

Subscapularis m

Teres major m

Semispinalis thoracis m

Erector spinae m

Trapezius m

Figure 1.1.15

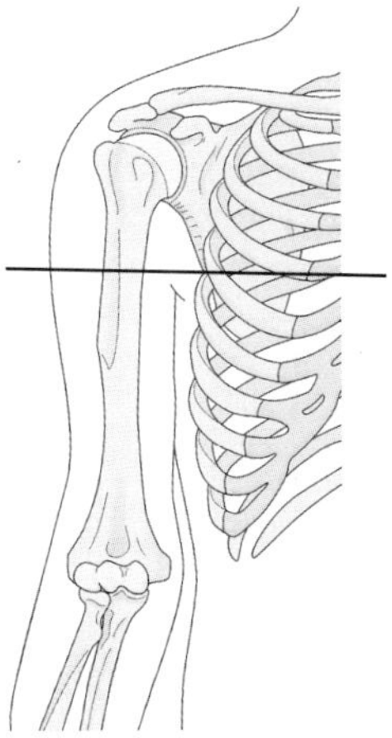

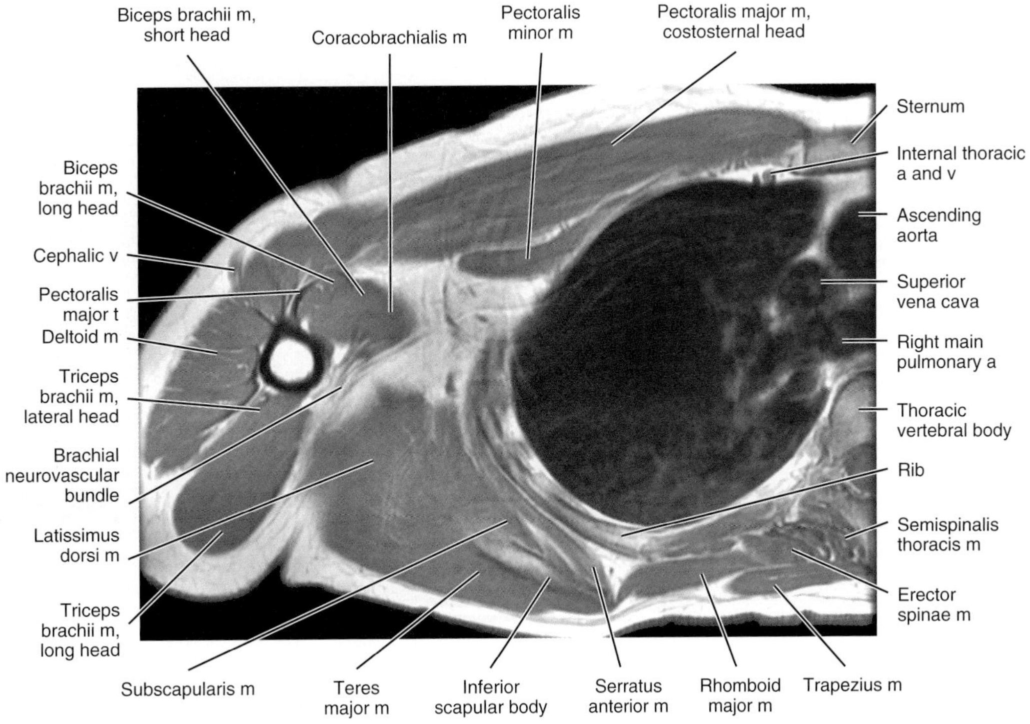

Biceps brachii m, short head
Coracobrachialis m
Pectoralis minor m
Pectoralis major m, costosternal head

Biceps brachii m, long head
Cephalic v
Pectoralis major t
Deltoid m
Triceps brachii m, lateral head
Brachial neurovascular bundle
Latissimus dorsi m
Triceps brachii m, long head

Sternum
Internal thoracic a and v
Ascending aorta
Superior vena cava
Right main pulmonary a
Thoracic vertebral body
Rib
Semispinalis thoracis m
Erector spinae m

Subscapularis m
Teres major m
Inferior scapular body
Serratus anterior m
Rhomboid major m
Trapezius m

Figure 1.1.16

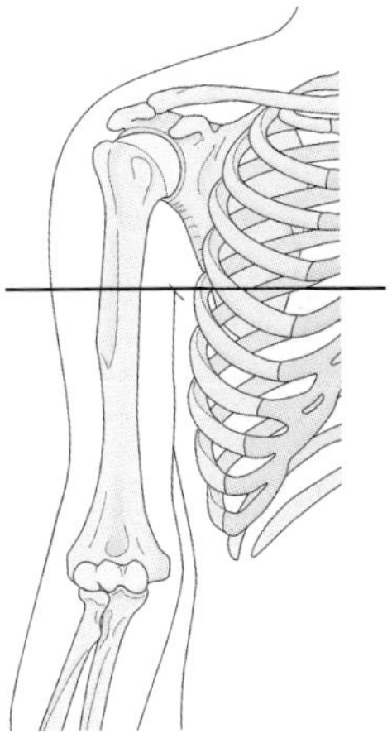

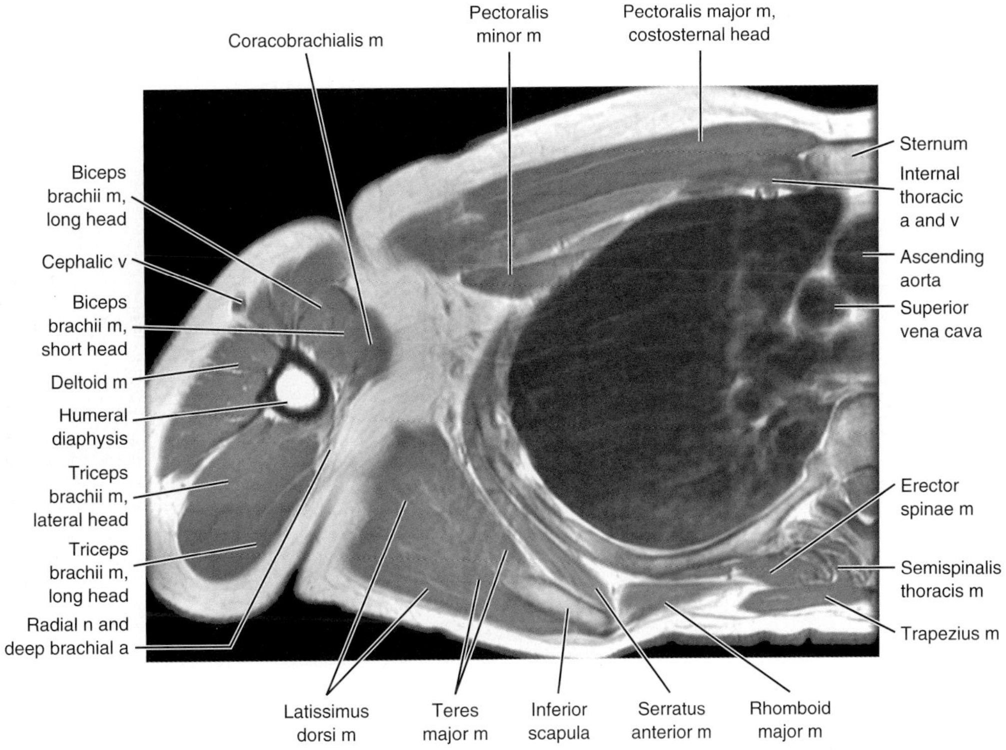

Coracobrachialis m
Pectoralis minor m
Pectoralis major m, costosternal head

Biceps brachii m, long head
Cephalic v
Biceps brachii m, short head
Deltoid m
Humeral diaphysis
Triceps brachii m, lateral head
Triceps brachii m, long head
Radial n and deep brachial a

Sternum
Internal thoracic a and v
Ascending aorta
Superior vena cava
Erector spinae m
Semispinalis thoracis m
Trapezius m

Latissimus dorsi m
Teres major m
Inferior scapula
Serratus anterior m
Rhomboid major m

Figure 1.1.17

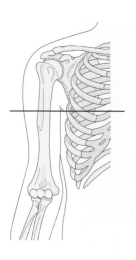

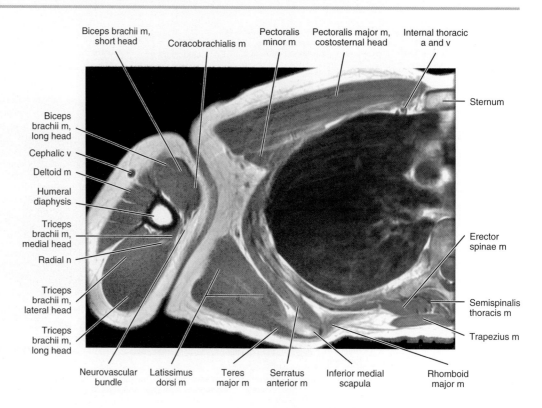

Biceps brachii m, short head

Coracobrachialis m

Pectoralis minor m

Pectoralis major m, costosternal head

Internal thoracic a and v

Biceps brachii m, long head

Cephalic v

Deltoid m

Humeral diaphysis

Triceps brachii m, medial head

Radial n

Triceps brachii m, lateral head

Triceps brachii m, long head

Neurovascular bundle

Latissimus dorsi m

Teres major m

Serratus anterior m

Inferior medial scapula

Rhomboid major m

Sternum

Erector spinae m

Semispinalis thoracis m

Trapezius m

Figure 1.1.18

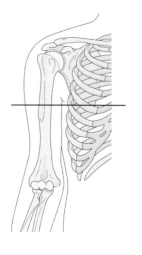

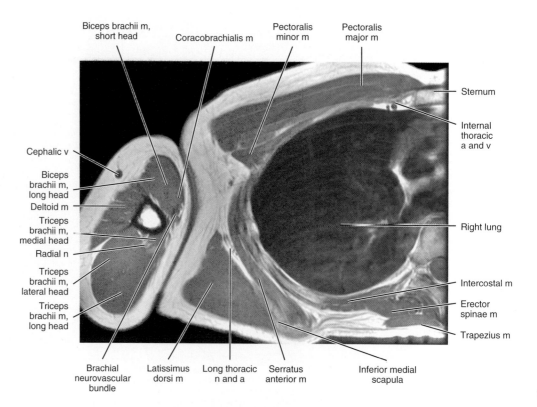

Biceps brachii m, short head

Coracobrachialis m

Pectoralis minor m

Pectoralis major m

Cephalic v

Biceps brachii m, long head

Deltoid m

Triceps brachii m, medial head

Radial n

Triceps brachii m, lateral head

Triceps brachii m, long head

Brachial neurovascular bundle

Latissimus dorsi m

Long thoracic n and a

Serratus anterior m

Inferior medial scapula

Sternum

Internal thoracic a and v

Right lung

Intercostal m

Erector spinae m

Trapezius m

Figure 1.1.19

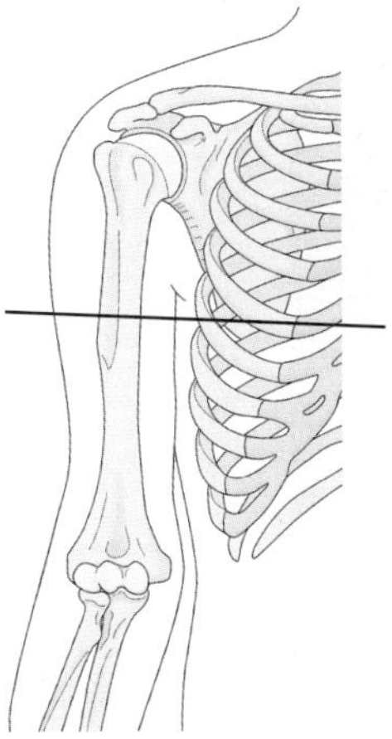

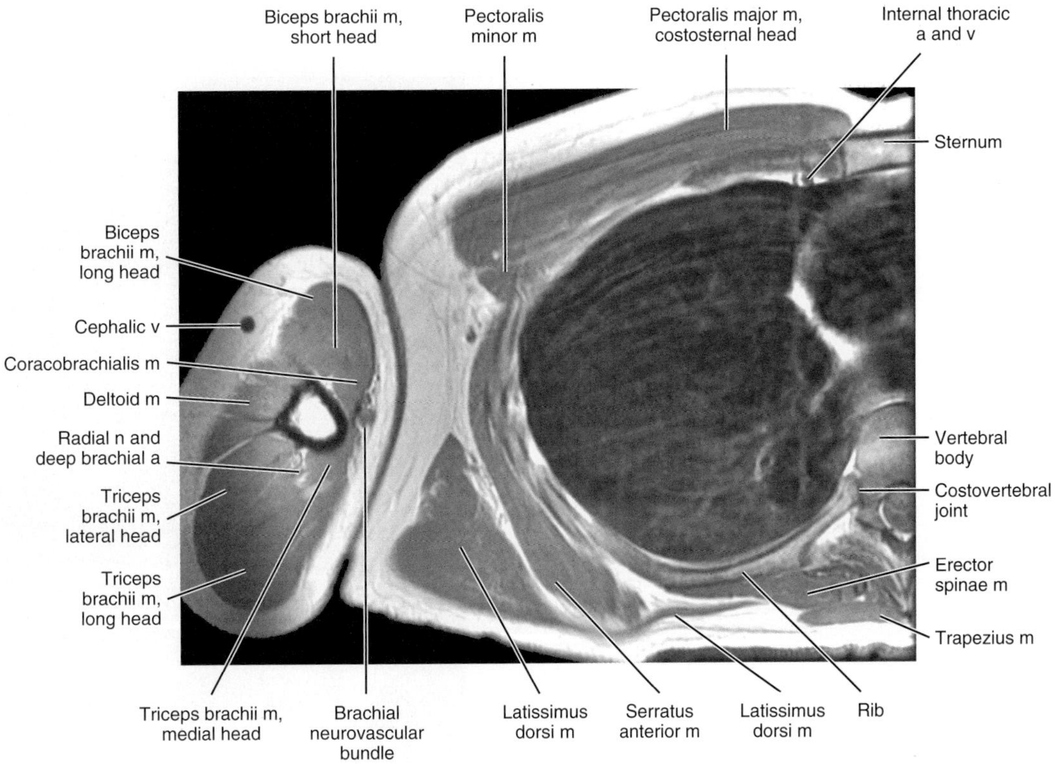
Biceps brachii m, short head
Pectoralis minor m
Pectoralis major m, costosternal head
Internal thoracic a and v
Sternum
Biceps brachii m, long head
Cephalic v
Coracobrachialis m
Deltoid m
Radial n and deep brachial a
Triceps brachii m, lateral head
Triceps brachii m, long head
Vertebral body
Costovertebral joint
Erector spinae m
Trapezius m
Triceps brachii m, medial head
Brachial neurovascular bundle
Latissimus dorsi m
Serratus anterior m
Latissimus dorsi m
Rib

SAGITTAL

Figure 1.2.1

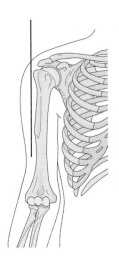

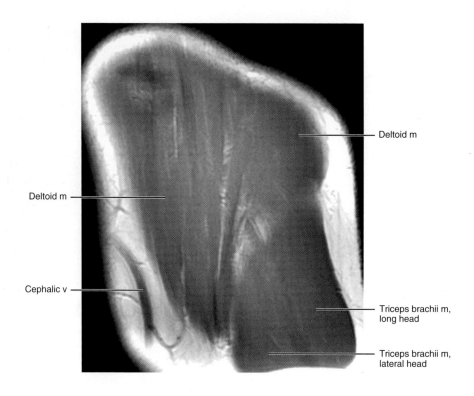

Deltoid m

Deltoid m

Cephalic v

Triceps brachii m, long head

Triceps brachii m, lateral head

Figure 1.2.2

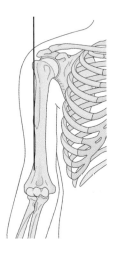

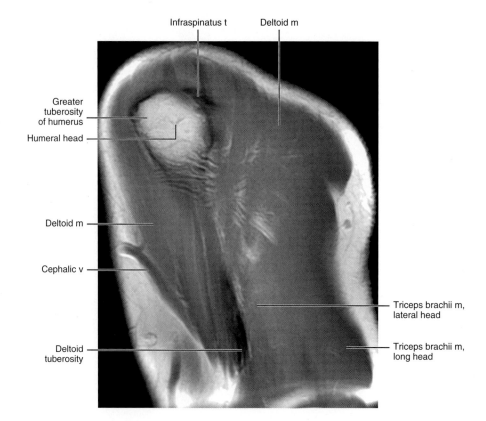

Infraspinatus t

Deltoid m

Greater tuberosity of humerus

Humeral head

Deltoid m

Cephalic v

Deltoid tuberosity

Triceps brachii m, lateral head

Triceps brachii m, long head

Figure 1.2.3

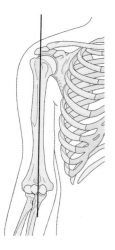

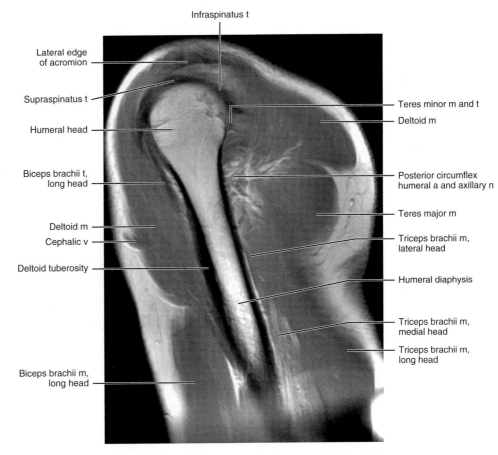

Infraspinatus t

Lateral edge of acromion

Supraspinatus t

Humeral head

Biceps brachii t, long head

Deltoid m

Cephalic v

Deltoid tuberosity

Biceps brachii m, long head

Teres minor m and t

Deltoid m

Posterior circumflex humeral a and axillary n

Teres major m

Triceps brachii m, lateral head

Humeral diaphysis

Triceps brachii m, medial head

Triceps brachii m, long head

Figure 1.2.4

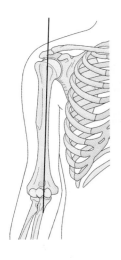

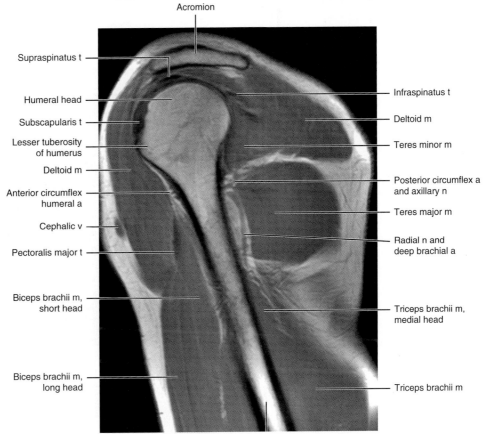

Acromion

Supraspinatus t

Humeral head

Subscapularis t

Lesser tuberosity of humerus

Deltoid m

Anterior circumflex humeral a

Cephalic v

Pectoralis major t

Biceps brachii m, short head

Biceps brachii m, long head

Infraspinatus t

Deltoid m

Teres minor m

Posterior circumflex a and axillary n

Teres major m

Radial n and deep brachial a

Triceps brachii m, medial head

Triceps brachii m

Figure 1.2.5

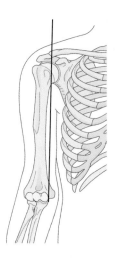

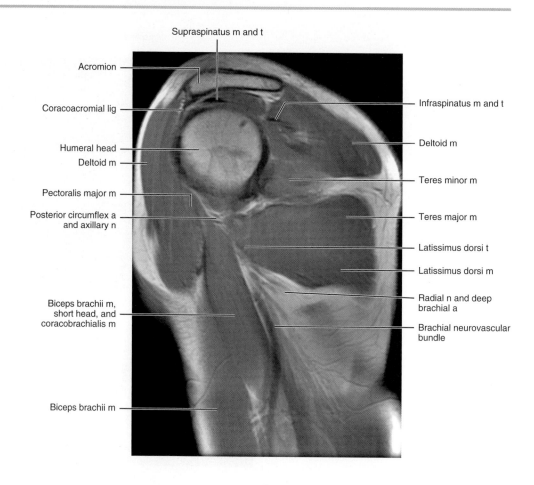

Supraspinatus m and t

Acromion

Coracoacromial lig

Humeral head

Deltoid m

Pectoralis major m

Posterior circumflex a
and axillary n

Biceps brachii m,
short head, and
coracobrachialis m

Biceps brachii m

Infraspinatus m and t

Deltoid m

Teres minor m

Teres major m

Latissimus dorsi t

Latissimus dorsi m

Radial n and deep
brachial a

Brachial neurovascular
bundle

Figure 1.2.6

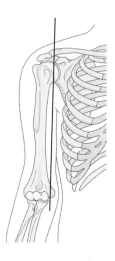

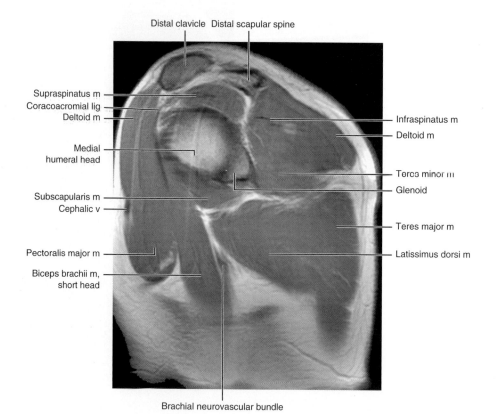

Distal clavicle   Distal scapular spine

Supraspinatus m

Coracoacromial lig

Deltoid m

Medial
humeral head

Subscapularis m

Cephalic v

Pectoralis major m

Biceps brachii m,
short head

Infraspinatus m

Deltoid m

Teres minor m

Glenoid

Teres major m

Latissimus dorsi m

Brachial neurovascular bundle

Figure 1.2.7

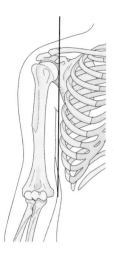

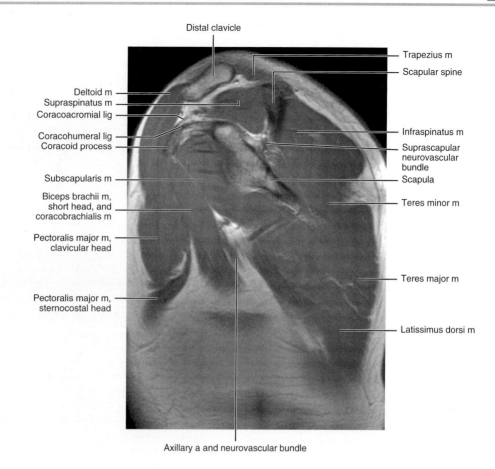

Distal clavicle

Trapezius m

Scapular spine

Deltoid m

Supraspinatus m

Coracoacromial lig

Coracohumeral lig

Coracoid process

Infraspinatus m

Suprascapular neurovascular bundle

Subscapularis m

Scapula

Biceps brachii m, short head, and coracobrachialis m

Teres minor m

Pectoralis major m, clavicular head

Pectoralis major m, sternocostal head

Teres major m

Latissimus dorsi m

Axillary a and neurovascular bundle

Figure 1.2.8

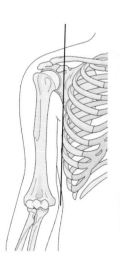

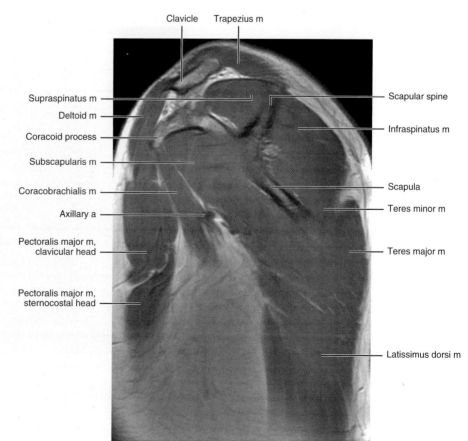

Clavicle   Trapezius m

Supraspinatus m

Deltoid m

Coracoid process

Subscapularis m

Coracobrachialis m

Axillary a

Scapular spine

Infraspinatus m

Scapula

Teres minor m

Pectoralis major m, clavicular head

Pectoralis major m, sternocostal head

Teres major m

Latissimus dorsi m

Figure 1.2.9

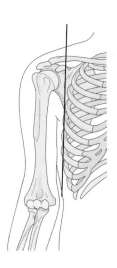

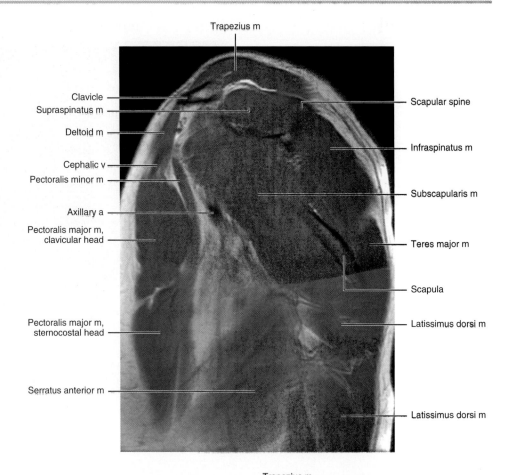

Trapezius m

Clavicle

Suprasinatus m

Deltoid m

Cephalic v

Pectoralis minor m

Axillary a

Pectoralis major m, clavicular head

Pectoralis major m, sternocostal head

Serratus anterior m

Scapular spine

Infraspinatus m

Subscapularis m

Teres major m

Scapula

Latissimus dorsi m

Latissimus dorsi m

Figure 1.2.10

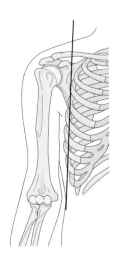

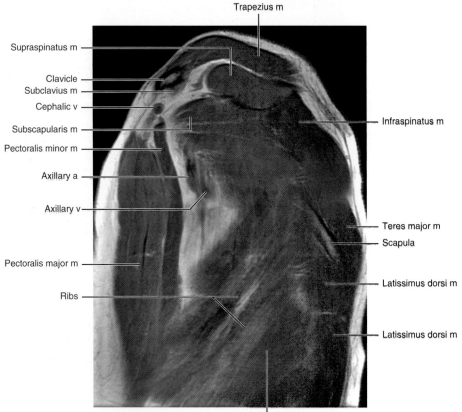

Trapezius m

Suprasinatus m

Clavicle

Subclavius m

Cephalic v

Subscapularis m

Pectoralis minor m

Axillary a

Axillary v

Pectoralis major m

Ribs

Infraspinatus m

Teres major m

Scapula

Latissimus dorsi m

Latissimus dorsi m

Serratus anterior m

Figure 1.2.11

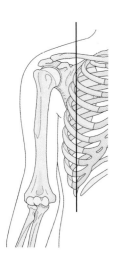

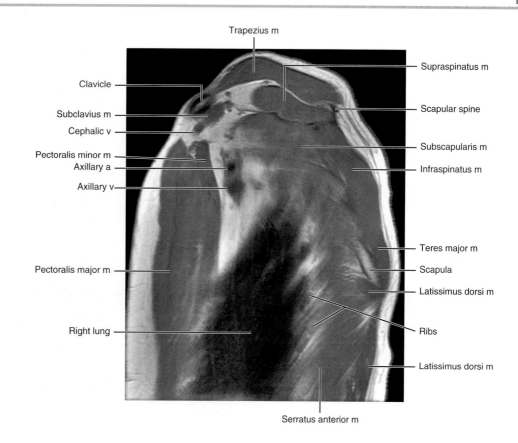

Trapezius m

Clavicle

Subclavius m

Cephalic v

Pectoralis minor m
Axillary a

Axillary v

Pectoralis major m

Right lung

Supraspinatus m

Scapular spine

Subscapularis m

Infraspinatus m

Teres major m

Scapula

Latissimus dorsi m

Ribs

Latissimus dorsi m

Serratus anterior m

Figure 1.2.12

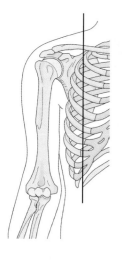

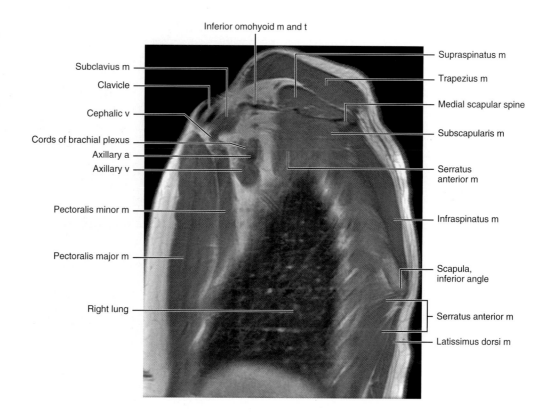

Inferior omohyoid m and t

Subclavius m

Clavicle

Cephalic v

Cords of brachial plexus
Axillary a
Axillary v

Pectoralis minor m

Pectoralis major m

Right lung

Supraspinatus m

Trapezius m

Medial scapular spine

Subscapularis m

Serratus
anterior m

Infraspinatus m

Scapula,
inferior angle

Serratus anterior m

Latissimus dorsi m

Figure 1.2.13

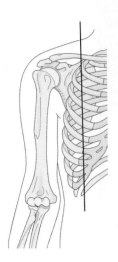

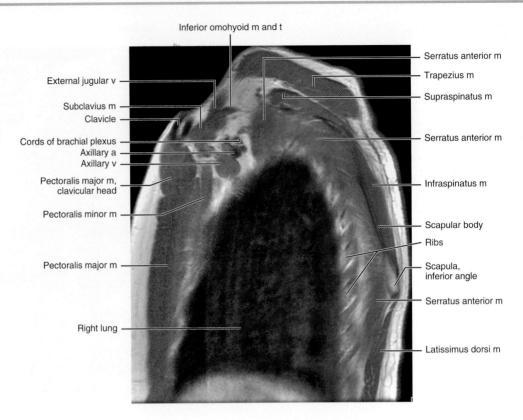

Inferior omohyoid m and t

External jugular v

Subclavius m

Clavicle

Cords of brachial plexus

Axillary a

Axillary v

Pectoralis major m, clavicular head

Pectoralis minor m

Pectoralis major m

Right lung

Serratus anterior m

Trapezius m

Supraspinatus m

Serratus anterior m

Infraspinatus m

Scapular body

Ribs

Scapula, inferior angle

Serratus anterior m

Latissimus dorsi m

Figure 1.2.14

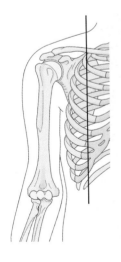

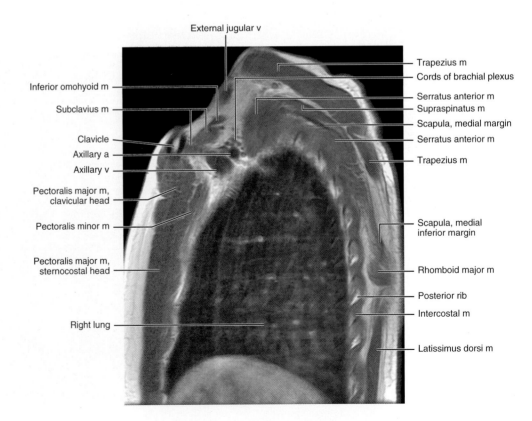

External jugular v

Inferior omohyoid m

Subclavius m

Clavicle

Axillary a

Axillary v

Pectoralis major m, clavicular head

Pectoralis minor m

Pectoralis major m, sternocostal head

Right lung

Trapezius m

Cords of brachial plexus

Serratus anterior m

Supraspinatus m

Scapula, medial margin

Serratus anterior m

Trapezius m

Scapula, medial inferior margin

Rhomboid major m

Posterior rib

Intercostal m

Latissimus dorsi m

Figure 1.2.15

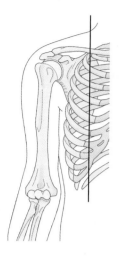

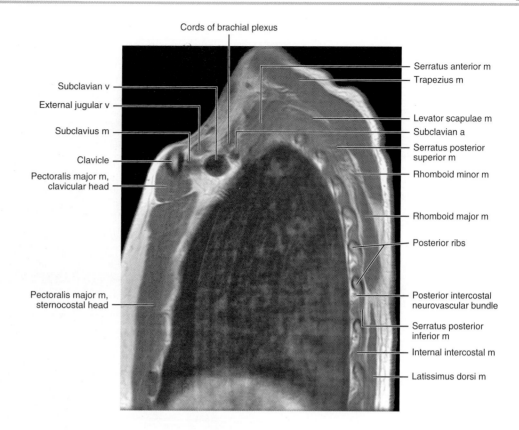

Cords of brachial plexus

Subclavian v

External jugular v

Subclavius m

Clavicle

Pectoralis major m, clavicular head

Pectoralis major m, sternocostal head

Serratus anterior m

Trapezius m

Levator scapulae m

Subclavian a

Serratus posterior superior m

Rhomboid minor m

Rhomboid major m

Posterior ribs

Posterior intercostal neurovascular bundle

Serratus posterior inferior m

Internal intercostal m

Latissimus dorsi m

Figure 1.2.16

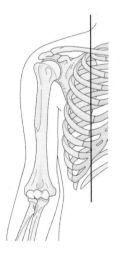

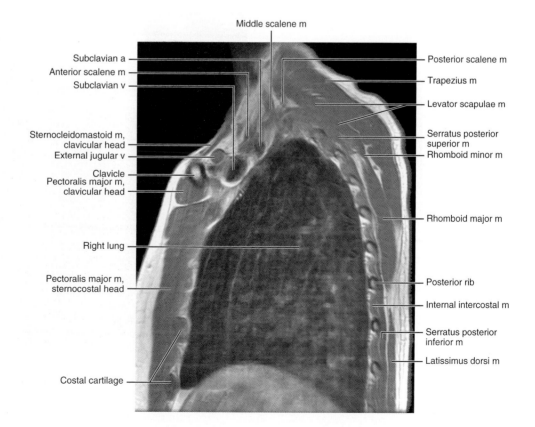

Middle scalene m

Subclavian a

Anterior scalene m

Subclavian v

Sternocleidomastoid m, clavicular head

External jugular v

Clavicle
Pectoralis major m, clavicular head

Right lung

Pectoralis major m, sternocostal head

Costal cartilage

Posterior scalene m

Trapezius m

Levator scapulae m

Serratus posterior superior m

Rhomboid minor m

Rhomboid major m

Posterior rib

Internal intercostal m

Serratus posterior inferior m

Latissimus dorsi m

Figure 1.2.17

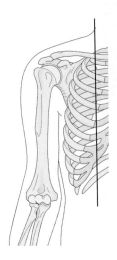

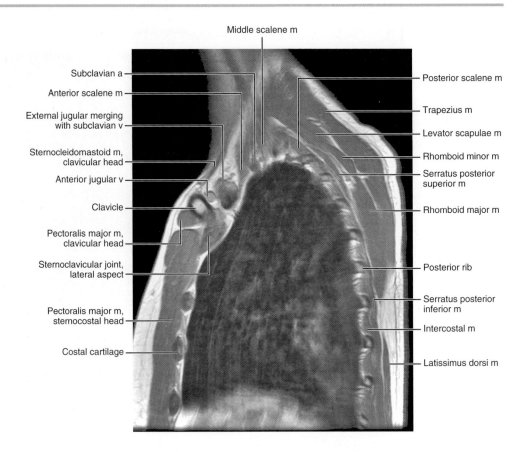

Middle scalene m

Subclavian a

Anterior scalene m

External jugular merging
with subclavian v

Sternocleidomastoid m,
clavicular head

Anterior jugular v

Clavicle

Pectoralis major m,
clavicular head

Sternoclavicular joint,
lateral aspect

Pectoralis major m,
sternocostal head

Costal cartilage

Posterior scalene m

Trapezius m

Levator scapulae m

Rhomboid minor m

Serratus posterior
superior m

Rhomboid major m

Posterior rib

Serratus posterior
inferior m

Intercostal m

Latissimus dorsi m

Figure 1.2.18

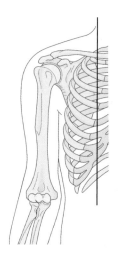

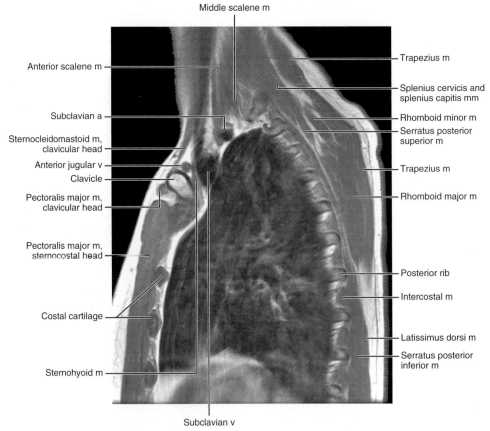

Middle scalene m

Anterior scalene m

Subclavian a

Sternocleidomastoid m,
clavicular head

Anterior jugular v

Clavicle

Pectoralis major m,
clavicular head

Pectoralis major m,
sternocostal head

Costal cartilage

Sternohyoid m

Trapezius m

Splenius cervicis and
splenius capitis mm

Rhomboid minor m

Serratus posterior
superior m

Trapezius m

Rhomboid major m

Posterior rib

Intercostal m

Latissimus dorsi m

Serratus posterior
inferior m

Subclavian v

Figure 1.2.19

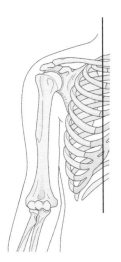

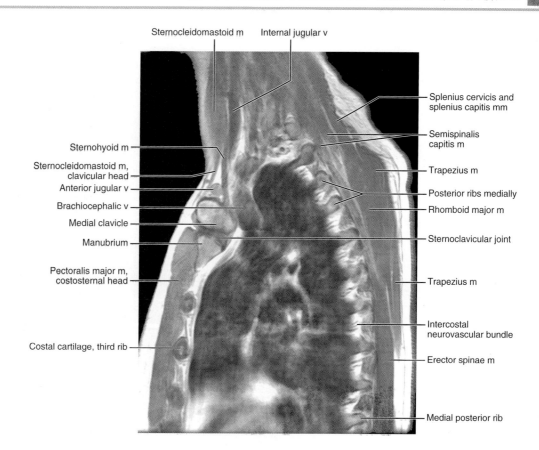

Sternocleidomastoid m

Internal jugular v

Splenius cervicis and splenius capitis mm

Semispinalis capitis m

Sternohyoid m

Trapezius m

Sternocleidomastoid m, clavicular head

Anterior jugular v

Posterior ribs medially

Brachiocephalic v

Rhomboid major m

Medial clavicle

Sternoclavicular joint

Manubrium

Pectoralis major m, costosternal head

Trapezius m

Intercostal neurovascular bundle

Erector spinae m

Costal cartilage, third rib

Medial posterior rib

CORONAL

Figure 1.3.1

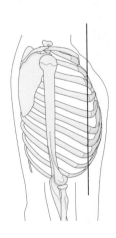

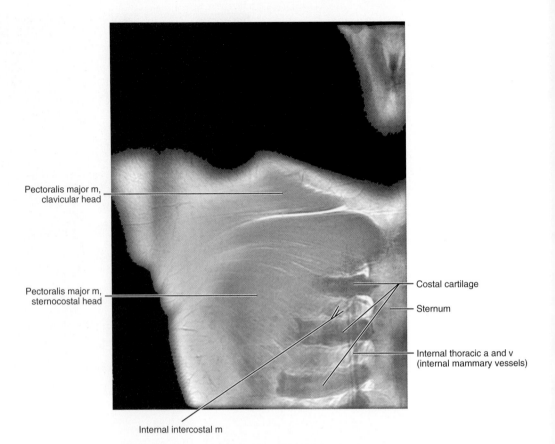

Pectoralis major m, clavicular head

Pectoralis major m, sternocostal head

Costal cartilage

Sternum

Internal thoracic a and v (internal mammary vessels)

Internal intercostal m

Figure 1.3.2

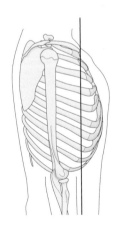

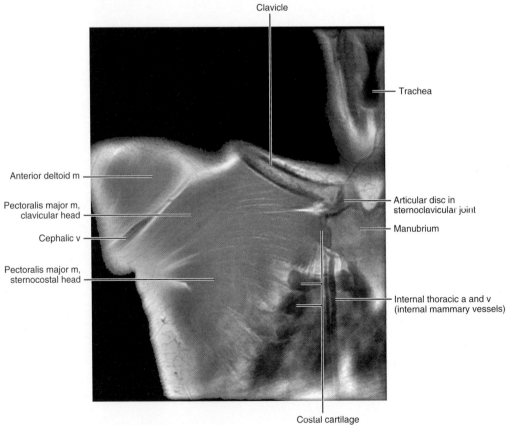

Clavicle

Trachea

Anterior deltoid m

Pectoralis major m, clavicular head

Cephalic v

Pectoralis major m, sternocostal head

Articular disc in sternoclavicular joint

Manubrium

Internal thoracic a and v (internal mammary vessels)

Costal cartilage

Figure 1.3.3

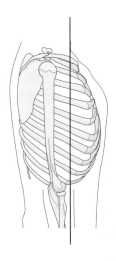

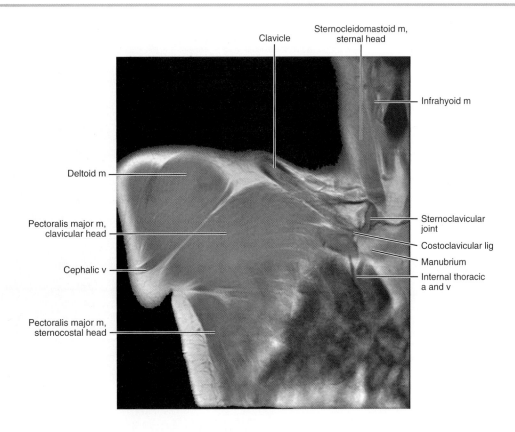

Clavicle

Sternocleidomastoid m, sternal head

Infrahyoid m

Deltoid m

Pectoralis major m, clavicular head

Cephalic v

Pectoralis major m, sternocostal head

Sternoclavicular joint

Costoclavicular lig

Manubrium

Internal thoracic a and v

Figure 1.3.4

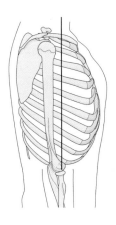

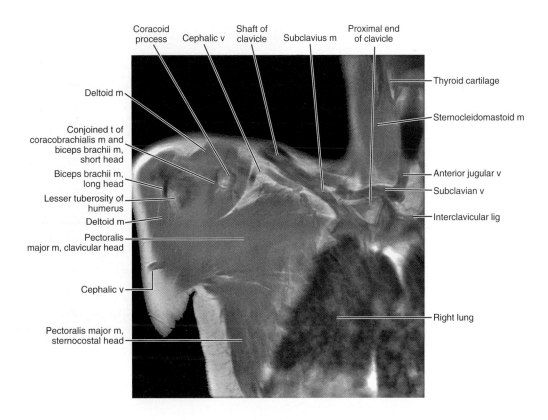

Coracoid process

Cephalic v

Shaft of clavicle

Subclavius m

Proximal end of clavicle

Deltoid m

Conjoined t of coracobrachialis m and biceps brachii m, short head

Biceps brachii m, long head

Lesser tuberosity of humerus

Deltoid m

Pectoralis major m, clavicular head

Cephalic v

Pectoralis major m, sternocostal head

Thyroid cartilage

Sternocleidomastoid m

Anterior jugular v

Subclavian v

Interclavicular lig

Right lung

Figure 1.3.5

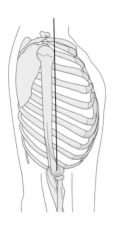

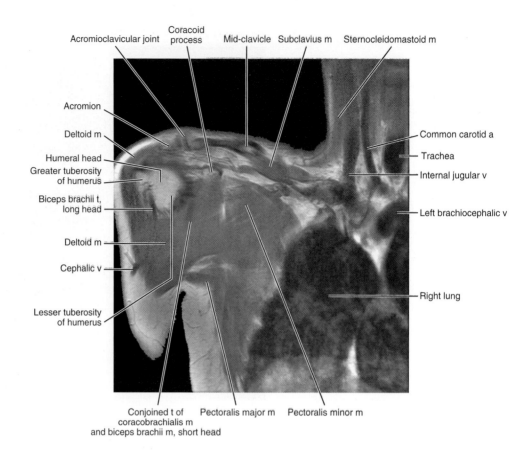

Acromioclavicular joint
Coracoid process
Mid-clavicle
Subclavius m
Sternocleidomastoid m

Acromion

Deltoid m

Humeral head
Greater tuberosity of humerus

Biceps brachii t, long head

Deltoid m

Cephalic v

Lesser tuberosity of humerus

Common carotid a

Trachea

Internal jugular v

Left brachiocephalic v

Right lung

Conjoined t of coracobrachialis m and biceps brachii m, short head
Pectoralis major m
Pectoralis minor m

Figure 1.3.6

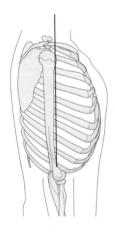

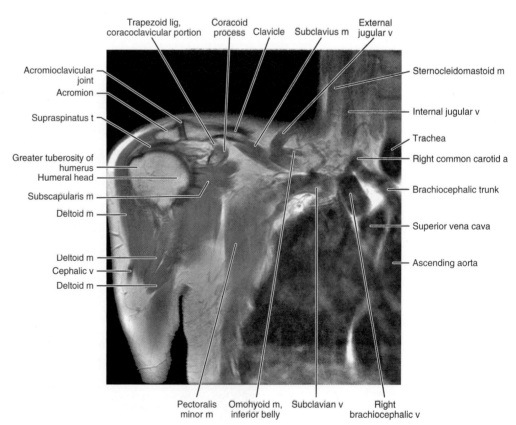

Trapezoid lig, coracoclavicular portion
Coracoid process
Clavicle
Subclavius m
External jugular v

Acromioclavicular joint

Acromion

Supraspinatus t

Greater tuberosity of humerus
Humeral head

Subscapularis m

Deltoid m

Deltoid m
Cephalic v
Deltoid m

Sternocleidomastoid m

Internal jugular v

Trachea

Right common carotid a

Brachiocephalic trunk

Superior vena cava

Ascending aorta

Pectoralis minor m
Omohyoid m, inferior belly
Subclavian v
Right brachiocephalic v

Figure 1.3.7

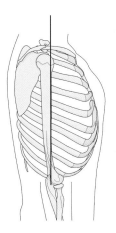

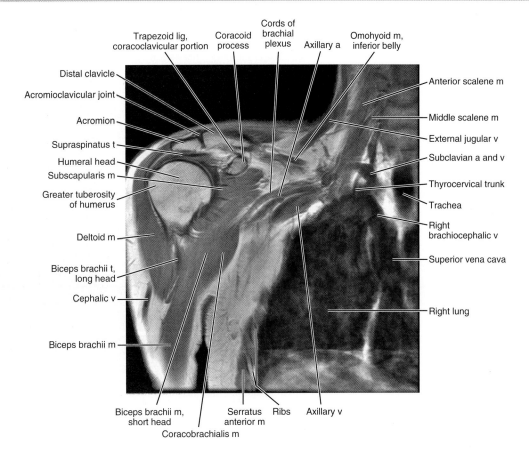

Trapezoid lig, coracoclavicular portion
Coracoid process
Cords of brachial plexus
Axillary a
Omohyoid m, inferior belly

Distal clavicle
Acromioclavicular joint
Acromion
Supraspinatus t
Humeral head
Subscapularis m
Greater tuberosity of humerus
Deltoid m
Biceps brachii t, long head
Cephalic v
Biceps brachii m

Anterior scalene m
Middle scalene m
External jugular v
Subclavian a and v
Thyrocervical trunk
Trachea
Right brachiocephalic v
Superior vena cava
Right lung

Biceps brachii m, short head
Serratus anterior m
Ribs
Axillary v
Coracobrachialis m

Figure 1.3.8

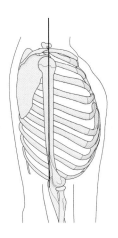

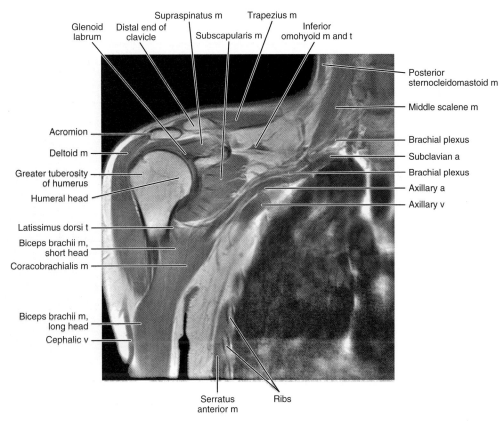

Glenoid labrum
Distal end of clavicle
Supraspinatus m
Subscapularis m
Trapezius m
Inferior omohyoid m and t

Acromion
Deltoid m
Greater tuberosity of humerus
Humeral head
Latissimus dorsi t
Biceps brachii m, short head
Coracobrachialis m
Biceps brachii m, long head
Cephalic v

Posterior sternocleidomastoid m
Middle scalene m
Brachial plexus
Subclavian a
Brachial plexus
Axillary a
Axillary v

Serratus anterior m
Ribs

Figure 1.3.9

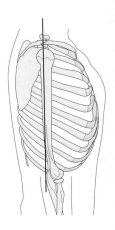

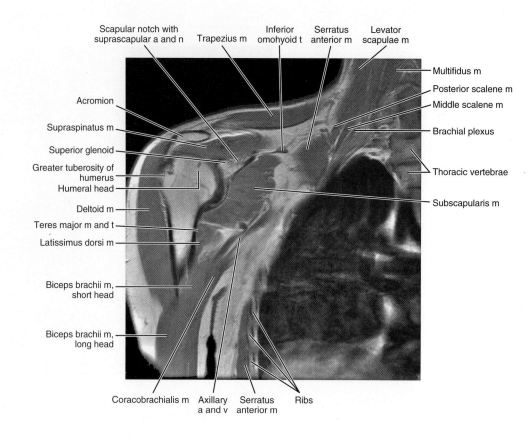

Scapular notch with suprascapular a and n
Trapezius m
Inferior omohyoid t
Serratus anterior m
Levator scapulae m
Acromion
Supraspinatus m
Superior glenoid
Greater tuberosity of humerus
Humeral head
Deltoid m
Teres major m and t
Latissimus dorsi m
Biceps brachii m, short head
Biceps brachii m, long head
Multifidus m
Posterior scalene m
Middle scalene m
Brachial plexus
Thoracic vertebrae
Subscapularis m
Coracobrachialis m
Axillary a and v
Serratus anterior m
Ribs

Figure 1.3.10

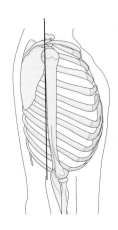

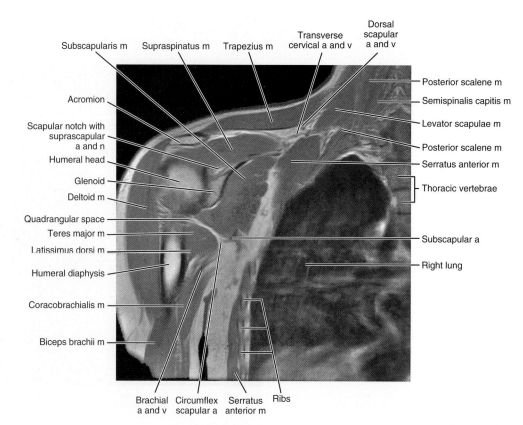

Subscapularis m
Supraspinatus m
Trapezius m
Transverse cervical a and v
Dorsal scapular a and v
Acromion
Scapular notch with suprascapular a and n
Humeral head
Glenoid
Deltoid m
Quadrangular space
Teres major m
Latissimus dorsi m
Humeral diaphysis
Coracobrachialis m
Biceps brachii m
Posterior scalene m
Semispinalis capitis m
Levator scapulae m
Posterior scalene m
Serratus anterior m
Thoracic vertebrae
Subscapular a
Right lung
Brachial a and v
Circumflex scapular a
Serratus anterior m
Ribs

Figure 1.3.11

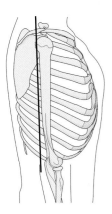

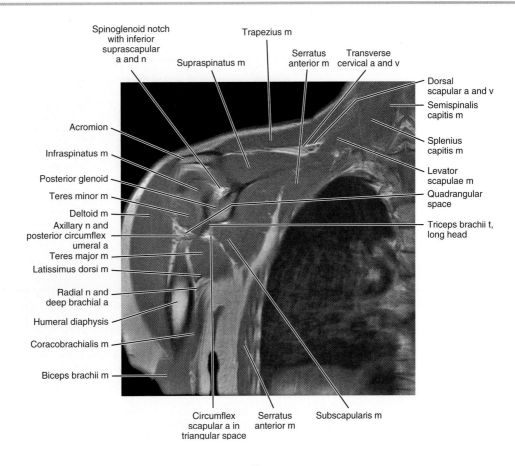

Spinoglenoid notch with inferior suprascapular a and n

Supraspinatus m

Trapezius m

Serratus anterior m

Transverse cervical a and v

Dorsal scapular a and v

Semispinalis capitis m

Splenius capitis m

Levator scapulae m

Quadrangular space

Triceps brachii t, long head

Acromion

Infraspinatus m

Posterior glenoid

Teres minor m

Deltoid m

Axillary n and posterior circumflex umeral a

Teres major m

Latissimus dorsi m

Radial n and deep brachial a

Humeral diaphysis

Coracobrachialis m

Biceps brachii m

Circumflex scapular a in triangular space

Serratus anterior m

Subscapularis m

Figure 1.3.12

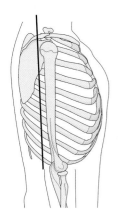

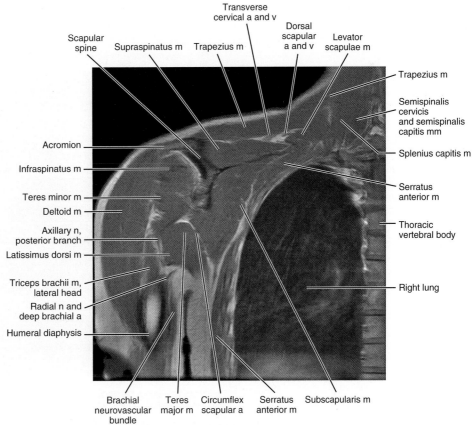

Scapular spine

Supraspinatus m

Trapezius m

Transverse cervical a and v

Dorsal scapular a and v

Levator scapulae m

Trapezius m

Semispinalis cervicis and semispinalis capitis mm

Splenius capitis m

Serratus anterior m

Thoracic vertebral body

Right lung

Acromion

Infraspinatus m

Teres minor m

Deltoid m

Axillary n, posterior branch

Latissimus dorsi m

Triceps brachii m, lateral head

Radial n and deep brachial a

Humeral diaphysis

Brachial neurovascular bundle

Teres major m

Circumflex scapular a

Serratus anterior m

Subscapularis m

Figure 1.3.13

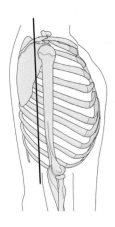

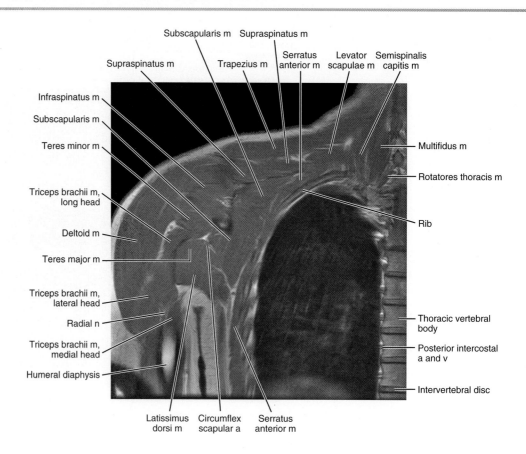

Subscapularis m   Supraspinatus m
Supraspinatus m   Trapezius m   Serratus anterior m   Levator scapulae m   Semispinalis capitis m

Infraspinatus m
Subscapularis m
Teres minor m
Triceps brachii m, long head
Deltoid m
Teres major m
Triceps brachii m, lateral head
Radial n
Triceps brachii m, medial head
Humeral diaphysis

Multifidus m
Rotatores thoracis m
Rib
Thoracic vertebral body
Posterior intercostal a and v
Intervertebral disc

Latissimus dorsi m   Circumflex scapular a   Serratus anterior m

Figure 1.3.14

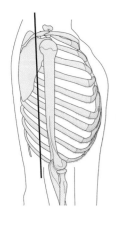

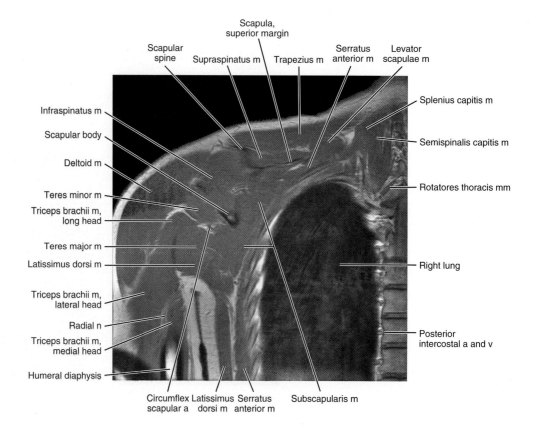

Scapula, superior margin
Scapular spine   Supraspinatus m   Trapezius m   Serratus anterior m   Levator scapulae m

Infraspinatus m
Scapular body
Deltoid m
Teres minor m
Triceps brachii m, long head
Teres major m
Latissimus dorsi m
Triceps brachii m, lateral head
Radial n
Triceps brachii m, medial head
Humeral diaphysis

Splenius capitis m
Semispinalis capitis m
Rotatores thoracis mm
Right lung
Posterior intercostal a and v

Circumflex scapular a   Latissimus dorsi m   Serratus anterior m   Subscapularis m

Figure 1.3.15

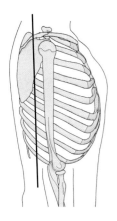

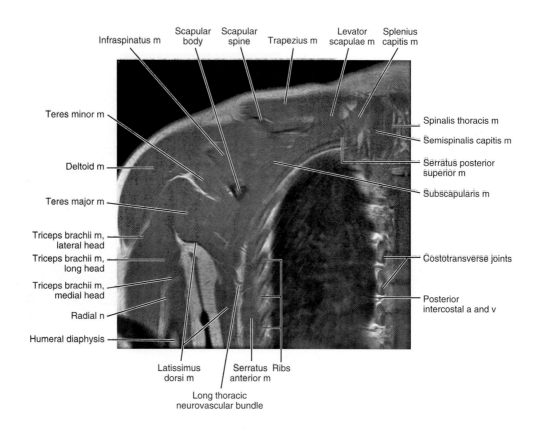

Infraspinatus m
Scapular body
Scapular spine
Trapezius m
Levator scapulae m
Splenius capitis m

Teres minor m

Deltoid m

Teres major m

Triceps brachii m, lateral head

Triceps brachii m, long head

Triceps brachii m, medial head

Radial n

Humeral diaphysis

Spinalis thoracis m

Semispinalis capitis m

Serratus posterior superior m

Subscapularis m

Costotransverse joints

Posterior intercostal a and v

Latissimus dorsi m

Serratus anterior m

Ribs

Long thoracic neurovascular bundle

Figure 1.3.16

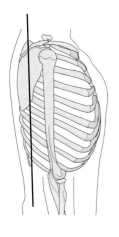

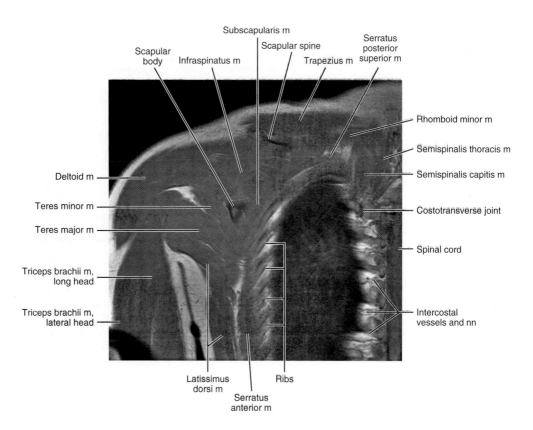

Subscapularis m
Scapular body
Infraspinatus m
Scapular spine
Trapezius m
Serratus posterior superior m

Deltoid m

Teres minor m

Teres major m

Triceps brachii m, long head

Triceps brachii m, lateral head

Rhomboid minor m

Semispinalis thoracis m

Semispinalis capitis m

Costotransverse joint

Spinal cord

Intercostal vessels and nn

Latissimus dorsi m

Serratus anterior m

Ribs

Figure 1.3.17

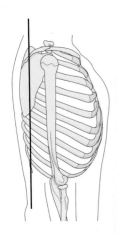

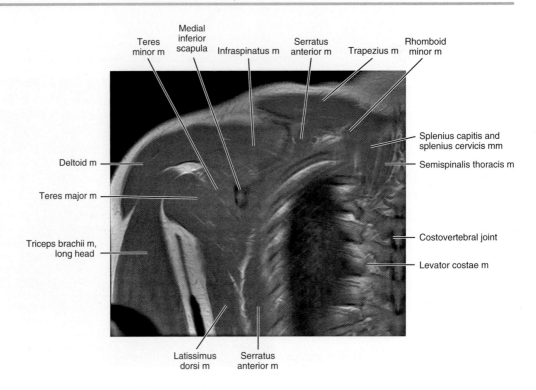

Teres minor m

Medial inferior scapula

Infraspinatus m

Serratus anterior m

Trapezius m

Rhomboid minor m

Deltoid m

Teres major m

Triceps brachii m, long head

Splenius capitis and splenius cervicis mm

Semispinalis thoracis m

Costovertebral joint

Levator costae m

Latissimus dorsi m

Serratus anterior m

Figure 1.3.18

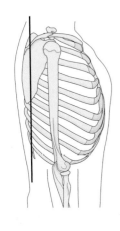

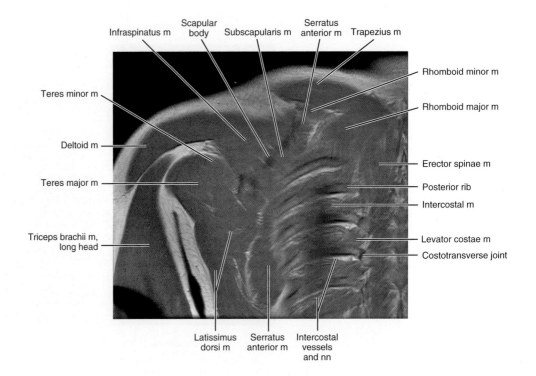

Infraspinatus m

Scapular body

Subscapularis m

Serratus anterior m

Trapezius m

Teres minor m

Deltoid m

Teres major m

Triceps brachii m, long head

Rhomboid minor m

Rhomboid major m

Erector spinae m

Posterior rib

Intercostal m

Levator costae m

Costotransverse joint

Latissimus dorsi m

Serratus anterior m

Intercostal vessels and nn

Figure 1.3.19

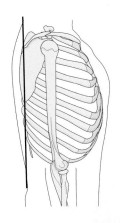

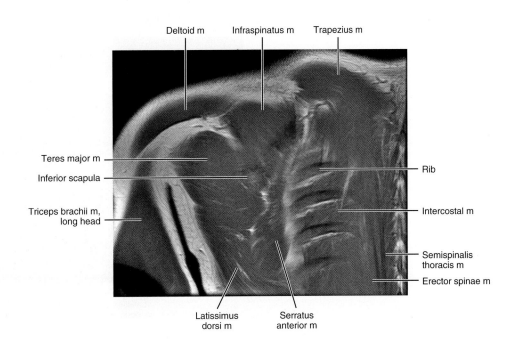

Deltoid m   Infraspinatus m   Trapezius m

Teres major m

Inferior scapula

Triceps brachii m,
long head

Rib

Intercostal m

Semispinalis
thoracis m

Erector spinae m

Latissimus
dorsi m

Serratus
anterior m

Figure 1.3.20

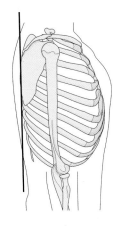

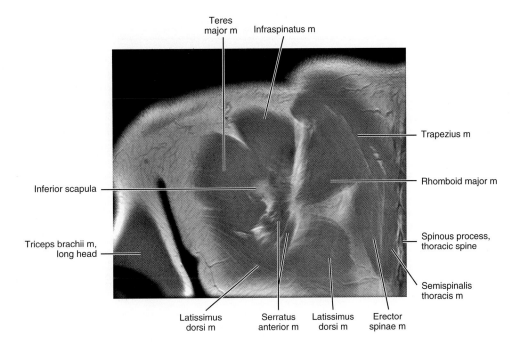

Teres
major m   Infraspinatus m

Inferior scapula

Triceps brachii m,
long head

Trapezius m

Rhomboid major m

Spinous process,
thoracic spine

Semispinalis
thoracis m

Latissimus
dorsi m

Serratus
anterior m

Latissimus
dorsi m

Erector
spinae m

Figure 1.3.21

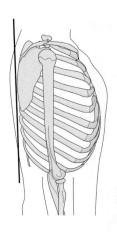

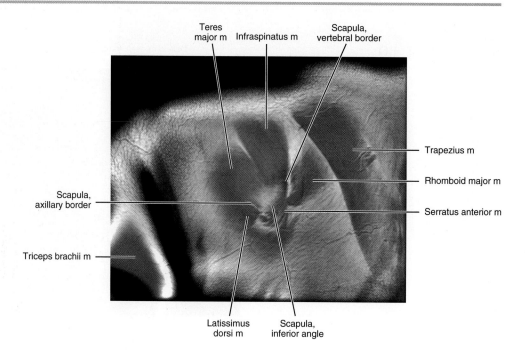

Teres major m

Infraspinatus m

Scapula, vertebral border

Trapezius m

Rhomboid major m

Serratus anterior m

Scapula, axillary border

Triceps brachii m

Latissimus dorsi m

Scapula, inferior angle

Chapter 2

MRI of the Shoulder

Table 1: Muscles of the Shoulder

MUSCLE	ORIGIN	INSERTION	NERVE SUPPLY
Pectoralis major	Medial half of the anterior surface of the clavicle, side and front of the sternum as far as the 6th costal cartilage, front and surfaces of the cartilage of the 2nd through 6th ribs, osseous ends of the 6th and 7th ribs, and aponeurosis of external abdominal oblique	Crest of the greater tubercle of the humerus, lateral lip of the intertubercular groove, deltoid tubercle, and fibrous periosteum of the intertubercular sulcus	Lateral and medial pectoral (C5 and C6 for the clavicular part, and C7, C8, and T1 for the sternocostal part)
Pectoralis minor	Aponeurotic slips from the 2nd through 5th ribs, near costal cartilages	Anterior half of the medial border and upper surface of the coracoid process of the scapula	Medial and lateral pectoral (C6, C7, C8)
Subclavius	First rib and its cartilage	Inferior surface of the clavicle between the costal and coracoid tuberosities	Nerve to subclavian (C5 or C5 and C6)
Deltoid	Lateral border and upper surface of the lateral third of the clavicle, the acromion, and the scapular spine	Deltoid tuberosity of the humerus	Axillary (C5, C6)
Supraspinatus	Supraspinous fossa and investing fascia	Shoulder capsule and superior facet of the greater tubercle of the humerus	Suprascapular (C4, C5, C6)
Infraspinatus	Infraspinous fossa, scapular spine, investing (deep) fascia, and adjacent aponeurotic septa	Shoulder capsule and middle facet of the greater tubercle of the humerus	Suprascapular (C4, C5, C6)
Teres minor	Upper two thirds of the axillary border of the scapula	Shoulder capsule and inferior facet of the greater tubercle of the humerus	Axillary (C4, C5, C6)
Subscapularis	Subscapularis fossa	Shoulder capsule and lesser tubercle of humerus and its shaft immediately below the tubercle	Two or three subscapular branches from posterior cord and upper and lower subscapular (C5, C6, C7)
Teres major	Inferior angle of the scapula	Medial lip of the intertubercular groove of the humerus	Lower subscapular (C6, C7)
Latissimus dorsi	Spine and interspinous ligaments of the lower five or six thoracic vertebrae, upper lumbar vertebrae, thoracodorsal fascia, posterior third of the crest of the ilium, and the lateral surface and upper edge of the lower three or four ribs	Muscle tendon inserts onto the ventral side of the lesser tubercle of the humerus and onto the floor of the intertubercular groove ventral to the tendon of the teres major. The tendon may extend to the greater tubercle of the humerus	Thoracodorsal (C6, C7, C8)

AXIAL
Figure 2.1.1

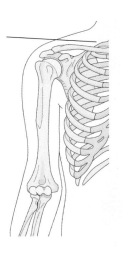

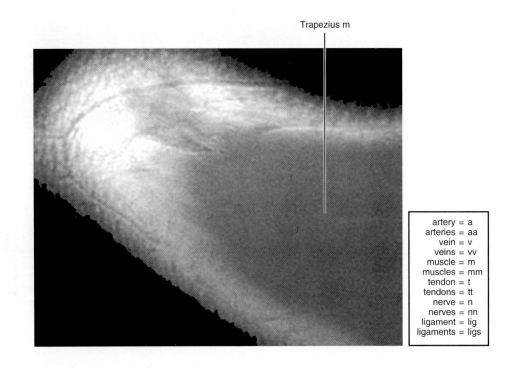

Trapezius m

artery = a
arteries = aa
vein = v
veins = vv
muscle = m
muscles = mm
tendon = t
tendons = tt
nerve = n
nerves = nn
ligament = lig
ligaments = ligs

Figure 2.1.2

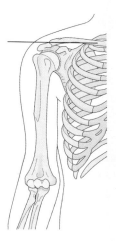

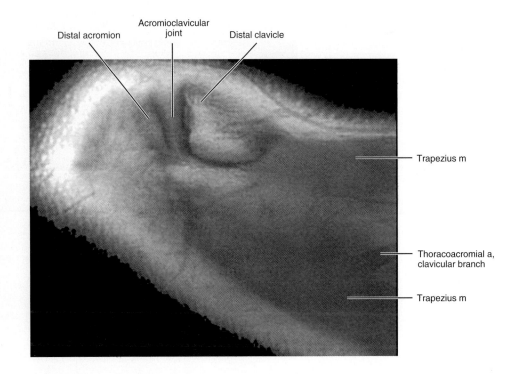

Distal acromion

Acromioclavicular joint

Distal clavicle

Trapezius m

Thoracoacromial a, clavicular branch

Trapezius m

Figure 2.1.3

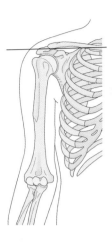

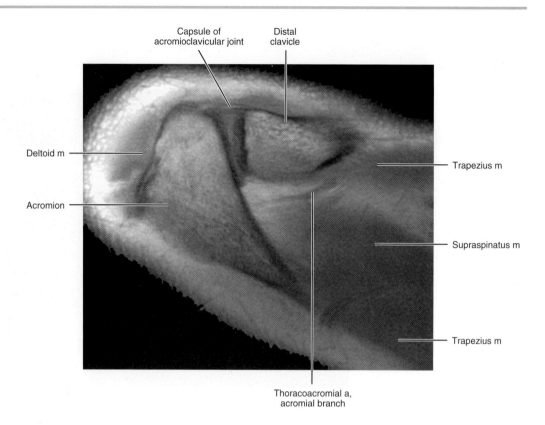

Capsule of acromioclavicular joint

Distal clavicle

Deltoid m

Acromion

Trapezius m

Supraspinatus m

Trapezius m

Thoracoacromial a, acromial branch

Figure 2.1.4

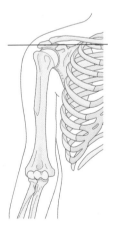

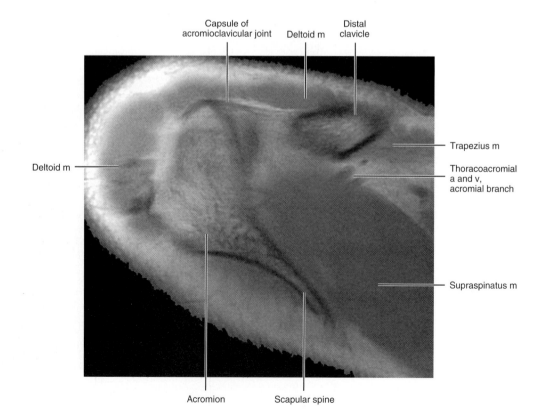

Capsule of acromioclavicular joint

Deltoid m

Distal clavicle

Deltoid m

Trapezius m

Thoracoacromial a and v, acromial branch

Supraspinatus m

Acromion

Scapular spine

Figure 2.1.5

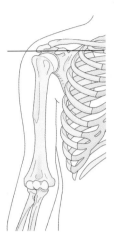

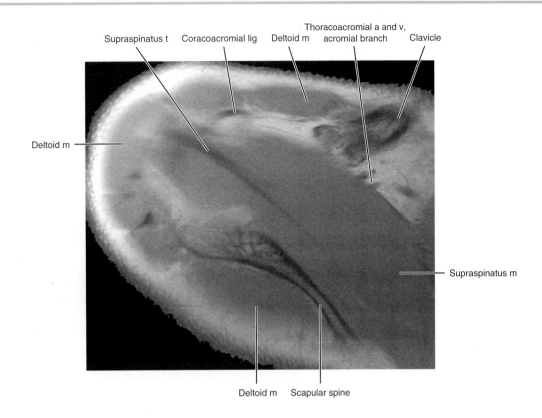

Supraspinatus t   Coracoacromial lig   Deltoid m   Thoracoacromial a and v, acromial branch   Clavicle

Deltoid m

Supraspinatus m

Deltoid m   Scapular spine

Figure 2.1.6

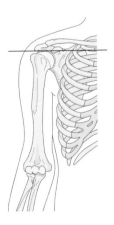

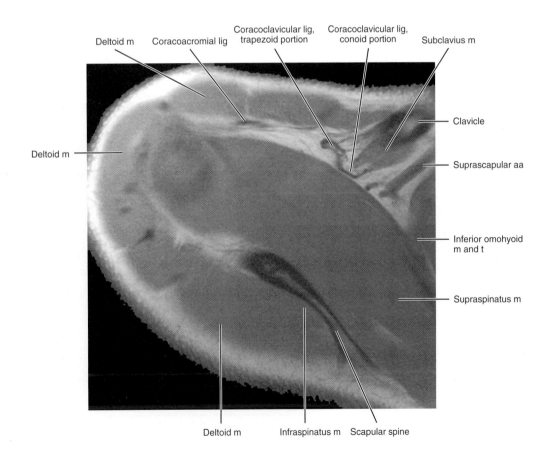

Deltoid m   Coracoacromial lig   Coracoclavicular lig, trapezoid portion   Coracoclavicular lig, conoid portion   Subclavius m

Deltoid m

Clavicle

Suprascapular aa

Inferior omohyoid m and t

Supraspinatus m

Deltoid m   Infraspinatus m   Scapular spine

Figure 2.1.7

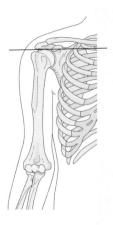

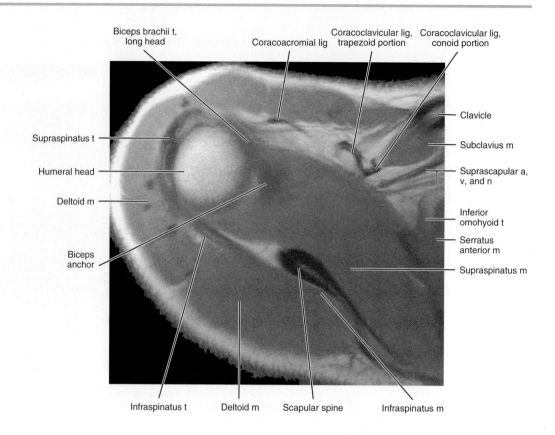

Biceps brachii t, long head

Coracoacromial lig

Coracoclavicular lig, trapezoid portion

Coracoclavicular lig, conoid portion

Clavicle

Subclavius m

Suprascapular a, v, and n

Inferior omohyoid t

Serratus anterior m

Supraspinatus m

Supraspinatus t

Humeral head

Deltoid m

Biceps anchor

Infraspinatus t   Deltoid m   Scapular spine   Infraspinatus m

Figure 2.1.8

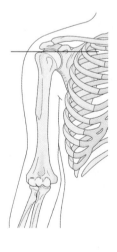

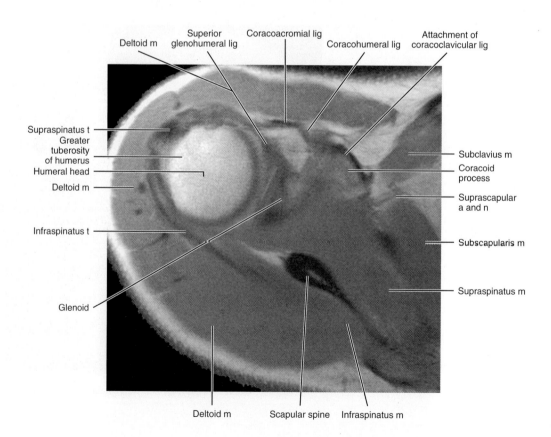

Deltoid m

Superior glenohumeral lig

Coracoacromial lig

Coracohumeral lig

Attachment of coracoclavicular lig

Supraspinatus t
Greater tuberosity of humerus

Humeral head

Deltoid m

Infraspinatus t

Glenoid

Subclavius m

Coracoid process

Suprascapular a and n

Subscapularis m

Supraspinatus m

Deltoid m   Scapular spine   Infraspinatus m

Figure 2.1.9

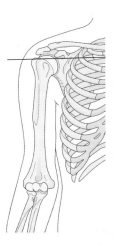

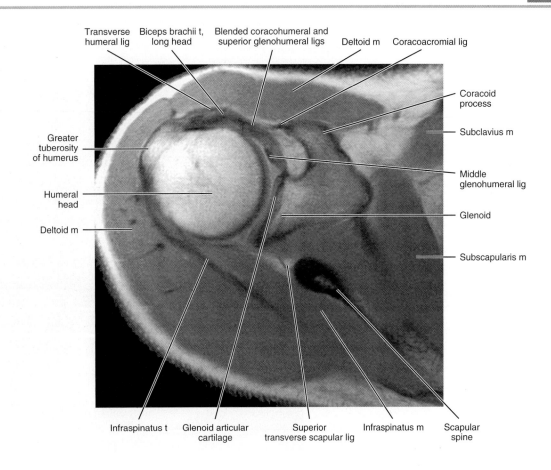

Transverse humeral lig | Biceps brachii t, long head | Blended coracohumeral and superior glenohumeral ligs | Deltoid m | Coracoacromial lig

Coracoid process

Subclavius m

Greater tuberosity of humerus

Middle glenohumeral lig

Humeral head

Glenoid

Deltoid m

Subscapularis m

Infraspinatus t | Glenoid articular cartilage | Superior transverse scapular lig | Infraspinatus m | Scapular spine

Figure 2.1.10

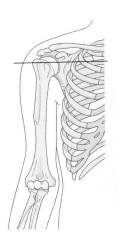

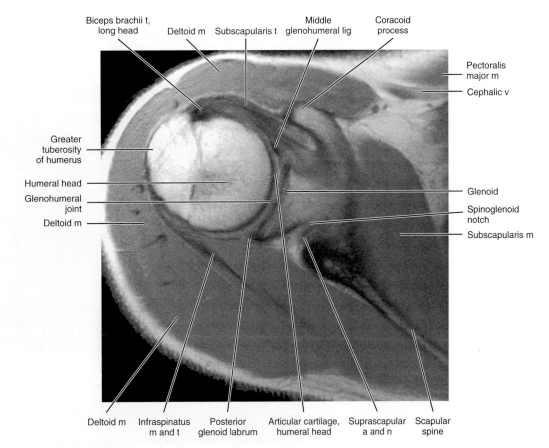

Biceps brachii t, long head | Deltoid m | Subscapularis t | Middle glenohumeral lig | Coracoid process

Pectoralis major m

Cephalic v

Greater tuberosity of humerus

Humeral head

Glenohumeral joint

Glenoid

Spinoglenoid notch

Deltoid m

Subscapularis m

Deltoid m | Infraspinatus m and t | Posterior glenoid labrum | Articular cartilage, humeral head | Suprascapular a and n | Scapular spine

Figure 2.1.11

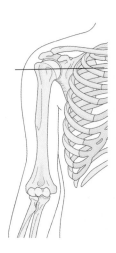

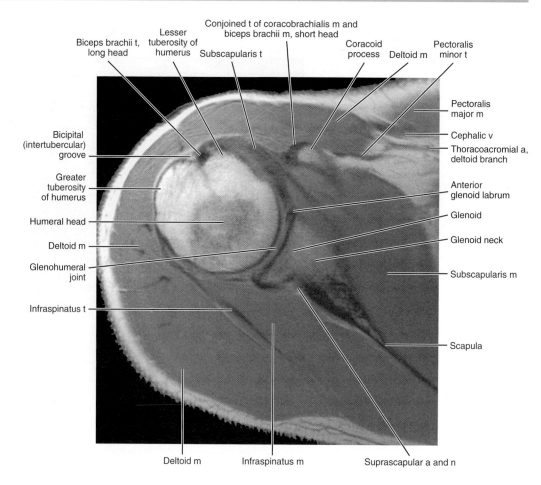

Biceps brachii t, long head

Lesser tuberosity of humerus

Subscapularis t

Conjoined t of coracobrachialis m and biceps brachii m, short head

Coracoid process

Deltoid m

Pectoralis minor t

Pectoralis major m

Cephalic v

Thoracoacromial a, deltoid branch

Anterior glenoid labrum

Glenoid

Glenoid neck

Subscapularis m

Scapula

Bicipital (intertubercular) groove

Greater tuberosity of humerus

Humeral head

Deltoid m

Glenohumeral joint

Infraspinatus t

Deltoid m

Infraspinatus m

Suprascapular a and n

Figure 2.1.12

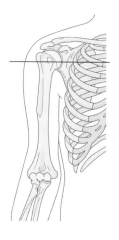

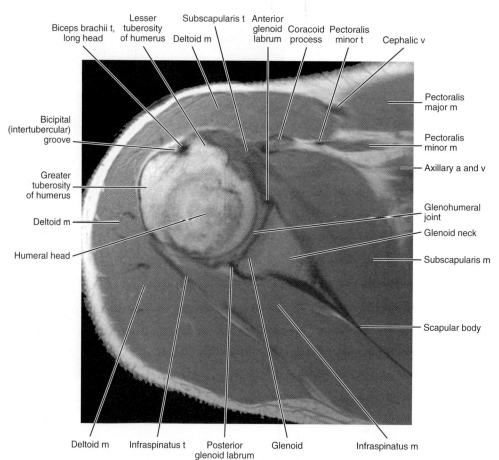

Biceps brachii t, long head

Lesser tuberosity of humerus

Subscapularis t

Deltoid m

Anterior glenoid labrum

Coracoid process

Pectoralis minor t

Cephalic v

Pectoralis major m

Pectoralis minor m

Axillary a and v

Glenohumeral joint

Glenoid neck

Subscapularis m

Scapular body

Bicipital (intertubercular) groove

Greater tuberosity of humerus

Deltoid m

Humeral head

Deltoid m

Infraspinatus t

Posterior glenoid labrum

Glenoid

Infraspinatus m

Figure 2.1.13

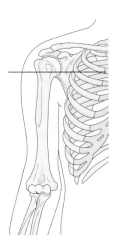

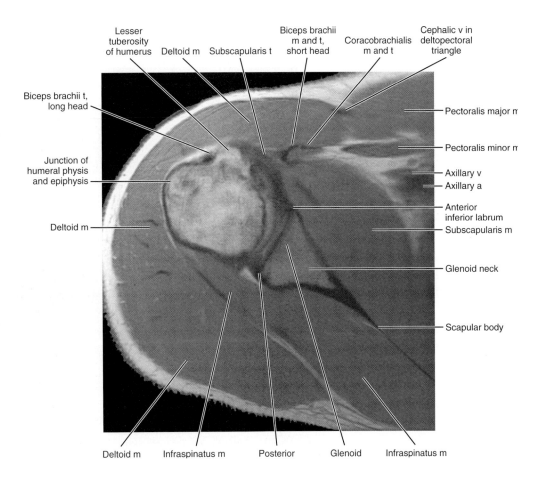

Lesser tuberosity of humerus

Deltoid m

Subscapularis t

Biceps brachii m and t, short head

Coracobrachialis m and t

Cephalic v in deltopectoral triangle

Biceps brachii t, long head

Junction of humeral physis and epiphysis

Deltoid m

Pectoralis major m

Pectoralis minor m

Axillary v

Axillary a

Anterior inferior labrum

Subscapularis m

Glenoid neck

Scapular body

Deltoid m   Infraspinatus m   Posterior   Glenoid   Infraspinatus m

Figure 2.1.14

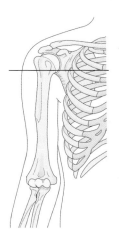

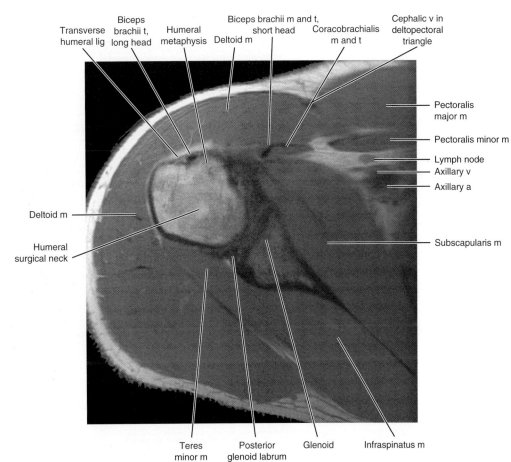

Transverse humeral lig

Biceps brachii t, long head

Humeral metaphysis

Deltoid m

Biceps brachii m and t, short head

Coracobrachialis m and t

Cephalic v in deltopectoral triangle

Deltoid m

Humeral surgical neck

Pectoralis major m

Pectoralis minor m

Lymph node

Axillary v

Axillary a

Subscapularis m

Teres minor m   Posterior glenoid labrum   Glenoid   Infraspinatus m

Figure 2.1.15

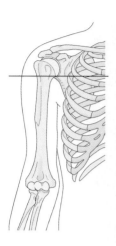

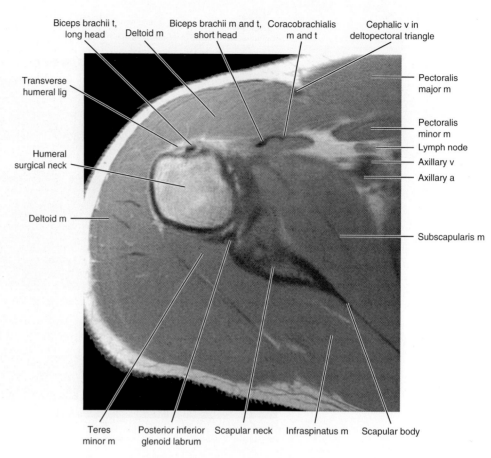

Biceps brachii t, long head
Deltoid m
Biceps brachii m and t, short head
Coracobrachialis m and t
Cephalic v in deltopectoral triangle
Transverse humeral lig
Humeral surgical neck
Deltoid m
Pectoralis major m
Pectoralis minor m
Lymph node
Axillary v
Axillary a
Subscapularis m

Teres minor m
Posterior inferior glenoid labrum
Scapular neck
Infraspinatus m
Scapular body

Figure 2.1.16

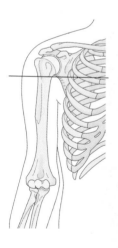

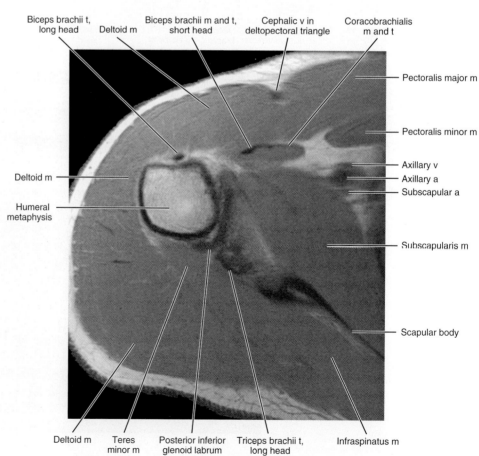

Biceps brachii t, long head
Deltoid m
Biceps brachii m and t, short head
Cephalic v in deltopectoral triangle
Coracobrachialis m and t
Deltoid m
Humeral metaphysis
Pectoralis major m
Pectoralis minor m
Axillary v
Axillary a
Subscapular a
Subscapularis m
Scapular body

Deltoid m
Teres minor m
Posterior inferior glenoid labrum
Triceps brachii t, long head
Infraspinatus m

Figure 2.1.17

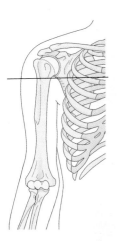

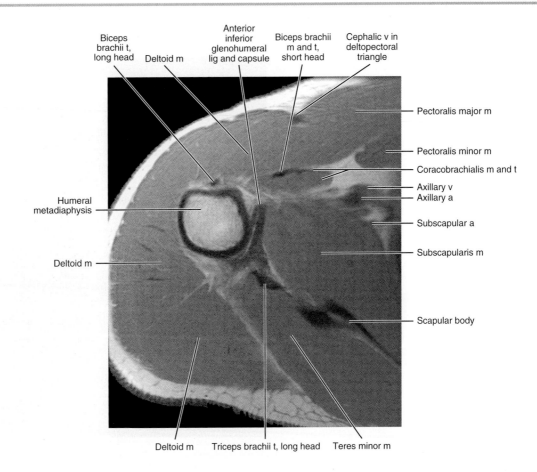

Biceps brachii t, long head — Deltoid m — Anterior inferior glenohumeral lig and capsule — Biceps brachii m and t, short head — Cephalic v in deltopectoral triangle

Pectoralis major m

Pectoralis minor m

Coracobrachialis m and t

Axillary v

Axillary a

Subscapular a

Subscapularis m

Scapular body

Humeral metadiaphysis

Deltoid m

Deltoid m   Triceps brachii t, long head   Teres minor m

Figure 2.1.18

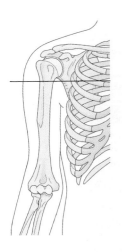

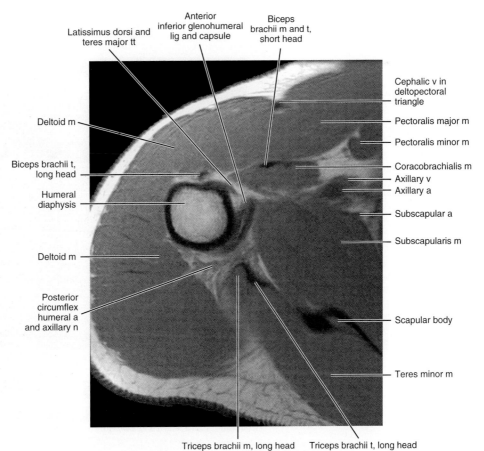

Latissimus dorsi and teres major tt — Anterior inferior glenohumeral lig and capsule — Biceps brachii m and t, short head

Cephalic v in deltopectoral triangle

Pectoralis major m

Pectoralis minor m

Coracobrachialis m

Axillary v

Axillary a

Subscapular a

Subscapularis m

Scapular body

Teres minor m

Deltoid m

Biceps brachii t, long head

Humeral diaphysis

Deltoid m

Posterior circumflex humeral a and axillary n

Triceps brachii m, long head   Triceps brachii t, long head

Figure 2.1.19

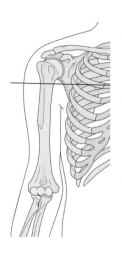

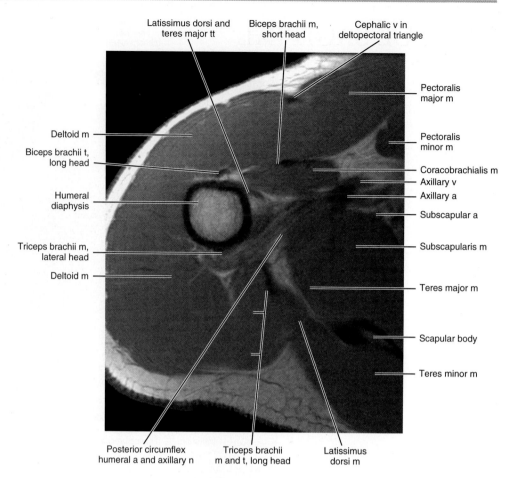

Latissimus dorsi and teres major tt

Biceps brachii m, short head

Cephalic v in deltopectoral triangle

Deltoid m

Biceps brachii t, long head

Humeral diaphysis

Triceps brachii m, lateral head

Deltoid m

Pectoralis major m

Pectoralis minor m

Coracobrachialis m

Axillary v

Axillary a

Subscapular a

Subscapularis m

Teres major m

Scapular body

Teres minor m

Posterior circumflex humeral a and axillary n

Triceps brachii m and t, long head

Latissimus dorsi m

Figure 2.1.20

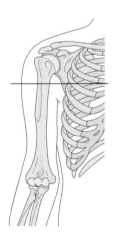

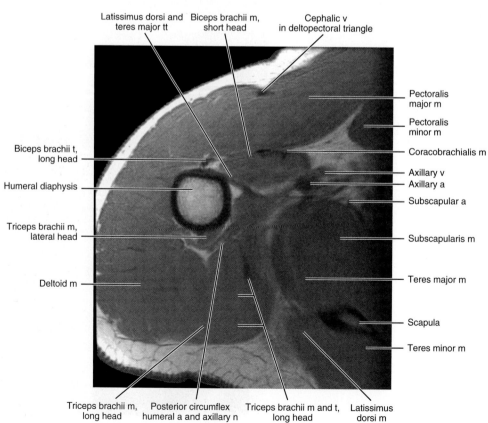

Latissimus dorsi and teres major tt

Biceps brachii m, short head

Cephalic v in deltopectoral triangle

Biceps brachii t, long head

Humeral diaphysis

Triceps brachii m, lateral head

Deltoid m

Pectoralis major m

Pectoralis minor m

Coracobrachialis m

Axillary v

Axillary a

Subscapular a

Subscapularis m

Teres major m

Scapula

Teres minor m

Triceps brachii m, long head

Posterior circumflex humeral a and axillary n

Triceps brachii m and t, long head

Latissimus dorsi m

OBLIQUE SAGITTAL

Figure 2.2.1

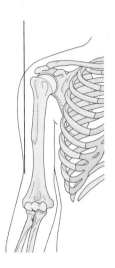

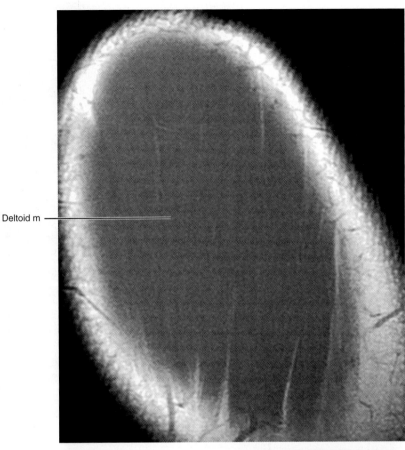

Deltoid m

Figure 2.2.2

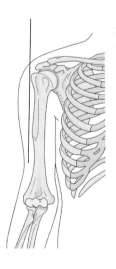

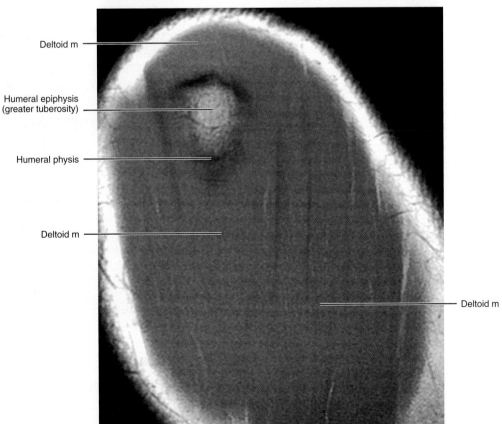

Deltoid m

Humeral epiphysis
(greater tuberosity)

Humeral physis

Deltoid m

Deltoid m

Figure 2.2.3

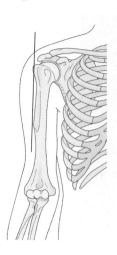

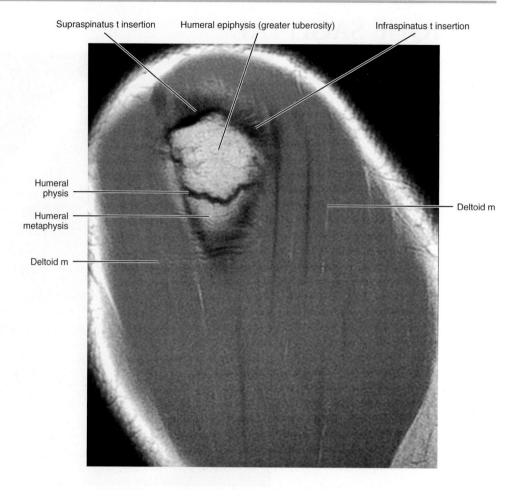

Supraspinatus t insertion   Humeral epiphysis (greater tuberosity)   Infraspinatus t insertion

Humeral physis

Humeral metaphysis

Deltoid m

Deltoid m

Figure 2.2.4

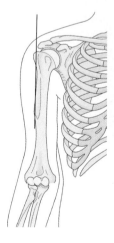

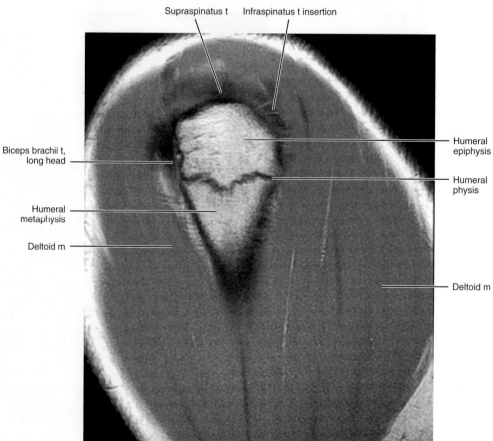

Supraspinatus t   Infraspinatus t insertion

Biceps brachii t, long head

Humeral metaphysis

Deltoid m

Humeral epiphysis

Humeral physis

Deltoid m

Figure 2.2.5

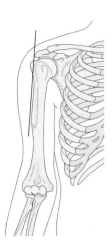

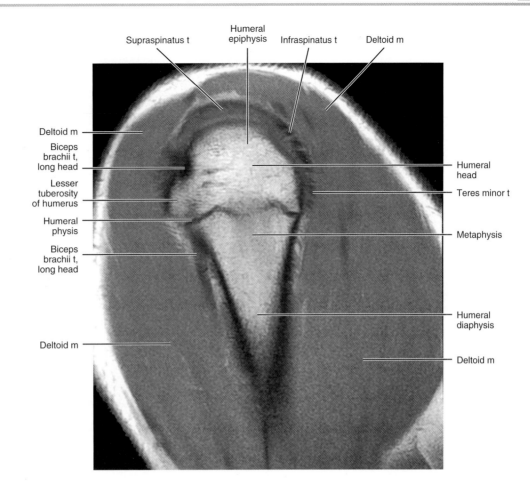

Supraspinatus t

Humeral epiphysis

Infraspinatus t

Deltoid m

Deltoid m

Biceps brachii t, long head

Lesser tuberosity of humerus

Humeral physis

Biceps brachii t, long head

Deltoid m

Humeral head

Teres minor t

Metaphysis

Humeral diaphysis

Deltoid m

Figure 2.2.6

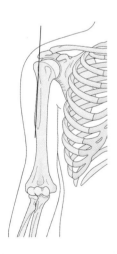

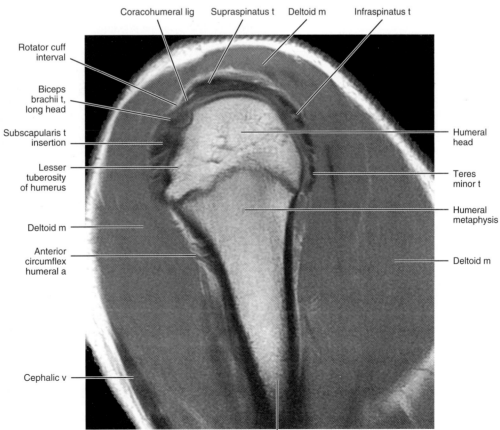

Coracohumeral lig

Supraspinatus t

Deltoid m

Infraspinatus t

Rotator cuff interval

Biceps brachii t, long head

Subscapularis t insertion

Lesser tuberosity of humerus

Deltoid m

Anterior circumflex humeral a

Cephalic v

Humeral head

Teres minor t

Humeral metaphysis

Deltoid m

Humeral diaphysis

Figure 2.2.7

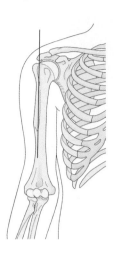

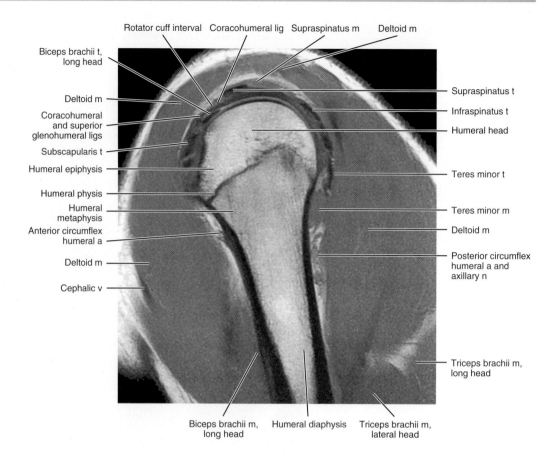

Rotator cuff interval   Coracohumeral lig   Supraspinatus m   Deltoid m

Biceps brachii t, long head

Deltoid m

Coracohumeral and superior glenohumeral ligs

Subscapularis t

Humeral epiphysis

Humeral physis

Humeral metaphysis

Anterior circumflex humeral a

Deltoid m

Cephalic v

Supraspinatus t

Infraspinatus t

Humeral head

Teres minor t

Teres minor m

Deltoid m

Posterior circumflex humeral a and axillary n

Triceps brachii m, long head

Biceps brachii m, long head   Humeral diaphysis   Triceps brachii m, lateral head

Figure 2.2.8

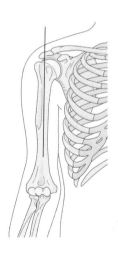

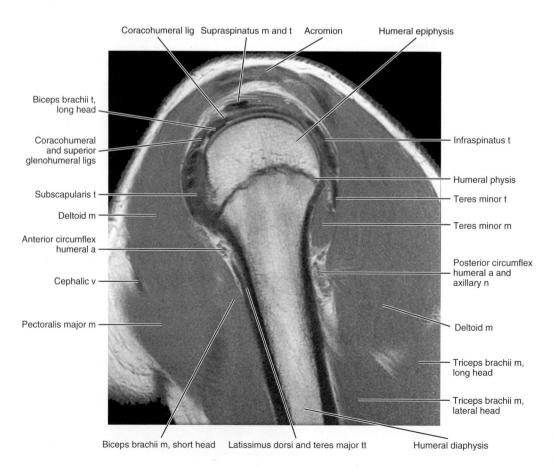

Coracohumeral lig   Supraspinatus m and t   Acromion   Humeral epiphysis

Biceps brachii t, long head

Coracohumeral and superior glenohumeral ligs

Subscapularis t

Deltoid m

Anterior circumflex humeral a

Cephalic v

Pectoralis major m

Infraspinatus t

Humeral physis

Teres minor t

Teres minor m

Posterior circumflex humeral a and axillary n

Deltoid m

Triceps brachii m, long head

Triceps brachii m, lateral head

Biceps brachii m, short head   Latissimus dorsi and teres major tt   Humeral diaphysis

Figure 2.2.9

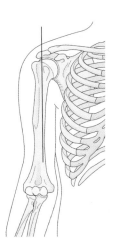

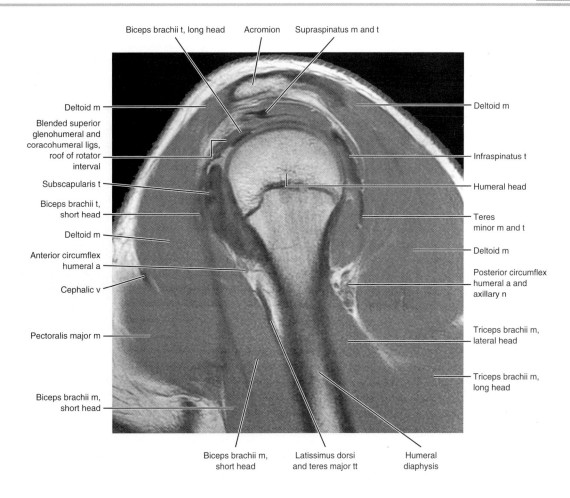

Biceps brachii t, long head — Acromion — Supraspinatus m and t

Deltoid m

Blended superior glenohumeral and coracohumeral ligs, roof of rotator interval

Subscapularis t

Biceps brachii t, short head

Deltoid m

Anterior circumflex humeral a

Cephalic v

Pectoralis major m

Biceps brachii m, short head

Deltoid m

Infraspinatus t

Humeral head

Teres minor m and t

Deltoid m

Posterior circumflex humeral a and axillary n

Triceps brachii m, lateral head

Triceps brachii m, long head

Biceps brachii m, short head — Latissimus dorsi and teres major tt — Humeral diaphysis

Figure 2.2.10

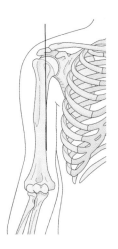

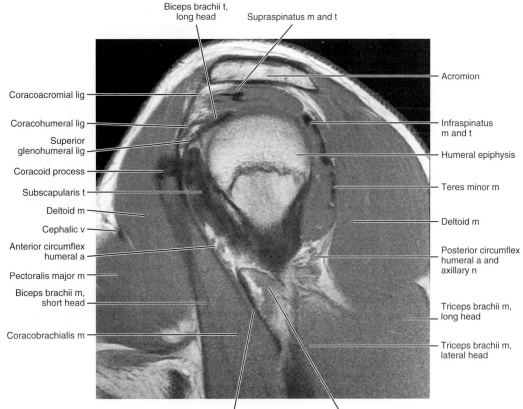

Biceps brachii t, long head — Supraspinatus m and t

Coracoacromial lig

Coracohumeral lig

Superior glenohumeral lig

Coracoid process

Subscapularis t

Deltoid m

Cephalic v

Anterior circumflex humeral a

Pectoralis major m

Biceps brachii m, short head

Coracobrachialis m

Acromion

Infraspinatus m and t

Humeral epiphysis

Teres minor m

Deltoid m

Posterior circumflex humeral a and axillary n

Triceps brachii m, long head

Triceps brachii m, lateral head

Latissimus dorsi and teres major tt — Teres major m

Figure 2.2.11

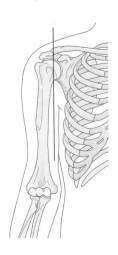

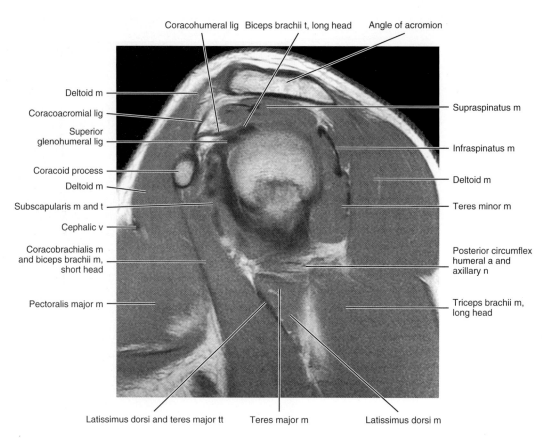

Coracohumeral lig
Biceps brachii t, long head
Angle of acromion
Deltoid m
Coracoacromial lig
Superior glenohumeral lig
Coracoid process
Deltoid m
Subscapularis m and t
Cephalic v
Coracobrachialis m and biceps brachii m, short head
Pectoralis major m
Supraspinatus m
Infraspinatus m
Deltoid m
Teres minor m
Posterior circumflex humeral a and axillary n
Triceps brachii m, long head
Latissimus dorsi and teres major tt
Teres major m
Latissimus dorsi m

Figure 2.2.12

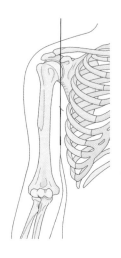

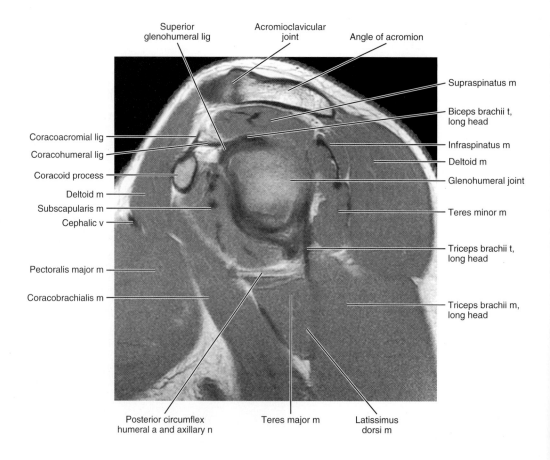

Superior glenohumeral lig
Acromioclavicular joint
Angle of acromion
Coracoacromial lig
Coracohumeral lig
Coracoid process
Deltoid m
Subscapularis m
Cephalic v
Pectoralis major m
Coracobrachialis m
Supraspinatus m
Biceps brachii t, long head
Infraspinatus m
Deltoid m
Glenohumeral joint
Teres minor m
Triceps brachii t, long head
Triceps brachii m, long head
Posterior circumflex humeral a and axillary n
Teres major m
Latissimus dorsi m

Figure 2.2.13

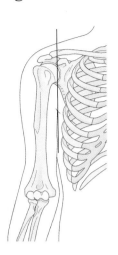

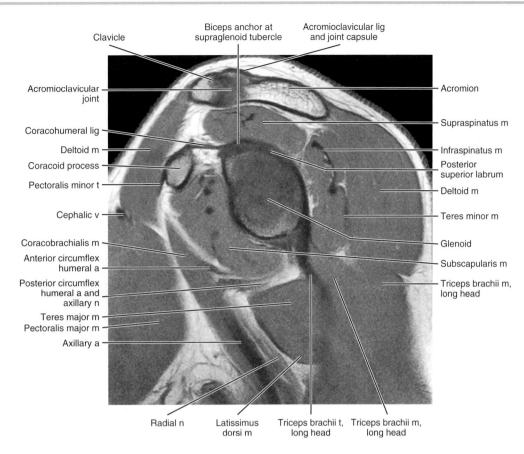

Clavicle

Biceps anchor at supraglenoid tubercle

Acromioclavicular lig and joint capsule

Acromioclavicular joint

Acromion

Coracohumeral lig

Supraspinatus m

Deltoid m

Infraspinatus m

Coracoid process

Posterior superior labrum

Pectoralis minor t

Deltoid m

Cephalic v

Teres minor m

Coracobrachialis m

Glenoid

Anterior circumflex humeral a

Subscapularis m

Posterior circumflex humeral a and axillary n

Triceps brachii m, long head

Teres major m
Pectoralis major m

Axillary a

Radial n   Latissimus dorsi m   Triceps brachii t, long head   Triceps brachii m, long head

Figure 2.2.14

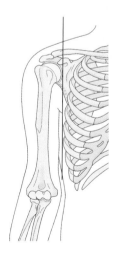

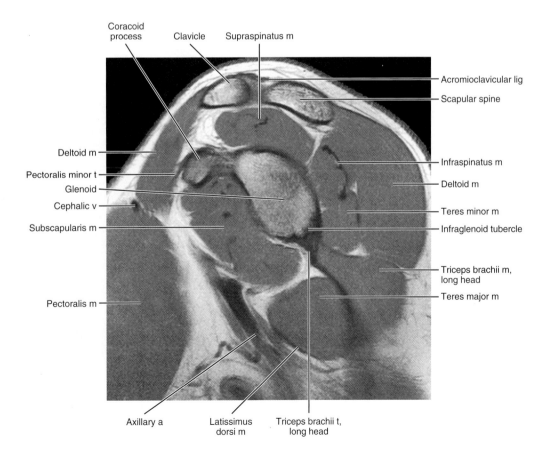

Coracoid process

Clavicle   Supraspinatus m

Acromioclavicular lig

Scapular spine

Deltoid m

Pectoralis minor t

Infraspinatus m

Glenoid

Deltoid m

Cephalic v

Teres minor m

Subscapularis m

Infraglenoid tubercle

Triceps brachii m, long head

Pectoralis m

Teres major m

Axillary a   Latissimus dorsi m   Triceps brachii t, long head

Figure 2.2.15

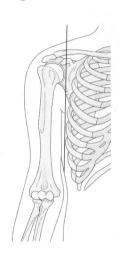

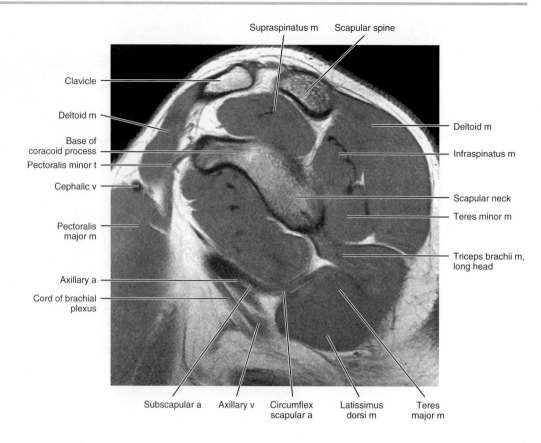

Supraspinatus m | Scapular spine
Clavicle
Deltoid m
Base of coracoid process
Pectoralis minor t
Cephalic v
Pectoralis major m
Axillary a
Cord of brachial plexus

Deltoid m
Infraspinatus m
Scapular neck
Teres minor m
Triceps brachii m, long head

Subscapular a | Axillary v | Circumflex scapular a | Latissimus dorsi m | Teres major m

Figure 2.2.16

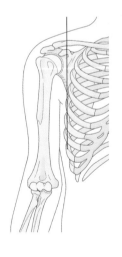

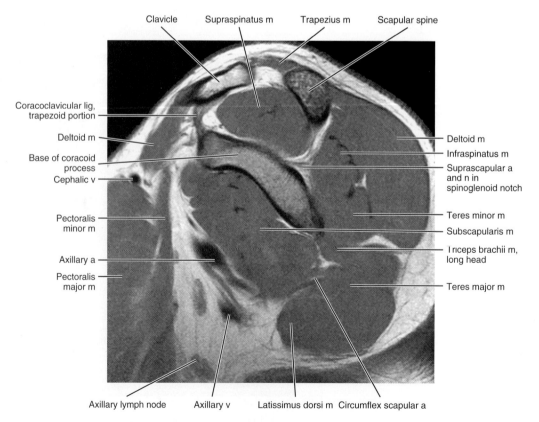

Clavicle | Supraspinatus m | Trapezius m | Scapular spine
Coracoclavicular lig, trapezoid portion
Deltoid m
Base of coracoid process
Cephalic v
Pectoralis minor m
Axillary a
Pectoralis major m

Deltoid m
Infraspinatus m
Suprascapular a and n in spinoglenoid notch
Teres minor m
Subscapularis m
Triceps brachii m, long head
Teres major m

Axillary lymph node | Axillary v | Latissimus dorsi m | Circumflex scapular a

Figure 2.2.17

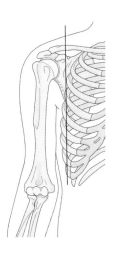

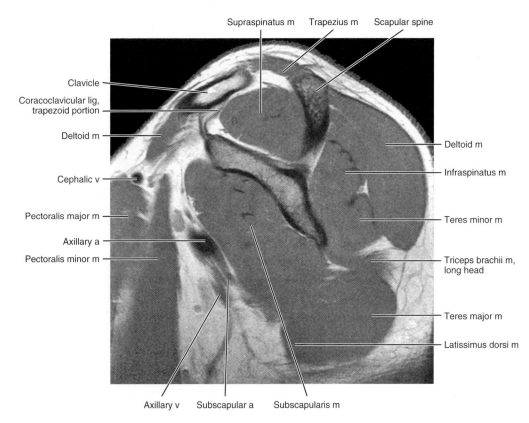

Supraspinatus m   Trapezius m   Scapular spine

Clavicle

Coracoclavicular lig, trapezoid portion

Deltoid m

Cephalic v

Pectoralis major m

Axillary a

Pectoralis minor m

Deltoid m

Infraspinatus m

Teres minor m

Triceps brachii m, long head

Teres major m

Latissimus dorsi m

Axillary v   Subscapular a   Subscapularis m

Figure 2.2.18

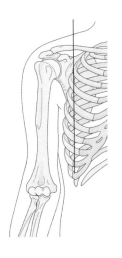

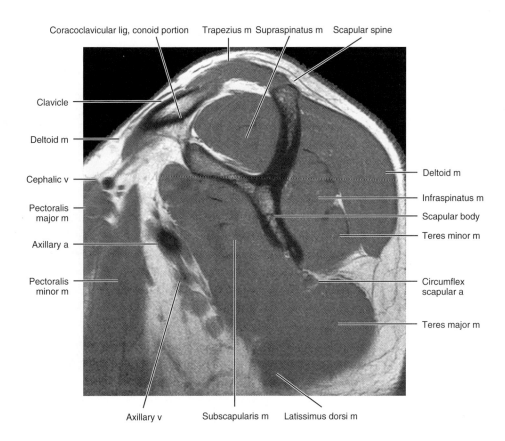

Coracoclavicular lig, conoid portion   Trapezius m   Suprasinatus m   Scapular spine

Clavicle

Deltoid m

Cephalic v

Pectoralis major m

Axillary a

Pectoralis minor m

Deltoid m

Infraspinatus m

Scapular body

Teres minor m

Circumflex scapular a

Teres major m

Axillary v   Subscapularis m   Latissimus dorsi m

Figure 2.2.19

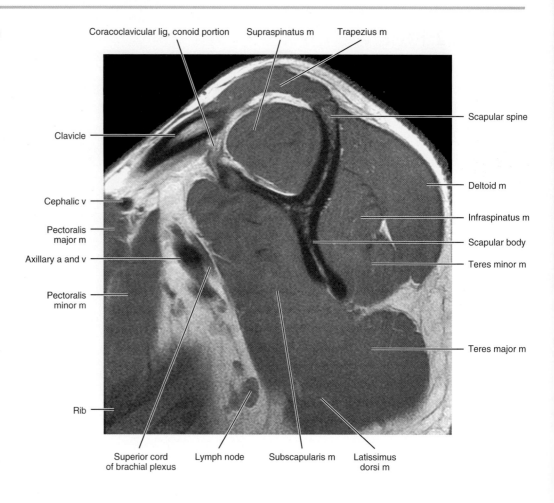

Coracoclavicular lig, conoid portion
Supraspinatus m
Trapezius m
Scapular spine
Clavicle
Deltoid m
Cephalic v
Infraspinatus m
Pectoralis major m
Scapular body
Axillary a and v
Teres minor m
Pectoralis minor m
Teres major m
Rib
Superior cord of brachial plexus
Lymph node
Subscapularis m
Latissimus dorsi m

Figure 2.2.20

Trapezius m
Supraspinatus m
Scapular spine
Clavicle
Deltoid m
Subclavius m
Cephalic v
Infraspinatus m
Axillary a
Scapular body
Pectoralis minor m
Teres minor m
Axillary v
Rib
Teres major m
Latissimus dorsi m
Long thoracic a and n
Subscapularis m

OBLIQUE CORONAL

Figure 2.3.1

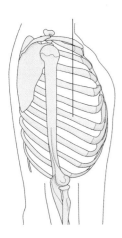

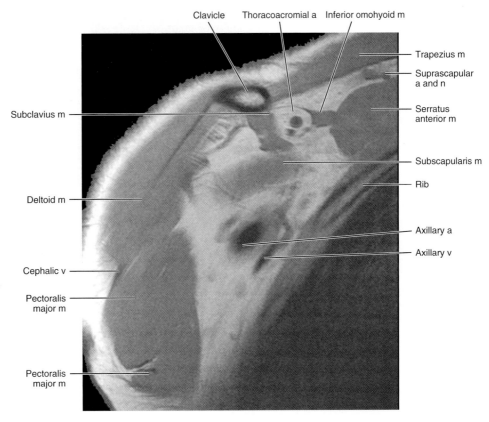

Clavicle · Thoracoacromial a · Inferior omohyoid m

Trapezius m

Suprascapular a and n

Subclavius m

Serratus anterior m

Subscapularis m

Rib

Deltoid m

Axillary a

Axillary v

Cephalic v

Pectoralis major m

Pectoralis major m

Figure 2.3.2

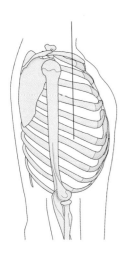

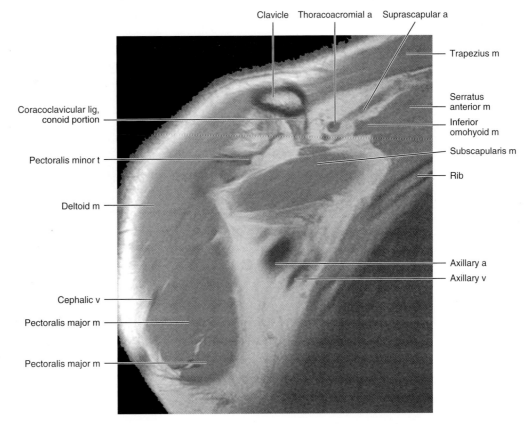

Clavicle · Thoracoacromial a · Suprascapular a

Trapezius m

Coracoclavicular lig, conoid portion

Serratus anterior m

Inferior omohyoid m

Pectoralis minor t

Subscapularis m

Rib

Deltoid m

Axillary a

Axillary v

Cephalic v

Pectoralis major m

Pectoralis major m

Figure 2.3.3

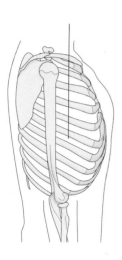

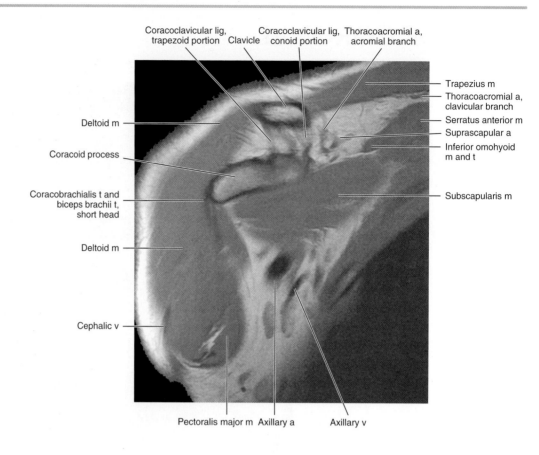

Coracoclavicular lig, trapezoid portion
Clavicle
Coracoclavicular lig, conoid portion
Thoracoacromial a, acromial branch

Trapezius m
Thoracoacromial a, clavicular branch
Serratus anterior m
Suprascapular a
Inferior omohyoid m and t

Deltoid m
Coracoid process
Coracobrachialis t and biceps brachii t, short head
Deltoid m
Cephalic v

Subscapularis m

Pectoralis major m   Axillary a   Axillary v

Figure 2.3.4

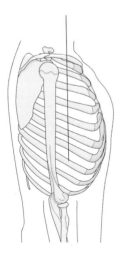

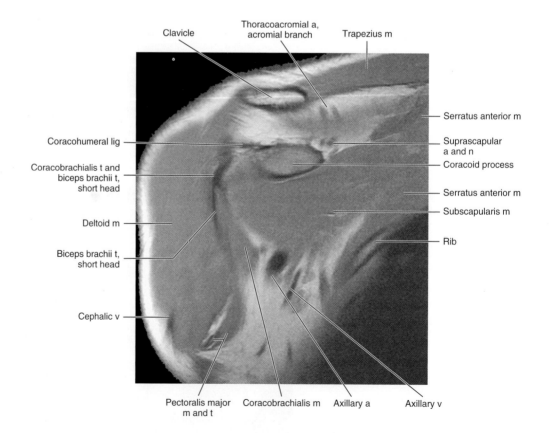

Clavicle
Thoracoacromial a, acromial branch
Trapezius m

Coracohumeral lig
Coracobrachialis t and biceps brachii t, short head
Deltoid m
Biceps brachii t, short head
Cephalic v

Serratus anterior m
Suprascapular a and n
Coracoid process
Serratus anterior m
Subscapularis m
Rib

Pectoralis major m and t   Coracobrachialis m   Axillary a   Axillary v

Figure 2.3.5

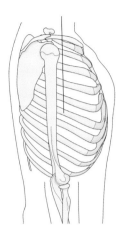

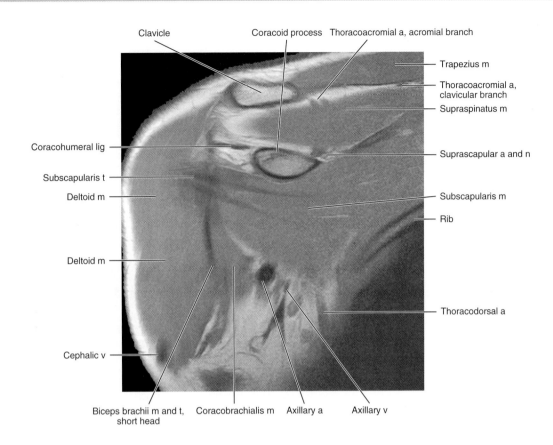

Clavicle · Coracoid process · Thoracoacromial a, acromial branch

Trapezius m

Thoracoacromial a, clavicular branch

Supraspinatus m

Coracohumeral lig

Suprascapular a and n

Subscapularis t

Deltoid m

Subscapularis m

Rib

Deltoid m

Thoracodorsal a

Cephalic v

Biceps brachii m and t, short head · Coracobrachialis m · Axillary a · Axillary v

Figure 2.3.6

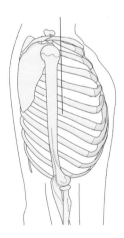

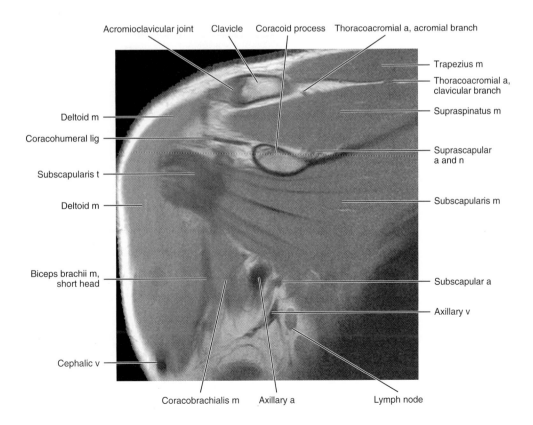

Acromioclavicular joint · Clavicle · Coracoid process · Thoracoacromial a, acromial branch

Trapezius m

Thoracoacromial a, clavicular branch

Deltoid m

Supraspinatus m

Coracohumeral lig

Suprascapular a and n

Subscapularis t

Deltoid m

Subscapularis m

Biceps brachii m, short head

Subscapular a

Axillary v

Cephalic v

Coracobrachialis m · Axillary a · Lymph node

Figure 2.3.7

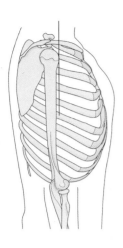

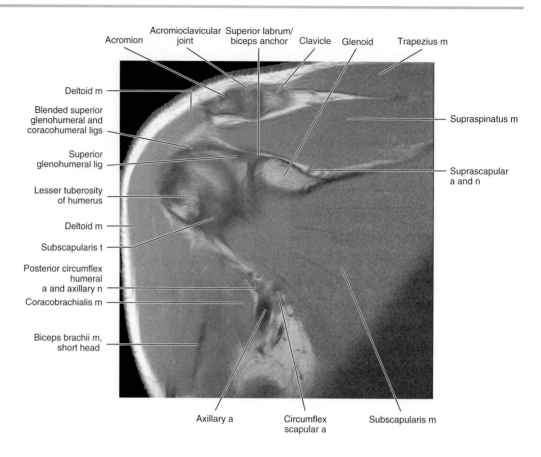

Acromion
Acromioclavicular joint
Superior labrum/biceps anchor
Clavicle
Glenoid
Trapezius m

Deltoid m

Blended superior glenohumeral and coracohumeral ligs

Superior glenohumeral lig

Lesser tuberosity of humerus

Deltoid m

Subscapularis t

Posterior circumflex humeral a and axillary n

Coracobrachialis m

Biceps brachii m, short head

Supraspinatus m

Suprascapular a and n

Axillary a
Circumflex scapular a
Subscapularis m

Figure 2.3.8

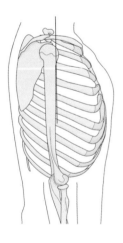

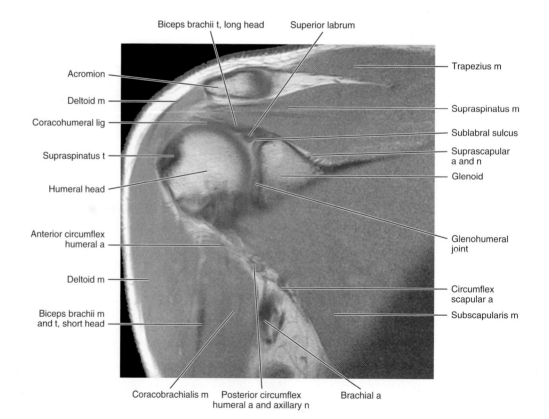

Biceps brachii t, long head
Superior labrum

Acromion

Deltoid m

Coracohumeral lig

Supraspinatus t

Humeral head

Anterior circumflex humeral a

Deltoid m

Biceps brachii m and t, short head

Trapezius m

Supraspinatus m

Sublabral sulcus

Suprascapular a and n

Glenoid

Glenohumeral joint

Circumflex scapular a

Subscapularis m

Coracobrachialis m
Posterior circumflex humeral a and axillary n
Brachial a

Figure 2.3.9

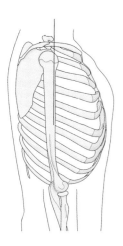

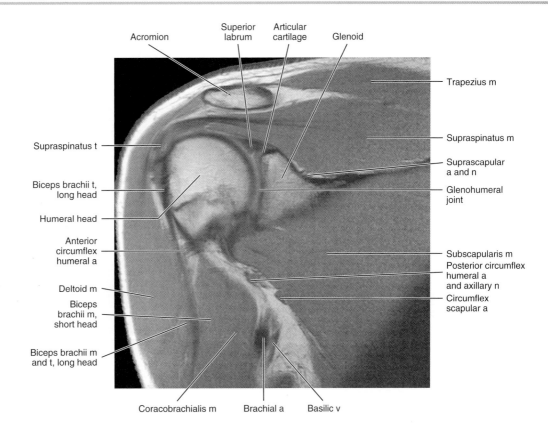

Acromion
Superior labrum
Articular cartilage
Glenoid
Trapezius m
Supraspinatus t
Supraspinatus m
Suprascapular a and n
Biceps brachii t, long head
Glenohumeral joint
Humeral head
Anterior circumflex humeral a
Subscapularis m
Posterior circumflex humeral a and axillary n
Deltoid m
Circumflex scapular a
Biceps brachii m, short head
Biceps brachii m and t, long head
Coracobrachialis m
Brachial a
Basilic v

Figure 2.3.10

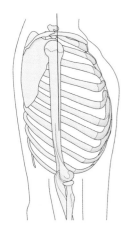

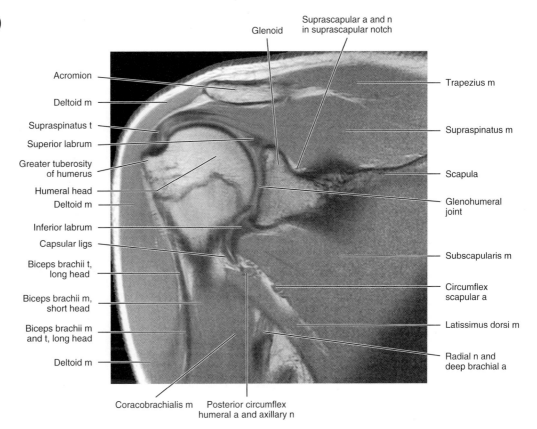

Glenoid
Suprascapular a and n in suprascapular notch
Acromion
Trapezius m
Deltoid m
Supraspinatus t
Supraspinatus m
Superior labrum
Greater tuberosity of humerus
Scapula
Humeral head
Deltoid m
Glenohumeral joint
Inferior labrum
Capsular ligs
Subscapularis m
Biceps brachii t, long head
Circumflex scapular a
Biceps brachii m, short head
Biceps brachii m and t, long head
Latissimus dorsi m
Deltoid m
Radial n and deep brachial a
Coracobrachialis m
Posterior circumflex humeral a and axillary n

Figure 2.3.11

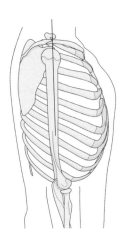

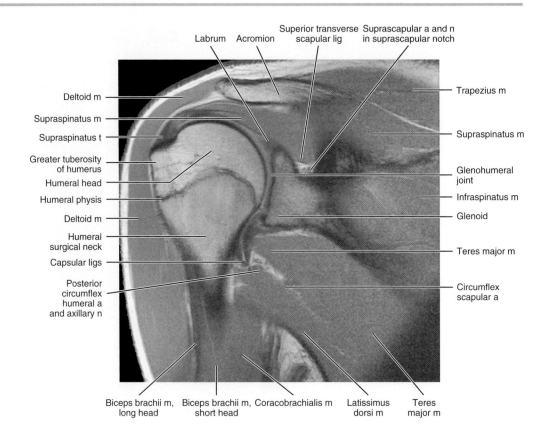

Labrum · Acromion · Superior transverse scapular lig · Suprascapular a and n in suprascapular notch

Deltoid m
Supraspinatus m
Supraspinatus t
Greater tuberosity of humerus
Humeral head
Humeral physis
Deltoid m
Humeral surgical neck
Capsular ligs
Posterior circumflex humeral a and axillary n

Trapezius m
Supraspinatus m
Glenohumeral joint
Infraspinatus m
Glenoid
Teres major m
Circumflex scapular a

Biceps brachii m, long head · Biceps brachii m, short head · Coracobrachialis m · Latissimus dorsi m · Teres major m

Figure 2.3.12

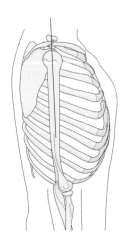

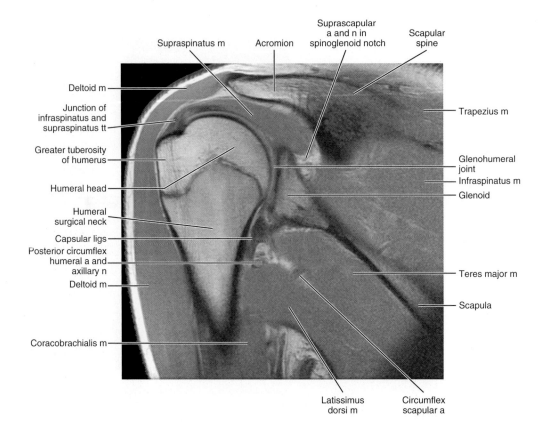

Supraspinatus m · Acromion · Suprascapular a and n in spinoglenoid notch · Scapular spine

Deltoid m
Junction of infraspinatus and supraspinatus tt
Greater tuberosity of humerus
Humeral head
Humeral surgical neck
Capsular ligs
Posterior circumflex humeral a and axillary n
Deltoid m
Coracobrachialis m

Trapezius m
Glenohumeral joint
Infraspinatus m
Glenoid
Teres major m
Scapula

Latissimus dorsi m · Circumflex scapular a

Figure 2.3.13

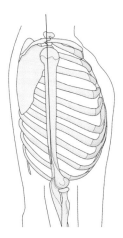

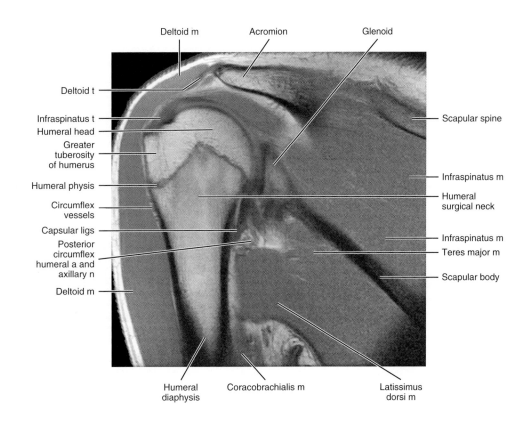

Deltoid m | Acromion | Glenoid

Deltoid t

Infraspinatus t
Humeral head
Greater tuberosity of humerus
Humeral physis
Circumflex vessels
Capsular ligs
Posterior circumflex humeral a and axillary n
Deltoid m

Scapular spine

Infraspinatus m
Humeral surgical neck

Infraspinatus m
Teres major m
Scapular body

Humeral diaphysis | Coracobrachialis m | Latissimus dorsi m

Figure 2.3.14

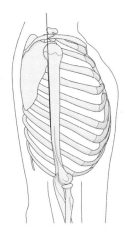

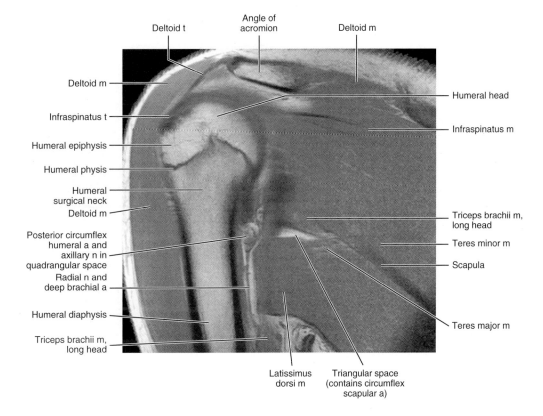

Deltoid t | Angle of acromion | Deltoid m

Deltoid m
Infraspinatus t
Humeral epiphysis
Humeral physis
Humeral surgical neck
Deltoid m
Posterior circumflex humeral a and axillary n in quadrangular space
Radial n and deep brachial a
Humeral diaphysis
Triceps brachii m, long head

Humeral head
Infraspinatus m

Triceps brachii m, long head
Teres minor m
Scapula

Teres major m

Latissimus dorsi m | Triangular space (contains circumflex scapular a)

Figure 2.3.15

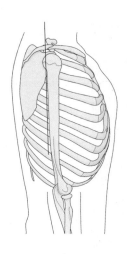

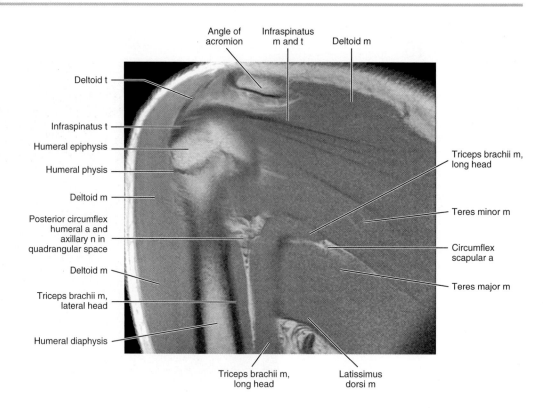

Deltoid t

Angle of acromion

Infraspinatus m and t

Deltoid m

Infraspinatus t

Humeral epiphysis

Humeral physis

Deltoid m

Posterior circumflex humeral a and axillary n in quadrangular space

Deltoid m

Triceps brachii m, lateral head

Humeral diaphysis

Triceps brachii m, long head

Teres minor m

Circumflex scapular a

Teres major m

Triceps brachii m, long head

Latissimus dorsi m

Figure 2.3.16

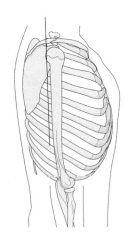

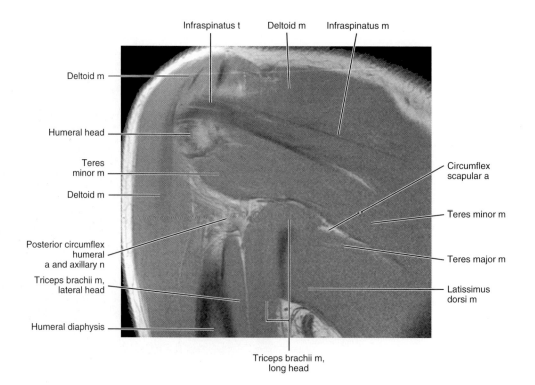

Infraspinatus t

Deltoid m

Infraspinatus m

Deltoid m

Humeral head

Teres minor m

Deltoid m

Posterior circumflex humeral a and axillary n

Triceps brachii m, lateral head

Humeral diaphysis

Circumflex scapular a

Teres minor m

Teres major m

Latissimus dorsi m

Triceps brachii m, long head

Figure 2.3.17

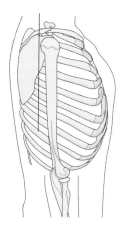

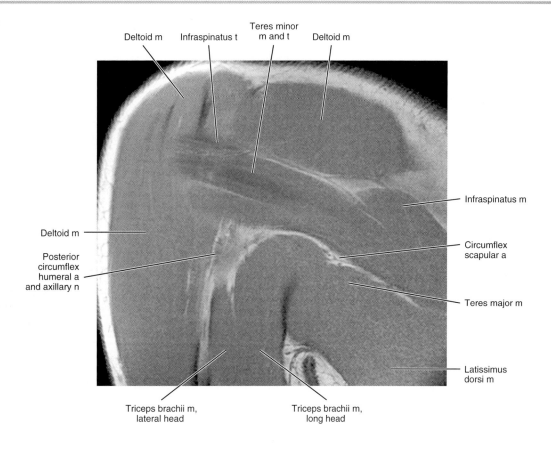

Deltoid m　Infraspinatus t　Teres minor m and t　Deltoid m

Infraspinatus m

Deltoid m

Circumflex scapular a

Posterior circumflex humeral a and axillary n

Teres major m

Latissimus dorsi m

Triceps brachii m, lateral head　Triceps brachii m, long head

Figure 2.3.18

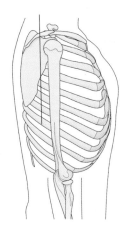

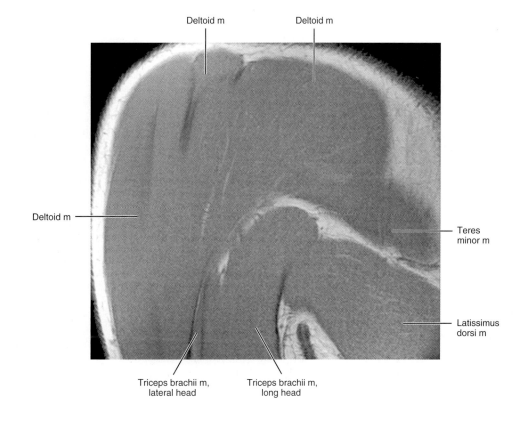

Deltoid m　Deltoid m

Deltoid m

Teres minor m

Latissimus dorsi m

Triceps brachii m, lateral head　Triceps brachii m, long head

Figure 2.3.19

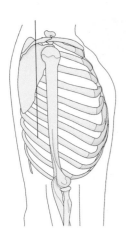

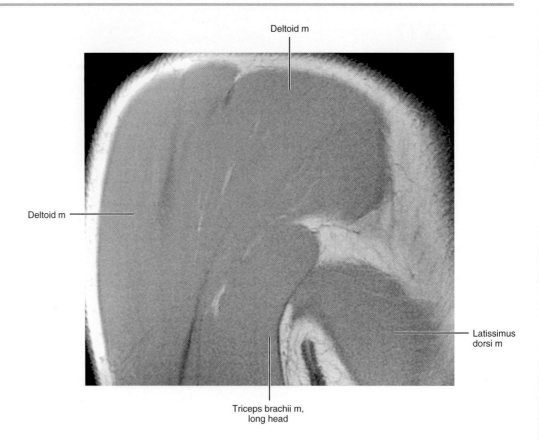

Deltoid m

Deltoid m

Latissimus dorsi m

Triceps brachii m, long head

Figure 2.3.20

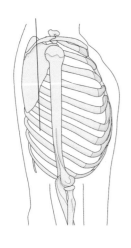

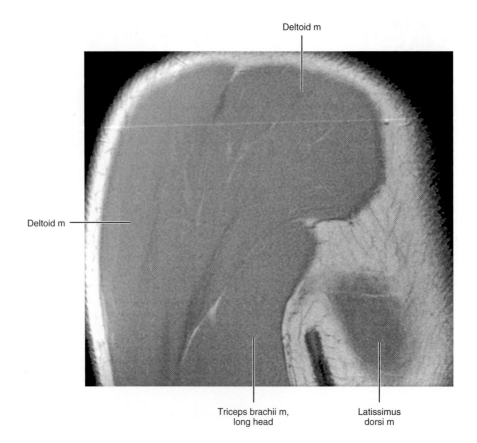

Deltoid m

Deltoid m

Triceps brachii m, long head

Latissimus dorsi m

Chapter 3

MR Arthrography
of the Shoulder

AXIAL

Figure 3.1.1

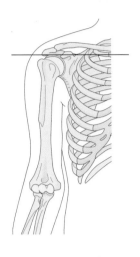

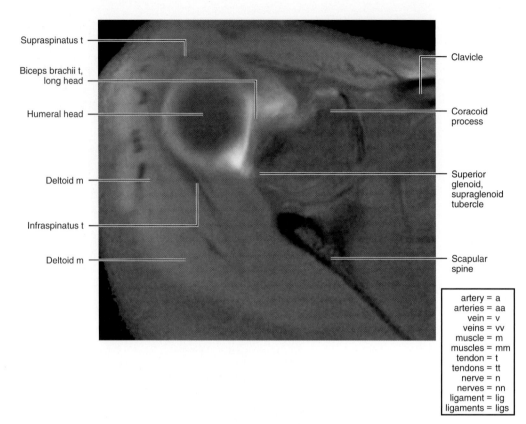

Supraspinatus t

Biceps brachii t, long head

Humeral head

Deltoid m

Infraspinatus t

Deltoid m

Clavicle

Coracoid process

Superior glenoid, supraglenoid tubercle

Scapular spine

| artery = a |
| arteries = aa |
| vein = v |
| veins = vv |
| muscle = m |
| muscles = mm |
| tendon = t |
| tendons = tt |
| nerve = n |
| nerves = nn |
| ligament = lig |
| ligaments = ligs |

Figure 3.1.2

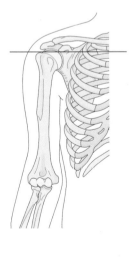

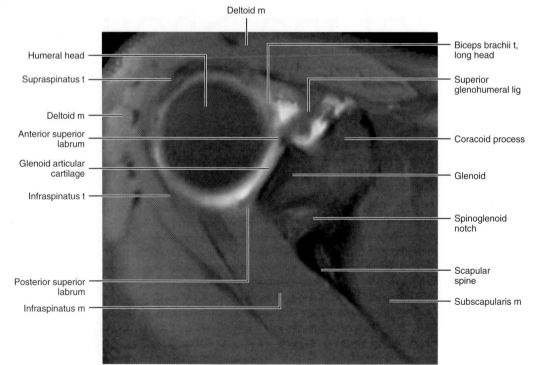

Deltoid m

Humeral head

Supraspinatus t

Deltoid m

Anterior superior labrum

Glenoid articular cartilage

Infraspinatus t

Posterior superior labrum

Infraspinatus m

Biceps brachii t, long head

Superior glenohumeral lig

Coracoid process

Glenoid

Spinoglenoid notch

Scapular spine

Subscapularis m

Figure 3.1.3

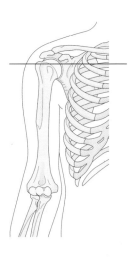

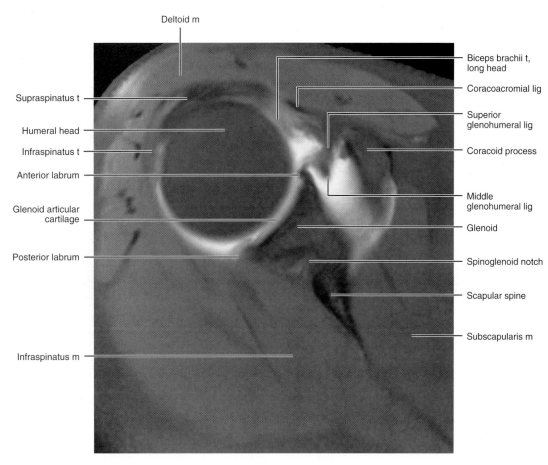

Deltoid m

Supraspinatus t

Humeral head

Infraspinatus t

Anterior labrum

Glenoid articular cartilage

Posterior labrum

Infraspinatus m

Biceps brachii t, long head

Coracoacromial lig

Superior glenohumeral lig

Coracoid process

Middle glenohumeral lig

Glenoid

Spinoglenoid notch

Scapular spine

Subscapularis m

Figure 3.1.4

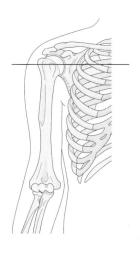

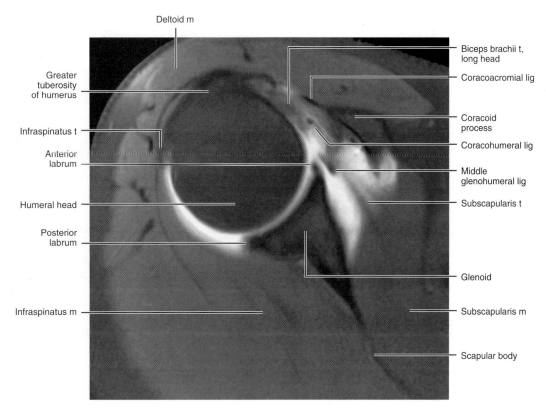

Deltoid m

Greater tuberosity of humerus

Infraspinatus t

Anterior labrum

Humeral head

Posterior labrum

Infraspinatus m

Biceps brachii t, long head

Coracoacromial lig

Coracoid process

Coracohumeral lig

Middle glenohumeral lig

Subscapularis t

Glenoid

Subscapularis m

Scapular body

Figure 3.1.5

Deltoid m

Biceps brachii t, long head

Coracoacromial lig

Greater tuberosity of humerus

Coracoid process

Subscapularis t

Superior subscapular recess

Humeral head

Anterior labrum

Middle glenohumeral lig

Infraspinatus t

Glenoid articular cartilage

Subscapularis m

Posterior labrum

Capsular insertion

Infraspinatus m

Scapular body

Figure 3.1.6

Bicipital (intertubercular) groove

Biceps brachii t, long head

Greater tuberosity of humerus

Coracoacromial lig

Lesser tuberosity of humerus

Pectoralis minor t

Subscapularis t

Coracoid process

Humeral head

Anterior labrum

Middle glenohumeral lig

Teres minor t

Articular cartilage

Posterior labrum

Glenoid

Deltoid m

Subscapularis m

Scapular body

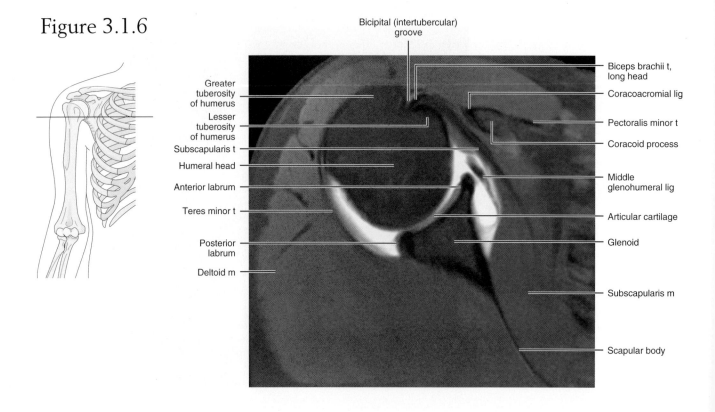

Figure 3.1.7

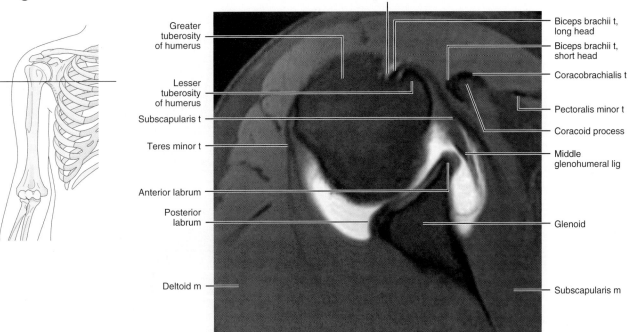

Bicipital (intertubercular) groove

Greater tuberosity of humerus

Lesser tuberosity of humerus

Subscapularis t

Teres minor t

Anterior labrum

Posterior labrum

Deltoid m

Biceps brachii t, long head

Biceps brachii t, short head

Coracobrachialis t

Pectoralis minor t

Coracoid process

Middle glenohumeral lig

Glenoid

Subscapularis m

Scapular body

Figure 3.1.8

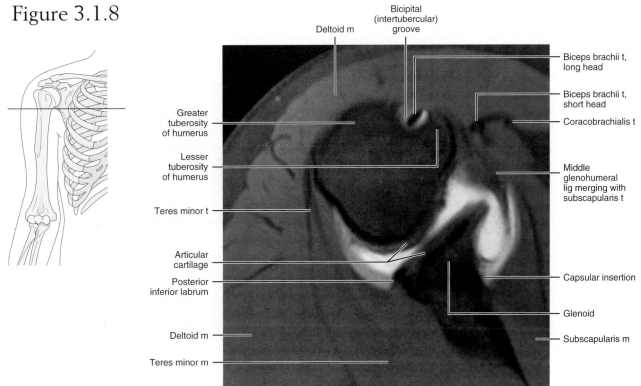

Deltoid m

Bicipital (intertubercular) groove

Greater tuberosity of humerus

Lesser tuberosity of humerus

Teres minor t

Articular cartilage

Posterior inferior labrum

Deltoid m

Teres minor m

Biceps brachii t, long head

Biceps brachii t, short head

Coracobrachialis t

Middle glenohumeral lig merging with subscapularis t

Capsular insertion

Glenoid

Subscapularis m

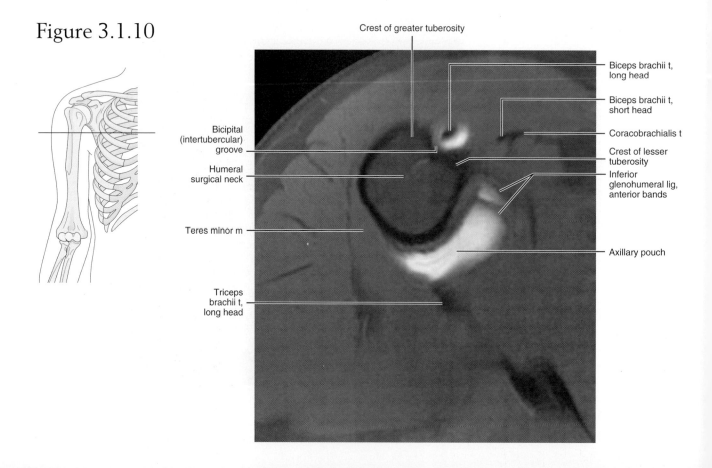

Figure 3.1.9

Crest of greater tuberosity
Biceps brachii t, long head
Biceps brachii t, short head
Coracobrachialis t
Bicipital (intertubercular) groove
Crest of lesser tuberosity
Humeral surgical neck
Inferior glenohumeral lig, anterior band
Teres minor m
Inferior glenoid, infraglenoid tubercle
Posterior inferior labrum

Figure 3.1.10

Crest of greater tuberosity
Biceps brachii t, long head
Biceps brachii t, short head
Coracobrachialis t
Bicipital (intertubercular) groove
Crest of lesser tuberosity
Humeral surgical neck
Inferior glenohumeral lig, anterior bands
Teres minor m
Axillary pouch
Triceps brachii t, long head

OBLIQUE SAGITTAL

Figure 3.2.1

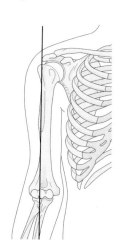

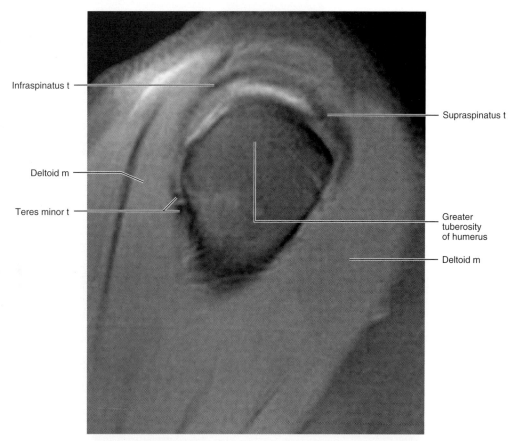

Infraspinatus t

Supraspinatus t

Deltoid m

Teres minor t

Greater tuberosity of humerus

Deltoid m

Figure 3.2.2

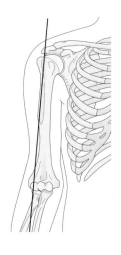

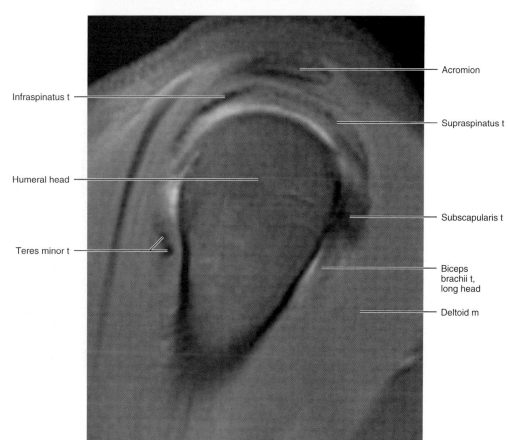

Infraspinatus t

Acromion

Supraspinatus t

Humeral head

Subscapularis t

Teres minor t

Biceps brachii t, long head

Deltoid m

Figure 3.2.3

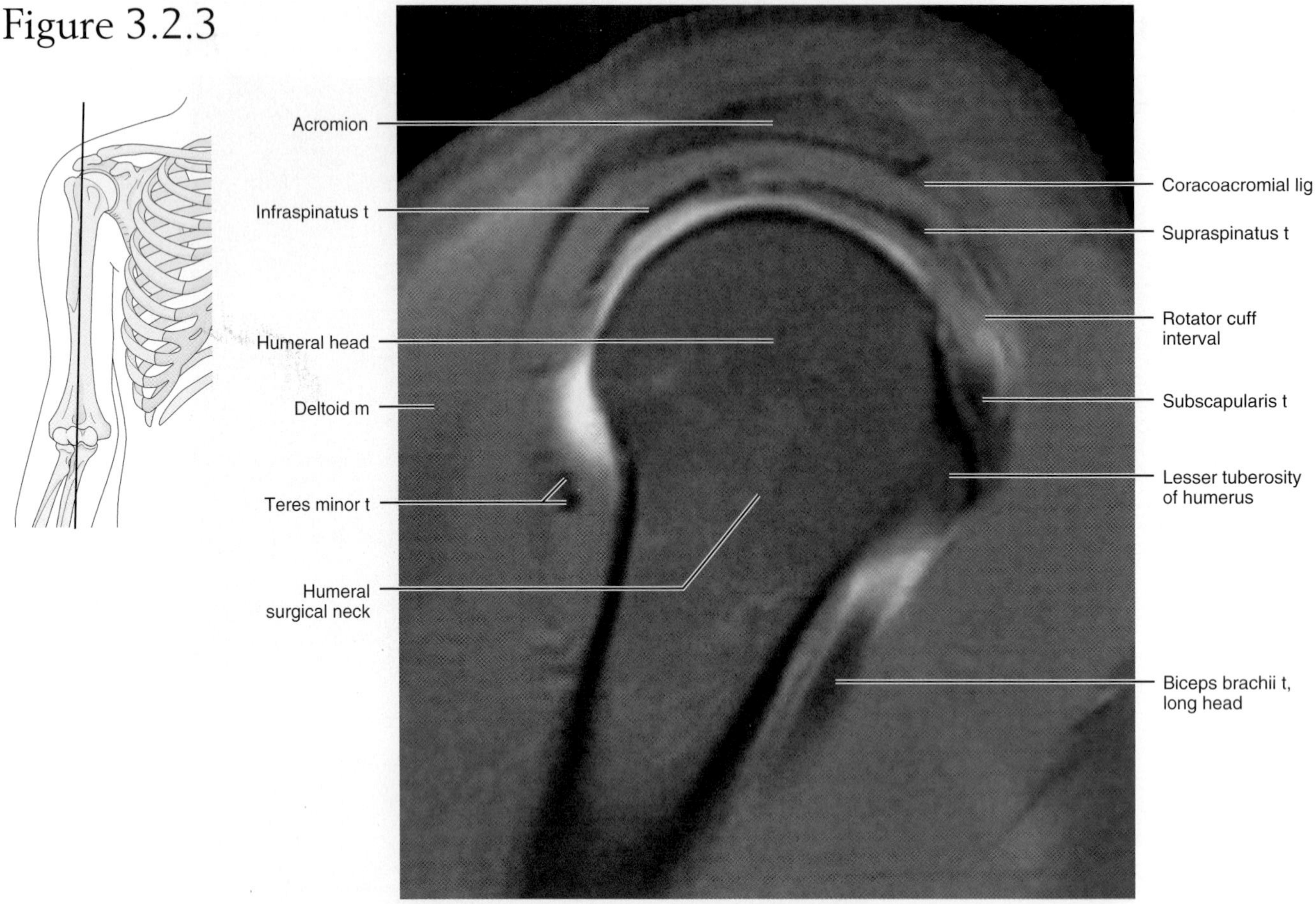

Acromion
Infraspinatus t
Humeral head
Deltoid m
Teres minor t
Humeral surgical neck

Coracoacromial lig
Supraspinatus t
Rotator cuff interval
Subscapularis t
Lesser tuberosity of humerus
Biceps brachii t, long head

Figure 3.2.4

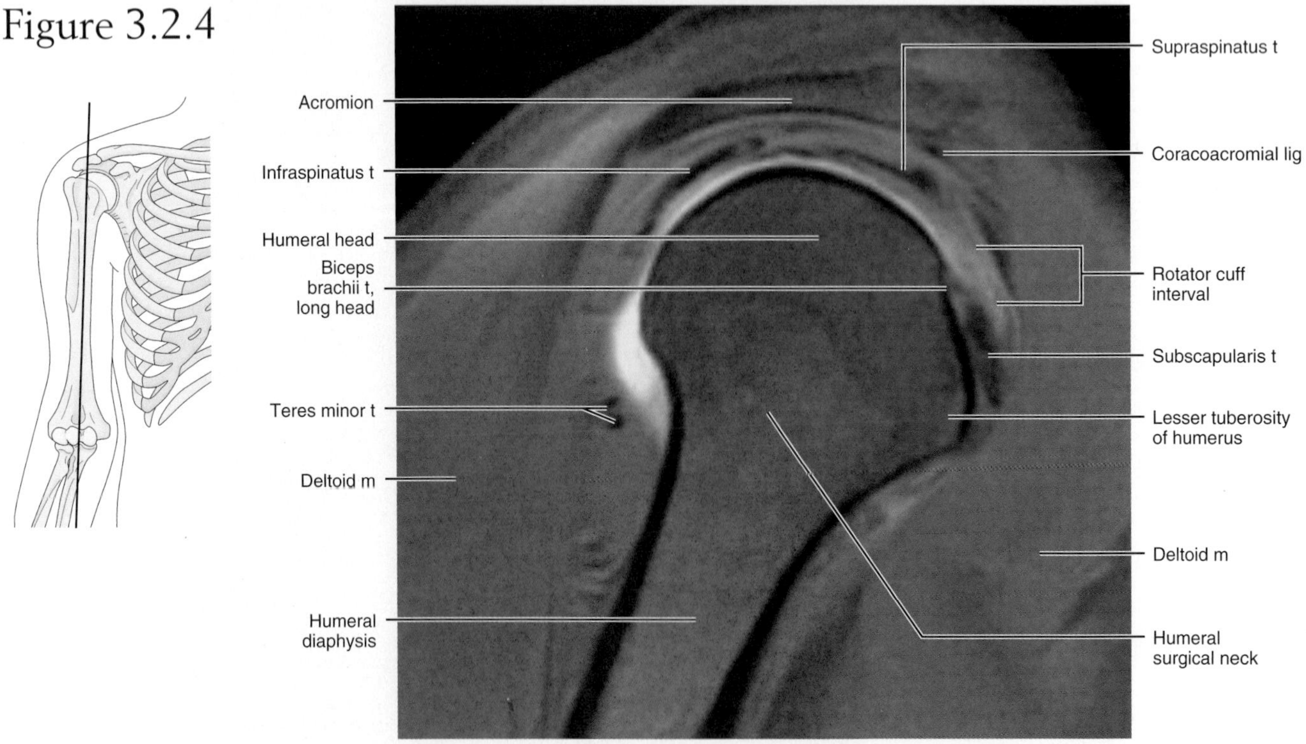

Acromion
Infraspinatus t
Humeral head
Biceps brachii t, long head
Teres minor t
Deltoid m
Humeral diaphysis

Supraspinatus t
Coracoacromial lig
Rotator cuff interval
Subscapularis t
Lesser tuberosity of humerus
Deltoid m
Humeral surgical neck

Figure 3.2.5

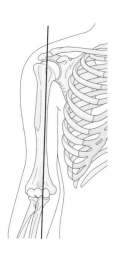

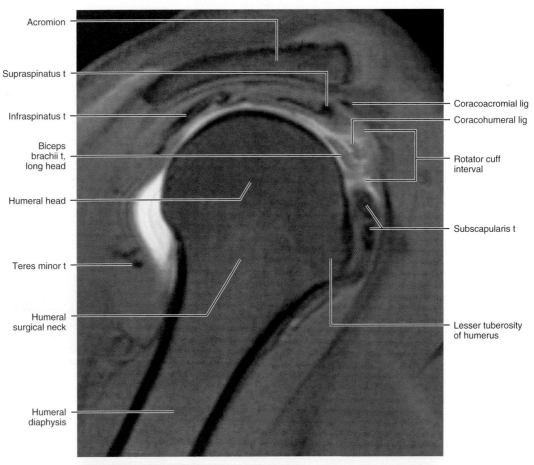

Acromion

Supraspinatus t

Infraspinatus t

Biceps brachii t, long head

Humeral head

Teres minor t

Humeral surgical neck

Humeral diaphysis

Coracoacromial lig

Coracohumeral lig

Rotator cuff interval

Subscapularis t

Lesser tuberosity of humerus

Figure 3.2.6

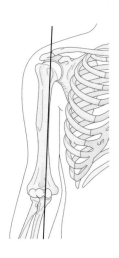

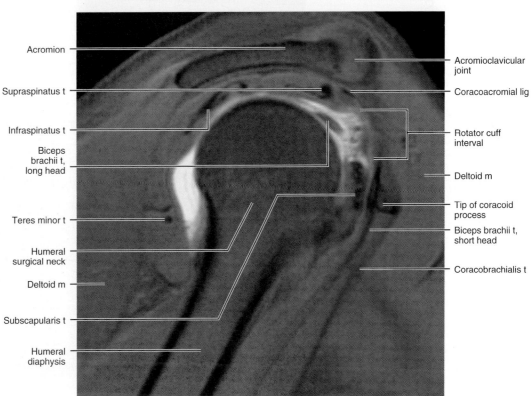

Acromion

Supraspinatus t

Infraspinatus t

Biceps brachii t, long head

Teres minor t

Humeral surgical neck

Deltoid m

Subscapularis t

Humeral diaphysis

Acromioclavicular joint

Coracoacromial lig

Rotator cuff interval

Deltoid m

Tip of coracoid process

Biceps brachii t, short head

Coracobrachialis t

Figure 3.2.7

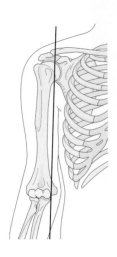

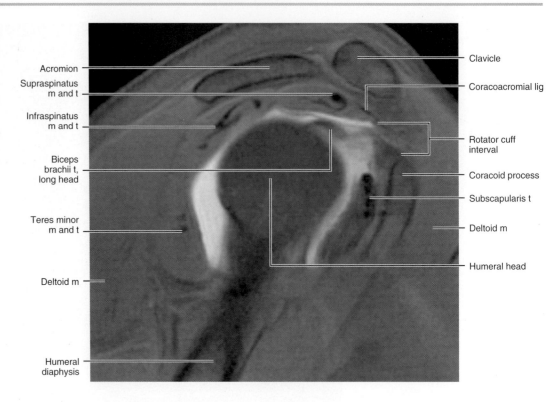

Acromion

Supraspinatus
m and t

Infraspinatus
m and t

Biceps
brachii t,
long head

Teres minor
m and t

Deltoid m

Humeral
diaphysis

Clavicle

Coracoacromial lig

Rotator cuff
interval

Coracoid process

Subscapularis t

Deltoid m

Humeral head

Figure 3.2.8

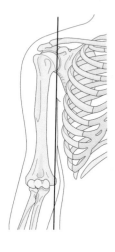

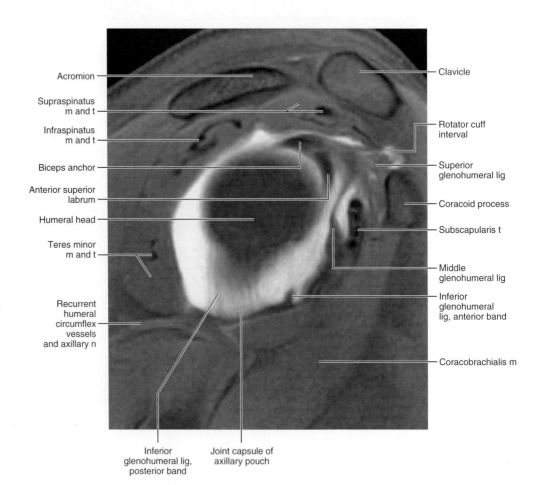

Acromion

Supraspinatus
m and t

Infraspinatus
m and t

Biceps anchor

Anterior superior
labrum

Humeral head

Teres minor
m and t

Recurrent
humeral
circumflex
vessels
and axillary n

Clavicle

Rotator cuff
interval

Superior
glenohumeral lig

Coracoid process

Subscapularis t

Middle
glenohumeral lig

Inferior
glenohumeral
lig, anterior band

Coracobrachialis m

Inferior
glenohumeral lig,
posterior band

Joint capsule of
axillary pouch

Figure 3.2.9

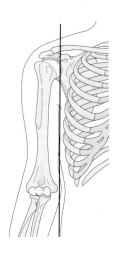

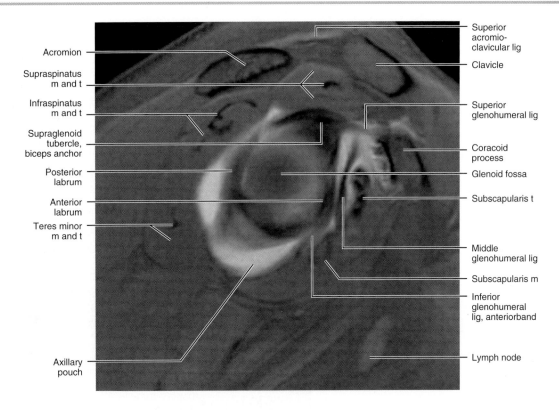

Acromion

Supraspinatus m and t

Infraspinatus m and t

Supraglenoid tubercle, biceps anchor

Posterior labrum

Anterior labrum

Teres minor m and t

Axillary pouch

Superior acromio-clavicular lig

Clavicle

Superior glenohumeral lig

Coracoid process

Glenoid fossa

Subscapularis t

Middle glenohumeral lig

Subscapularis m

Inferior glenohumeral lig, anteriorband

Lymph node

Figure 3.2.10

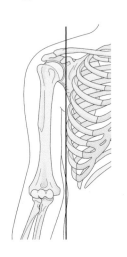

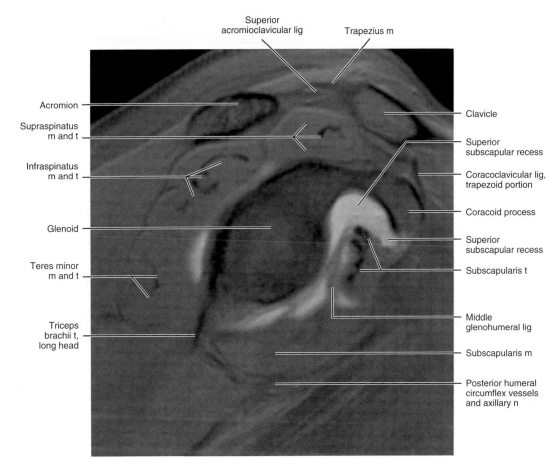

Superior acromioclavicular lig

Trapezius m

Acromion

Supraspinatus m and t

Infraspinatus m and t

Glenoid

Teres minor m and t

Triceps brachii t, long head

Clavicle

Superior subscapular recess

Coracoclavicular lig, trapezoid portion

Coracoid process

Superior subscapular recess

Subscapularis t

Middle glenohumeral lig

Subscapularis m

Posterior humeral circumflex vessels and axillary n

Figure 3.2.11

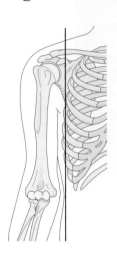

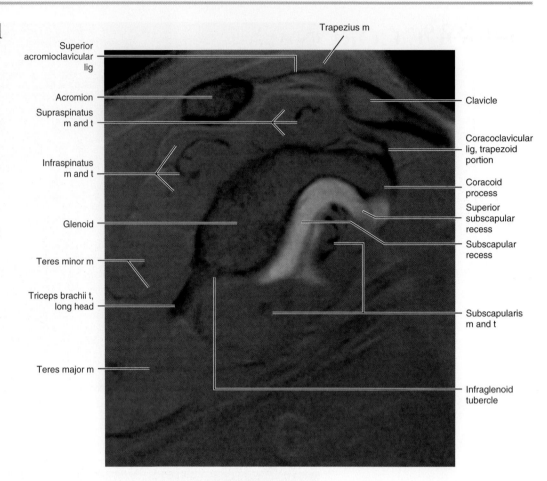

Trapezius m

Superior acromioclavicular lig

Acromion

Supraspinatus m and t

Infraspinatus m and t

Glenoid

Teres minor m

Triceps brachii t, long head

Teres major m

Clavicle

Coracoclavicular lig, trapezoid portion

Coracoid process

Superior subscapular recess

Subscapular recess

Subscapularis m and t

Infraglenoid tubercle

OBLIQUE CORONAL

Figure 3.3.1

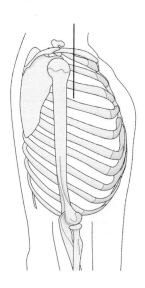

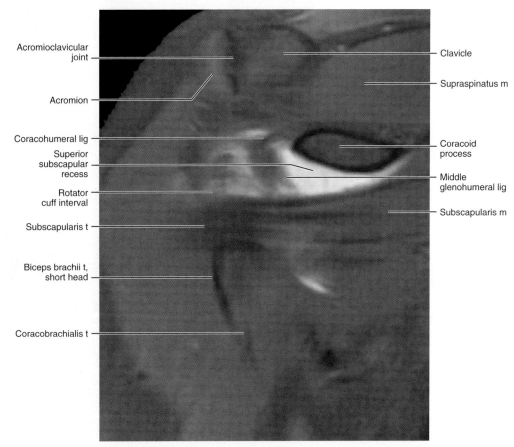

Acromioclavicular joint

Acromion

Coracohumeral lig

Superior subscapular recess

Rotator cuff interval

Subscapularis t

Biceps brachii t, short head

Coracobrachialis t

Clavicle

Supraspinatus m

Coracoid process

Middle glenohumeral lig

Subscapularis m

Figure 3.3.2

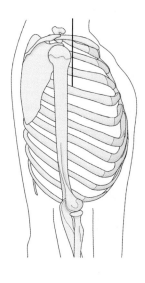

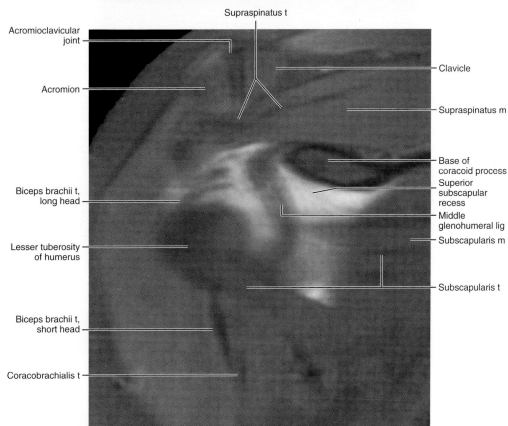

Supraspinatus t

Acromioclavicular joint

Acromion

Biceps brachii t, long head

Lesser tuberosity of humerus

Biceps brachii t, short head

Coracobrachialis t

Clavicle

Supraspinatus m

Base of coracoid process

Superior subscapular recess

Middle glenohumeral lig

Subscapularis m

Subscapularis t

Figure 3.3.3

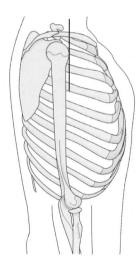

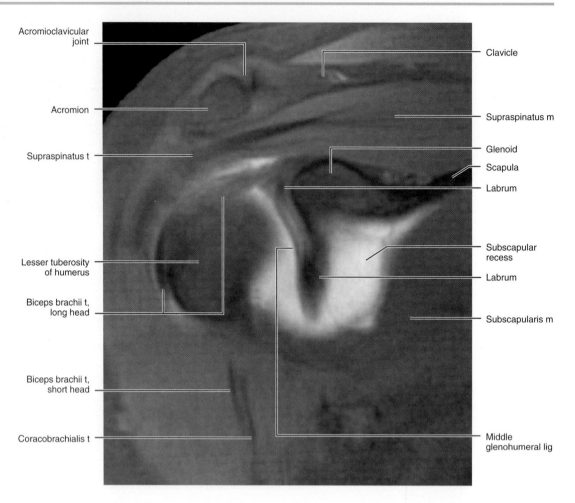

Acromioclavicular joint

Acromion

Supraspinatus t

Lesser tuberosity of humerus

Biceps brachii t, long head

Biceps brachii t, short head

Coracobrachialis t

Clavicle

Supraspinatus m

Glenoid

Scapula

Labrum

Subscapular recess

Labrum

Subscapularis m

Middle glenohumeral lig

Figure 3.3.4

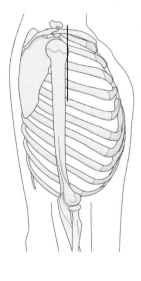

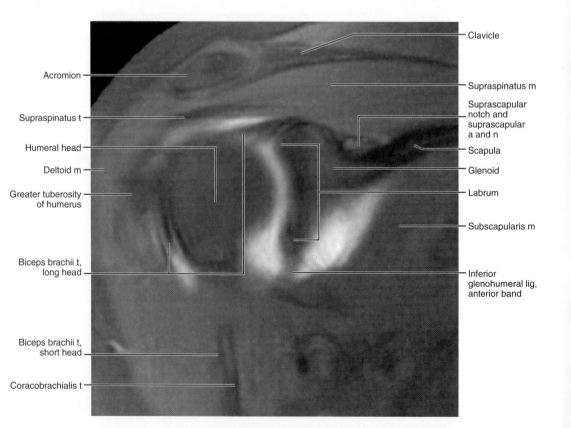

Acromion

Supraspinatus t

Humeral head

Deltoid m

Greater tuberosity of humerus

Biceps brachii t, long head

Biceps brachii t, short head

Coracobrachialis t

Clavicle

Supraspinatus m

Suprascapular notch and suprascapular a and n

Scapula

Glenoid

Labrum

Subscapularis m

Inferior glenohumeral lig, anterior band

Figure 3.3.5

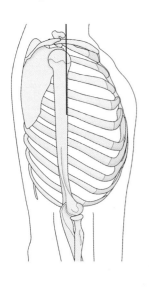

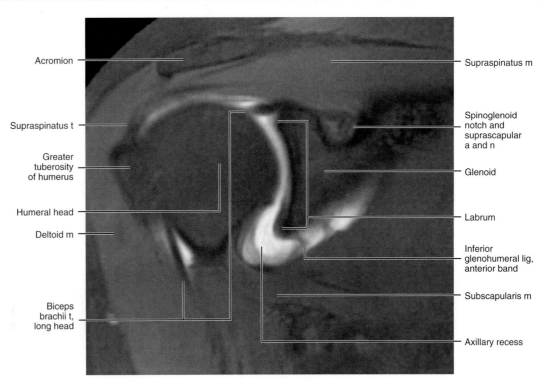

Acromion

Supraspinatus t

Greater
tuberosity
of humerus

Humeral head

Deltoid m

Biceps
brachii t,
long head

Supraspinatus m

Spinoglenoid
notch and
suprascapular
a and n

Glenoid

Labrum

Inferior
glenohumeral lig,
anterior band

Subscapularis m

Axillary recess

Figure 3.3.6

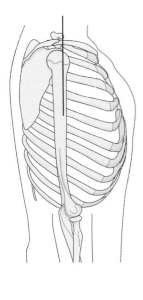

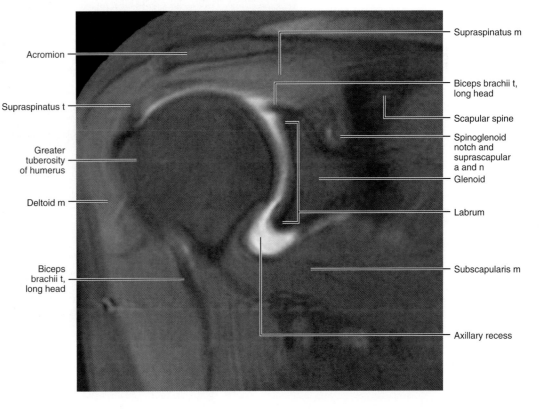

Acromion

Supraspinatus t

Greater
tuberosity
of humerus

Deltoid m

Biceps
brachii t,
long head

Supraspinatus m

Biceps brachii t,
long head

Scapular spine

Spinoglenoid
notch and
suprascapular
a and n

Glenoid

Labrum

Subscapularis m

Axillary recess

Figure 3.3.7

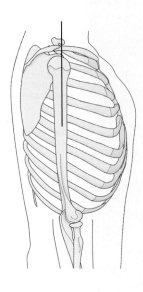

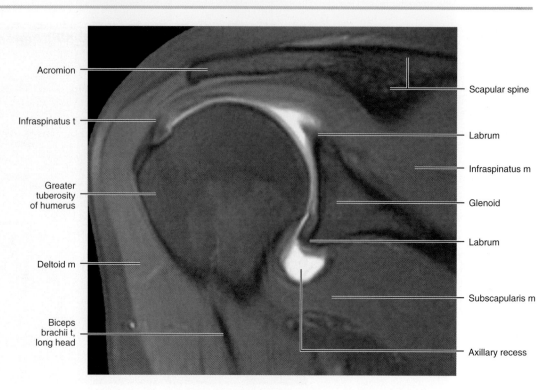

Acromion

Infraspinatus t

Greater tuberosity of humerus

Deltoid m

Biceps brachii t, long head

Scapular spine

Labrum

Infraspinatus m

Glenoid

Labrum

Subscapularis m

Axillary recess

Figure 3.3.8

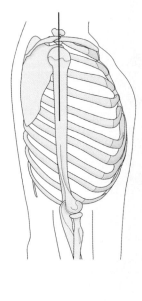

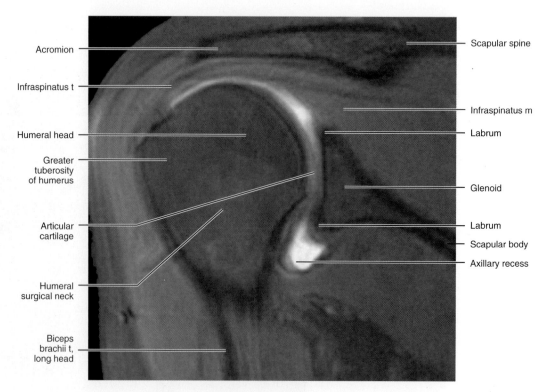

Acromion

Infraspinatus t

Humeral head

Greater tuberosity of humerus

Articular cartilage

Humeral surgical neck

Biceps brachii t, long head

Scapular spine

Infraspinatus m

Labrum

Glenoid

Labrum

Scapular body

Axillary recess

Figure 3.3.9

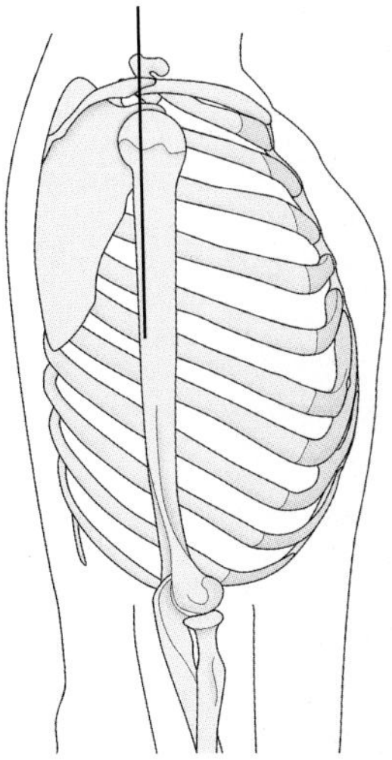

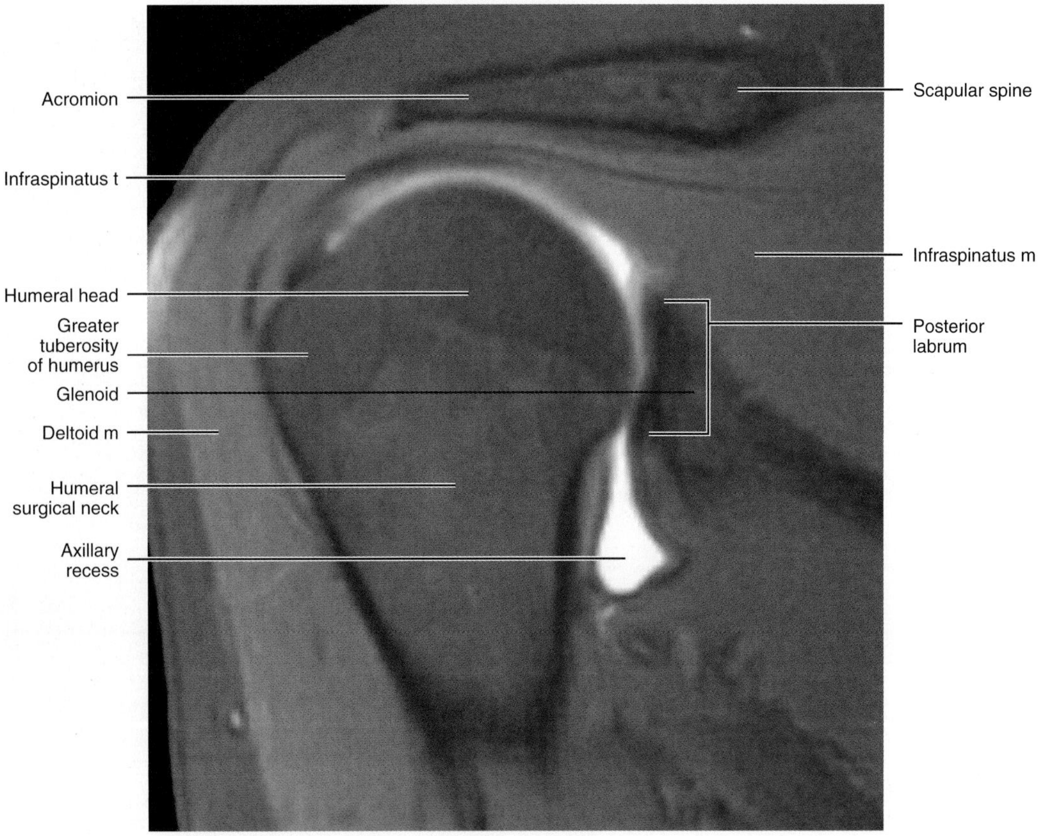

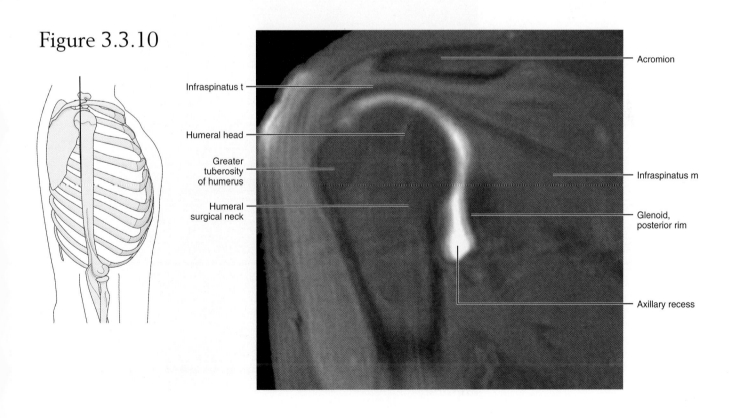

Acromion

Infraspinatus t

Humeral head

Greater tuberosity of humerus

Glenoid

Deltoid m

Humeral surgical neck

Axillary recess

Scapular spine

Infraspinatus m

Posterior labrum

Figure 3.3.10

Infraspinatus t

Humeral head

Greater tuberosity of humerus

Humeral surgical neck

Acromion

Infraspinatus m

Glenoid, posterior rim

Axillary recess

Figure 3.3.11

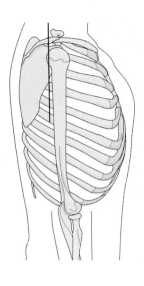

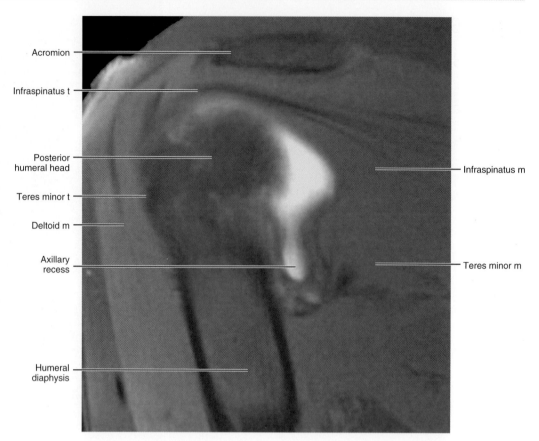

Acromion

Infraspinatus t

Posterior
humeral head

Teres minor t

Deltoid m

Axillary
recess

Humeral
diaphysis

Infraspinatus m

Teres minor m

Figure 3.3.12

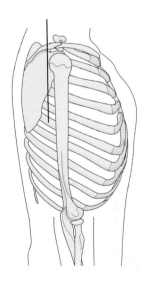

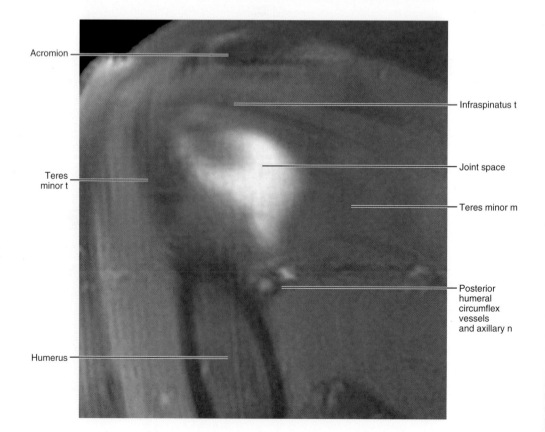

Acromion

Teres
minor t

Humerus

Infraspinatus t

Joint space

Teres minor m

Posterior
humeral
circumflex
vessels
and axillary n

ABER*

Figure 3.4.1

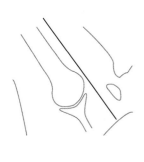

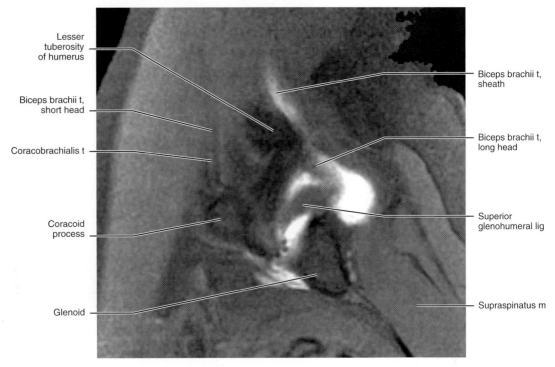

Lesser tuberosity of humerus

Biceps brachii t, short head

Coracobrachialis t

Coracoid process

Glenoid

Biceps brachii t, sheath

Biceps brachii t, long head

Superior glenohumeral lig

Supraspinatus m

Figure 3.4.2

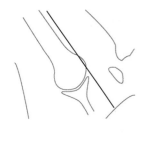

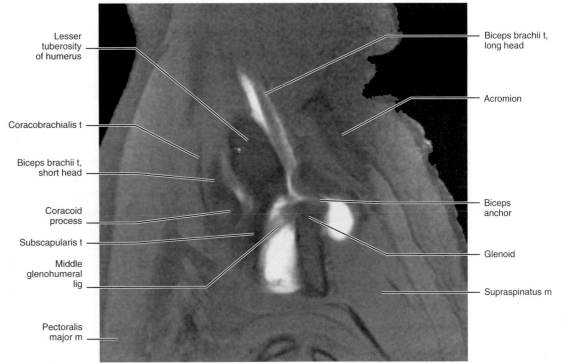

Lesser tuberosity of humerus

Coracobrachialis t

Biceps brachii t, short head

Coracoid process

Subscapularis t

Middle glenohumeral lig

Pectoralis major m

Biceps brachii t, long head

Acromion

Biceps anchor

Glenoid

Supraspinatus m

*ABER = abduction and external rotation

Figure 3.4.3

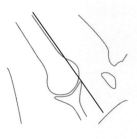

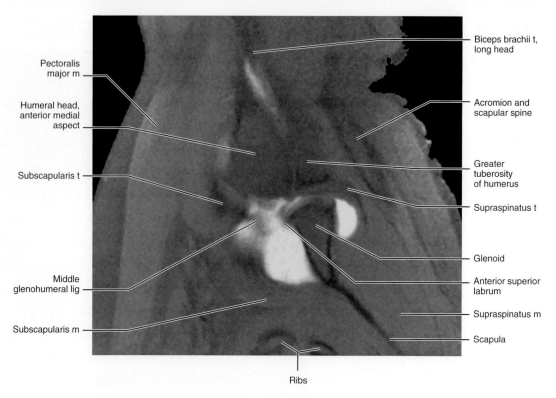

Pectoralis major m

Humeral head, anterior medial aspect

Subscapularis t

Middle glenohumeral lig

Subscapularis m

Biceps brachii t, long head

Acromion and scapular spine

Greater tuberosity of humerus

Supraspinatus t

Glenoid

Anterior superior labrum

Supraspinatus m

Scapula

Ribs

Figure 3.4.4

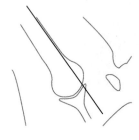

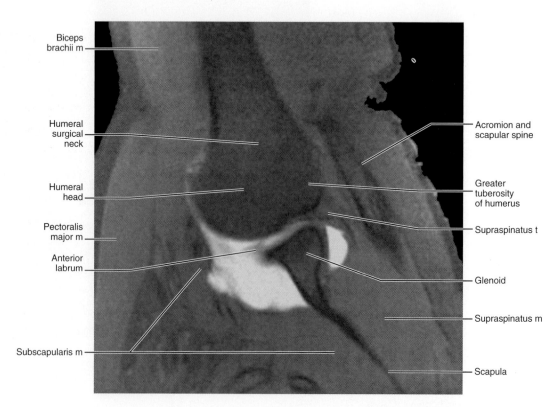

Biceps brachii m

Humeral surgical neck

Humeral head

Pectoralis major m

Anterior labrum

Subscapularis m

Acromion and scapular spine

Greater tuberosity of humerus

Supraspinatus t

Glenoid

Supraspinatus m

Scapula

Figure 3.4.5

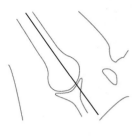

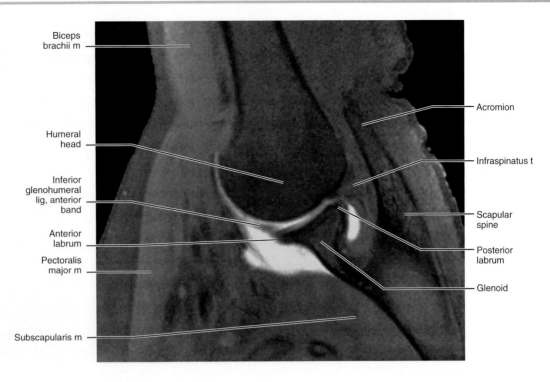

Biceps brachii m

Humeral head

Inferior glenohumeral lig, anterior band

Anterior labrum

Pectoralis major m

Subscapularis m

Acromion

Infraspinatus t

Scapular spine

Posterior labrum

Glenoid

Figure 3.4.6

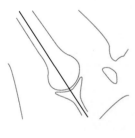

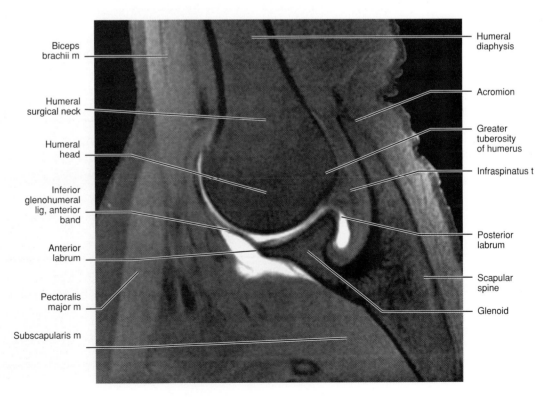

Biceps brachii m

Humeral surgical neck

Humeral head

Inferior glenohumeral lig, anterior band

Anterior labrum

Pectoralis major m

Subscapularis m

Humeral diaphysis

Acromion

Greater tuberosity of humerus

Infraspinatus t

Posterior labrum

Scapular spine

Glenoid

Figure 3.4.7

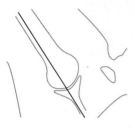

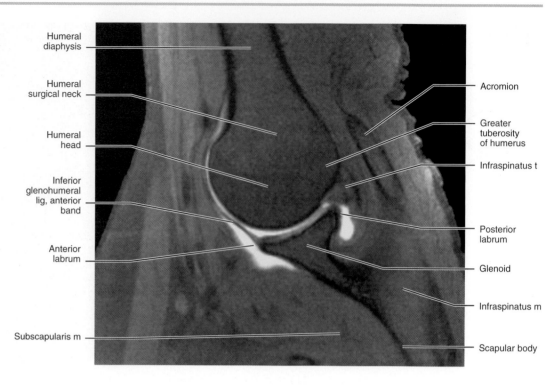

Humeral diaphysis

Humeral surgical neck

Humeral head

Inferior glenohumeral lig, anterior band

Anterior labrum

Subscapularis m

Acromion

Greater tuberosity of humerus

Infraspinatus t

Posterior labrum

Glenoid

Infraspinatus m

Scapular body

Figure 3.4.8

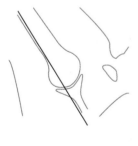

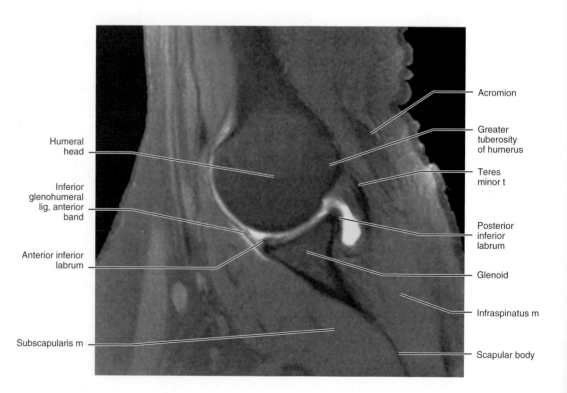

Humeral head

Inferior glenohumeral lig, anterior band

Anterior inferior labrum

Subscapularis m

Acromion

Greater tuberosity of humerus

Teres minor t

Posterior inferior labrum

Glenoid

Infraspinatus m

Scapular body

Figure 3.4.9

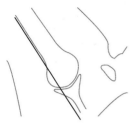

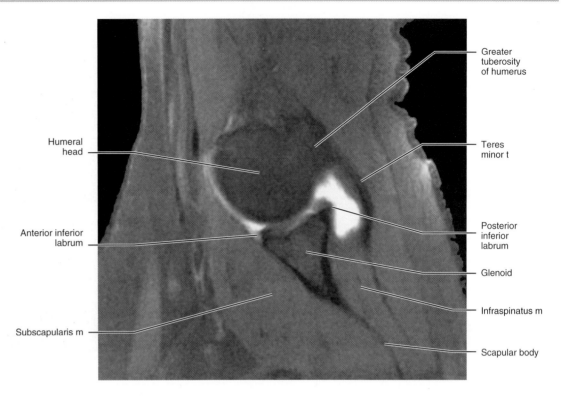

Greater
tuberosity
of humerus

Humeral
head

Teres
minor t

Posterior
inferior
labrum

Anterior inferior
labrum

Glenoid

Infraspinatus m

Subscapularis m

Scapular body

Figure 3.4.10

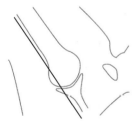

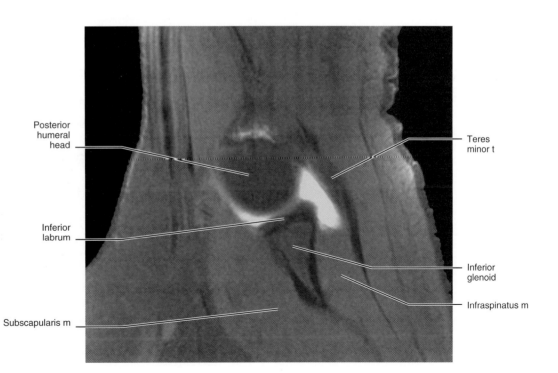

Posterior
humeral
head

Teres
minor t

Inferior
labrum

Inferior
glenoid

Infraspinatus m

Subscapularis m

Figure 3.4.11

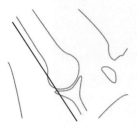

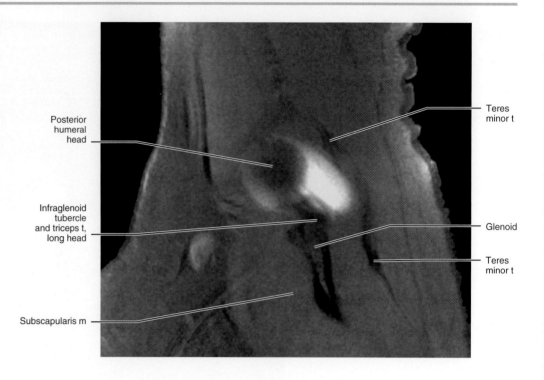

Posterior humeral head

Teres minor t

Infraglenoid tubercle and triceps t, long head

Glenoid

Teres minor t

Subscapularis m

Chapter 4

MRI of the Arm

Table 2: Muscles of the Arm

MUSCLE	ORIGIN	INSERTION	NERVE SUPPLY
Coracobrachialis	Coracoid process	Shaft of the humerus above the middle of the bone	Musculocutaneous (C5, C6, C7)
Biceps brachii	Short head, coracoid process; long head, supraglenoid tubercle; superior part of glenoid labrum	Tuberosity of the radius and by aponeurotic expansion to the fascia on the ulnar side of the forearm	Musculocutaneous (C5, C6)
Brachialis	Distal half of anterior surface of humerus	Capsule of the elbow joint and ulnar tuberosity	Musculocutaneous (C5, C6)
Triceps	Long head, infraglenoid tuberosity of the scapula; lateral head, from the posterior surface of the humerus; medial head, from the posterior surface of the humerus below the radial groove and dorsal surfaces of the medial and lateral intermuscular septa	Primary tendon inserts onto the olecranon process of the ulna and laterally, by expansion over the anconeus, into the dorsal fascia of the forearm	Radial (C6, C7, C8)

AXIAL
Figure 4.1.1

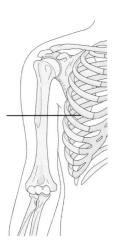

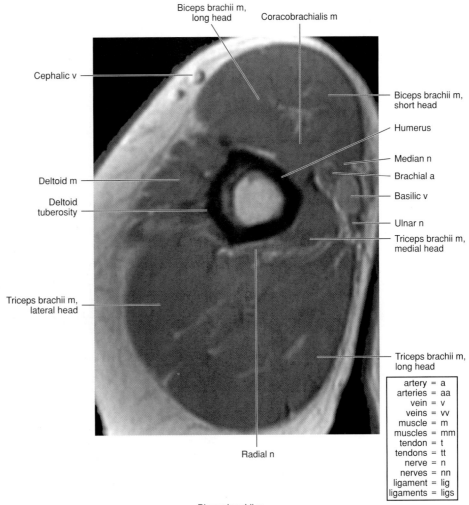

Biceps brachii m, long head

Coracobrachialis m

Cephalic v

Biceps brachii m, short head

Humerus

Median n

Brachial a

Deltoid m

Basilic v

Deltoid tuberosity

Ulnar n

Triceps brachii m, medial head

Triceps brachii m, lateral head

Triceps brachii m, long head

Radial n

artery	= a
arteries	= aa
vein	= v
veins	= vv
muscle	= m
muscles	= mm
tendon	= t
tendons	= tt
nerve	= n
nerves	= nn
ligament	= lig
ligaments	= ligs

Figure 4.1.2

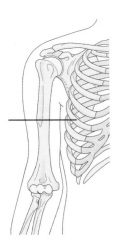

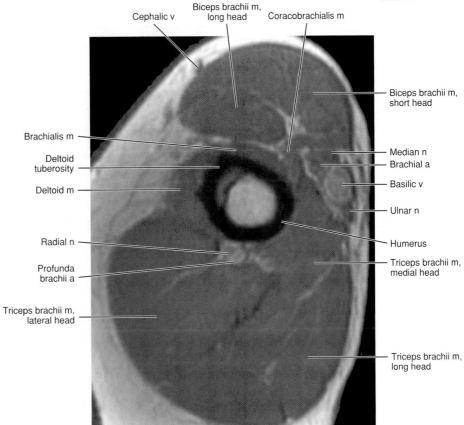

Cephalic v

Biceps brachii m, long head

Coracobrachialis m

Biceps brachii m, short head

Brachialis m

Median n

Deltoid tuberosity

Brachial a

Deltoid m

Basilic v

Ulnar n

Radial n

Humerus

Profunda brachii a

Triceps brachii m, medial head

Triceps brachii m, lateral head

Triceps brachii m, long head

Figure 4.1.3

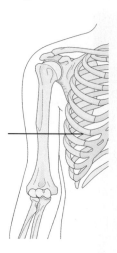

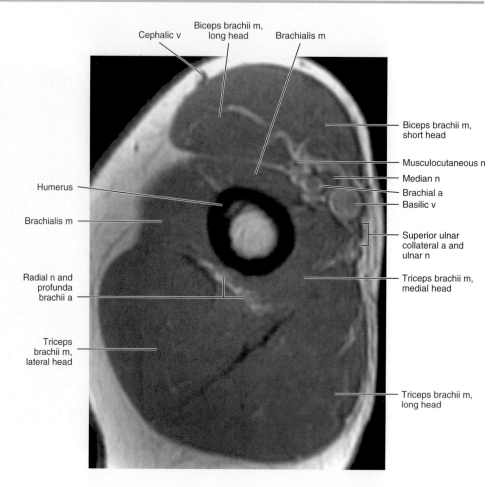

Cephalic v

Biceps brachii m, long head

Brachialis m

Biceps brachii m, short head

Musculocutaneous n

Median n

Brachial a

Basilic v

Superior ulnar collateral a and ulnar n

Triceps brachii m, medial head

Triceps brachii m, long head

Humerus

Brachialis m

Radial n and profunda brachii a

Triceps brachii m, lateral head

Figure 4.1.4

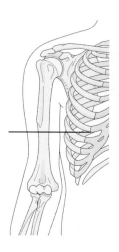

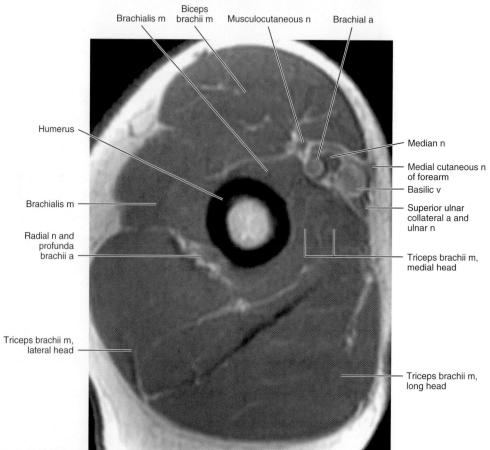

Brachialis m

Biceps brachii m

Musculocutaneous n

Brachial a

Median n

Medial cutaneous n of forearm

Basilic v

Superior ulnar collateral a and ulnar n

Triceps brachii m, medial head

Humerus

Brachialis m

Radial n and profunda brachii a

Triceps brachii m, lateral head

Triceps brachii m, long head

Figure 4.1.5

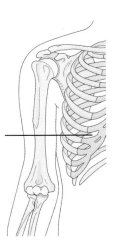

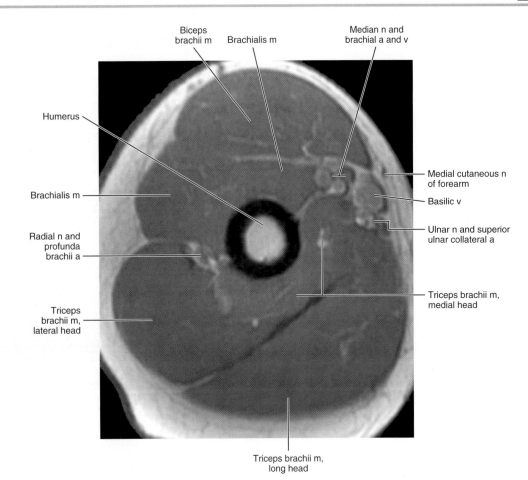

Biceps brachii m

Brachialis m

Median n and brachial a and v

Humerus

Medial cutaneous n of forearm

Brachialis m

Basilic v

Ulnar n and superior ulnar collateral a

Radial n and profunda brachii a

Triceps brachii m, medial head

Triceps brachii m, lateral head

Triceps brachii m, long head

Figure 4.1.6

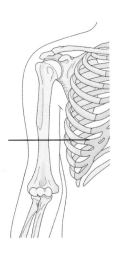

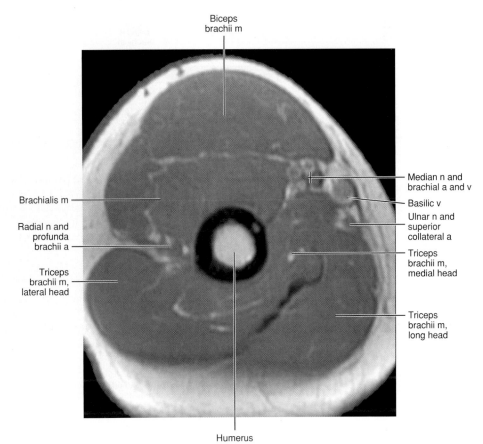

Biceps brachii m

Median n and brachial a and v

Brachialis m

Basilic v

Ulnar n and superior collateral a

Radial n and profunda brachii a

Triceps brachii m, medial head

Triceps brachii m, lateral head

Triceps brachii m, long head

Humerus

Figure 4.1.7

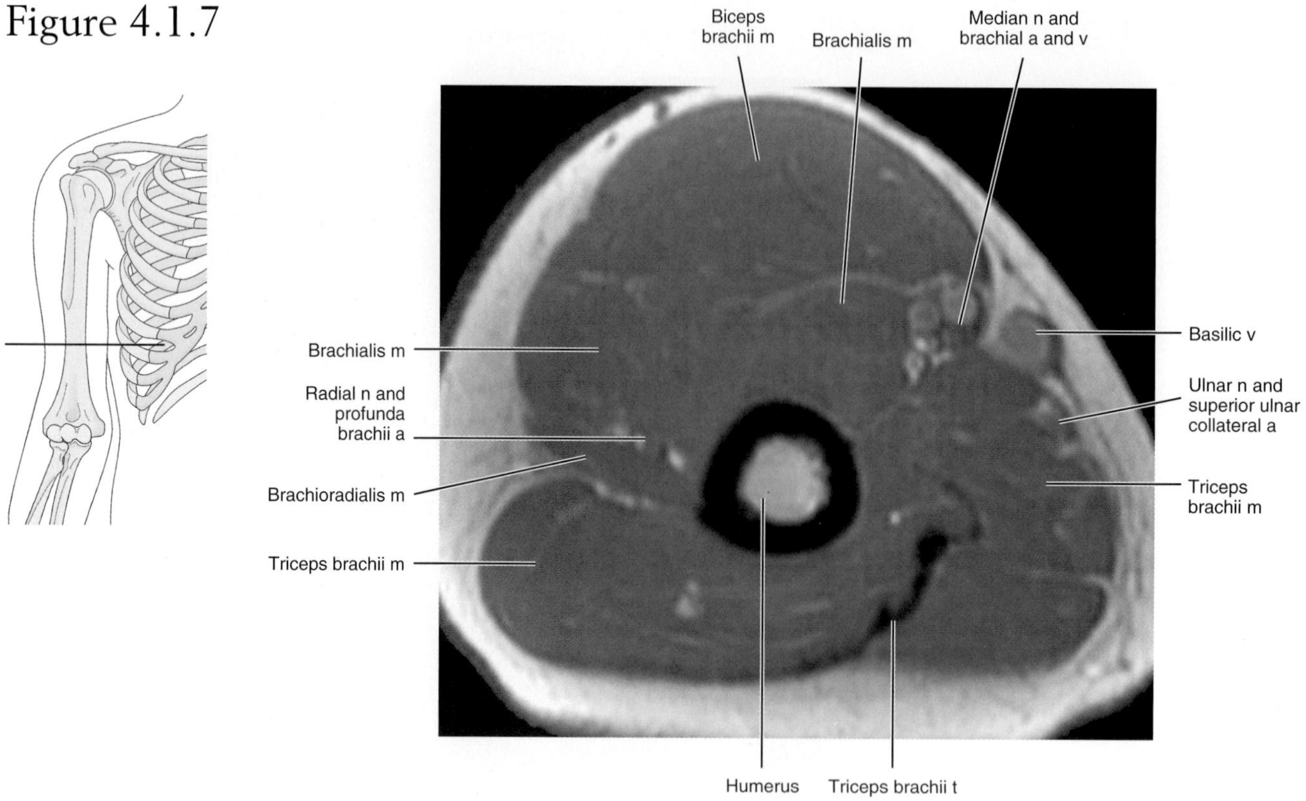

Biceps brachii m

Brachialis m

Median n and brachial a and v

Brachialis m

Radial n and profunda brachii a

Brachioradialis m

Triceps brachii m

Basilic v

Ulnar n and superior ulnar collateral a

Triceps brachii m

Humerus   Triceps brachii t

Figure 4.1.8

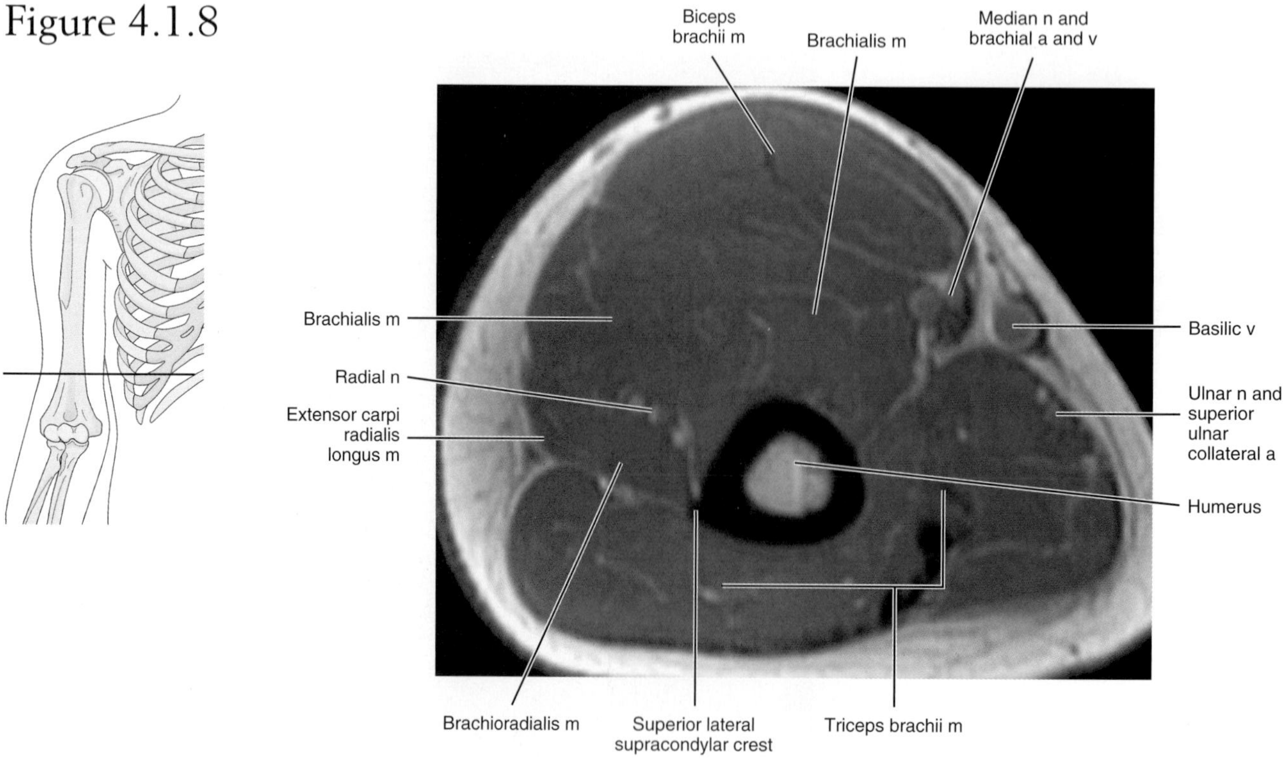

Biceps brachii m

Brachialis m

Median n and brachial a and v

Brachialis m

Radial n

Extensor carpi radialis longus m

Basilic v

Ulnar n and superior ulnar collateral a

Humerus

Brachioradialis m

Superior lateral supracondylar crest

Triceps brachii m

Figure 4.1.9

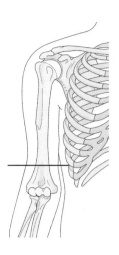

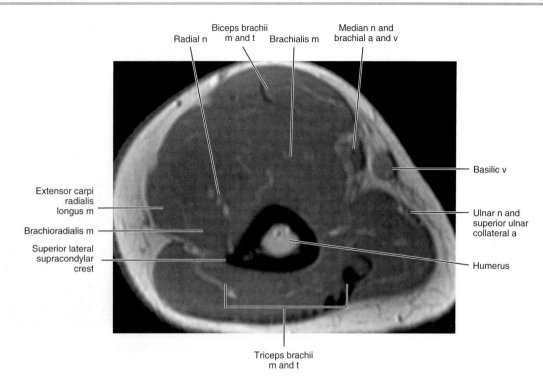

Radial n

Biceps brachii
m and t

Brachialis m

Median n and
brachial a and v

Extensor carpi
radialis
longus m

Brachioradialis m

Superior lateral
supracondylar
crest

Basilic v

Ulnar n and
superior ulnar
collateral a

Humerus

Triceps brachii
m and t

Figure 4.1.10

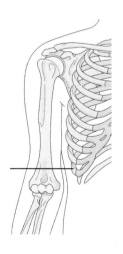

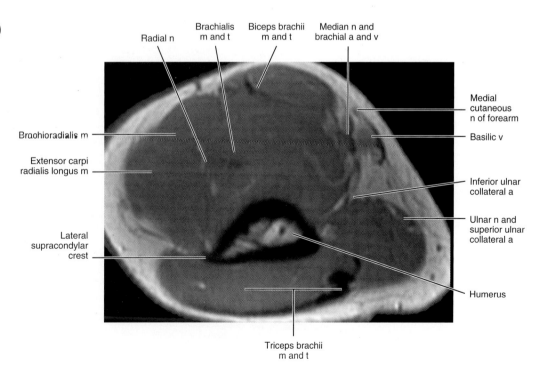

Radial n

Brachialis
m and t

Biceps brachii
m and t

Median n and
brachial a and v

Brachioradialis m

Extensor carpi
radialis longus m

Lateral
supracondylar
crest

Medial
cutaneous
n of forearm

Basilic v

Inferior ulnar
collateral a

Ulnar n and
superior ulnar
collateral a

Humerus

Triceps brachii
m and t

Figure 4.1.11

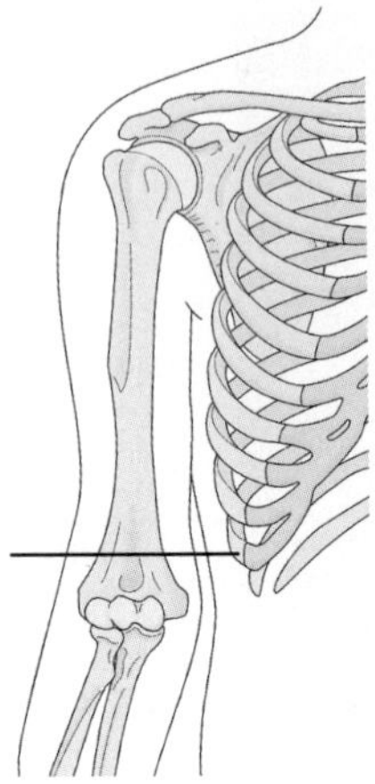

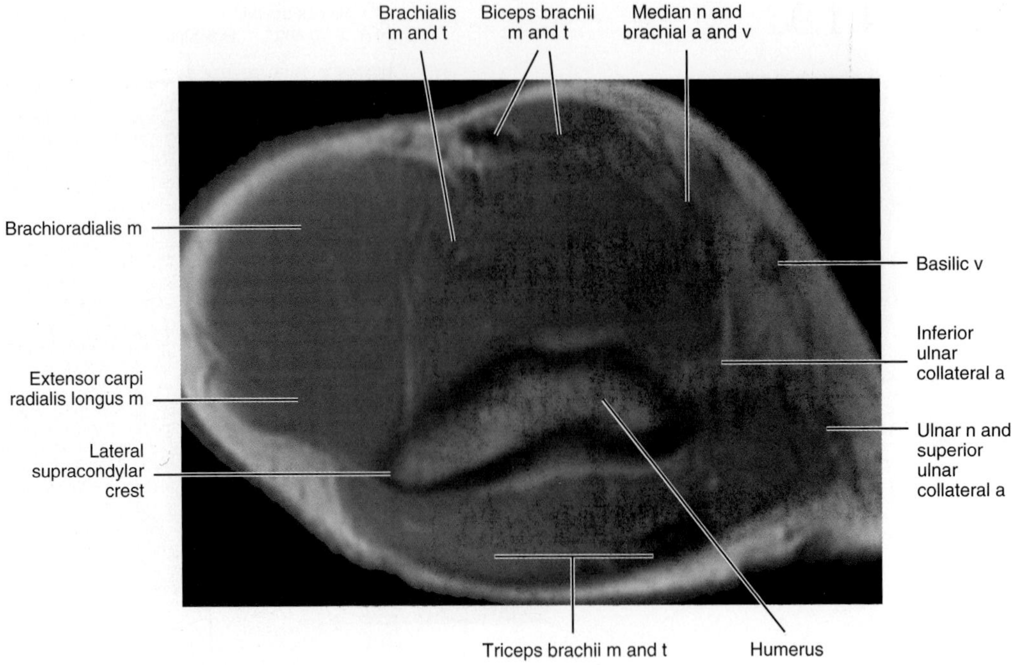

Brachialis m and t

Biceps brachii m and t

Median n and brachial a and v

Brachioradialis m

Basilic v

Extensor carpi radialis longus m

Inferior ulnar collateral a

Lateral supracondylar crest

Ulnar n and superior ulnar collateral a

Triceps brachii m and t

Humerus

SAGITTAL

Figure 4.2.1

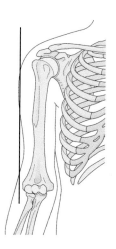

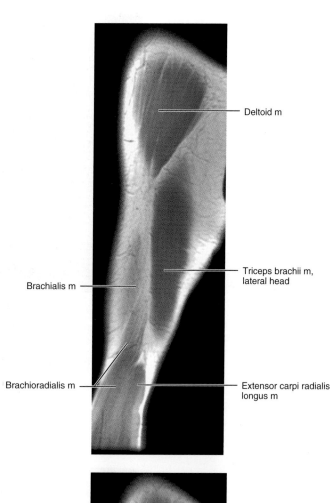

Deltoid m

Triceps brachii m,
lateral head

Brachialis m

Brachioradialis m

Extensor carpi radialis
longus m

Figure 4.2.2

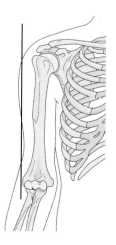

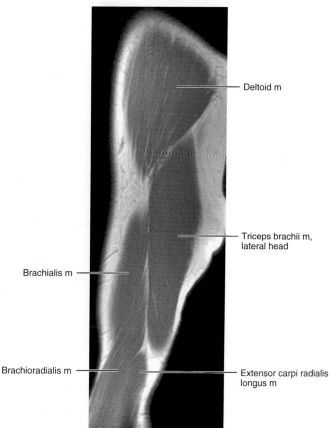

Deltoid m

Triceps brachii m,
lateral head

Brachialis m

Brachioradialis m

Extensor carpi radialis
longus m

Figure 4.2.3

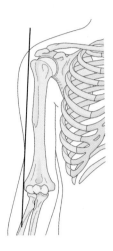

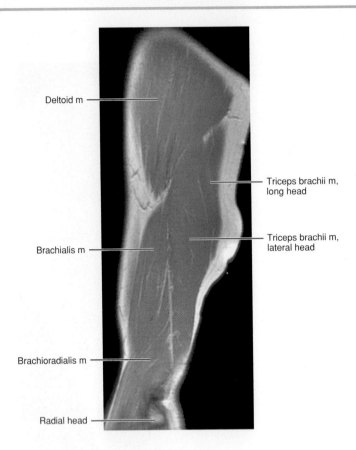

Deltoid m

Triceps brachii m, long head

Triceps brachii m, lateral head

Brachialis m

Brachioradialis m

Radial head

Figure 4.2.4

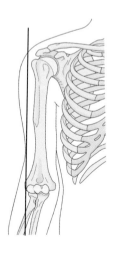

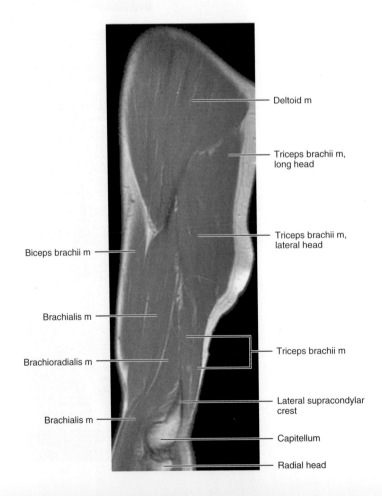

Deltoid m

Triceps brachii m, long head

Triceps brachii m, lateral head

Biceps brachii m

Triceps brachii m

Brachialis m

Brachioradialis m

Lateral supracondylar crest

Brachialis m

Capitellum

Radial head

Figure 4.2.5

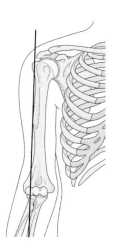

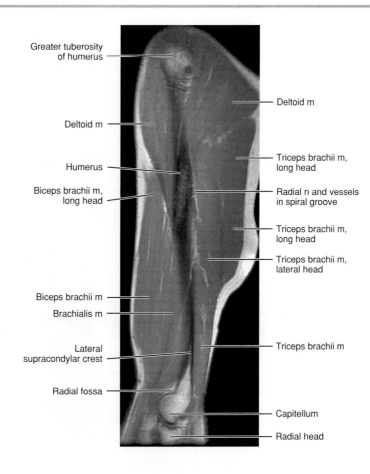

Greater tuberosity of humerus

Deltoid m

Deltoid m

Humerus

Triceps brachii m, long head

Biceps brachii m, long head

Radial n and vessels in spiral groove

Triceps brachii m, long head

Triceps brachii m, lateral head

Biceps brachii m

Brachialis m

Triceps brachii m

Lateral supracondylar crest

Radial fossa

Capitellum

Radial head

Figure 4.2.6

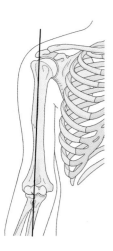

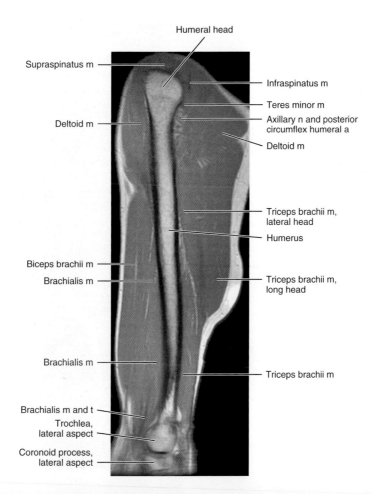

Humeral head

Supraspinatus m

Infraspinatus m

Teres minor m

Deltoid m

Axillary n and posterior circumflex humeral a

Deltoid m

Triceps brachii m, lateral head

Humerus

Biceps brachii m

Brachialis m

Triceps brachii m, long head

Brachialis m

Triceps brachii m

Brachialis m and t

Trochlea, lateral aspect

Coronoid process, lateral aspect

Figure 4.2.7

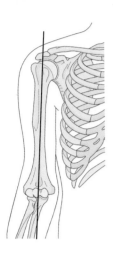

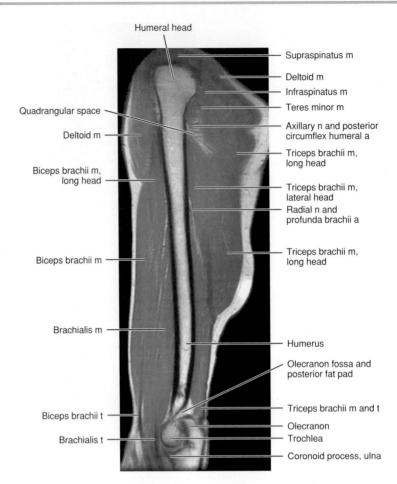

Humeral head

Supraspinatus m

Deltoid m

Infraspinatus m

Teres minor m

Quadrangular space

Deltoid m

Axillary n and posterior circumflex humeral a

Triceps brachii m, long head

Biceps brachii m, long head

Triceps brachii m, lateral head

Radial n and profunda brachii a

Triceps brachii m, long head

Biceps brachii m

Brachialis m

Humerus

Olecranon fossa and posterior fat pad

Triceps brachii m and t

Biceps brachii t

Olecranon

Brachialis t

Trochlea

Coronoid process, ulna

Figure 4.2.8

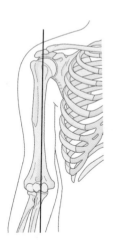

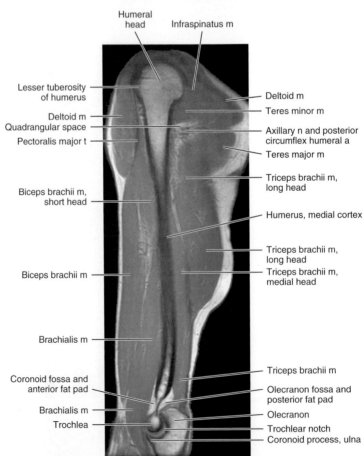

Humeral head

Infraspinatus m

Lesser tuberosity of humerus

Deltoid m

Teres minor m

Deltoid m

Quadrangular space

Axillary n and posterior circumflex humeral a

Pectoralis major t

Teres major m

Triceps brachii m, long head

Biceps brachii m, short head

Humerus, medial cortex

Triceps brachii m, long head

Biceps brachii m

Triceps brachii m, medial head

Brachialis m

Triceps brachii m

Coronoid fossa and anterior fat pad

Olecranon fossa and posterior fat pad

Brachialis m

Olecranon

Trochlea

Trochlear notch

Coronoid process, ulna

Figure 4.2.9

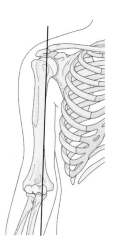

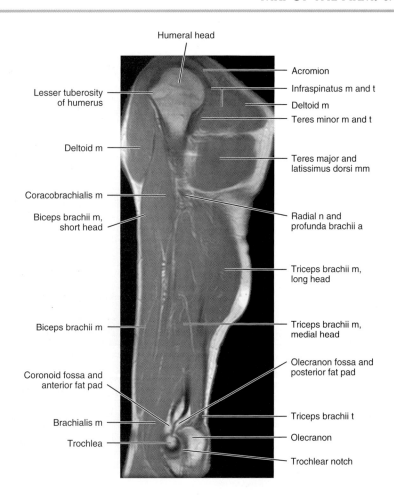

Humeral head

Acromion

Lesser tuberosity of humerus

Infraspinatus m and t

Deltoid m

Teres minor m and t

Deltoid m

Teres major and latissimus dorsi mm

Coracobrachialis m

Radial n and profunda brachii a

Biceps brachii m, short head

Triceps brachii m, long head

Biceps brachii m

Triceps brachii m, medial head

Olecranon fossa and posterior fat pad

Coronoid fossa and anterior fat pad

Brachialis m

Triceps brachii t

Trochlea

Olecranon

Trochlear notch

Figure 4.2.10

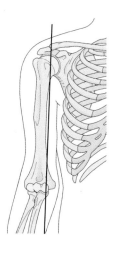

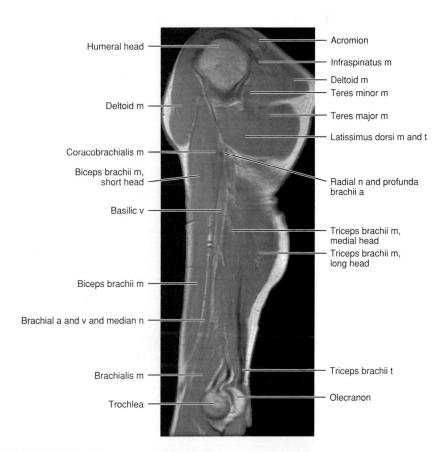

Humeral head

Acromion

Infraspinatus m

Deltoid m

Deltoid m

Teres minor m

Teres major m

Coracobrachialis m

Latissimus dorsi m and t

Biceps brachii m, short head

Radial n and profunda brachii a

Basilic v

Triceps brachii m, medial head

Triceps brachii m, long head

Biceps brachii m

Brachial a and v and median n

Brachialis m

Triceps brachii t

Trochlea

Olecranon

Figure 4.2.11

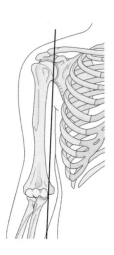

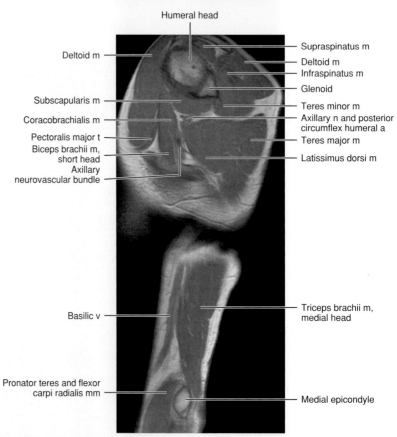

Supraspinatus m and t

Deltoid m

Subscapularis m

Pectoralis major t

Coracobrachialis m

Biceps m,
short head

Basilic v

Biceps brachii m

Pronator teres and flexor
carpi radialis mm

Trochlea

Acromion

Deltoid m

Infraspinatus m

Teres minor m

Axillary n and posterior
circumflex humeral a

Teres major m

Latissimus dorsi t and m

Triceps brachii m,
long head

Triceps brachii m,
medial head

Figure 4.2.12

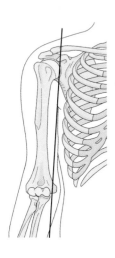

Humeral head

Deltoid m

Subscapularis m

Coracobrachialis m

Pectoralis major t

Biceps brachii m,
short head

Axillary
neurovascular bundle

Basilic v

Pronator teres and flexor
carpi radialis mm

Supraspinatus m

Deltoid m

Infraspinatus m

Glenoid

Teres minor m

Axillary n and posterior
circumflex humeral a

Teres major m

Latissimus dorsi m

Triceps brachii m,
medial head

Medial epicondyle

Figure 4.2.13

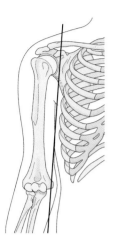

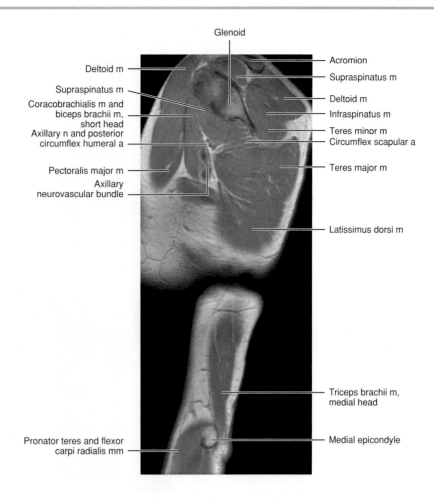

Glenoid

Deltoid m

Supraspinatus m

Coracobrachialis m and
biceps brachii m,
short head

Axillary n and posterior
circumflex humeral a

Pectoralis major m

Axillary
neurovascular bundle

Pronator teres and flexor
carpi radialis mm

Acromion

Supraspinatus m

Deltoid m

Infraspinatus m

Teres minor m

Circumflex scapular a

Teres major m

Latissimus dorsi m

Triceps brachii m,
medial head

Medial epicondyle

CORONAL

Figure 4.3.1

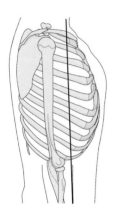

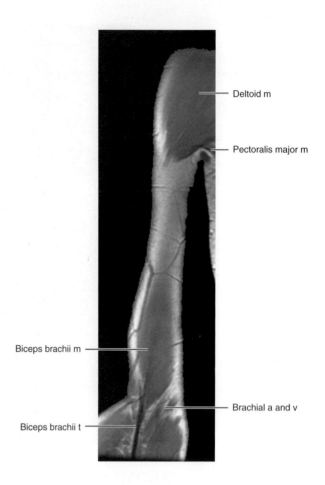

Deltoid m

Pectoralis major m

Biceps brachii m

Brachial a and v

Biceps brachii t

Figure 4.3.2

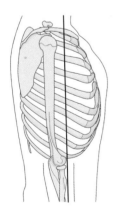

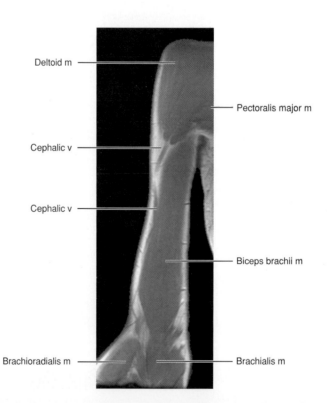

Deltoid m

Pectoralis major m

Cephalic v

Cephalic v

Biceps brachii m

Brachioradialis m

Brachialis m

Figure 4.3.3

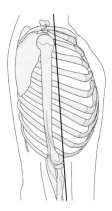

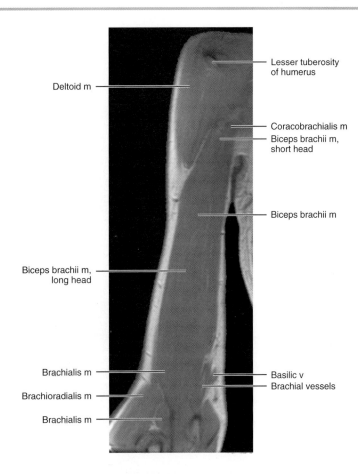

Deltoid m

Lesser tuberosity of humerus

Coracobrachialis m

Biceps brachii m, short head

Biceps brachii m

Biceps brachii m, long head

Brachialis m

Basilic v
Brachial vessels

Brachioradialis m

Brachialis m

Figure 4.3.4

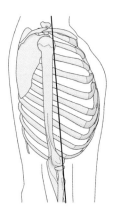

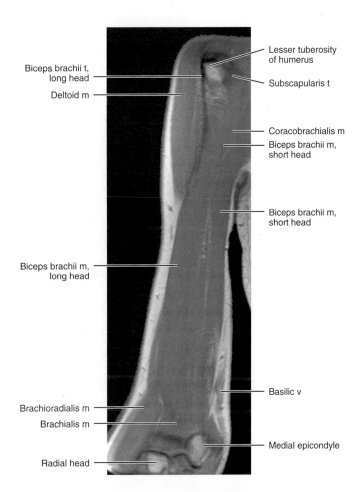

Biceps brachii t, long head

Lesser tuberosity of humerus

Deltoid m

Subscapularis t

Coracobrachialis m

Biceps brachii m, short head

Biceps brachii m, short head

Biceps brachii m, long head

Basilic v

Brachioradialis m

Brachialis m

Medial epicondyle

Radial head

Figure 4.3.5

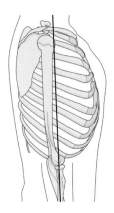

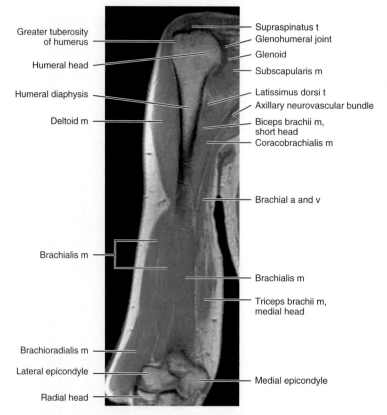

Greater tuberosity of humerus

Deltoid m

Biceps brachii m

Brachialis m

Brachioradialis m

Lateral epicondyle

Radial head

Lesser tuberosity of humerus

Subscapularis m

Biceps brachii t, long head

Biceps brachii m, short head

Coracobrachialis m

Biceps brachii m, long head

Brachial neurovascular bundle

Basilic v

Medial epicondyle

Common flexor t

Ulnar collateral lig, anterior band

Coronoid process, ulna

Figure 4.3.6

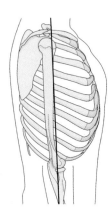

Greater tuberosity of humerus

Humeral head

Humeral diaphysis

Deltoid m

Brachialis m

Brachioradialis m

Lateral epicondyle

Radial head

Supraspinatus t

Glenohumeral joint

Glenoid

Subscapularis m

Latissimus dorsi t

Axillary neurovascular bundle

Biceps brachii m, short head

Coracobrachialis m

Brachial a and v

Brachialis m

Triceps brachii m, medial head

Medial epicondyle

Figure 4.3.7

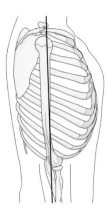

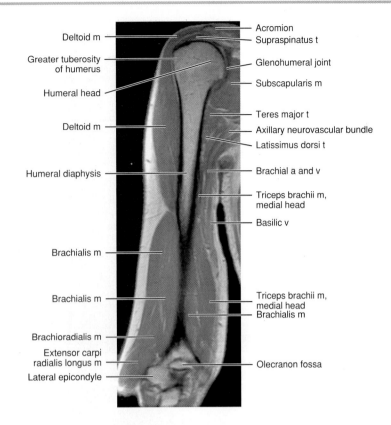

Deltoid m
Greater tuberosity of humerus
Humeral head
Deltoid m
Humeral diaphysis
Brachialis m
Brachialis m
Brachioradialis m
Extensor carpi radialis longus m
Lateral epicondyle

Acromion
Supraspinatus t
Glenohumeral joint
Subscapularis m
Teres major t
Axillary neurovascular bundle
Latissimus dorsi t
Brachial a and v
Triceps brachii m, medial head
Basilic v
Triceps brachii m, medial head
Brachialis m
Olecranon fossa

Figure 4.3.8

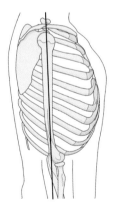

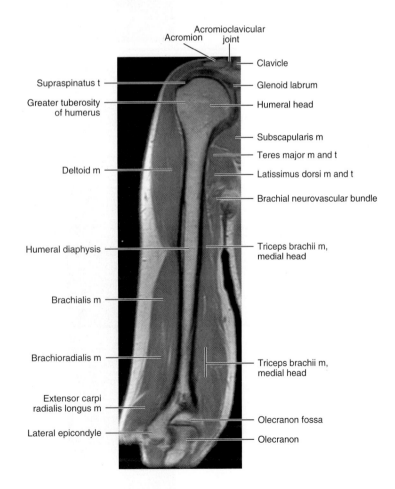

Supraspinatus t
Greater tuberosity of humerus
Deltoid m
Humeral diaphysis
Brachialis m
Brachioradialis m
Extensor carpi radialis longus m
Lateral epicondyle

Acromioclavicular joint
Acromion
Clavicle
Glenoid labrum
Humeral head
Subscapularis m
Teres major m and t
Latissimus dorsi m and t
Brachial neurovascular bundle
Triceps brachii m, medial head
Triceps brachii m, medial head
Olecranon fossa
Olecranon

Figure 4.3.9

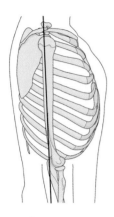

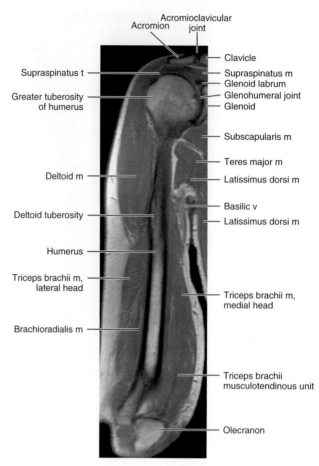

Acromioclavicular joint
Acromion
Clavicle
Supraspinatus t
Supraspinatus m
Glenoid labrum
Greater tuberosity of humerus
Glenohumeral joint
Glenoid
Subscapularis m
Teres major m
Deltoid m
Latissimus dorsi m
Deltoid tuberosity
Basilic v
Latissimus dorsi m
Humerus
Triceps brachii m, lateral head
Triceps brachii m, medial head
Brachioradialis m
Triceps brachii musculotendinous unit
Olecranon

Figure 4.3.10

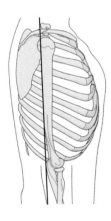

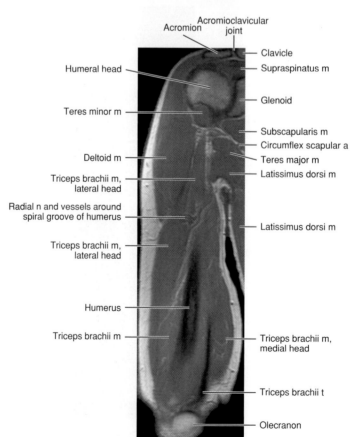

Acromioclavicular joint
Acromion
Clavicle
Humeral head
Supraspinatus m
Teres minor m
Glenoid
Subscapularis m
Circumflex scapular a
Deltoid m
Teres major m
Triceps brachii m, lateral head
Latissimus dorsi m
Radial n and vessels around spiral groove of humerus
Latissimus dorsi m
Triceps brachii m, lateral head
Humerus
Triceps brachii m
Triceps brachii m, medial head
Triceps brachii t
Olecranon

Figure 4.3.11

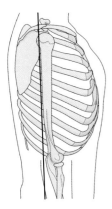

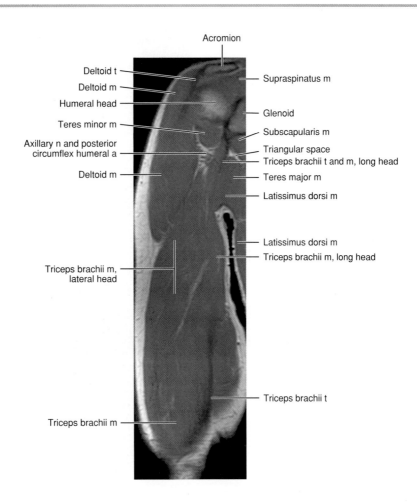

Acromion

Deltoid t

Deltoid m

Humeral head

Teres minor m

Axillary n and posterior
circumflex humeral a

Deltoid m

Triceps brachii m,
lateral head

Triceps brachii m

Supraspinatus m

Glenoid

Subscapularis m

Triangular space

Triceps brachii t and m, long head

Teres major m

Latissimus dorsi m

Latissimus dorsi m

Triceps brachii m, long head

Triceps brachii t

Figure 4.3.12

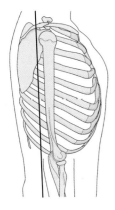

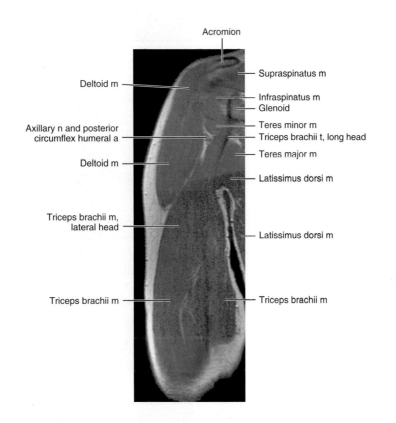

Acromion

Deltoid m

Axillary n and posterior
circumflex humeral a

Deltoid m

Triceps brachii m,
lateral head

Triceps brachii m

Supraspinatus m

Infraspinatus m

Glenoid

Teres minor m

Triceps brachii t, long head

Teres major m

Latissimus dorsi m

Latissimus dorsi m

Triceps brachii m

Figure 4.3.13

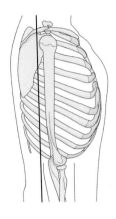

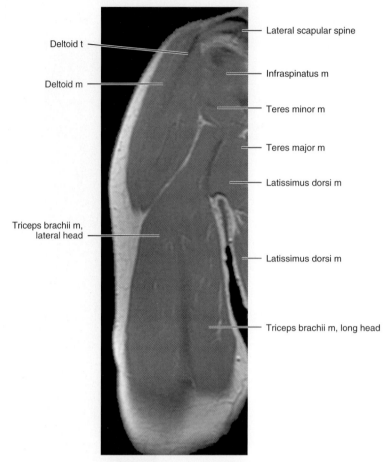

Deltoid t

Deltoid m

Triceps brachii m, lateral head

Lateral scapular spine

Infraspinatus m

Teres minor m

Teres major m

Latissimus dorsi m

Latissimus dorsi m

Triceps brachii m, long head

Figure 4.3.14

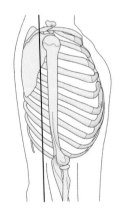

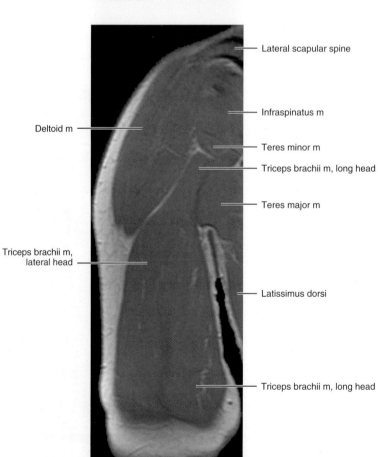

Deltoid m

Triceps brachii m, lateral head

Lateral scapular spine

Infraspinatus m

Teres minor m

Triceps brachii m, long head

Teres major m

Latissimus dorsi

Triceps brachii m, long head

Figure 4.3.15

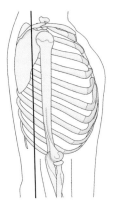

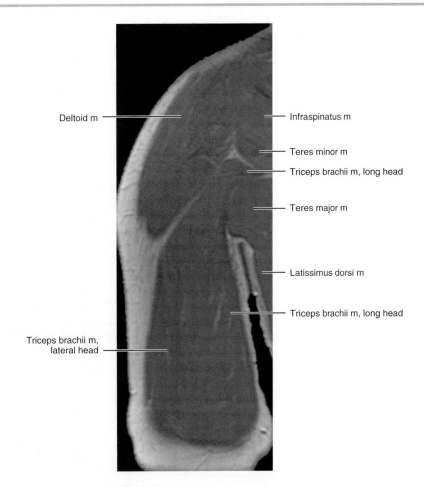

Deltoid m

Infraspinatus m

Teres minor m

Triceps brachii m, long head

Teres major m

Latissimus dorsi m

Triceps brachii m, long head

Triceps brachii m, lateral head

Figure 4.3.16

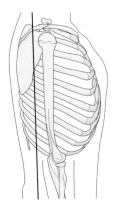

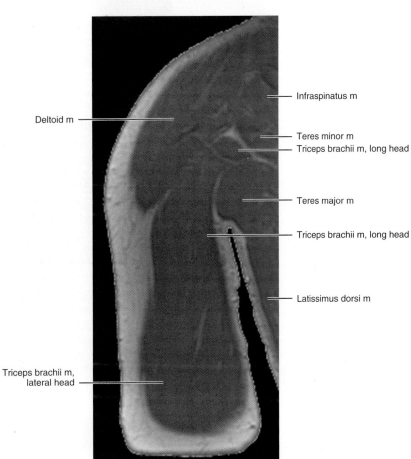

Deltoid m

Infraspinatus m

Teres minor m

Triceps brachii m, long head

Teres major m

Triceps brachii m, long head

Latissimus dorsi m

Triceps brachii m, lateral head

Figure 4.3.17

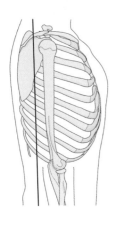

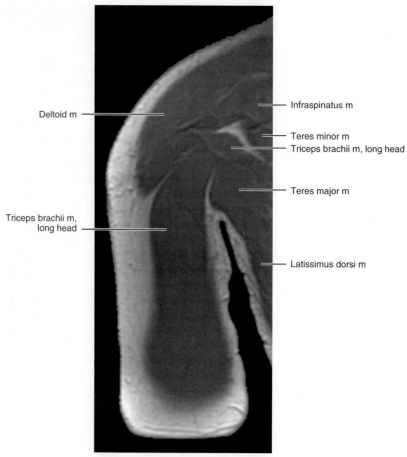

Deltoid m

Infraspinatus m

Teres minor m
Triceps brachii m, long head

Teres major m

Triceps brachii m, long head

Latissimus dorsi m

Figure 4.3.18

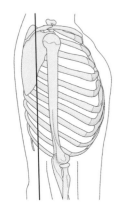

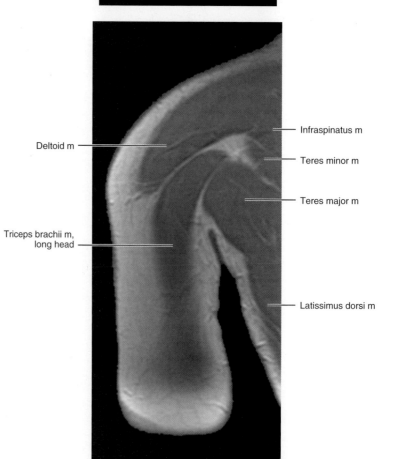

Deltoid m

Infraspinatus m

Teres minor m

Teres major m

Triceps brachii m, long head

Latissimus dorsi m

Chapter 5

MRI of the Elbow

AXIAL

Figure 5.1.1

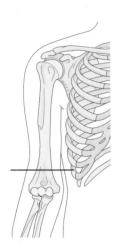

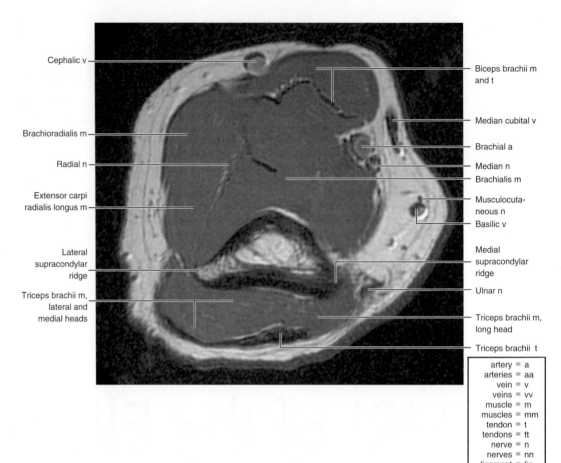

Cephalic v

Brachioradialis m

Radial n

Extensor carpi radialis longus m

Lateral supracondylar ridge

Triceps brachii m, lateral and medial heads

Biceps brachii m and t

Median cubital v

Brachial a

Median n

Brachialis m

Musculocutaneous n

Basilic v

Medial supracondylar ridge

Ulnar n

Triceps brachii m, long head

Triceps brachii t

artery = a
arteries = aa
vein = v
veins = vv
muscle = m
muscles = mm
tendon = t
tendons = tt
nerve = n
nerves = nn
ligament = lig
ligaments = ligs

Figure 5.1.2

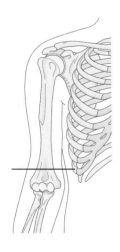

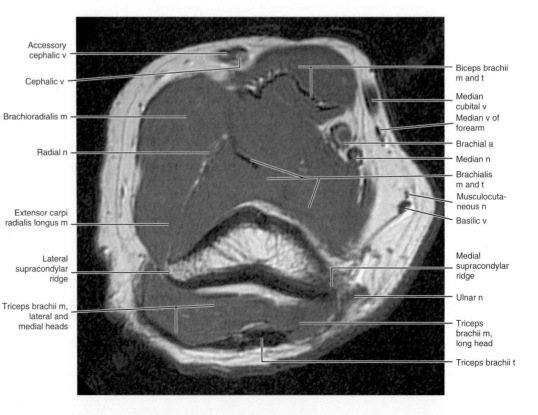

Accessory cephalic v

Cephalic v

Brachioradialis m

Radial n

Extensor carpi radialis longus m

Lateral supracondylar ridge

Triceps brachii m, lateral and medial heads

Biceps brachii m and t

Median cubital v

Median v of forearm

Brachial a

Median n

Brachialis m and t

Musculocutaneous n

Basilic v

Medial supracondylar ridge

Ulnar n

Triceps brachii m, long head

Triceps brachii t

Figure 5.1.3

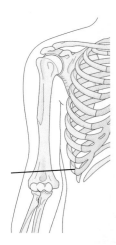

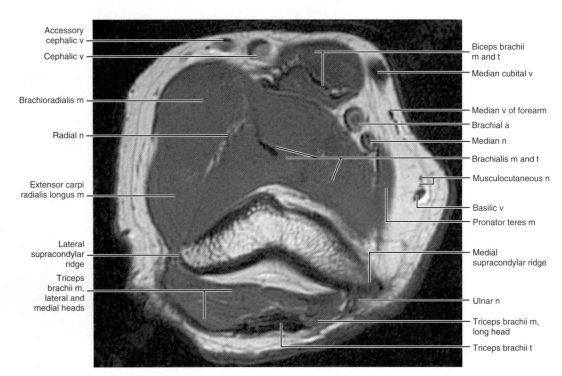

Accessory cephalic v
Cephalic v
Brachioradialis m
Radial n
Extensor carpi radialis longus m
Lateral supracondylar ridge
Triceps brachii m, lateral and medial heads

Biceps brachii m and t
Median cubital v
Median v of forearm
Brachial a
Median n
Brachialis m and t
Musculocutaneous n
Basilic v
Pronator teres m
Medial supracondylar ridge
Ulnar n
Triceps brachii m, long head
Triceps brachii t

Figure 5.1.4

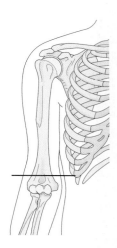

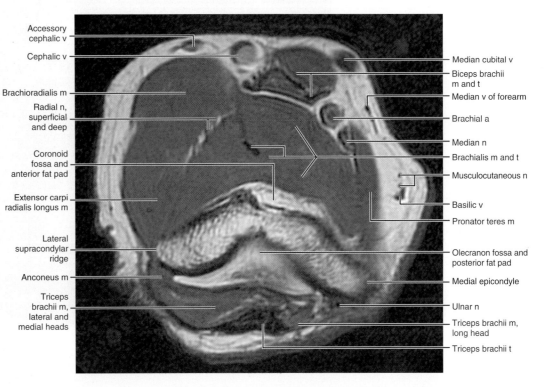

Accessory cephalic v
Cephalic v
Brachioradialis m
Radial n, superficial and deep
Coronoid fossa and anterior fat pad
Extensor carpi radialis longus m
Lateral supracondylar ridge
Anconeus m
Triceps brachii m, lateral and medial heads

Median cubital v
Biceps brachii m and t
Median v of forearm
Brachial a
Median n
Brachialis m and t
Musculocutaneous n
Basilic v
Pronator teres m
Olecranon fossa and posterior fat pad
Medial epicondyle
Ulnar n
Triceps brachii m, long head
Triceps brachii t

Figure 5.1.5

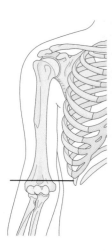

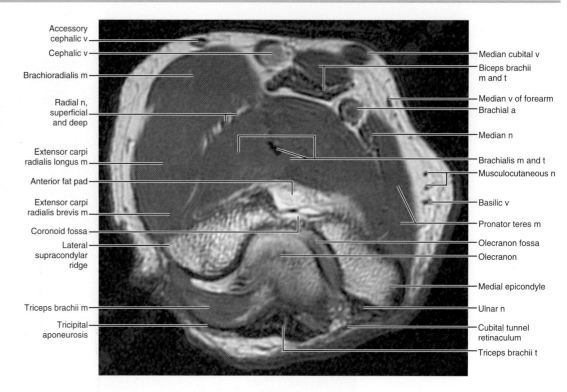

Accessory cephalic v
Cephalic v
Brachioradialis m
Radial n, superficial and deep
Extensor carpi radialis longus m
Anterior fat pad
Extensor carpi radialis brevis m
Coronoid fossa
Lateral supracondylar ridge
Triceps brachii m
Tricipital aponeurosis

Median cubital v
Biceps brachii m and t
Median v of forearm
Brachial a
Median n
Brachialis m and t
Musculocutaneous n
Basilic v
Pronator teres m
Olecranon fossa
Olecranon
Medial epicondyle
Ulnar n
Cubital tunnel retinaculum
Triceps brachii t

Figure 5.1.6

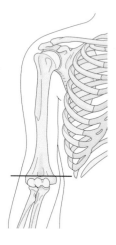

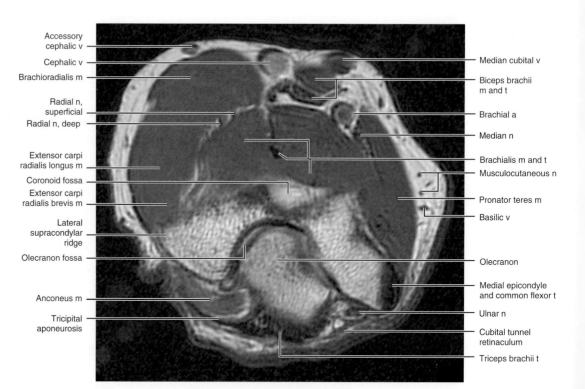

Accessory cephalic v
Cephalic v
Brachioradialis m
Radial n, superficial
Radial n, deep
Extensor carpi radialis longus m
Coronoid fossa
Extensor carpi radialis brevis m
Lateral supracondylar ridge
Olecranon fossa
Anconeus m
Tricipital aponeurosis

Median cubital v
Biceps brachii m and t
Brachial a
Median n
Brachialis m and t
Musculocutaneous n
Pronator teres m
Basilic v
Olecranon
Medial epicondyle and common flexor t
Ulnar n
Cubital tunnel retinaculum
Triceps brachii t

Figure 5.1.7

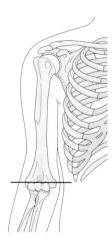

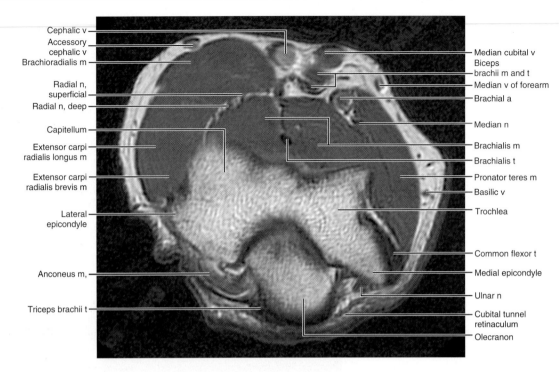

Cephalic v
Accessory cephalic v
Brachioradialis m,
Radial n, superficial
Radial n, deep
Capitellum
Extensor carpi radialis longus m
Extensor carpi radialis brevis m
Lateral epicondyle
Anconeus m,
Triceps brachii t

Median cubital v
Biceps brachii m and t
Median v of forearm
Brachial a
Median n
Brachialis m
Brachialis t
Pronator teres m
Basilic v
Trochlea
Common flexor t
Medial epicondyle
Ulnar n
Cubital tunnel retinaculum
Olecranon

Figure 5.1.8

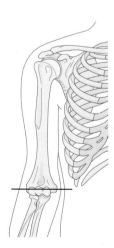

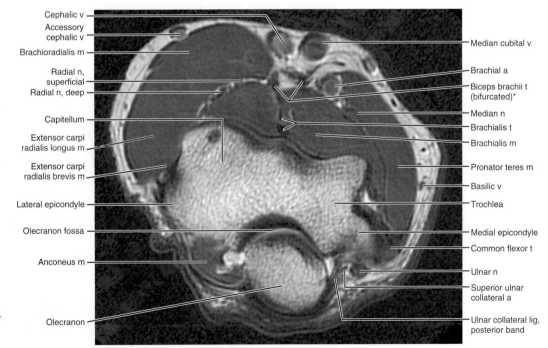

Cephalic v
Accessory cephalic v
Brachioradialis m
Radial n, superficial
Radial n, deep
Capitellum
Extensor carpi radialis longus m
Extensor carpi radialis brevis m
Lateral epicondyle
Olecranon fossa
Anconeus m
Olecranon

Median cubital v
Brachial a
Biceps brachii t (bifurcated)*
Median n
Brachialis t
Brachialis m
Pronator teres m
Basilic v
Trochlea
Medial epicondyle
Common flexor t
Ulnar n
Superior ulnar collateral a
Ulnar collateral lig, posterior band

*Data from Sassmannshausen G, Mair SD, Blazar PE. Rupture of a bifurcated distal biceps tendon. A case report. J Bone Joint Surg [Am] 2004;86:2737-2740.

Figure 5.1.9

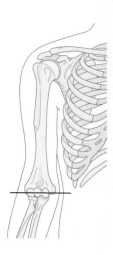

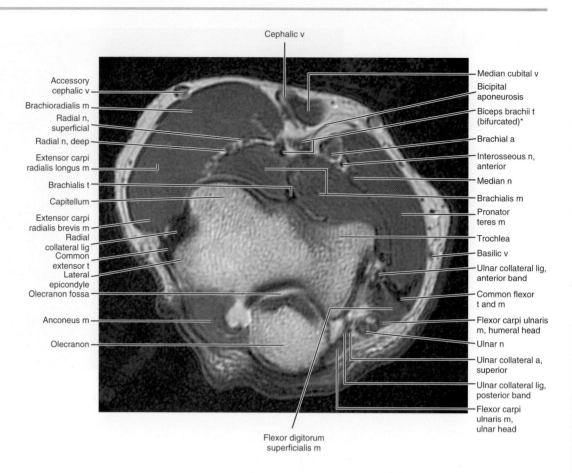

Cephalic v

Accessory cephalic v

Brachioradialis m

Radial n, superficial

Radial n, deep

Extensor carpi radialis longus m

Brachialis t

Capitellum

Extensor carpi radialis brevis m

Radial collateral lig

Common extensor t

Lateral epicondyle

Olecranon fossa

Anconeus m

Olecranon

Median cubital v

Bicipital aponeurosis

Biceps brachii t (bifurcated)*

Brachial a

Interosseous n, anterior

Median n

Brachialis m

Pronator teres m

Trochlea

Basilic v

Ulnar collateral lig, anterior band

Common flexor t and m

Flexor carpi ulnaris m, humeral head

Ulnar n

Ulnar collateral a, superior

Ulnar collateral lig, posterior band

Flexor carpi ulnaris m, ulnar head

Flexor digitorum superficialis m

*Data from Sassmannshausen G, Mair SD, Blazar PE. Rupture of a bifurcated distal biceps tendon. A case report. J Bone Joint Surg [Am] 2004;86:2737-2740.

Figure 5.1.10

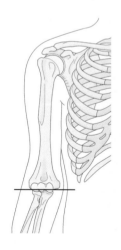

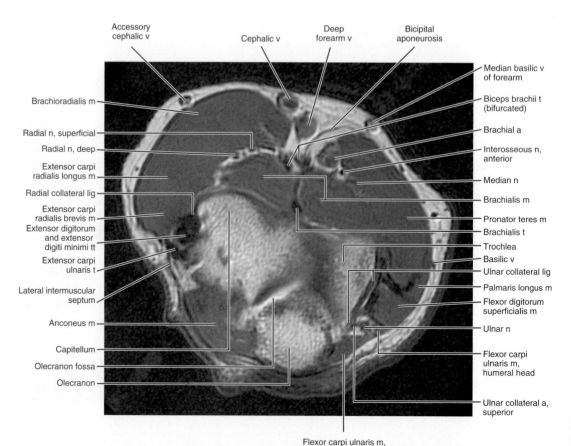

Accessory cephalic v

Cephalic v

Deep forearm v

Bicipital aponeurosis

Brachioradialis m

Radial n, superficial

Radial n, deep

Extensor carpi radialis longus m

Radial collateral lig

Extensor carpi radialis brevis m

Extensor digitorum and extensor digiti minimi tt

Extensor carpi ulnaris t

Lateral intermuscular septum

Anconeus m

Capitellum

Olecranon fossa

Olecranon

Median basilic v of forearm

Biceps brachii t (bifurcated)

Brachial a

Interosseous n, anterior

Median n

Brachialis m

Pronator teres m

Brachialis t

Trochlea

Basilic v

Ulnar collateral lig

Palmaris longus m

Flexor digitorum superficialis m

Ulnar n

Flexor carpi ulnaris m, humeral head

Ulnar collateral a, superior

Flexor carpi ulnaris m, ulnar head

Figure 5.1.11

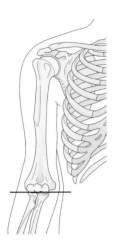

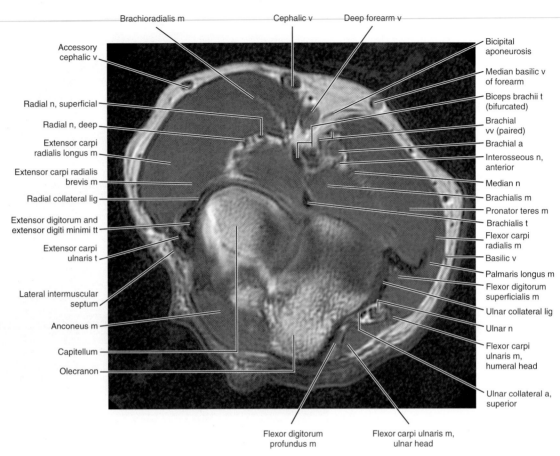

Accessory cephalic v

Radial n, superficial

Radial n, deep

Extensor carpi radialis longus m

Extensor carpi radialis brevis m

Radial collateral lig

Extensor digitorum and extensor digiti minimi tt

Extensor carpi ulnaris t

Lateral intermuscular septum

Anconeus m

Capitellum

Olecranon

Brachioradialis m

Cephalic v

Deep forearm v

Bicipital aponeurosis

Median basilic v of forearm

Biceps brachii t (bifurcated)

Brachial vv (paired)

Brachial a

Interosseous n, anterior

Median n

Brachialis m

Pronator teres m

Brachialis t

Flexor carpi radialis m

Basilic v

Palmaris longus m

Flexor digitorum superficialis m

Ulnar collateral lig

Ulnar n

Flexor carpi ulnaris m, humeral head

Ulnar collateral a, superior

Flexor digitorum profundus m

Flexor carpi ulnaris m, ulnar head

Figure 5.1.12

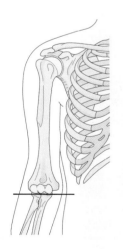

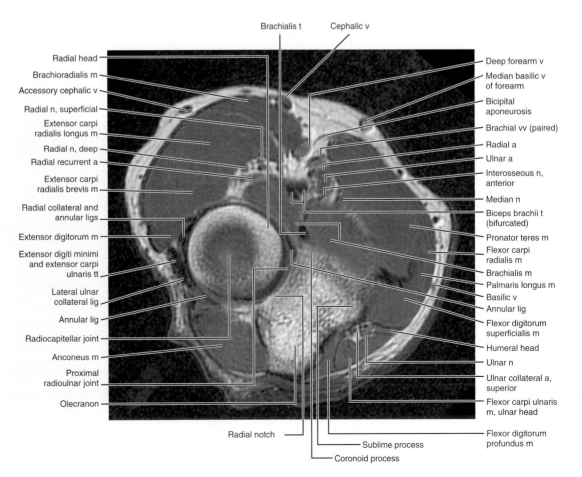

Radial head

Brachioradialis m

Accessory cephalic v

Radial n, superficial

Extensor carpi radialis longus m

Radial n, deep

Radial recurrent a

Extensor carpi radialis brevis m

Radial collateral and annular ligs

Extensor digitorum m

Extensor digiti minimi and extensor carpi ulnaris tt

Lateral ulnar collateral lig

Annular lig

Radiocapitellar joint

Anconeus m

Proximal radioulnar joint

Olecranon

Brachialis t

Cephalic v

Deep forearm v

Median basilic v of forearm

Bicipital aponeurosis

Brachial vv (paired)

Radial a

Ulnar a

Interosseous n, anterior

Median n

Biceps brachii t (bifurcated)

Pronator teres m

Flexor carpi radialis m

Brachialis m

Palmaris longus m

Basilic v

Annular lig

Flexor digitorum superficialis m

Humeral head

Ulnar n

Ulnar collateral a, superior

Flexor carpi ulnaris m, ulnar head

Flexor digitorum profundus m

Radial notch

Sublime process

Coronoid process

Figure 5.1.13

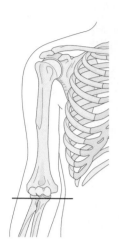

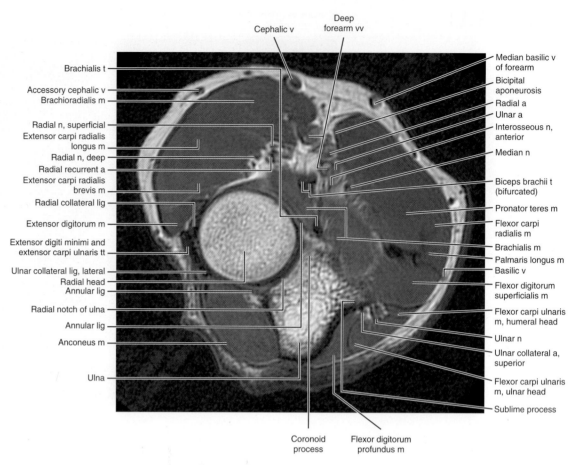

Cephalic v
Deep forearm vv

Brachialis t
Accessory cephalic v
Brachioradialis m

Radial n, superficial
Extensor carpi radialis longus m
Radial n, deep
Radial recurrent a
Extensor carpi radialis brevis m
Radial collateral lig
Extensor digitorum m
Extensor digiti minimi and extensor carpi ulnaris tt
Ulnar collateral lig, lateral
Radial head
Annular lig
Radial notch of ulna
Annular lig
Anconeus m
Ulna

Median basilic v of forearm
Bicipital aponeurosis
Radial a
Ulnar a
Interosseous n, anterior
Median n
Biceps brachii t (bifurcated)
Pronator teres m
Flexor carpi radialis m
Brachialis m
Palmaris longus m
Basilic v
Flexor digitorum superficialis m
Flexor carpi ulnaris m, humeral head
Ulnar n
Ulnar collateral a, superior
Flexor carpi ulnaris m, ulnar head
Sublime process

Coronoid process
Flexor digitorum profundus m

Figure 5.1.14

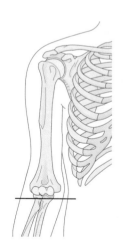

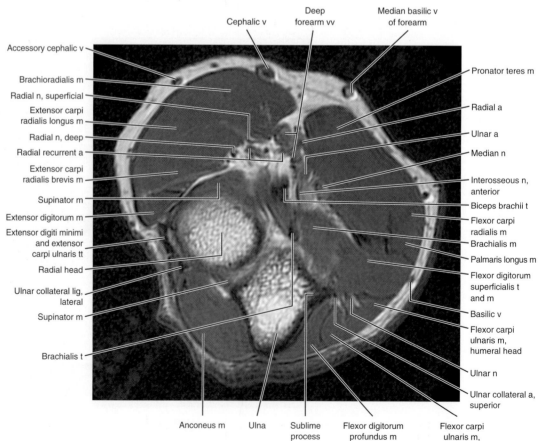

Cephalic v
Deep forearm vv
Median basilic v of forearm

Accessory cephalic v
Brachioradialis m
Radial n, superficial
Extensor carpi radialis longus m
Radial n, deep
Radial recurrent a
Extensor carpi radialis brevis m
Supinator m
Extensor digitorum m
Extensor digiti minimi and extensor carpi ulnaris tt
Radial head
Ulnar collateral lig, lateral
Supinator m
Brachialis t

Pronator teres m
Radial a
Ulnar a
Median n
Interosseous n, anterior
Biceps brachii t
Flexor carpi radialis m
Brachialis m
Palmaris longus m
Flexor digitorum superficialis t and m
Basilic v
Flexor carpi ulnaris m, humeral head
Ulnar n
Ulnar collateral a, superior

Anconeus m
Ulna
Sublime process
Flexor digitorum profundus m
Flexor carpi ulnaris m, ulnar head

Figure 5.1.15

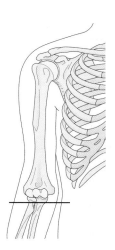

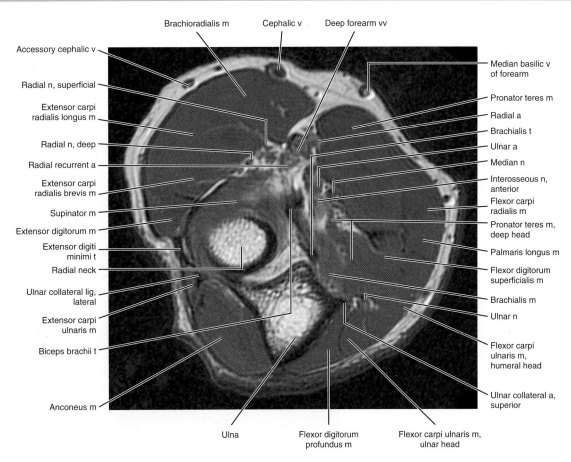

Accessory cephalic v
Radial n, superficial
Extensor carpi radialis longus m
Radial n, deep
Radial recurrent a
Extensor carpi radialis brevis m
Supinator m
Extensor digitorum m
Extensor digiti minimi t
Radial neck
Ulnar collateral lig, lateral
Extensor carpi ulnaris m
Biceps brachii t
Anconeus m

Brachioradialis m
Cephalic v
Deep forearm vv

Median basilic v of forearm
Pronator teres m
Radial a
Brachialis t
Ulnar a
Median n
Interosseous n, anterior
Flexor carpi radialis m
Pronator teres m, deep head
Palmaris longus m
Flexor digitorum superficialis m
Brachialis m
Ulnar n
Flexor carpi ulnaris m, humeral head
Ulnar collateral a, superior

Ulna
Flexor digitorum profundus m
Flexor carpi ulnaris m, ulnar head

Figure 5.1.16

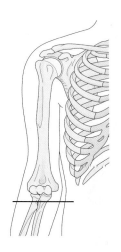

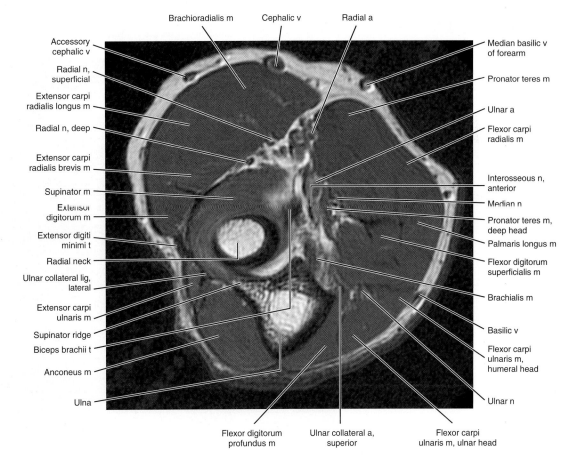

Accessory cephalic v
Radial n, superficial
Extensor carpi radialis longus m
Radial n, deep
Extensor carpi radialis brevis m
Supinator m
Extensor digitorum m
Extensor digiti minimi t
Radial neck
Ulnar collateral lig, lateral
Extensor carpi ulnaris m
Supinator ridge
Biceps brachii t
Anconeus m
Ulna

Brachioradialis m
Cephalic v
Radial a

Median basilic v of forearm
Pronator teres m
Ulnar a
Flexor carpi radialis m
Interosseous n, anterior
Median n
Pronator teres m, deep head
Palmaris longus m
Flexor digitorum superficialis m
Brachialis m
Basilic v
Flexor carpi ulnaris m, humeral head
Ulnar n

Flexor digitorum profundus m
Ulnar collateral a, superior
Flexor carpi ulnaris m, ulnar head

Figure 5.1.17

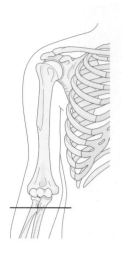

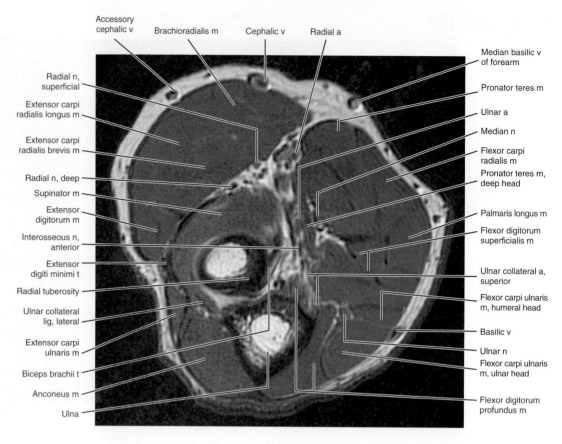

Accessory cephalic v — Brachioradialis m — Cephalic v — Radial a

Radial n, superficial

Extensor carpi radialis longus m

Extensor carpi radialis brevis m

Radial n, deep

Supinator m

Extensor digitorum m

Interosseous n, anterior

Extensor digiti minimi t

Radial tuberosity

Ulnar collateral lig, lateral

Extensor carpi ulnaris m

Biceps brachii t

Anconeus m

Ulna

Median basilic v of forearm

Pronator teres m

Ulnar a

Median n

Flexor carpi radialis m

Pronator teres m, deep head

Palmaris longus m

Flexor digitorum superficialis m

Ulnar collateral a, superior

Flexor carpi ulnaris m, humeral head

Basilic v

Ulnar n

Flexor carpi ulnaris m, ulnar head

Flexor digitorum profundus m

Figure 5.1.18

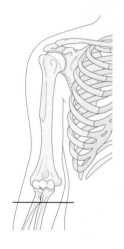

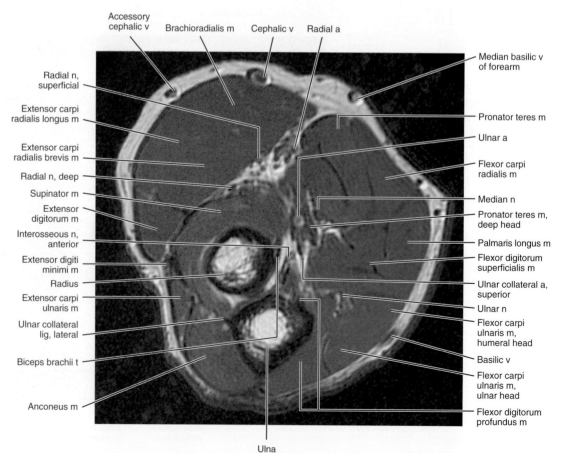

Accessory cephalic v — Brachioradialis m — Cephalic v — Radial a

Radial n, superficial

Extensor carpi radialis longus m

Extensor carpi radialis brevis m

Radial n, deep

Supinator m

Extensor digitorum m

Interosseous n, anterior

Extensor digiti minimi m

Radius

Extensor carpi ulnaris m

Ulnar collateral lig, lateral

Biceps brachii t

Anconeus m

Ulna

Median basilic v of forearm

Pronator teres m

Ulnar a

Flexor carpi radialis m

Median n

Pronator teres m, deep head

Palmaris longus m

Flexor digitorum superficialis m

Ulnar collateral a, superior

Ulnar n

Flexor carpi ulnaris m, humeral head

Basilic v

Flexor carpi ulnaris m, ulnar head

Flexor digitorum profundus m

Figure 5.1.19

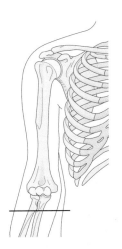

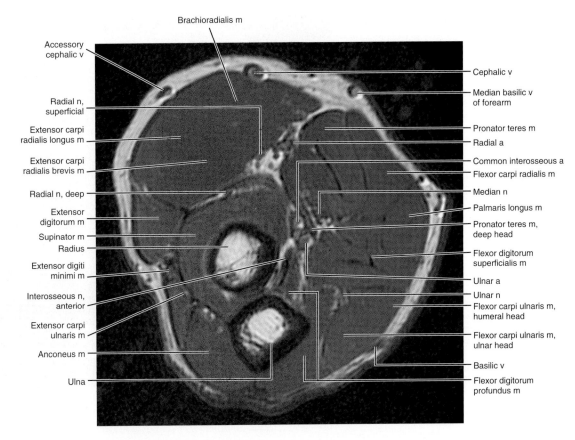

Brachioradialis m

Accessory cephalic v

Radial n, superficial

Extensor carpi radialis longus m

Extensor carpi radialis brevis m

Radial n, deep

Extensor digitorum m

Supinator m

Radius

Extensor digiti minimi m

Interosseous n, anterior

Extensor carpi ulnaris m

Anconeus m

Ulna

Cephalic v

Median basilic v of forearm

Pronator teres m

Radial a

Common interosseous a

Flexor carpi radialis m

Median n

Palmaris longus m

Pronator teres m, deep head

Flexor digitorum superficialis m

Ulnar a

Ulnar n

Flexor carpi ulnaris m, humeral head

Flexor carpi ulnaris m, ulnar head

Basilic v

Flexor digitorum profundus m

Figure 5.1.20

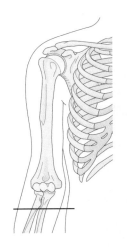

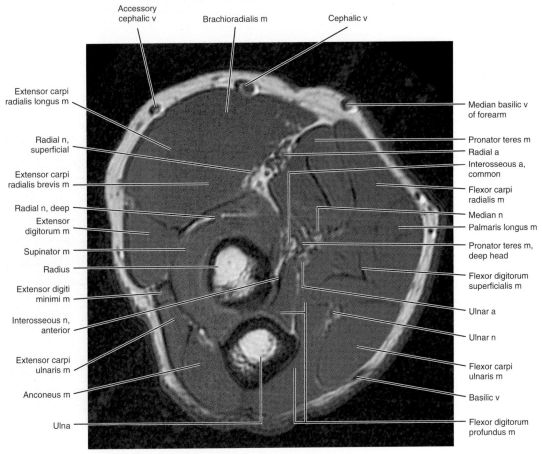

Accessory cephalic v

Brachioradialis m

Cephalic v

Extensor carpi radialis longus m

Radial n, superficial

Extensor carpi radialis brevis m

Radial n, deep

Extensor digitorum m

Supinator m

Radius

Extensor digiti minimi m

Interosseous n, anterior

Extensor carpi ulnaris m

Anconeus m

Ulna

Median basilic v of forearm

Pronator teres m

Radial a

Interosseous a, common

Flexor carpi radialis m

Median n

Palmaris longus m

Pronator teres m, deep head

Flexor digitorum superficialis m

Ulnar a

Ulnar n

Flexor carpi ulnaris m

Basilic v

Flexor digitorum profundus m

Figure 5.1.21

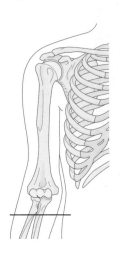

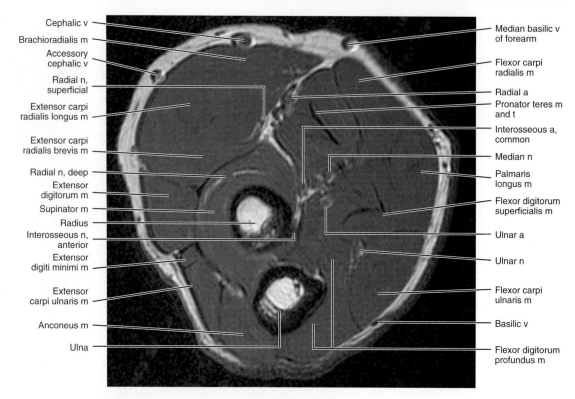

Cephalic v
Brachioradialis m
Accessory cephalic v
Radial n, superficial
Extensor carpi radialis longus m
Extensor carpi radialis brevis m
Radial n, deep
Extensor digitorum m
Supinator m
Radius
Interosseous n, anterior
Extensor digiti minimi m
Extensor carpi ulnaris m
Anconeus m
Ulna

Median basilic v of forearm
Flexor carpi radialis m
Radial a
Pronator teres m and t
Interosseous a, common
Median n
Palmaris longus m
Flexor digitorum superficialis m
Ulnar a
Ulnar n
Flexor carpi ulnaris m
Basilic v
Flexor digitorum profundus m

Figure 5.1.22

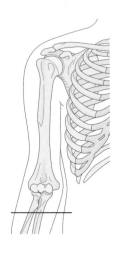

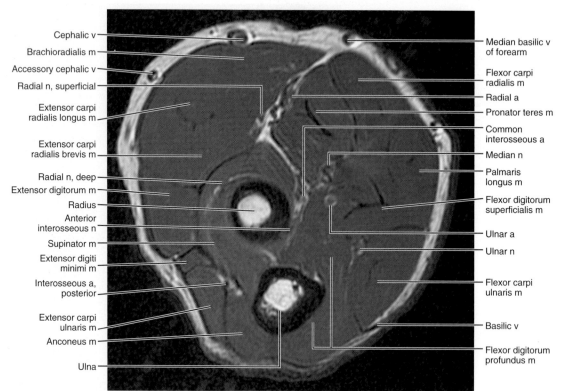

Cephalic v
Brachioradialis m
Accessory cephalic v
Radial n, superficial
Extensor carpi radialis longus m
Extensor carpi radialis brevis m
Radial n, deep
Extensor digitorum m
Radius
Anterior interosseous n
Supinator m
Extensor digiti minimi m
Interosseous a, posterior
Extensor carpi ulnaris m
Anconeus m
Ulna

Median basilic v of forearm
Flexor carpi radialis m
Radial a
Pronator teres m
Common interosseous a
Median n
Palmaris longus m
Flexor digitorum superficialis m
Ulnar a
Ulnar n
Flexor carpi ulnaris m
Basilic v
Flexor digitorum profundus m

Figure 5.1.23

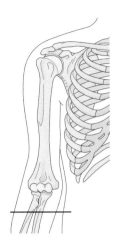

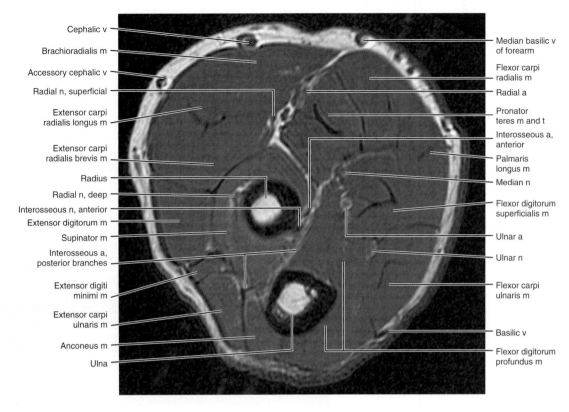

Cephalic v
Brachioradialis m
Accessory cephalic v
Radial n, superficial
Extensor carpi radialis longus m
Extensor carpi radialis brevis m
Radius
Radial n, deep
Interosseous n, anterior
Extensor digitorum m
Supinator m
Interosseous a, posterior branches
Extensor digiti minimi m
Extensor carpi ulnaris m
Anconeus m
Ulna

Median basilic v of forearm
Flexor carpi radialis m
Radial a
Pronator teres m and t
Interosseous a, anterior
Palmaris longus m
Median n
Flexor digitorum superficialis m
Ulnar a
Ulnar n
Flexor carpi ulnaris m
Basilic v
Flexor digitorum profundus m

Figure 5.1.24

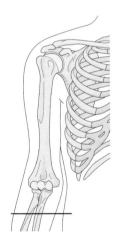

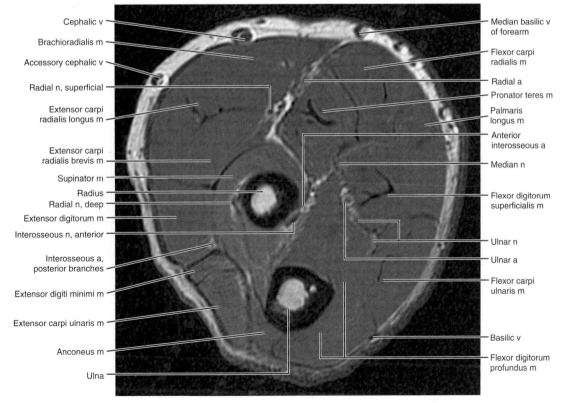

Cephalic v
Brachioradialis m
Accessory cephalic v
Radial n, superficial
Extensor carpi radialis longus m
Extensor carpi radialis brevis m
Supinator m
Radius
Radial n, deep
Extensor digitorum m
Interosseous n, anterior
Interosseous a, posterior branches
Extensor digiti minimi m
Extensor carpi ulnaris m
Anconeus m
Ulna

Median basilic v of forearm
Flexor carpi radialis m
Radial a
Pronator teres m
Palmaris longus m
Anterior interosseous a
Median n
Flexor digitorum superficialis m
Ulnar n
Ulnar a
Flexor carpi ulnaris m
Basilic v
Flexor digitorum profundus m

Figure 5.1.25

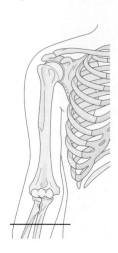

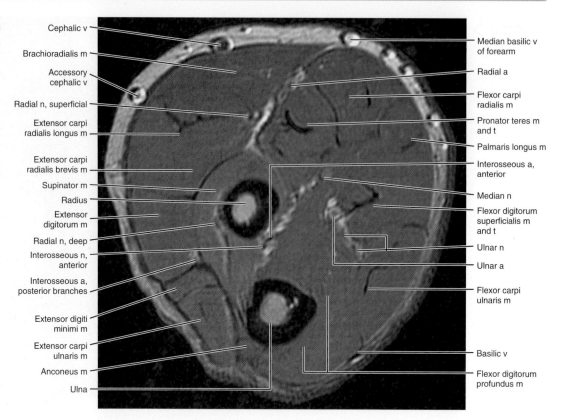

Cephalic v

Brachioradialis m

Accessory cephalic v

Radial n, superficial

Extensor carpi radialis longus m

Extensor carpi radialis brevis m

Supinator m

Radius

Extensor digitorum m

Radial n, deep

Interosseous n, anterior

Interosseous a, posterior branches

Extensor digiti minimi m

Extensor carpi ulnaris m

Anconeus m

Ulna

Median basilic v of forearm

Radial a

Flexor carpi radialis m

Pronator teres m and t

Palmaris longus m

Interosseous a, anterior

Median n

Flexor digitorum superficialis m and t

Ulnar n

Ulnar a

Flexor carpi ulnaris m

Basilic v

Flexor digitorum profundus m

SAGITTAL

Figure 5.2.1

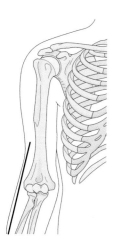

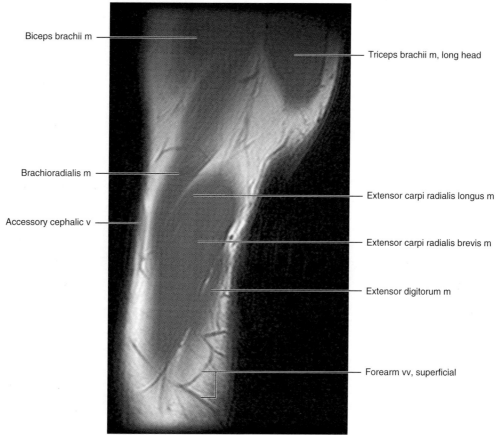

Biceps brachii m

Triceps brachii m, long head

Brachioradialis m

Extensor carpi radialis longus m

Accessory cephalic v

Extensor carpi radialis brevis m

Extensor digitorum m

Forearm vv, superficial

Figure 5.2.2

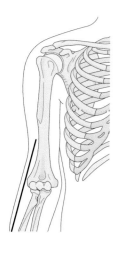

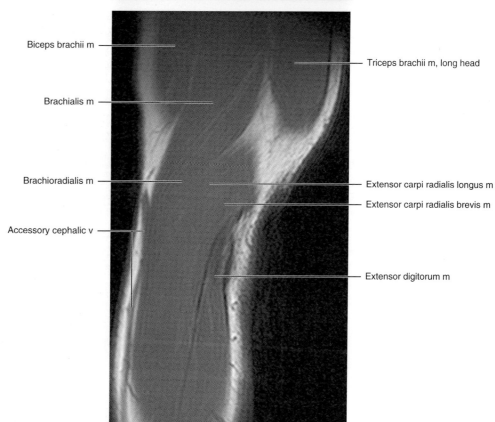

Biceps brachii m

Triceps brachii m, long head

Brachialis m

Brachioradialis m

Extensor carpi radialis longus m

Extensor carpi radialis brevis m

Accessory cephalic v

Extensor digitorum m

Figure 5.2.3

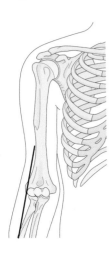

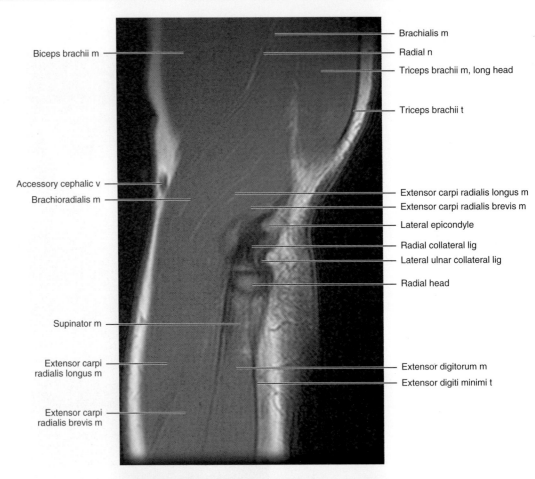

Biceps brachii m

Accessory cephalic v

Brachioradialis m

Supinator m

Extensor carpi radialis longus m

Extensor carpi radialis brevis m

Brachialis m

Radial n

Triceps brachii m, long head

Triceps brachii t

Extensor carpi radialis longus m

Extensor carpi radialis brevis m

Lateral epicondyle

Radial collateral lig

Lateral ulnar collateral lig

Radial head

Extensor digitorum m

Extensor digiti minimi t

Figure 5.2.4

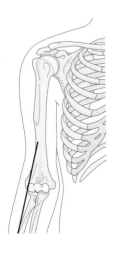

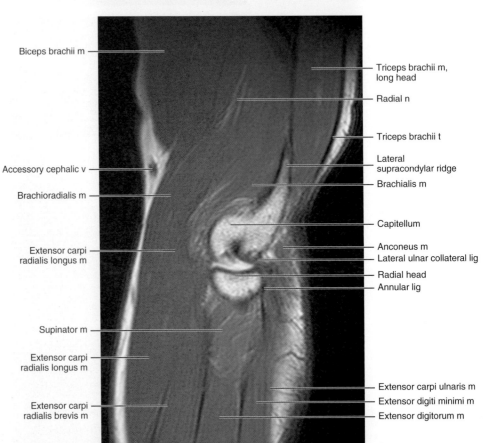

Biceps brachii m

Accessory cephalic v

Brachioradialis m

Extensor carpi radialis longus m

Supinator m

Extensor carpi radialis longus m

Extensor carpi radialis brevis m

Triceps brachii m, long head

Radial n

Triceps brachii t

Lateral supracondylar ridge

Brachialis m

Capitellum

Anconeus m

Lateral ulnar collateral lig

Radial head

Annular lig

Extensor carpi ulnaris m

Extensor digiti minimi m

Extensor digitorum m

Figure 5.2.5

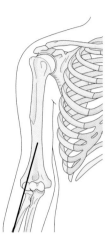

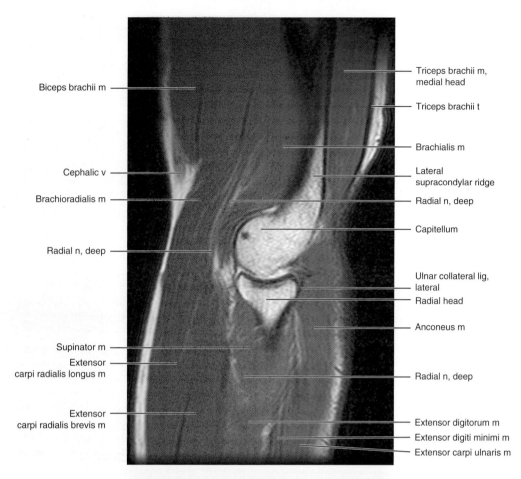

Biceps brachii m

Cephalic v

Brachioradialis m

Radial n, deep

Supinator m

Extensor
carpi radialis longus m

Extensor
carpi radialis brevis m

Triceps brachii m,
medial head

Triceps brachii t

Brachialis m

Lateral
supracondylar ridge

Radial n, deep

Capitellum

Ulnar collateral lig,
lateral

Radial head

Anconeus m

Radial n, deep

Extensor digitorum m

Extensor digiti minimi m

Extensor carpi ulnaris m

Figure 5.2.6

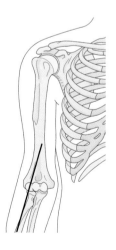

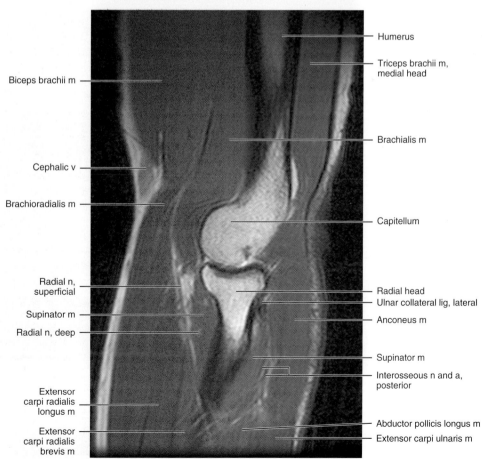

Biceps brachii m

Cephalic v

Brachioradialis m

Radial n,
superficial

Supinator m

Radial n, deep

Extensor
carpi radialis
longus m

Extensor
carpi radialis
brevis m

Humerus

Triceps brachii m,
medial head

Brachialis m

Capitellum

Radial head

Ulnar collateral lig, lateral

Anconeus m

Supinator m

Interosseous n and a,
posterior

Abductor pollicis longus m

Extensor carpi ulnaris m

Figure 5.2.7

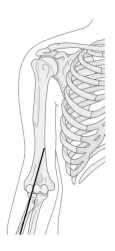

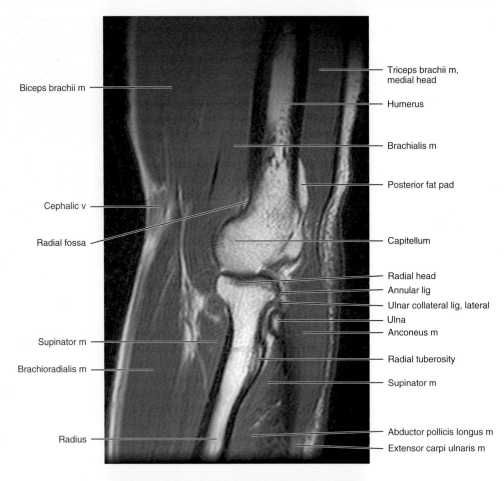

Biceps brachii m

Cephalic v

Radial fossa

Supinator m

Brachioradialis m

Radius

Triceps brachii m, medial head

Humerus

Brachialis m

Posterior fat pad

Capitellum

Radial head
Annular lig
Ulnar collateral lig, lateral
Ulna
Anconeus m

Radial tuberosity

Supinator m

Abductor pollicis longus m
Extensor carpi ulnaris m

Figure 5.2.8

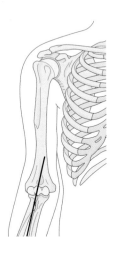

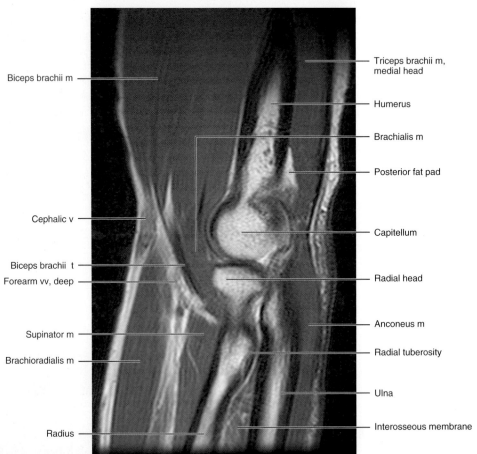

Biceps brachii m

Cephalic v

Biceps brachii t
Forearm vv, deep

Supinator m

Brachioradialis m

Radius

Triceps brachii m, medial head

Humerus

Brachialis m

Posterior fat pad

Capitellum

Radial head

Anconeus m

Radial tuberosity

Ulna

Interosseous membrane

Figure 5.2.9

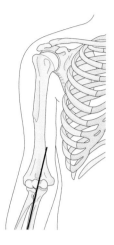

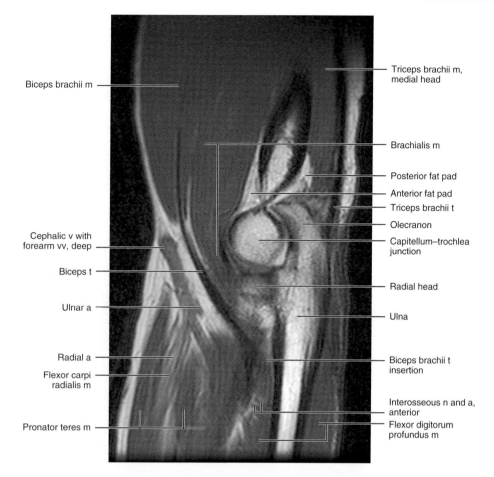

Biceps brachii m

Triceps brachii m, medial head

Brachialis m

Posterior fat pad

Anterior fat pad

Triceps brachii t

Olecranon

Capitellum–trochlea junction

Cephalic v with forearm vv, deep

Biceps t

Radial head

Ulnar a

Ulna

Radial a

Biceps brachii t insertion

Flexor carpi radialis m

Pronator teres m

Interosseous n and a, anterior

Flexor digitorum profundus m

Figure 5.2.10

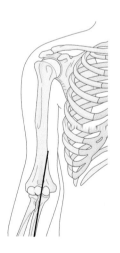

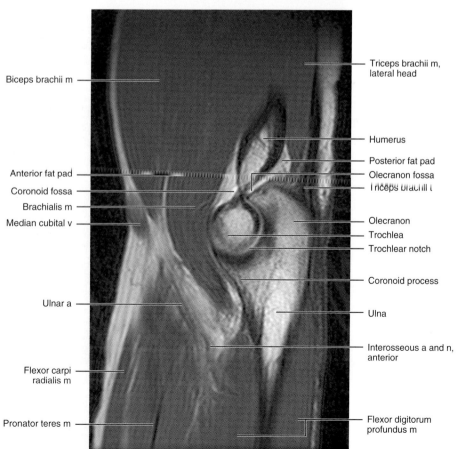

Biceps brachii m

Triceps brachii m, lateral head

Humerus

Posterior fat pad

Olecranon fossa

Triceps brachii t

Anterior fat pad

Coronoid fossa

Brachialis m

Median cubital v

Olecranon

Trochlea

Trochlear notch

Coronoid process

Ulnar a

Ulna

Interosseous a and n, anterior

Flexor carpi radialis m

Pronator teres m

Flexor digitorum profundus m

Figure 5.2.11

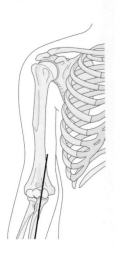

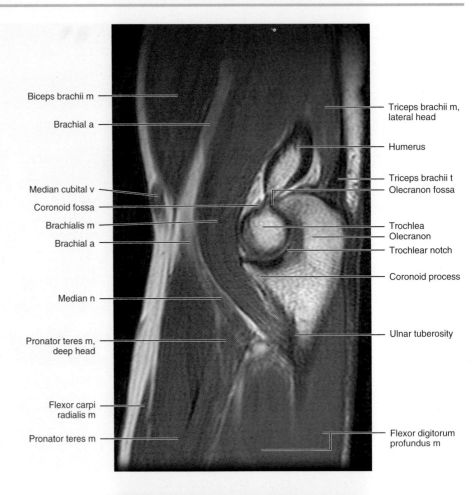

Biceps brachii m

Brachial a

Median cubital v

Coronoid fossa

Brachialis m

Brachial a

Median n

Pronator teres m, deep head

Flexor carpi radialis m

Pronator teres m

Triceps brachii m, lateral head

Humerus

Triceps brachii t

Olecranon fossa

Trochlea

Olecranon

Trochlear notch

Coronoid process

Ulnar tuberosity

Flexor digitorum profundus m

Figure 5.2.12

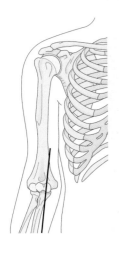

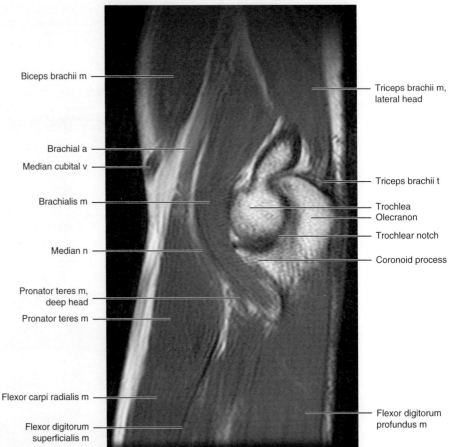

Biceps brachii m

Brachial a

Median cubital v

Brachialis m

Median n

Pronator teres m, deep head

Pronator teres m

Flexor carpi radialis m

Flexor digitorum superficialis m

Triceps brachii m, lateral head

Triceps brachii t

Trochlea

Olecranon

Trochlear notch

Coronoid process

Flexor digitorum profundus m

Figure 5.2.13

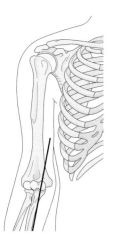

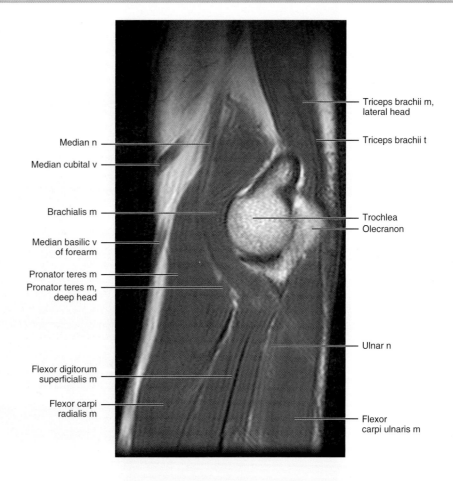

Median n

Median cubital v

Brachialis m

Median basilic v
of forearm

Pronator teres m

Pronator teres m,
deep head

Flexor digitorum
superficialis m

Flexor carpi
radialis m

Triceps brachii m,
lateral head

Triceps brachii t

Trochlea

Olecranon

Ulnar n

Flexor
carpi ulnaris m

Figure 5.2.14

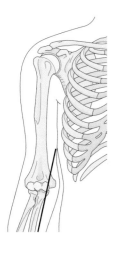

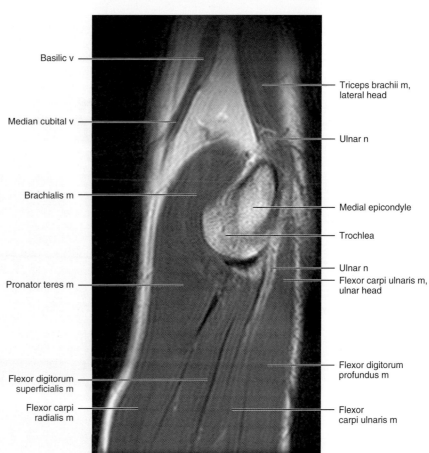

Basilic v

Median cubital v

Brachialis m

Pronator teres m

Flexor digitorum
superficialis m

Flexor carpi
radialis m

Triceps brachii m,
lateral head

Ulnar n

Medial epicondyle

Trochlea

Ulnar n

Flexor carpi ulnaris m,
ulnar head

Flexor digitorum
profundus m

Flexor
carpi ulnaris m

Figure 5.2.15

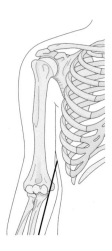

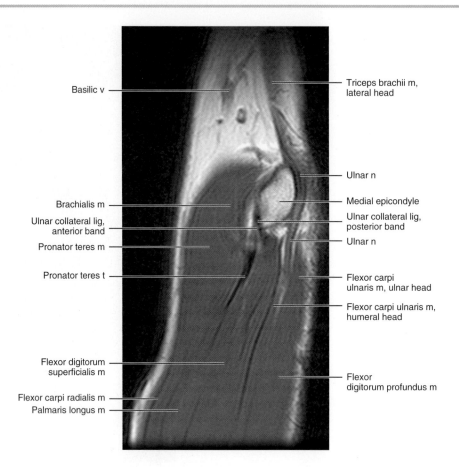

Basilic v

Brachialis m

Ulnar collateral lig,
anterior band

Pronator teres m

Pronator teres t

Flexor digitorum
superficialis m

Flexor carpi radialis m

Palmaris longus m

Triceps brachii m,
lateral head

Ulnar n

Medial epicondyle

Ulnar collateral lig,
posterior band

Ulnar n

Flexor carpi
ulnaris m, ulnar head

Flexor carpi ulnaris m,
humeral head

Flexor
digitorum profundus m

Figure 5.2.16

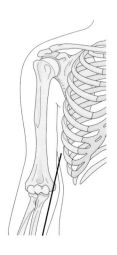

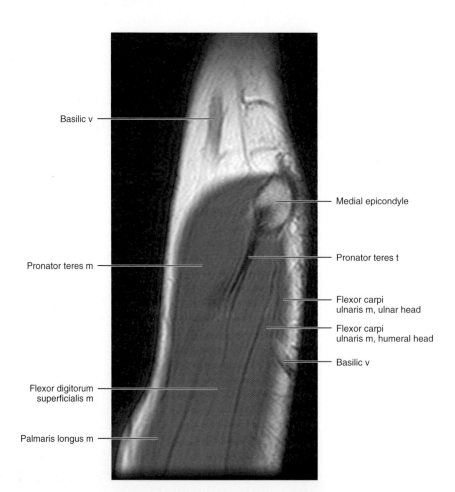

Basilic v

Pronator teres m

Flexor digitorum
superficialis m

Palmaris longus m

Medial epicondyle

Pronator teres t

Flexor carpi
ulnaris m, ulnar head

Flexor carpi
ulnaris m, humeral head

Basilic v

Figure 5.2.17

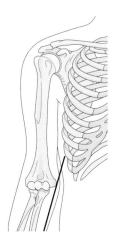

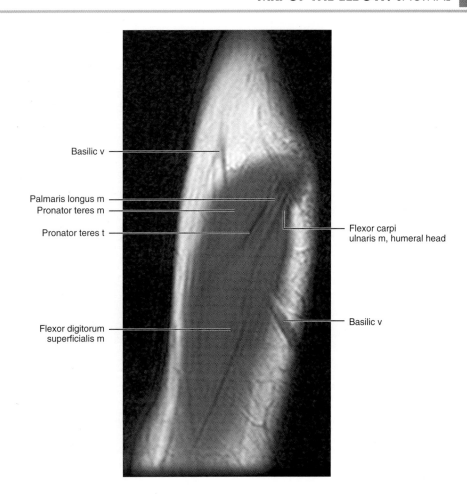

Basilic v

Palmaris longus m

Pronator teres m

Pronator teres t

Flexor carpi
ulnaris m, humeral head

Flexor digitorum
superficialis m

Basilic v

CORONAL
Figure 5.3.1

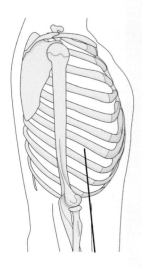

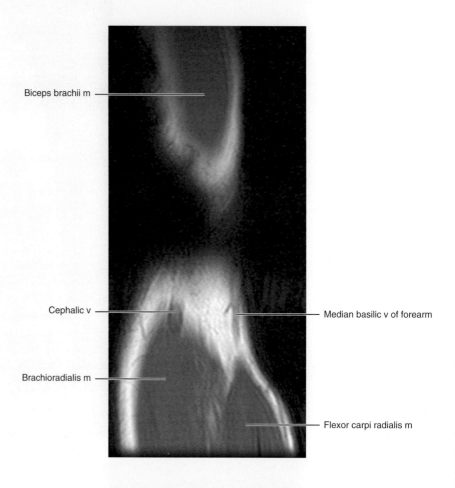

Biceps brachii m

Cephalic v

Median basilic v of forearm

Brachioradialis m

Flexor carpi radialis m

Figure 5.3.2

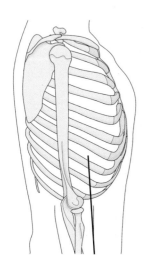

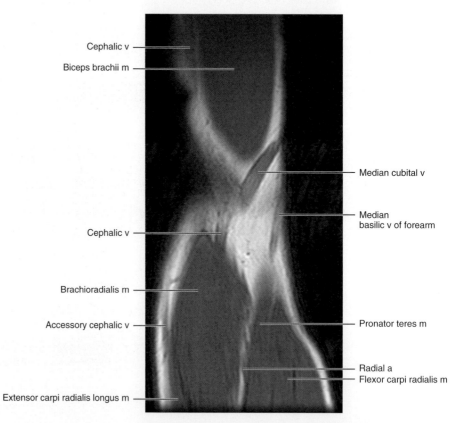

Cephalic v

Biceps brachii m

Median cubital v

Median
basilic v of forearm

Cephalic v

Brachioradialis m

Pronator teres m

Accessory cephalic v

Radial a
Flexor carpi radialis m

Extensor carpi radialis longus m

Figure 5.3.3

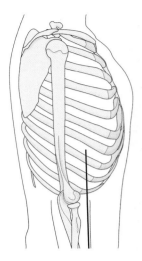

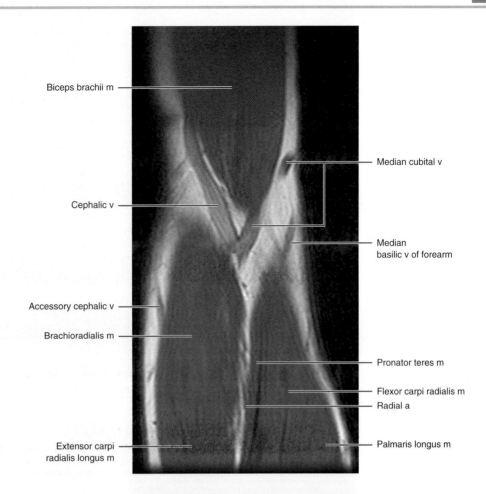

Biceps brachii m

Median cubital v

Cephalic v

Median basilic v of forearm

Accessory cephalic v

Brachioradialis m

Pronator teres m

Flexor carpi radialis m

Radial a

Extensor carpi radialis longus m

Palmaris longus m

Figure 5.3.4

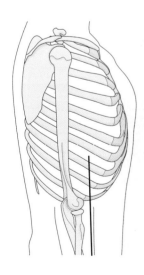

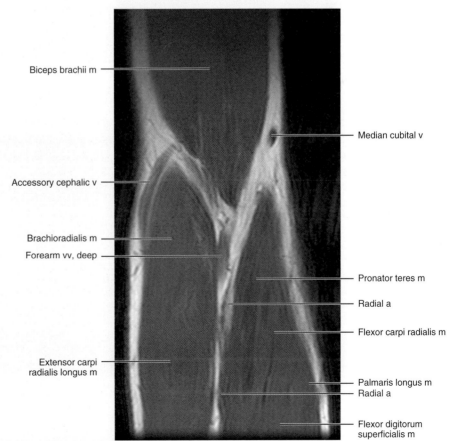

Biceps brachii m

Median cubital v

Accessory cephalic v

Brachioradialis m

Forearm vv, deep

Pronator teres m

Radial a

Flexor carpi radialis m

Extensor carpi radialis longus m

Palmaris longus m

Radial a

Flexor digitorum superficialis m

Figure 5.3.5

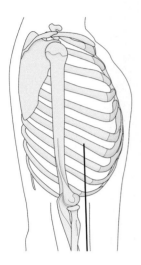

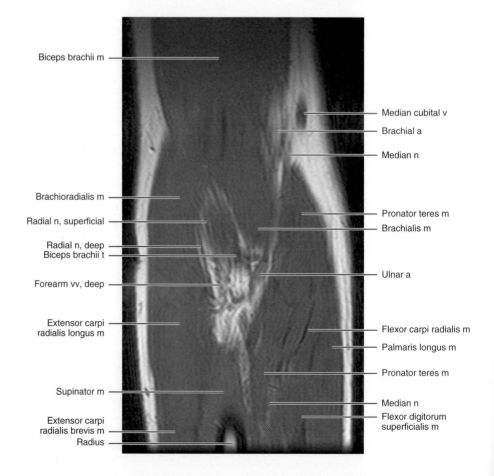

Biceps brachii m

Median cubital v

Brachial a
Biceps brachii t — Brachialis m and t
Brachioradialis m — Pronator teres m

Radial a

Forearm vv, deep

Radial n, superficial

Flexor carpi radialis m

Extensor carpi
radialis longus m — Palmaris longus m
Pronator teres m

Supinator m — Median n
Extensor carpi — Flexor digitorum
radialis brevis m — superficialis m

Figure 5.3.6

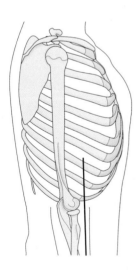

Biceps brachii m

Median cubital v
Brachial a

Median n

Brachioradialis m

Radial n, superficial — Pronator teres m
Brachialis m

Radial n, deep
Biceps brachii t

Forearm vv, deep — Ulnar a

Extensor carpi
radialis longus m — Flexor carpi radialis m
Palmaris longus m

Pronator teres m

Supinator m

Median n
Extensor carpi — Flexor digitorum
radialis brevis m — superficialis m
Radius

Figure 5.3.7

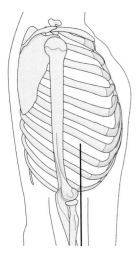

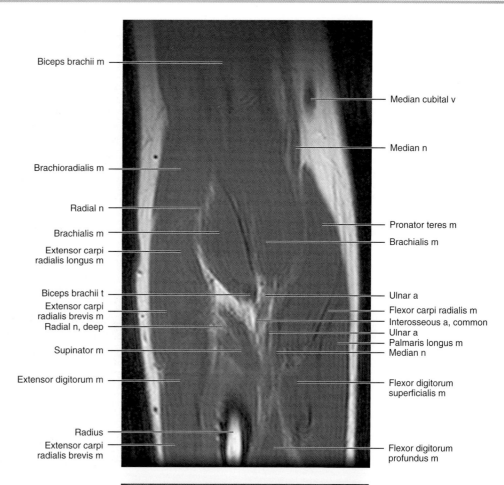

Biceps brachii m

Median cubital v

Median n

Brachioradialis m

Radial n

Pronator teres m

Brachialis m

Brachialis m

Extensor carpi
radialis longus m

Biceps brachii t

Ulnar a

Extensor carpi
radialis brevis m

Flexor carpi radialis m

Interosseous a, common

Radial n, deep

Ulnar a

Supinator m

Palmaris longus m

Median n

Extensor digitorum m

Flexor digitorum
superficialis m

Radius

Extensor carpi
radialis brevis m

Flexor digitorum
profundus m

Figure 5.3.8

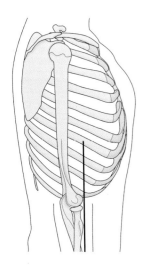

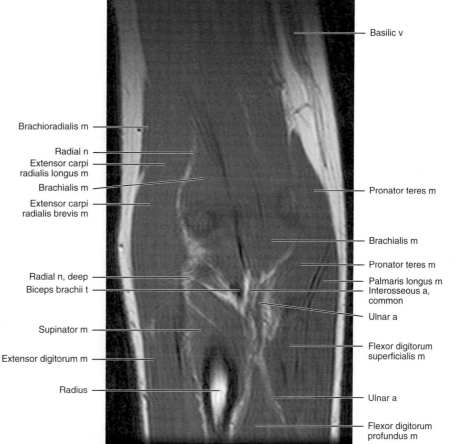

Basilic v

Brachioradialis m

Radial n

Extensor carpi
radialis longus m

Brachialis m

Pronator teres m

Extensor carpi
radialis brevis m

Brachialis m

Pronator teres m

Radial n, deep

Palmaris longus m

Biceps brachii t

Interosseous a,
common

Ulnar a

Supinator m

Flexor digitorum
superficialis m

Extensor digitorum m

Radius

Ulnar a

Flexor digitorum
profundus m

Figure 5.3.9

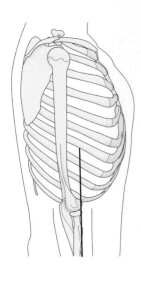

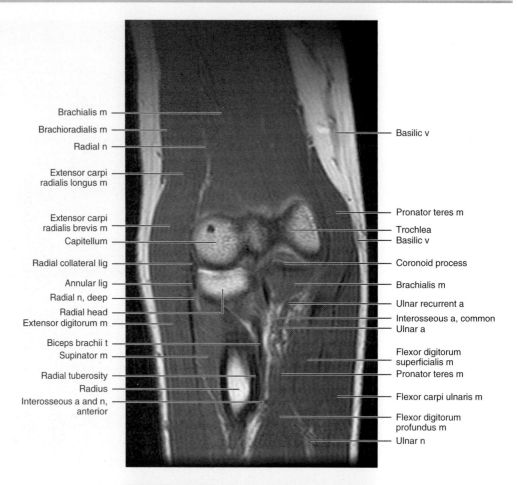

Brachialis m

Brachioradialis m

Radial n

Extensor carpi
radialis longus m

Extensor carpi
radialis brevis m

Capitellum

Radial collateral lig

Annular lig

Radial n, deep

Radial head

Extensor digitorum m

Biceps brachii t

Supinator m

Radial tuberosity

Radius

Interosseous a and n,
anterior

Basilic v

Pronator teres m

Trochlea

Basilic v

Coronoid process

Brachialis m

Ulnar recurrent a

Interosseous a, common

Ulnar a

Flexor digitorum
superficialis m

Pronator teres m

Flexor carpi ulnaris m

Flexor digitorum
profundus m

Ulnar n

Figure 5.3.10

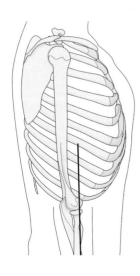

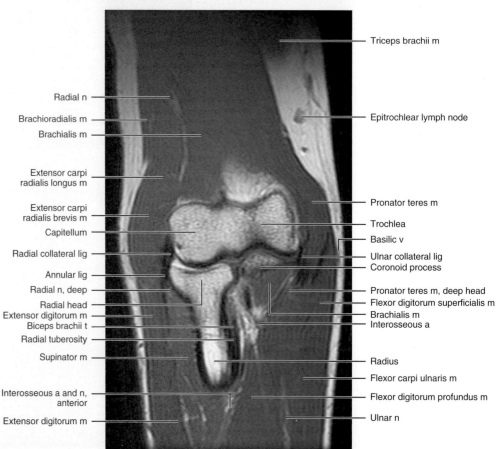

Radial n

Brachioradialis m

Brachialis m

Extensor carpi
radialis longus m

Extensor carpi
radialis brevis m

Capitellum

Radial collateral lig

Annular lig

Radial n, deep

Radial head

Extensor digitorum m

Biceps brachii t

Radial tuberosity

Supinator m

Interosseous a and n,
anterior

Extensor digitorum m

Triceps brachii m

Epitrochlear lymph node

Pronator teres m

Trochlea

Basilic v

Ulnar collateral lig

Coronoid process

Pronator teres m, deep head

Flexor digitorum superficialis m

Brachialis m

Interosseous a

Radius

Flexor carpi ulnaris m

Flexor digitorum profundus m

Ulnar n

Figure 5.3.11

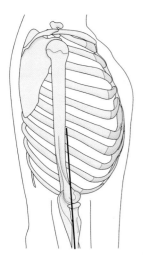

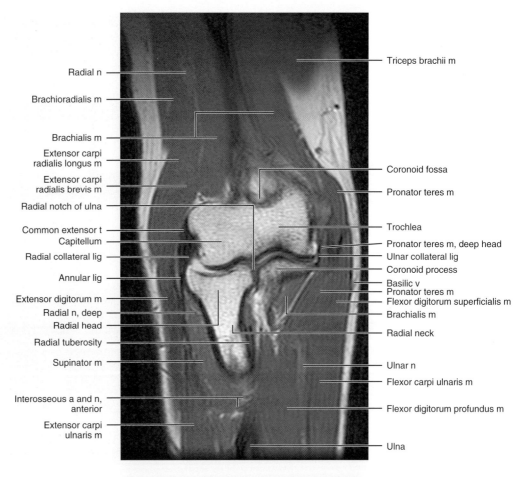

Radial n

Brachioradialis m

Brachialis m

Extensor carpi radialis longus m

Extensor carpi radialis brevis m

Radial notch of ulna

Common extensor t
Capitellum

Radial collateral lig

Annular lig

Extensor digitorum m
Radial n, deep
Radial head

Radial tuberosity

Supinator m

Interosseous a and n, anterior

Extensor carpi ulnaris m

Triceps brachii m

Coronoid fossa

Pronator teres m

Trochlea
Pronator teres m, deep head
Ulnar collateral lig
Coronoid process
Basilic v
Pronator teres m
Flexor digitorum superficialis m
Brachialis m

Radial neck

Ulnar n

Flexor carpi ulnaris m

Flexor digitorum profundus m

Ulna

Figure 5.3.12

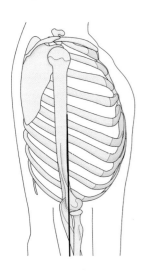

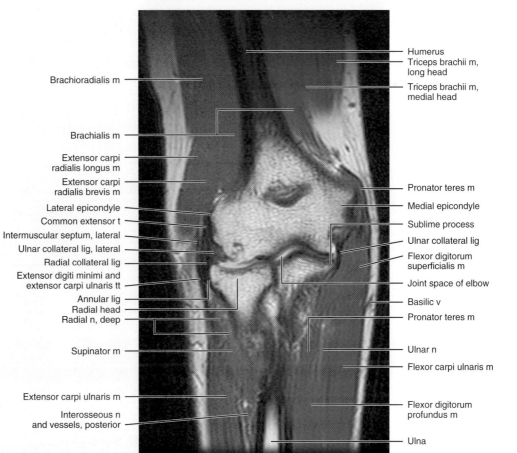

Brachioradialis m

Brachialis m

Extensor carpi radialis longus m

Extensor carpi radialis brevis m

Lateral epicondyle
Common extensor t
Intermuscular septum, lateral
Ulnar collateral lig, lateral
Radial collateral lig
Extensor digiti minimi and extensor carpi ulnaris tt
Annular lig
Radial head
Radial n, deep

Supinator m

Extensor carpi ulnaris m

Interosseous n and vessels, posterior

Humerus
Triceps brachii m, long head
Triceps brachii m, medial head

Pronator teres m

Medial epicondyle

Sublime process

Ulnar collateral lig

Flexor digitorum superficialis m

Joint space of elbow

Basilic v

Pronator teres m

Ulnar n

Flexor carpi ulnaris m

Flexor digitorum profundus m

Ulna

Figure 5.3.13

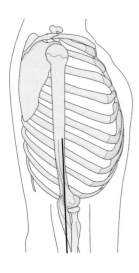

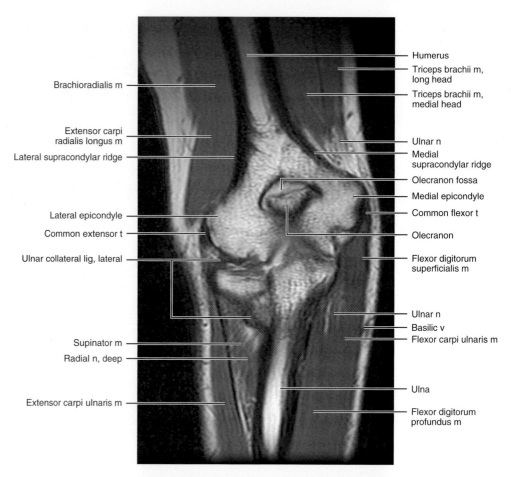

Brachioradialis m

Extensor carpi radialis longus m

Lateral supracondylar ridge

Lateral epicondyle

Common extensor t

Ulnar collateral lig, lateral

Supinator m

Radial n, deep

Extensor carpi ulnaris m

Humerus

Triceps brachii m, long head

Triceps brachii m, medial head

Ulnar n

Medial supracondylar ridge

Olecranon fossa

Medial epicondyle

Common flexor t

Olecranon

Flexor digitorum superficialis m

Ulnar n

Basilic v

Flexor carpi ulnaris m

Ulna

Flexor digitorum profundus m

Figure 5.3.14

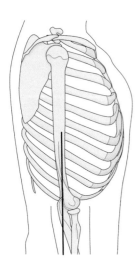

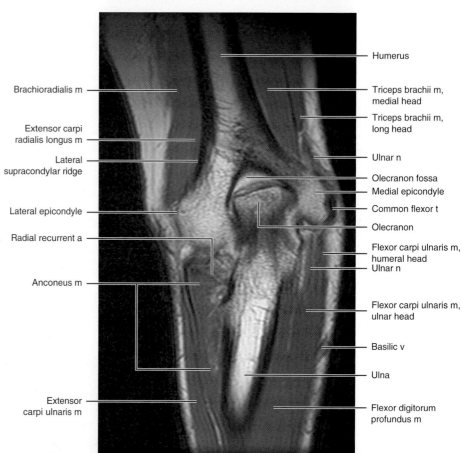

Brachioradialis m

Extensor carpi radialis longus m

Lateral supracondylar ridge

Lateral epicondyle

Radial recurrent a

Anconeus m

Extensor carpi ulnaris m

Humerus

Triceps brachii m, medial head

Triceps brachii m, long head

Ulnar n

Olecranon fossa

Medial epicondyle

Common flexor t

Olecranon

Flexor carpi ulnaris m, humeral head

Ulnar n

Flexor carpi ulnaris m, ulnar head

Basilic v

Ulna

Flexor digitorum profundus m

Figure 5.3.15

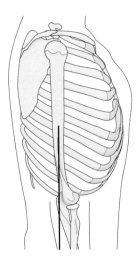

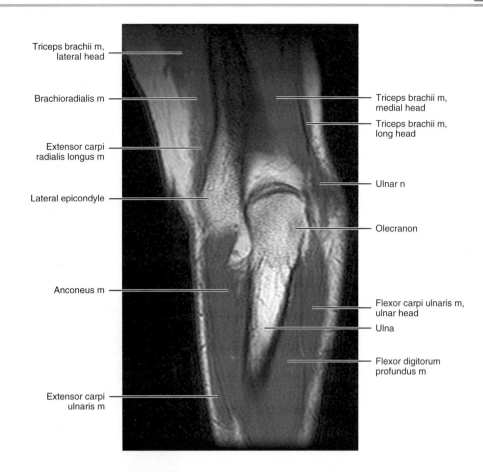

Triceps brachii m, lateral head

Brachioradialis m

Extensor carpi radialis longus m

Lateral epicondyle

Anconeus m

Extensor carpi ulnaris m

Triceps brachii m, medial head

Triceps brachii m, long head

Ulnar n

Olecranon

Flexor carpi ulnaris m, ulnar head

Ulna

Flexor digitorum profundus m

Figure 5.3.16

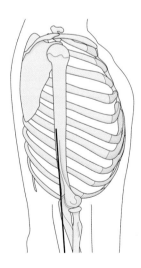

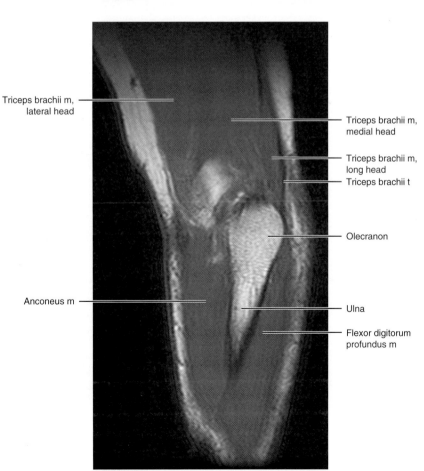

Triceps brachii m, lateral head

Anconeus m

Triceps brachii m, medial head

Triceps brachii m, long head

Triceps brachii t

Olecranon

Ulna

Flexor digitorum profundus m

Figure 5.3.17

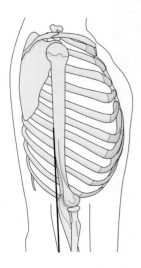

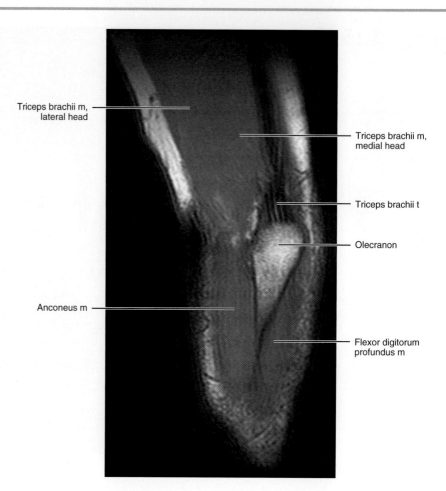

Triceps brachii m, lateral head

Triceps brachii m, medial head

Triceps brachii t

Olecranon

Anconeus m

Flexor digitorum profundus m

Chapter 6

MRI of the Forearm

Table 3: Muscles of the Forearm

MUSCLE	ORIGIN	INSERTION	NERVE SUPPLY
Anconeus	Posterior surface of the lateral epicondyle, and adjacent part of the elbow joint capsular ligament	Onto the radial side of the olecranon and adjacent part onto the shaft of the ulna	Nerve to anconeus (C7, C8, T1)
Brachioradialis	Upper two thirds of the lateral epicondylar ridge of the humerus and the anterior surface of the lateral intermuscular septum	Lateral side of the base of the styloid process of the radius	Radial (C5, C6, C7)
Extensor carpi radialis longus	Lower third of the lateral epicondylar ridge, lateral intermuscular septum, and extensor tendons from the lateral epicondyle	Lateral part of the base of the second metacarpal	Radial (C5, C6, C7)
Extensor carpi radialis brevis	Common extensor tendon from the lateral epicondyle, intermuscular septa, and radial collateral ligament of the elbow joint	Back of the base of the third metacarpal	Radial or deep radial (posterior interosseus) (C7, C8)
Extensor digitorum	Common extensor tendon	Dorsal digital fibrous expansion covering the dorsum of the proximal phalanx and sides of its base, base of the middle and distal phalanges	Deep radial (posterior interosseus) (C7, C8)
Extensor digiti minimi	Intermuscular septa, overlying fascia, and common extensor tendon	Base of the proximal phalanx of the little finger	Deep radial (posterior interosseus) (C7, C8)
Extensor carpi ulnaris	Two heads: (1) distal dorsal part of the epicondyle, and (2) proximal three fourths of the dorsal border of the ulna	Onto a tubercle at the base of the fifth metacarpal	Deep radial (posterior interosseus) (C7, C8)
Supinator	Dorsal aspect of the lateral epicondyle, ulnar depression distal to the radial notch, and supinator crest	Lateral surface of the radius between the anterior and posterior oblique lines	Deep radial (posterior interosseous) (C5, C6)
Abductor pollicis longus	Lateral edge of the proximal part of the middle third of the ulna, adjacent interosseous membrane, dorsal surface of the radius, and occasionally, the intermuscular septa	Radial side of the ventral aspect of the base of the first metacarpal	Deep radial (posterior interosseus) (C7, C8)
Extensor pollicis brevis	Distal end of the middle third of the radius in its dorsal surface, interosseous membrane, and occasionally, the ulna	Base of the proximal phalanx of the thumb or into the capsule of the metacarpophalangeal joint	Deep radial (posterior interosseus) (C7, C8)

Table 3: Muscles of the Forearm—Cont'd

MUSCLE	ORIGIN	INSERTION	NERVE SUPPLY
Extensor pollicis longus	Middle third of the dorsal surface of the ulna adjacent to the interosseous membrane	Base of the distal phalanx of the thumb	Deep radial (posterior interosseus) (C7, C8)
Extensor indicis	Proximal part of the distal third of the posterior surface of the ulna interosseous membrane	Dorsal aponeurosis on the ulnar side of the index finger, adjacent to the base of the proximal phalanx	Deep radial (posterior interosseus) (C7, C8)
Pronator teres	Two heads: (1) humeral head (superior half of the ventral surface of the medial epicondyle), and (2) ulnar head (medial border of the coronoid process)	Onto the middle third of lateral surface of the radius	Median (C6, C7)
Flexor carpi radialis	Medial epicondyle of the humerus	Base of the second metacarpal and usually, base of the third metacarpal	Median (C6, C7)
Palmaris longus	Medial epicondyle	Flexor retinaculum and palmar aponeurosis	Median (C7, C8)
Flexor carpi ulnaris	Two heads: (1) medial epicondyle, and (2) medial side of the olecranon, upper two thirds of the dorsal border of the ulna	Primarily onto the pisiform	Ulnar (C7, C8)
Flexor digitorum superficialis	Two heads: (1) ulnar (medial epicondyle, ventral surface of the epicondyle, ulnar collateral ligament, ulnar tuberosity, medial border of coronoid process), and (2) radial (anterior oblique line and ventral border below the radial oblique line)	Ventral surface of the shaft of the middle phalanx of each finger	Median (C7, C8, T1)
Flexor digitorum profundus	Proximal three fourths of the medial and anterior surface of the ulna and interosseous membrane	Bases of the distal phalanges of the second to fifth digits	Median, anterior interosseous branch (C8, T1)
Flexor pollicis longus	Ventral surface of the radius, oblique line, and adjacent interosseus membrane	Base of the distal phalanx of the thumb	Median, anterior interosseous branch (C8, T1)
Pronator quadratus	Medial side, ventral surface of the distal fourth of the ulna	Distal quarter of the ventral surface of the radius	Median, anterior interosseous branch (C8, T1)

AXIAL

Figure 6.1.1

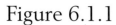

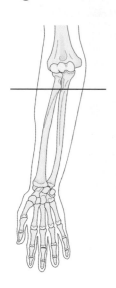

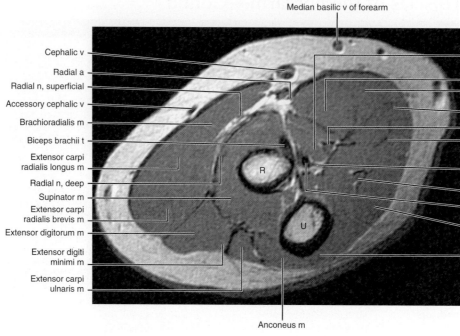

Median basilic v of forearm

Cephalic v
Radial a
Radial n, superficial
Accessory cephalic v
Brachioradialis m
Biceps brachii t
Extensor carpi radialis longus m
Radial n, deep
Supinator m
Extensor carpi radialis brevis m
Extensor digitorum m
Extensor digiti minimi m
Extensor carpi ulnaris m

Pronator teres m, deep head
Pronator teres m
Flexor carpi radialis m
Palmaris longus m
Median n
Flexor digitorum superficialis m
Interosseous n, anterior
Ulnar n
Ulnar a
Flexor carpi ulnaris m
Flexor digitorum profundus m

Anconeus m

R
U

artery = a
arteries = aa
vein = v
veins = vv
muscle = m
muscles = mm
tendon = t
tendons = tt
nerve = n
nerves = nn
ligament = lig
ligaments = ligs
radius = R
ulna = U

Figure 6.1.2

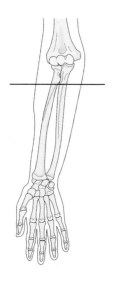

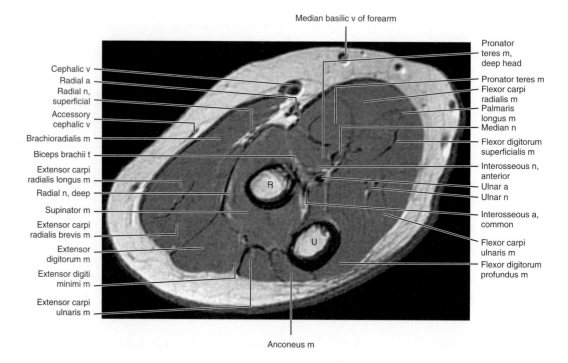

Median basilic v of forearm

Cephalic v
Radial a
Radial n, superficial
Accessory cephalic v
Brachioradialis m
Biceps brachii t
Extensor carpi radialis longus m
Radial n, deep
Supinator m
Extensor carpi radialis brevis m
Extensor digitorum m
Extensor digiti minimi m
Extensor carpi ulnaris m

Pronator teres m, deep head
Pronator teres m
Flexor carpi radialis m
Palmaris longus m
Median n
Flexor digitorum superficialis m
Interosseous n, anterior
Ulnar a
Ulnar n
Interosseous a, common
Flexor carpi ulnaris m
Flexor digitorum profundus m

Anconeus m

R
U

Figure 6.1.3

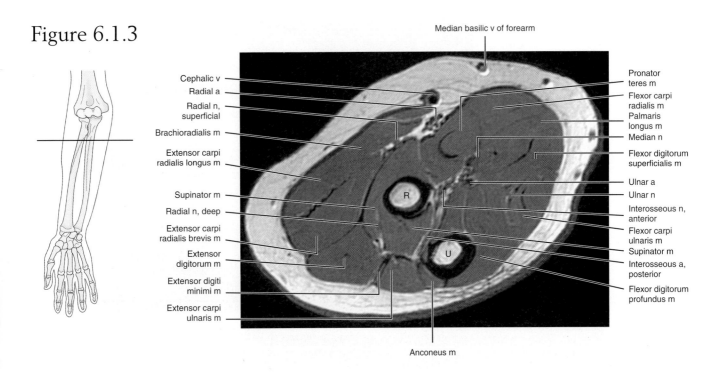

Median basilic v of forearm

Cephalic v
Radial a
Radial n, superficial
Brachioradialis m
Extensor carpi radialis longus m
Supinator m
Radial n, deep
Extensor carpi radialis brevis m
Extensor digitorum m
Extensor digiti minimi m
Extensor carpi ulnaris m

R
U

Pronator teres m
Flexor carpi radialis m
Palmaris longus m
Median n
Flexor digitorum superficialis m
Ulnar a
Ulnar n
Interosseous n, anterior
Flexor carpi ulnaris m
Supinator m
Interosseous a, posterior
Flexor digitorum profundus m

Anconeus m

Figure 6.1.4

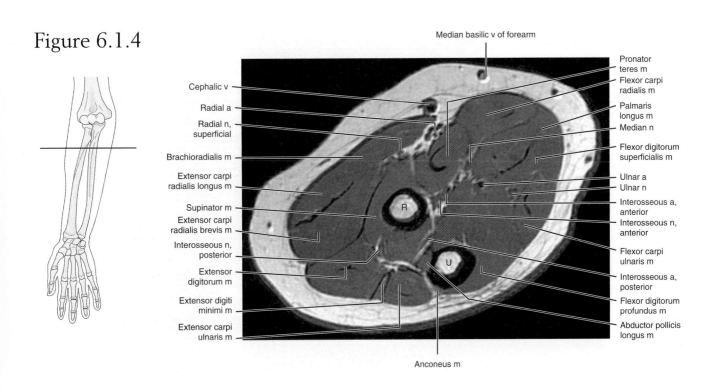

Median basilic v of forearm

Cephalic v
Radial a
Radial n, superficial
Brachioradialis m
Extensor carpi radialis longus m
Supinator m
Extensor carpi radialis brevis m
Interosseous n, posterior
Extensor digitorum m
Extensor digiti minimi m
Extensor carpi ulnaris m

R
U

Pronator teres m
Flexor carpi radialis m
Palmaris longus m
Median n
Flexor digitorum superficialis m
Ulnar a
Ulnar n
Interosseous a, anterior
Interosseous n, anterior
Flexor carpi ulnaris m
Interosseous a, posterior
Flexor digitorum profundus m
Abductor pollicis longus m

Anconeus m

Figure 6.1.5

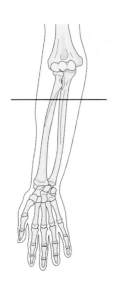

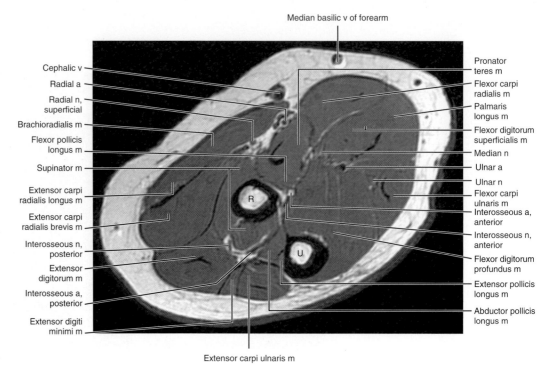

Median basilic v of forearm

Cephalic v

Radial a

Radial n,
superficial

Brachioradialis m

Flexor pollicis
longus m

Supinator m

Extensor carpi
radialis longus m

Extensor carpi
radialis brevis m

Interosseous n,
posterior

Extensor
digitorum m

Interosseous a,
posterior

Extensor digiti
minimi m

Pronator
teres m

Flexor carpi
radialis m

Palmaris
longus m

Flexor digitorum
superficialis m

Median n

Ulnar a

Ulnar n

Flexor carpi
ulnaris m

Interosseous a,
anterior

Interosseous n,
anterior

Flexor digitorum
profundus m

Extensor pollicis
longus m

Abductor pollicis
longus m

Extensor carpi ulnaris m

Figure 6.1.6

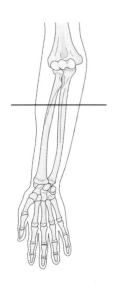

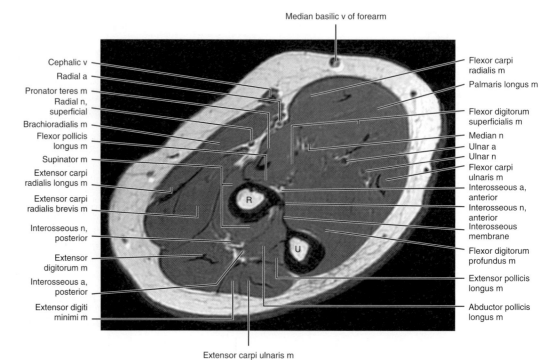

Median basilic v of forearm

Cephalic v

Radial a

Pronator teres m

Radial n,
superficial

Brachioradialis m

Flexor pollicis
longus m

Supinator m

Extensor carpi
radialis longus m

Extensor carpi
radialis brevis m

Interosseous n,
posterior

Extensor
digitorum m

Interosseous a,
posterior

Extensor digiti
minimi m

Flexor carpi
radialis m

Palmaris longus m

Flexor digitorum
superficialis m

Median n

Ulnar a

Ulnar n

Flexor carpi
ulnaris m

Interosseous a,
anterior

Interosseous n,
anterior

Interosseous
membrane

Flexor digitorum
profundus m

Extensor pollicis
longus m

Abductor pollicis
longus m

Extensor carpi ulnaris m

Figure 6.1.7

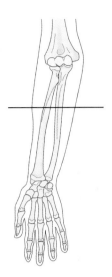

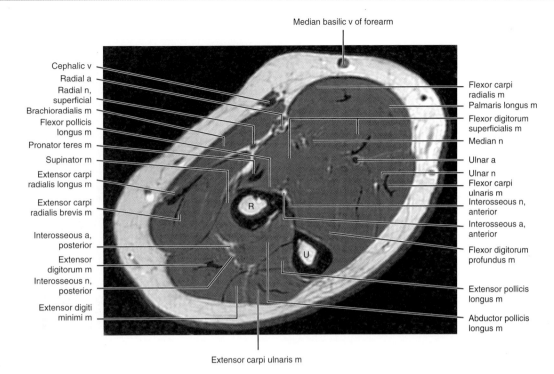

Median basilic v of forearm

Cephalic v
Radial a
Radial n, superficial
Brachioradialis m
Flexor pollicis longus m
Pronator teres m
Supinator m
Extensor carpi radialis longus m
Extensor carpi radialis brevis m
Interosseous a, posterior
Extensor digitorum m
Interosseous n, posterior
Extensor digiti minimi m

Flexor carpi radialis m
Palmaris longus m
Flexor digitorum superficialis m
Median n
Ulnar a
Ulnar n
Flexor carpi ulnaris m
Interosseous n, anterior
Interosseous a, anterior
Flexor digitorum profundus m
Extensor pollicis longus m
Abductor pollicis longus m

Extensor carpi ulnaris m

Figure 6.1.8

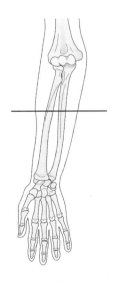

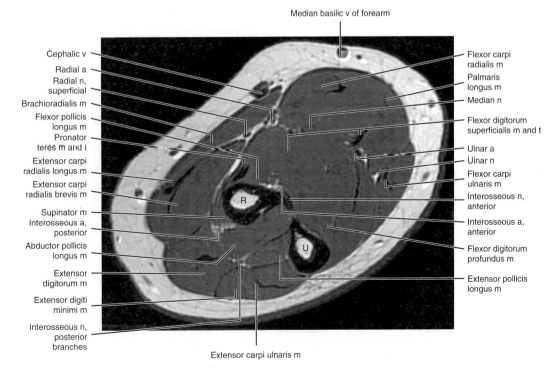

Median basilic v of forearm

Cephalic v
Radial a
Radial n, superficial
Brachioradialis m
Flexor pollicis longus m
Pronator teres m and t
Extensor carpi radialis longus m
Extensor carpi radialis brevis m
Supinator m
Interosseous a, posterior
Abductor pollicis longus m
Extensor digitorum m
Extensor digiti minimi m
Interosseous n, posterior branches

Flexor carpi radialis m
Palmaris longus m
Median n
Flexor digitorum superficialis m and t
Ulnar a
Ulnar n
Flexor carpi ulnaris m
Interosseous n, anterior
Interosseous a, anterior
Flexor digitorum profundus m
Extensor pollicis longus m

Extensor carpi ulnaris m

Figure 6.1.9

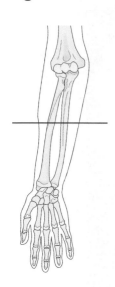

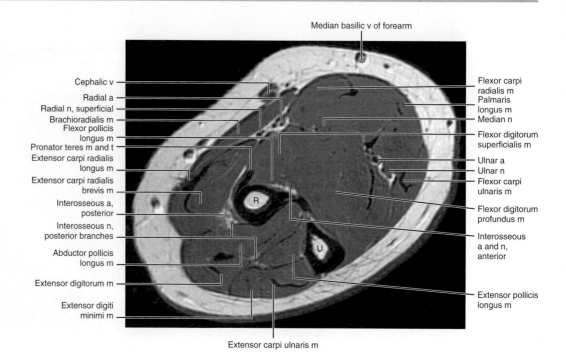

Median basilic v of forearm

Cephalic v

Radial a

Radial n, superficial

Brachioradialis m
Flexor pollicis
longus m

Pronator teres m and t

Extensor carpi radialis
longus m

Extensor carpi radialis
brevis m

Interosseous a,
posterior

Interosseous n,
posterior branches

Abductor pollicis
longus m

Extensor digitorum m

Extensor digiti
minimi m

Flexor carpi
radialis m
Palmaris
longus m
Median n

Flexor digitorum
superficialis m

Ulnar a
Ulnar n
Flexor carpi
ulnaris m

Flexor digitorum
profundus m

Interosseous
a and n,
anterior

Extensor pollicis
longus m

Extensor carpi ulnaris m

Figure 6.1.10

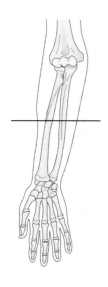

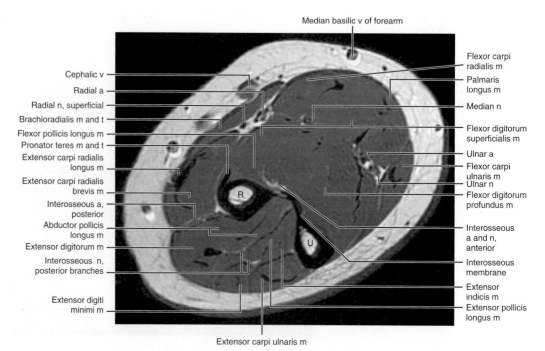

Median basilic v of forearm

Cephalic v

Radial a

Radial n, superficial

Brachioradialis m and t

Flexor pollicis longus m

Pronator teres m and t

Extensor carpi radialis
longus m

Extensor carpi radialis
brevis m

Interosseous a,
posterior

Abductor pollicis
longus m

Extensor digitorum m

Interosseous n,
posterior branches

Extensor digiti
minimi m

Flexor carpi
radialis m
Palmaris
longus m

Median n

Flexor digitorum
superficialis m

Ulnar a
Flexor carpi
ulnaris m
Ulnar n
Flexor digitorum
profundus m

Interosseous
a and n,
anterior

Interosseous
membrane

Extensor
indicis m
Extensor pollicis
longus m

Extensor carpi ulnaris m

Figure 6.1.11

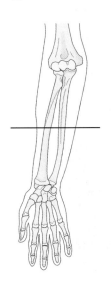

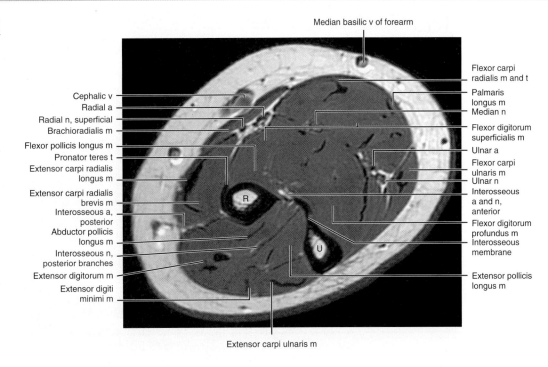

Median basilic v of forearm

Cephalic v
Radial a
Radial n, superficial
Brachioradialis m
Flexor pollicis longus m
Pronator teres t
Extensor carpi radialis longus m
Extensor carpi radialis brevis m
Interosseous a, posterior
Abductor pollicis longus m
Interosseous n, posterior branches
Extensor digitorum m
Extensor digiti minimi m

Flexor carpi radialis m and t
Palmaris longus m
Median n
Flexor digitorum superficialis m
Ulnar a
Flexor carpi ulnaris m
Ulnar n
Interosseous a and n, anterior
Flexor digitorum profundus m
Interosseous membrane
Extensor pollicis longus m

R
U

Extensor carpi ulnaris m

Figure 6.1.12

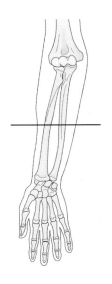

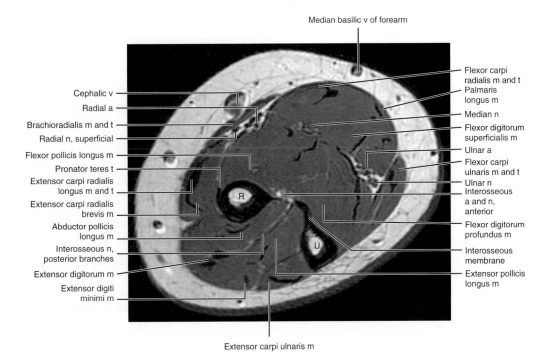

Median basilic v of forearm

Cephalic v
Radial a
Brachioradialis m and t
Radial n, superficial
Flexor pollicis longus m
Pronator teres t
Extensor carpi radialis longus m and t
Extensor carpi radialis brevis m
Abductor pollicis longus m
Interosseous n, posterior branches
Extensor digitorum m
Extensor digiti minimi m

Flexor carpi radialis m and t
Palmaris longus m
Median n
Flexor digitorum superficialis m
Ulnar a
Flexor carpi ulnaris m and t
Ulnar n
Interosseous a and n, anterior
Flexor digitorum profundus m
Interosseous membrane
Extensor pollicis longus m

R
U

Extensor carpi ulnaris m

Figure 6.1.13

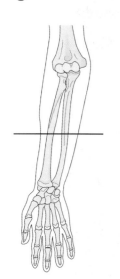

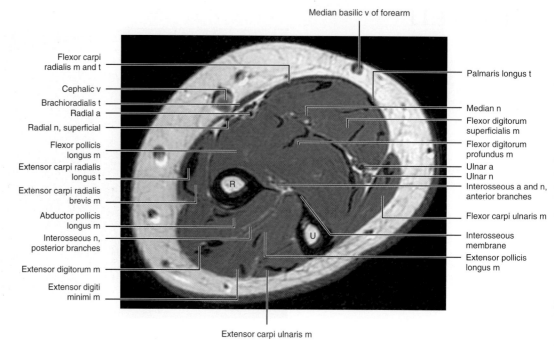

Median basilic v of forearm

Flexor carpi radialis m and t

Cephalic v

Brachioradialis t

Radial a

Radial n, superficial

Flexor pollicis longus m

Extensor carpi radialis longus t

Extensor carpi radialis brevis m

Abductor pollicis longus m

Interosseous n, posterior branches

Extensor digitorum m

Extensor digiti minimi m

Palmaris longus t

Median n

Flexor digitorum superficialis m

Flexor digitorum profundus m

Ulnar a

Ulnar n

Interosseous a and n, anterior branches

Flexor carpi ulnaris m

Interosseous membrane

Extensor pollicis longus m

Extensor carpi ulnaris m

Figure 6.1.14

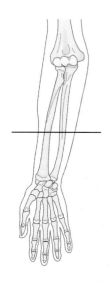

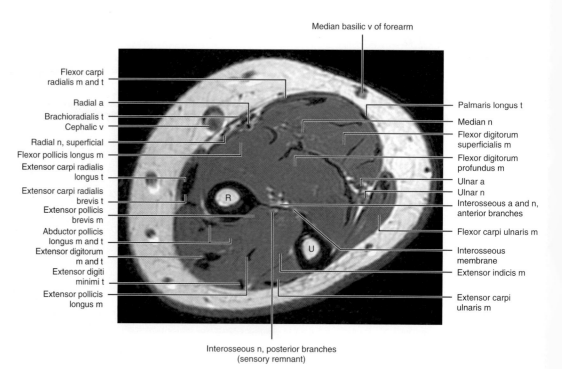

Median basilic v of forearm

Flexor carpi radialis m and t

Radial a

Brachioradialis t

Cephalic v

Radial n, superficial

Flexor pollicis longus m

Extensor carpi radialis longus t

Extensor carpi radialis brevis t

Extensor pollicis brevis m

Abductor pollicis longus m and t

Extensor digitorum m and t

Extensor digiti minimi t

Extensor pollicis longus m

Palmaris longus t

Median n

Flexor digitorum superficialis m

Flexor digitorum profundus m

Ulnar a

Ulnar n

Interosseous a and n, anterior branches

Flexor carpi ulnaris m

Interosseous membrane

Extensor indicis m

Extensor carpi ulnaris m

Interosseous n, posterior branches (sensory remnant)

Figure 6.1.15

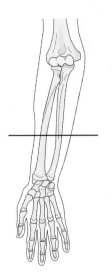

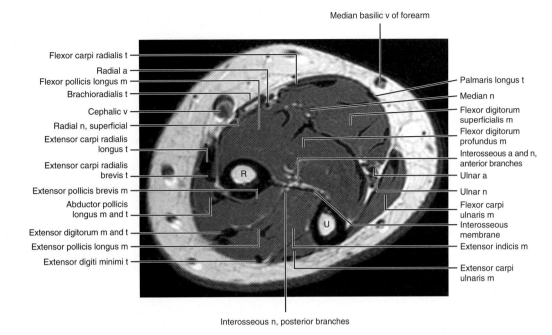

Median basilic v of forearm

Flexor carpi radialis t
Radial a
Flexor pollicis longus m
Brachioradialis t
Cephalic v
Radial n, superficial
Extensor carpi radialis longus t
Extensor carpi radialis brevis t
Extensor pollicis brevis m
Abductor pollicis longus m and t
Extensor digitorum m and t
Extensor pollicis longus m
Extensor digiti minimi t

Palmaris longus t
Median n
Flexor digitorum superficialis m
Flexor digitorum profundus m
Interosseous a and n, anterior branches
Ulnar a
Ulnar n
Flexor carpi ulnaris m
Interosseous membrane
Extensor indicis m
Extensor carpi ulnaris m

Interosseous n, posterior branches

Figure 6.1.16

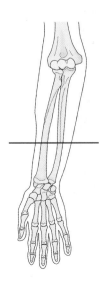

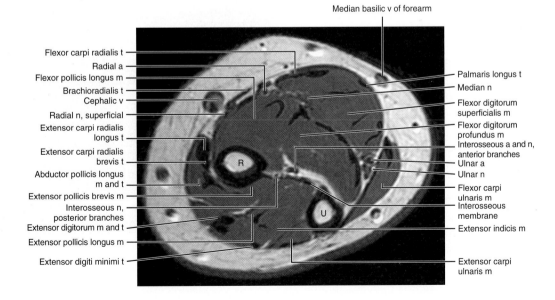

Median basilic v of forearm

Flexor carpi radialis t
Radial a
Flexor pollicis longus m
Brachioradialis t
Cephalic v
Radial n, superficial
Extensor carpi radialis longus t
Extensor carpi radialis brevis t
Abductor pollicis longus m and t
Extensor pollicis brevis m
Interosseous n, posterior branches
Extensor digitorum m and t
Extensor pollicis longus m
Extensor digiti minimi t

Palmaris longus t
Median n
Flexor digitorum superficialis m
Flexor digitorum profundus m
Interosseous a and n, anterior branches
Ulnar a
Ulnar n
Flexor carpi ulnaris m
Interosseous membrane
Extensor indicis m
Extensor carpi ulnaris m

Figure 6.1.17

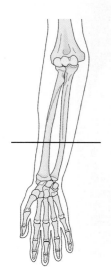

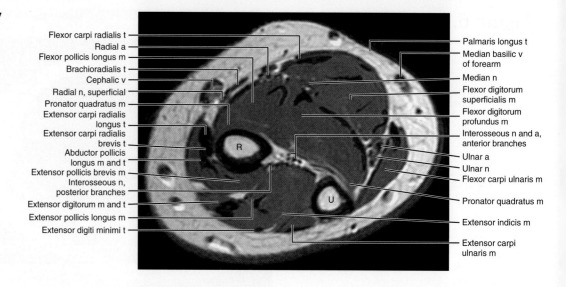

Flexor carpi radialis t
Radial a
Flexor pollicis longus m
Brachioradialis t
Cephalic v
Radial n, superficial
Pronator quadratus m
Extensor carpi radialis longus t
Extensor carpi radialis brevis t
Abductor pollicis longus m and t
Extensor pollicis brevis m
Interosseous n, posterior branches
Extensor digitorum m and t
Extensor pollicis longus m
Extensor digiti minimi t

Palmaris longus t
Median basilic v of forearm
Median n
Flexor digitorum superficialis m
Flexor digitorum profundus m
Interosseous n and a, anterior branches
Ulnar a
Ulnar n
Flexor carpi ulnaris m
Pronator quadratus m
Extensor indicis m
Extensor carpi ulnaris m

Figure 6.1.18

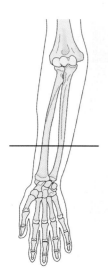

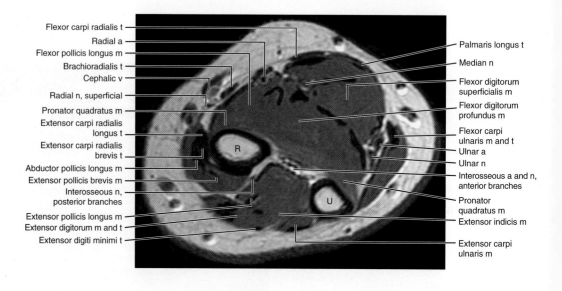

Flexor carpi radialis t
Radial a
Flexor pollicis longus m
Brachioradialis t
Cephalic v
Radial n, superficial
Pronator quadratus m
Extensor carpi radialis longus t
Extensor carpi radialis brevis t
Abductor pollicis longus m
Extensor pollicis brevis m
Interosseous n, posterior branches
Extensor pollicis longus m
Extensor digitorum m and t
Extensor digiti minimi t

Palmaris longus t
Median n
Flexor digitorum superficialis m
Flexor digitorum profundus m
Flexor carpi ulnaris m and t
Ulnar a
Ulnar n
Interosseous a and n, anterior branches
Pronator quadratus m
Extensor indicis m
Extensor carpi ulnaris m

Figure 6.1.19

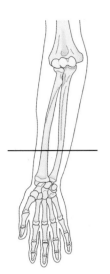

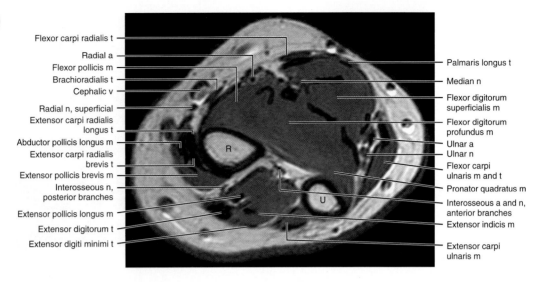

Flexor carpi radialis t
Radial a
Flexor pollicis m
Brachioradialis t
Cephalic v
Radial n, superficial
Extensor carpi radialis longus t
Abductor pollicis longus m
Extensor carpi radialis brevis t
Extensor pollicis brevis m
Interosseous n, posterior branches
Extensor pollicis longus m
Extensor digitorum t
Extensor digiti minimi t

Palmaris longus t
Median n
Flexor digitorum superficialis m
Flexor digitorum profundus m
Ulnar a
Ulnar n
Flexor carpi ulnaris m and t
Pronator quadratus m
Interosseous a and n, anterior branches
Extensor indicis m
Extensor carpi ulnaris m

R
U

Figure 6.1.20

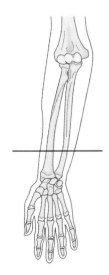

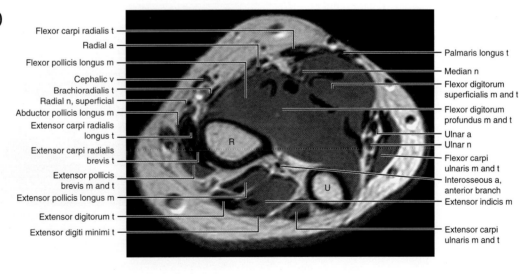

Flexor carpi radialis t
Radial a
Flexor pollicis longus m
Cephalic v
Brachioradialis t
Radial n, superficial
Abductor pollicis longus m
Extensor carpi radialis longus t
Extensor carpi radialis brevis t
Extensor pollicis brevis m and t
Extensor pollicis longus m
Extensor digitorum t
Extensor digiti minimi t

Palmaris longus t
Median n
Flexor digitorum superficialis m and t
Flexor digitorum profundus m and t
Ulnar a
Ulnar n
Flexor carpi ulnaris m and t
Interosseous a, anterior branch
Extensor indicis m
Extensor carpi ulnaris m and t

R
U

Figure 6.1.21

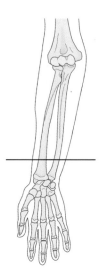

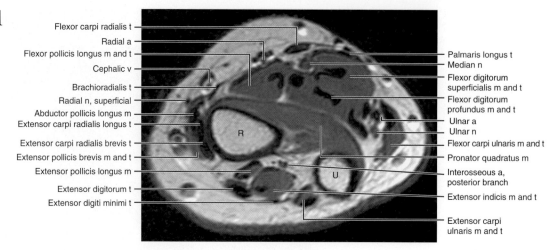

Flexor carpi radialis t
Radial a
Flexor pollicis longus m and t
Cephalic v
Brachioradialis t
Radial n, superficial
Abductor pollicis longus m
Extensor carpi radialis longus t
Extensor carpi radialis brevis t
Extensor pollicis brevis m and t
Extensor pollicis longus m
Extensor digitorum t
Extensor digiti minimi t

Palmaris longus t
Median n
Flexor digitorum superficialis m and t
Flexor digitorum profundus m and t
Ulnar a
Ulnar n
Flexor carpi ulnaris m and t
Pronator quadratus m
Interosseous a, posterior branch
Extensor indicis m and t
Extensor carpi ulnaris m and t

R
U

Figure 6.1.22

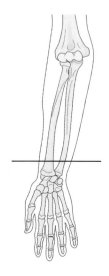

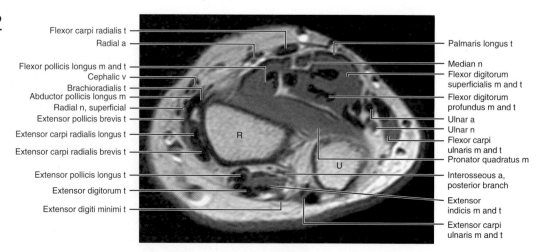

Flexor carpi radialis t
Radial a
Flexor pollicis longus m and t
Cephalic v
Brachioradialis t
Abductor pollicis longus m
Radial n, superficial
Extensor pollicis brevis t
Extensor carpi radialis longus t
Extensor carpi radialis brevis t
Extensor pollicis longus t
Extensor digitorum t
Extensor digiti minimi t

Palmaris longus t
Median n
Flexor digitorum superficialis m and t
Flexor digitorum profundus m and t
Ulnar a
Ulnar n
Flexor carpi ulnaris m and t
Pronator quadratus m
Interosseous a, posterior branch
Extensor indicis m and t
Extensor carpi ulnaris m and t

R
U

SAGITTAL
Figure 6.2.1

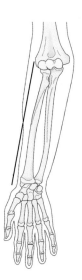

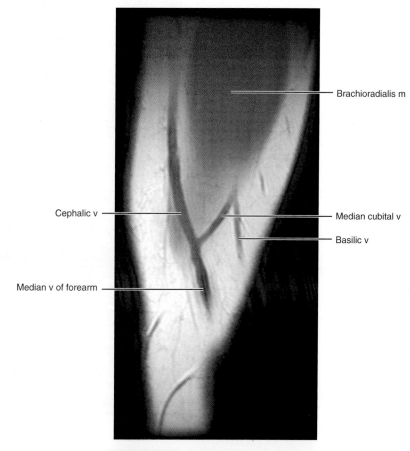

Brachioradialis m

Cephalic v

Median cubital v

Basilic v

Median v of forearm

Figure 6.2.2

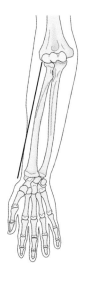

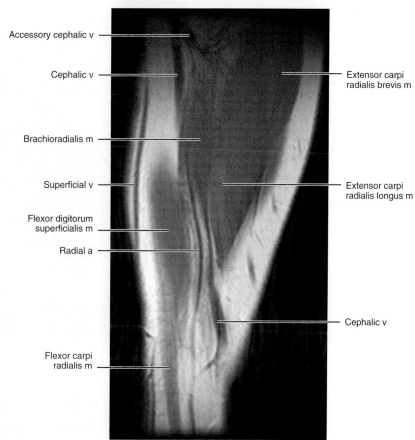

Accessory cephalic v

Cephalic v

Extensor carpi radialis brevis m

Brachioradialis m

Superficial v

Extensor carpi radialis longus m

Flexor digitorum superficialis m

Radial a

Cephalic v

Flexor carpi radialis m

Figure 6.2.3

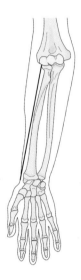

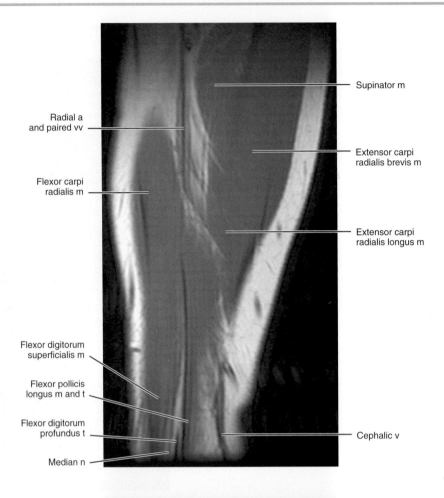

Radial a
and paired vv

Flexor carpi
radialis m

Flexor digitorum
superficialis m

Flexor pollicis
longus m and t

Flexor digitorum
profundus t

Median n

Supinator m

Extensor carpi
radialis brevis m

Extensor carpi
radialis longus m

Cephalic v

Figure 6.2.4

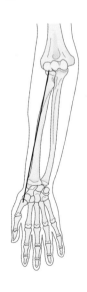

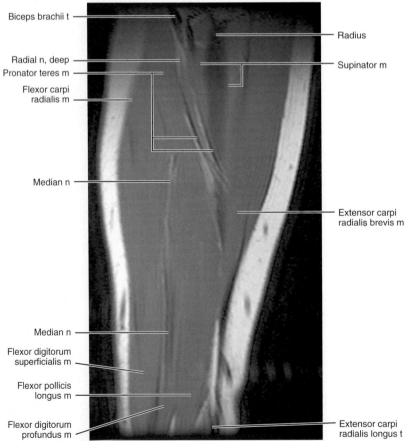

Biceps brachii t

Radial n, deep

Pronator teres m

Flexor carpi
radialis m

Median n

Median n

Flexor digitorum
superficialis m

Flexor pollicis
longus m

Flexor digitorum
profundus m

Radius

Supinator m

Extensor carpi
radialis brevis m

Extensor carpi
radialis longus t

Figure 6.2.5

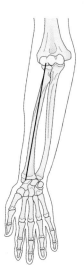

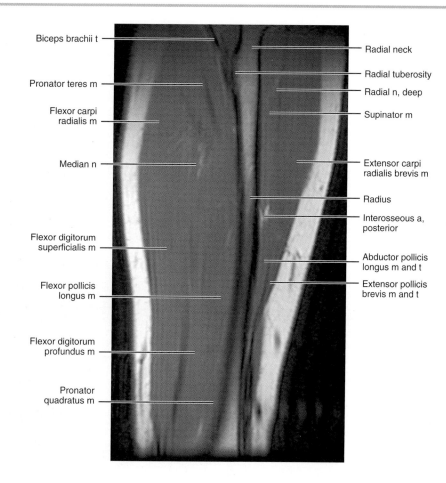

Biceps brachii t

Pronator teres m

Flexor carpi
radialis m

Median n

Flexor digitorum
superficialis m

Flexor pollicis
longus m

Flexor digitorum
profundus m

Pronator
quadratus m

Radial neck

Radial tuberosity

Radial n, deep

Supinator m

Extensor carpi
radialis brevis m

Radius

Interosseous a,
posterior

Abductor pollicis
longus m and t

Extensor pollicis
brevis m and t

Figure 6.2.6

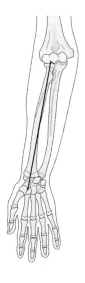

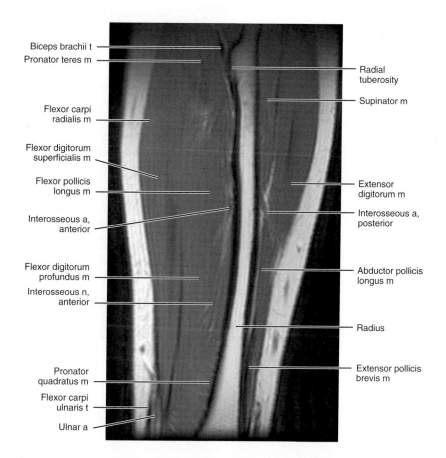

Biceps brachii t
Pronator teres m

Flexor carpi
radialis m

Flexor digitorum
superficialis m

Flexor pollicis
longus m

Interosseous a,
anterior

Flexor digitorum
profundus m

Interosseous n,
anterior

Pronator
quadratus m

Flexor carpi
ulnaris t

Ulnar a

Radial
tuberosity

Supinator m

Extensor
digitorum m

Interosseous a,
posterior

Abductor pollicis
longus m

Radius

Extensor pollicis
brevis m

Figure 6.2.7

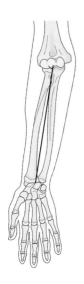

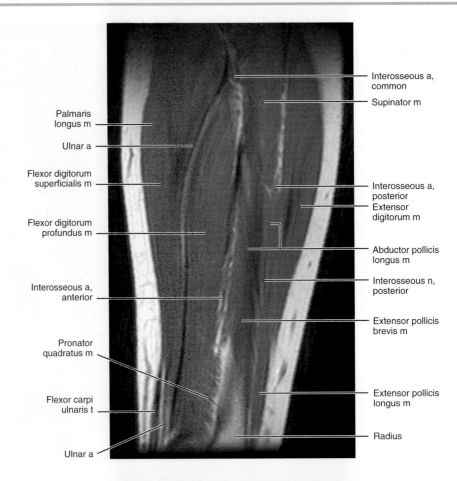

Palmaris longus m

Ulnar a

Flexor digitorum superficialis m

Flexor digitorum profundus m

Interosseous a, anterior

Pronator quadratus m

Flexor carpi ulnaris t

Ulnar a

Interosseous a, common

Supinator m

Interosseous a, posterior

Extensor digitorum m

Abductor pollicis longus m

Interosseous n, posterior

Extensor pollicis brevis m

Extensor pollicis longus m

Radius

Figure 6.2.8

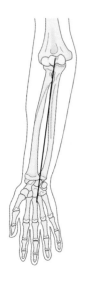

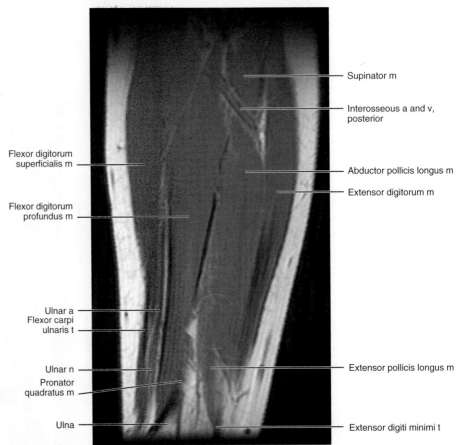

Flexor digitorum superficialis m

Flexor digitorum profundus m

Ulnar a
Flexor carpi ulnaris t

Ulnar n
Pronator quadratus m

Ulna

Supinator m

Interosseous a and v, posterior

Abductor pollicis longus m

Extensor digitorum m

Extensor pollicis longus m

Extensor digiti minimi t

Figure 6.2.9

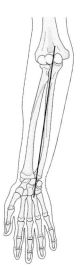

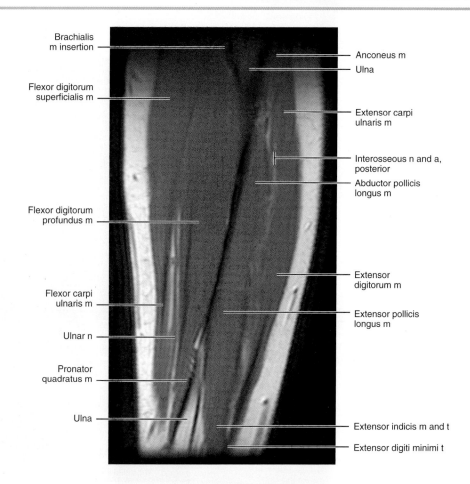

Brachialis m insertion

Flexor digitorum superficialis m

Flexor digitorum profundus m

Flexor carpi ulnaris m

Ulnar n

Pronator quadratus m

Ulna

Anconeus m

Ulna

Extensor carpi ulnaris m

Interosseous n and a, posterior

Abductor pollicis longus m

Extensor digitorum m

Extensor pollicis longus m

Extensor indicis m and t

Extensor digiti minimi t

Figure 6.2.10

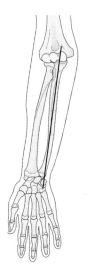

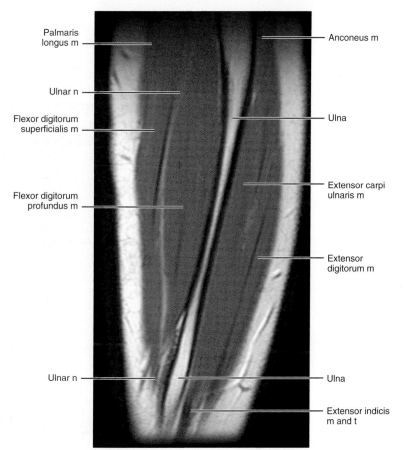

Palmaris longus m

Ulnar n

Flexor digitorum superficialis m

Flexor digitorum profundus m

Ulnar n

Anconeus m

Ulna

Extensor carpi ulnaris m

Extensor digitorum m

Ulna

Extensor indicis m and t

Figure 6.2.11

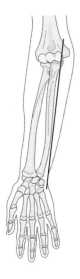

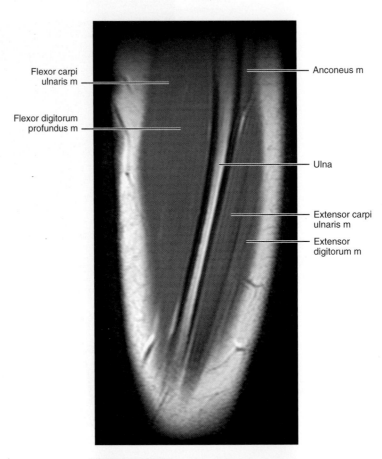

Flexor carpi ulnaris m

Flexor digitorum profundus m

Anconeus m

Ulna

Extensor carpi ulnaris m

Extensor digitorum m

Figure 6.2.12

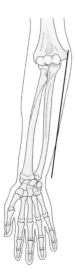

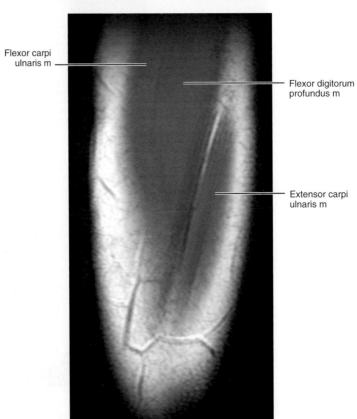

Flexor carpi ulnaris m

Flexor digitorum profundus m

Extensor carpi ulnaris m

CORONAL
Figure 6.3.1

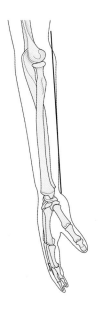

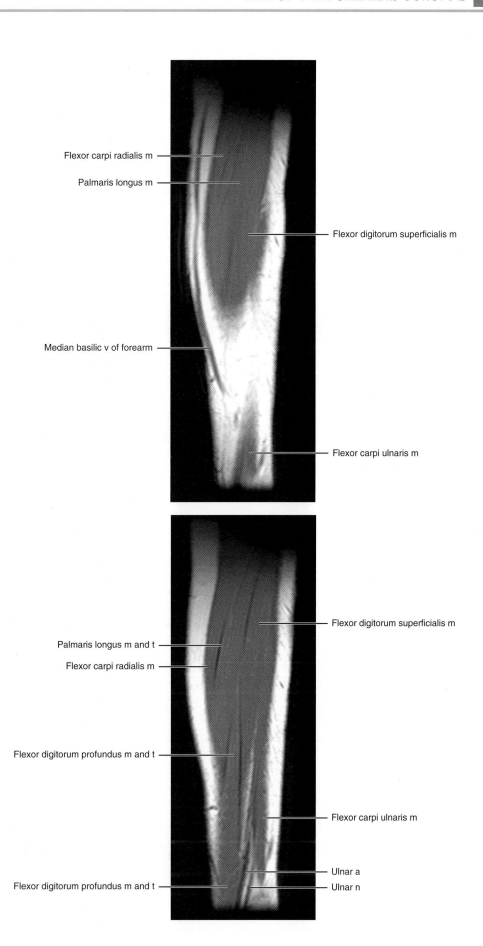

Flexor carpi radialis m

Palmaris longus m

Flexor digitorum superficialis m

Median basilic v of forearm

Flexor carpi ulnaris m

Figure 6.3.2

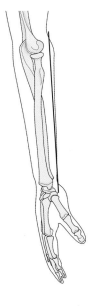

Flexor digitorum superficialis m

Palmaris longus m and t

Flexor carpi radialis m

Flexor digitorum profundus m and t

Flexor carpi ulnaris m

Ulnar a

Ulnar n

Flexor digitorum profundus m and t

Figure 6.3.3

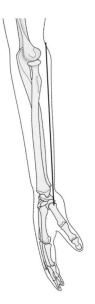

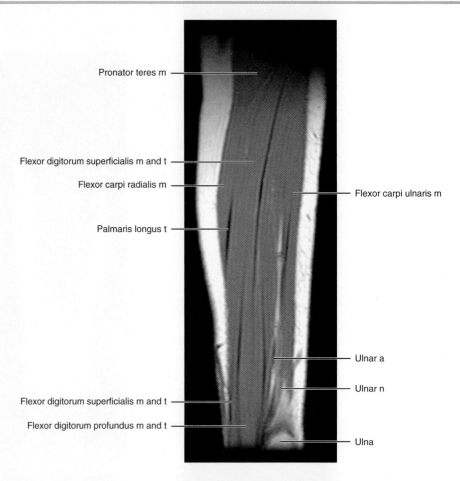

Pronator teres m

Flexor digitorum superficialis m and t

Flexor carpi radialis m

Palmaris longus t

Flexor carpi ulnaris m

Flexor digitorum superficialis m and t

Flexor digitorum profundus m and t

Ulnar a

Ulnar n

Ulna

Figure 6.3.4

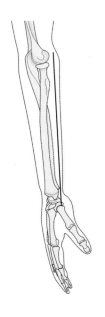

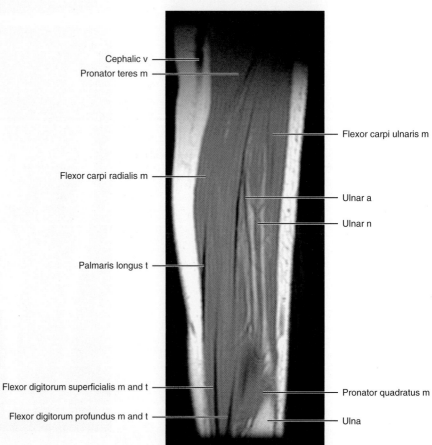

Cephalic v

Pronator teres m

Flexor carpi radialis m

Flexor carpi ulnaris m

Ulnar a

Ulnar n

Palmaris longus t

Flexor digitorum superficialis m and t

Flexor digitorum profundus m and t

Pronator quadratus m

Ulna

Figure 6.3.5

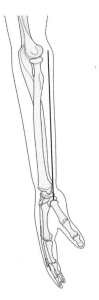

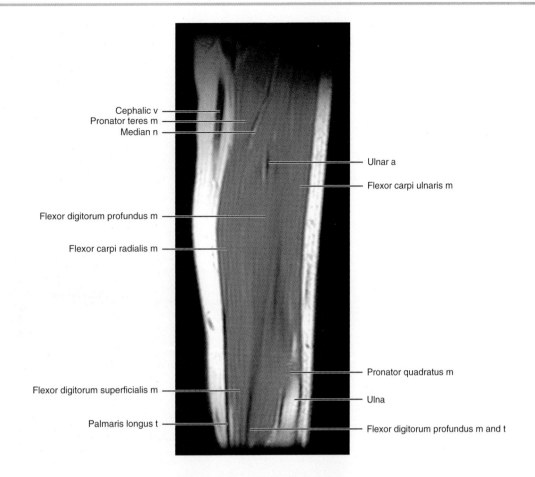

Cephalic v
Pronator teres m
Median n

Ulnar a
Flexor carpi ulnaris m

Flexor digitorum profundus m

Flexor carpi radialis m

Pronator quadratus m

Flexor digitorum superficialis m

Ulna

Palmaris longus t

Flexor digitorum profundus m and t

Figure 6.3.6

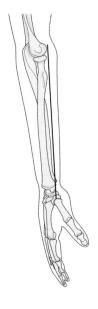

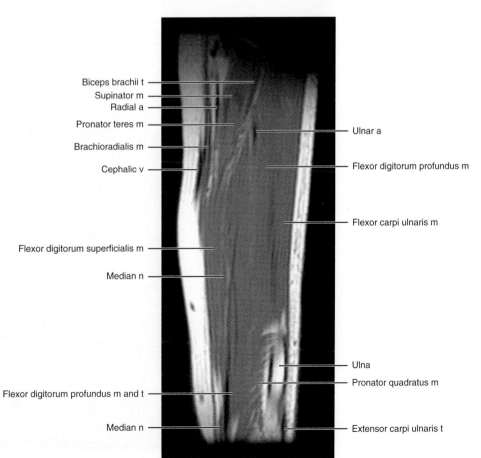

Biceps brachii t
Supinator m
Radial a
Pronator teres m

Brachioradialis m

Cephalic v

Ulnar a

Flexor digitorum profundus m

Flexor digitorum superficialis m

Flexor carpi ulnaris m

Median n

Flexor digitorum profundus m and t

Ulna
Pronator quadratus m

Median n

Extensor carpi ulnaris t

Figure 6.3.7

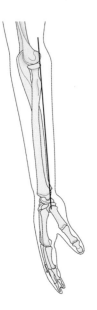

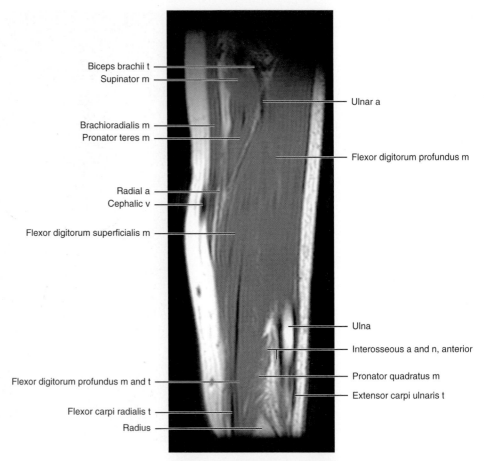

Biceps brachii t
Supinator m
Ulnar a
Brachioradialis m
Pronator teres m
Flexor digitorum profundus m
Radial a
Cephalic v
Flexor digitorum superficialis m
Ulna
Interosseous a and n, anterior
Flexor digitorum profundus m and t
Pronator quadratus m
Extensor carpi ulnaris t
Flexor carpi radialis t
Radius

Figure 6.3.8

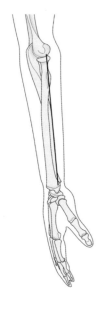

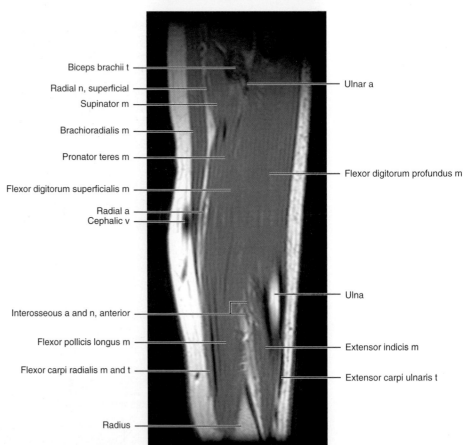

Biceps brachii t
Radial n, superficial
Ulnar a
Supinator m
Brachioradialis m
Pronator teres m
Flexor digitorum profundus m
Flexor digitorum superficialis m
Radial a
Cephalic v
Ulna
Interosseous a and n, anterior
Flexor pollicis longus m
Extensor indicis m
Flexor carpi radialis m and t
Extensor carpi ulnaris t
Radius

Figure 6.3.9

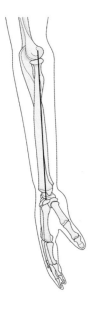

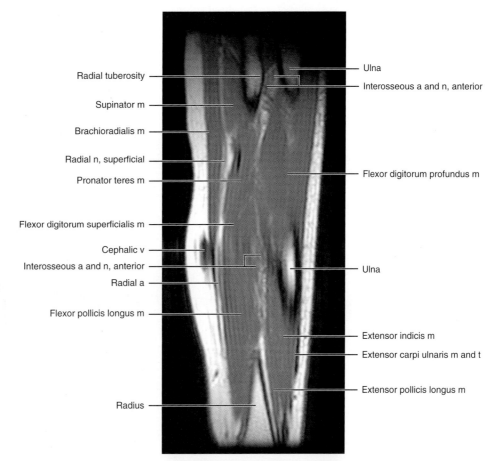

Radial tuberosity

Supinator m

Brachioradialis m

Radial n, superficial

Pronator teres m

Flexor digitorum superficialis m

Cephalic v

Interosseous a and n, anterior

Radial a

Flexor pollicis longus m

Radius

Ulna

Interosseous a and n, anterior

Flexor digitorum profundus m

Ulna

Extensor indicis m

Extensor carpi ulnaris m and t

Extensor pollicis longus m

Figure 6.3.10

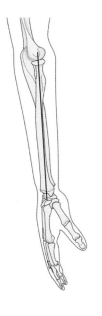

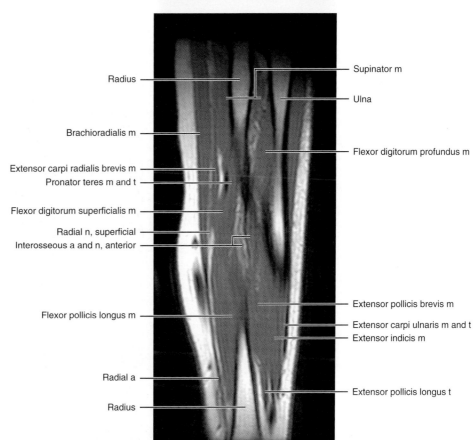

Radius

Brachioradialis m

Extensor carpi radialis brevis m

Pronator teres m and t

Flexor digitorum superficialis m

Radial n, superficial

Interosseous a and n, anterior

Flexor pollicis longus m

Radial a

Radius

Supinator m

Ulna

Flexor digitorum profundus m

Extensor pollicis brevis m

Extensor carpi ulnaris m and t

Extensor indicis m

Extensor pollicis longus t

Figure 6.3.11

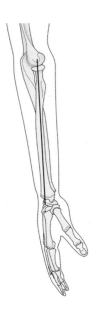

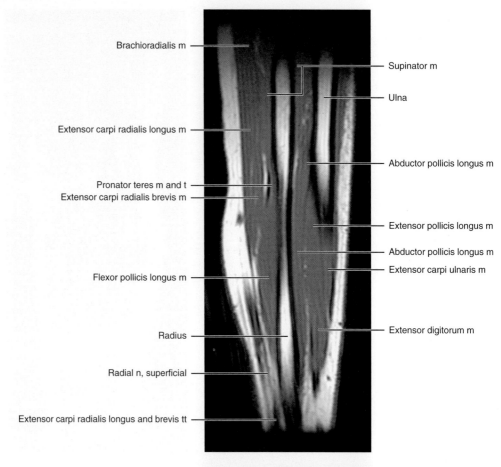

Brachioradialis m

Supinator m

Ulna

Extensor carpi radialis longus m

Abductor pollicis longus m

Pronator teres m and t
Extensor carpi radialis brevis m

Extensor pollicis longus m

Abductor pollicis longus m
Extensor carpi ulnaris m

Flexor pollicis longus m

Extensor digitorum m

Radius

Radial n, superficial

Extensor carpi radialis longus and brevis tt

Figure 6.3.12

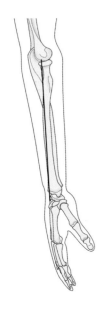

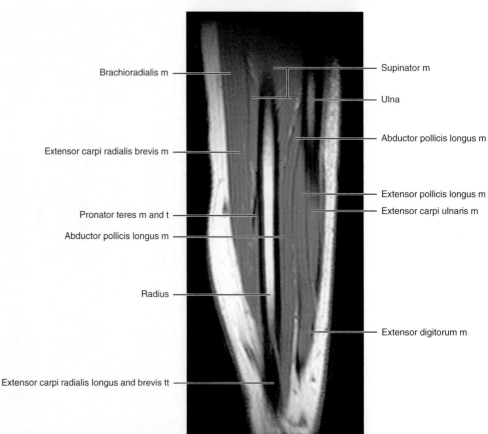

Brachioradialis m

Supinator m

Ulna

Extensor carpi radialis brevis m

Abductor pollicis longus m

Extensor pollicis longus m
Extensor carpi ulnaris m

Pronator teres m and t

Abductor pollicis longus m

Radius

Extensor digitorum m

Extensor carpi radialis longus and brevis tt

Figure 6.3.13

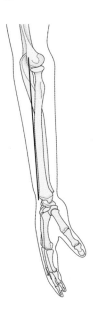

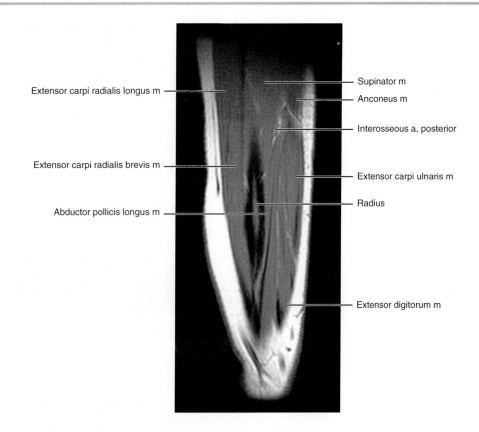

Extensor carpi radialis longus m —

Extensor carpi radialis brevis m —

Abductor pollicis longus m —

— Supinator m
— Anconeus m
— Interosseous a, posterior
— Extensor carpi ulnaris m
— Radius
— Extensor digitorum m

Figure 6.3.14

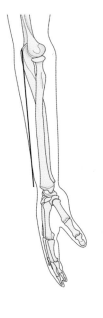

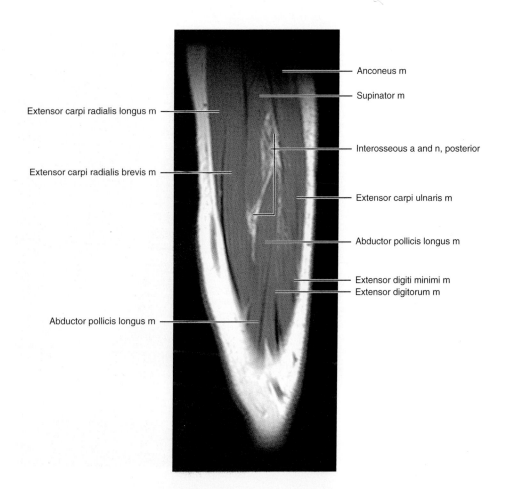

Extensor carpi radialis longus m —

Extensor carpi radialis brevis m —

Abductor pollicis longus m —

— Anconeus m
— Supinator m
— Interosseous a and n, posterior
— Extensor carpi ulnaris m
— Abductor pollicis longus m
— Extensor digiti minimi m
— Extensor digitorum m

Figure 6.3.15

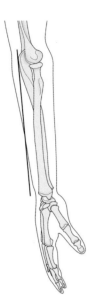

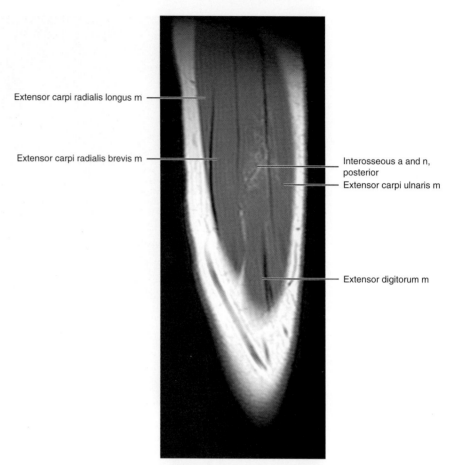

Extensor carpi radialis longus m

Extensor carpi radialis brevis m

Interosseous a and n, posterior

Extensor carpi ulnaris m

Extensor digitorum m

Figure 6.3.16

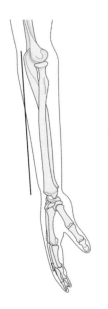

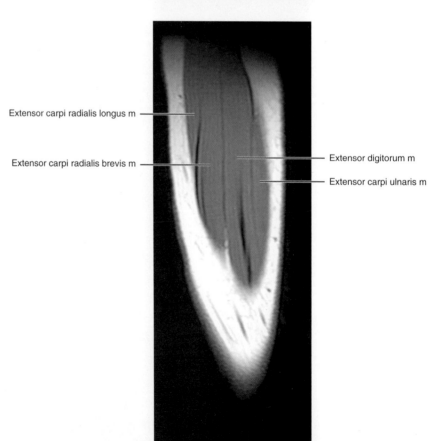

Extensor carpi radialis longus m

Extensor carpi radialis brevis m

Extensor digitorum m

Extensor carpi ulnaris m

Chapter 7

MRI of the Wrist

AXIAL

Figure 7.1.1

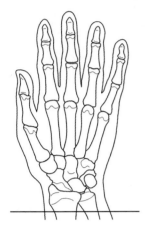

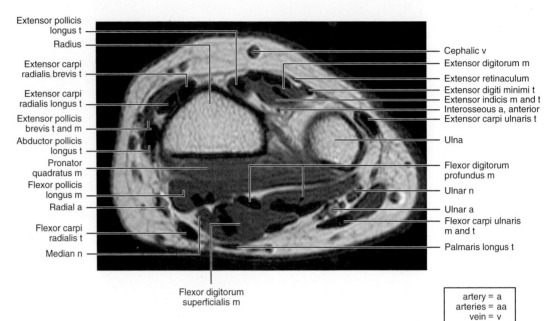

Extensor pollicis longus t
Radius
Extensor carpi radialis brevis t
Extensor carpi radialis longus t
Extensor pollicis brevis t and m
Abductor pollicis longus t
Pronator quadratus m
Flexor pollicis longus m
Radial a
Flexor carpi radialis t
Median n

Cephalic v
Extensor digitorum m
Extensor retinaculum
Extensor digiti minimi t
Extensor indicis m and t
Interosseous a, anterior
Extensor carpi ulnaris t
Ulna
Flexor digitorum profundus m
Ulnar n
Ulnar a
Flexor carpi ulnaris m and t
Palmaris longus t

Flexor digitorum superficialis m

artery = a
arteries = aa
vein = v
veins = vv
muscle = m
muscles = mm
tendon = t
tendons = tt
nerve = n
nerves = nn
ligament = lig
ligaments = ligs

Figure 7.1.2

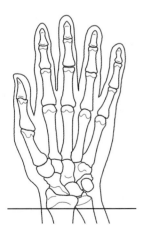

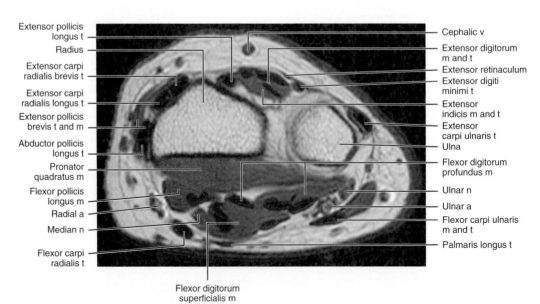

Extensor pollicis longus t
Radius
Extensor carpi radialis brevis t
Extensor carpi radialis longus t
Extensor pollicis brevis t and m
Abductor pollicis longus t
Pronator quadratus m
Flexor pollicis longus m
Radial a
Median n
Flexor carpi radialis t

Cephalic v
Extensor digitorum m and t
Extensor retinaculum
Extensor digiti minimi t
Extensor indicis m and t
Extensor carpi ulnaris t
Ulna
Flexor digitorum profundus m
Ulnar n
Ulnar a
Flexor carpi ulnaris m and t
Palmaris longus t

Flexor digitorum superficialis m

Figure 7.1.3

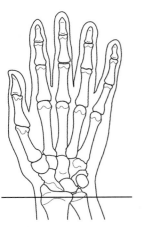

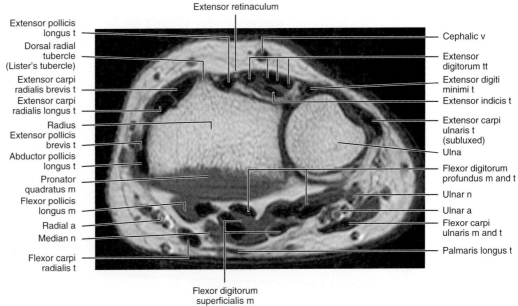

Extensor retinaculum

Extensor pollicis longus t

Dorsal radial tubercle (Lister's tubercle)

Extensor carpi radialis brevis t

Extensor carpi radialis longus t

Radius

Extensor pollicis brevis t

Abductor pollicis longus t

Pronator quadratus m

Flexor pollicis longus m

Radial a

Median n

Flexor carpi radialis t

Cephalic v

Extensor digitorum tt

Extensor digiti minimi t

Extensor indicis t

Extensor carpi ulnaris t (subluxed)

Ulna

Flexor digitorum profundus m and t

Ulnar n

Ulnar a

Flexor carpi ulnaris m and t

Palmaris longus t

Flexor digitorum superficialis m

Figure 7.1.4

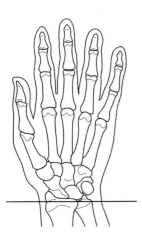

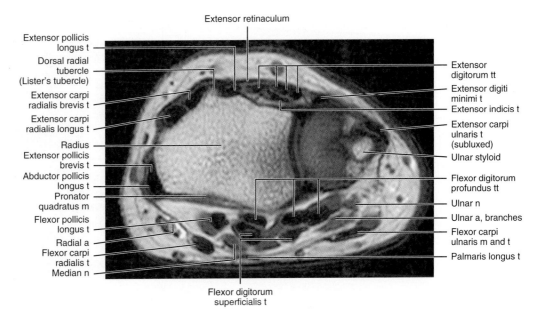

Extensor retinaculum

Extensor pollicis longus t

Dorsal radial tubercle (Lister's tubercle)

Extensor carpi radialis brevis t

Extensor carpi radialis longus t

Radius

Extensor pollicis brevis t

Abductor pollicis longus t

Pronator quadratus m

Flexor pollicis longus t

Radial a

Flexor carpi radialis t

Median n

Extensor digitorum tt

Extensor digiti minimi t

Extensor indicis t

Extensor carpi ulnaris t (subluxed)

Ulnar styloid

Flexor digitorum profundus tt

Ulnar n

Ulnar a, branches

Flexor carpi ulnaris m and t

Palmaris longus t

Flexor digitorum superficialis t

Figure 7.1.5

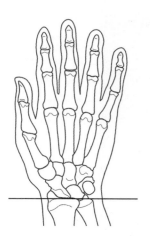

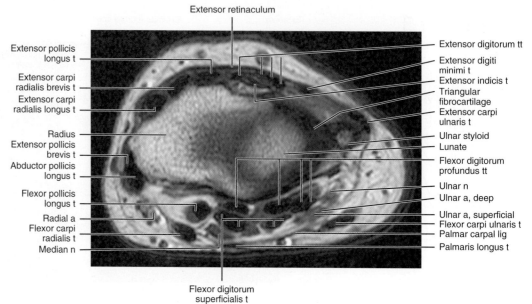

Extensor retinaculum

Extensor pollicis longus t

Extensor carpi radialis brevis t

Extensor carpi radialis longus t

Radius

Extensor pollicis brevis t

Abductor pollicis longus t

Flexor pollicis longus t

Radial a

Flexor carpi radialis t

Median n

Extensor digitorum tt

Extensor digiti minimi t

Extensor indicis t

Triangular fibrocartilage

Extensor carpi ulnaris t

Ulnar styloid

Lunate

Flexor digitorum profundus tt

Ulnar n

Ulnar a, deep

Ulnar a, superficial

Flexor carpi ulnaris t

Palmar carpal lig

Palmaris longus t

Flexor digitorum superficialis t

Figure 7.1.6

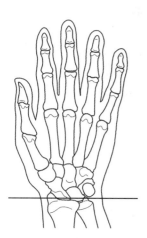

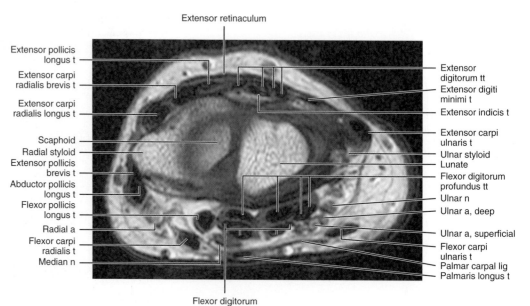

Extensor retinaculum

Extensor pollicis longus t

Extensor carpi radialis brevis t

Extensor carpi radialis longus t

Scaphoid

Radial styloid

Extensor pollicis brevis t

Abductor pollicis longus t

Flexor pollicis longus t

Radial a

Flexor carpi radialis t

Median n

Extensor digitorum tt

Extensor digiti minimi t

Extensor indicis t

Extensor carpi ulnaris t

Ulnar styloid

Lunate

Flexor digitorum profundus tt

Ulnar n

Ulnar a, deep

Ulnar a, superficial

Flexor carpi ulnaris t

Palmar carpal lig

Palmaris longus t

Flexor digitorum superficialis t

Figure 7.1.7

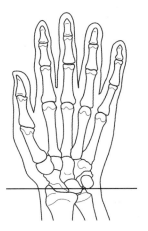

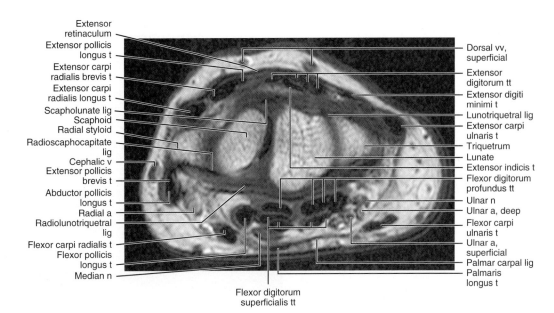

Extensor retinaculum
Extensor pollicis longus t
Extensor carpi radialis brevis t
Extensor carpi radialis longus t
Scapholunate lig
Scaphoid
Radial styloid
Radioscaphocapitate lig
Cephalic v
Extensor pollicis brevis t
Abductor pollicis longus t
Radial a
Radiolunotriquetral lig
Flexor carpi radialis t
Flexor pollicis longus t
Median n

Dorsal vv, superficial
Extensor digitorum tt
Extensor digiti minimi t
Lunotriquetral lig
Extensor carpi ulnaris t
Triquetrum
Lunate
Extensor indicis t
Flexor digitorum profundus tt
Ulnar n
Ulnar a, deep
Flexor carpi ulnaris t
Ulnar a, superficial
Palmar carpal lig
Palmaris longus t

Flexor digitorum superficialis tt

Figure 7.1.8

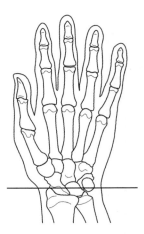

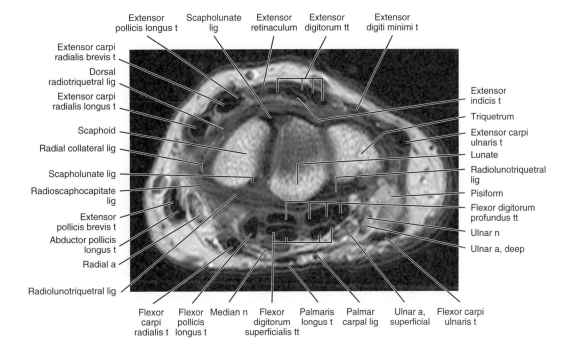

Extensor pollicis longus t
Scapholunate lig
Extensor retinaculum
Extensor digitorum tt
Extensor digiti minimi t

Extensor carpi radialis brevis t
Dorsal radiotriquetral lig
Extensor carpi radialis longus t
Scaphoid
Radial collateral lig
Scapholunate lig
Radioscaphocapitate lig
Extensor pollicis brevis t
Abductor pollicis longus t
Radial a
Radiolunotriquetral lig

Extensor indicis t
Triquetrum
Extensor carpi ulnaris t
Lunate
Radiolunotriquetral lig
Pisiform
Flexor digitorum profundus tt
Ulnar n
Ulnar a, deep

Flexor carpi radialis t
Flexor pollicis longus t
Median n
Flexor digitorum superficialis tt
Palmaris longus t
Palmar carpal lig
Ulnar a, superficial
Flexor carpi ulnaris t

Figure 7.1.9

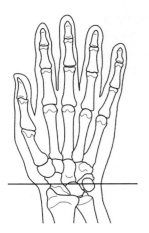

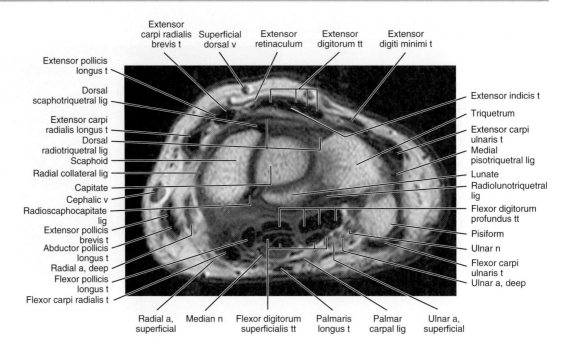

Extensor pollicis longus t
Dorsal scaphotriquetral lig
Extensor carpi radialis longus t
Dorsal radiotriquetral lig
Scaphoid
Radial collateral lig
Capitate
Cephalic v
Radioscaphocapitate lig
Extensor pollicis brevis t
Abductor pollicis longus t
Radial a, deep
Flexor pollicis longus t
Flexor carpi radialis t

Extensor carpi radialis brevis t
Superficial dorsal v
Extensor retinaculum
Extensor digitorum tt
Extensor digiti minimi t

Extensor indicis t
Triquetrum
Extensor carpi ulnaris t
Medial pisotriquetral lig
Lunate
Radiolunotriquetral lig
Flexor digitorum profundus tt
Pisiform
Ulnar n
Flexor carpi ulnaris t
Ulnar a, deep

Radial a, superficial
Median n
Flexor digitorum superficialis tt
Palmaris longus t
Palmar carpal lig
Ulnar a, superficial

Figure 7.1.10

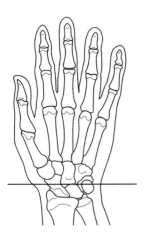

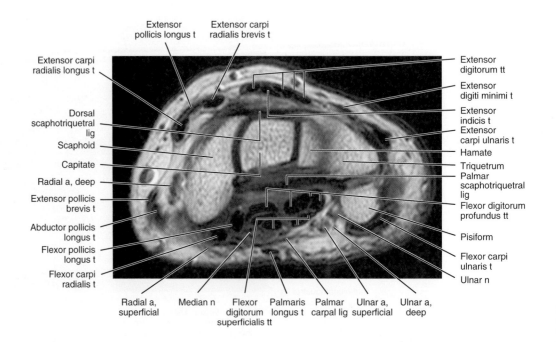

Extensor carpi radialis longus t

Dorsal scaphotriquetral lig
Scaphoid
Capitate
Radial a, deep
Extensor pollicis brevis t
Abductor pollicis longus t
Flexor pollicis longus t
Flexor carpi radialis t

Extensor pollicis longus t
Extensor carpi radialis brevis t

Extensor digitorum tt
Extensor digiti minimi t
Extensor indicis t
Extensor carpi ulnaris t
Hamate
Triquetrum
Palmar scaphotriquetral lig
Flexor digitorum profundus tt
Pisiform
Flexor carpi ulnaris t
Ulnar n

Radial a, superficial
Median n
Flexor digitorum superficialis tt
Palmaris longus t
Palmar carpal lig
Ulnar a, superficial
Ulnar a, deep

Figure 7.1.11

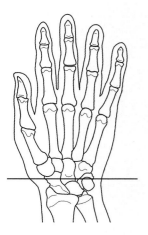

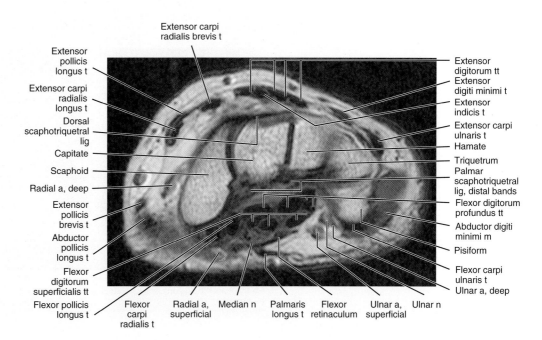

Extensor carpi
radialis brevis t

Extensor
pollicis
longus t

Extensor carpi
radialis
longus t

Dorsal
scaphotriquetral
lig

Capitate

Scaphoid

Radial a, deep

Extensor
pollicis
brevis t

Abductor
pollicis
longus t

Flexor
digitorum
superficialis tt

Flexor pollicis
longus t

Extensor
digitorum tt

Extensor
digiti minimi t

Extensor
indicis t

Extensor carpi
ulnaris t

Hamate

Triquetrum

Palmar
scaphotriquetral
lig, distal bands

Flexor digitorum
profundus tt

Abductor digiti
minimi m

Pisiform

Flexor carpi
ulnaris t

Ulnar a, deep

Flexor
carpi
radialis t

Radial a,
superficial

Median n

Palmaris
longus t

Flexor
retinaculum

Ulnar a,
superficial

Ulnar n

Figure 7.1.12

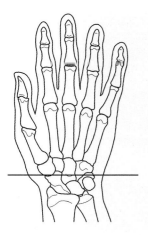

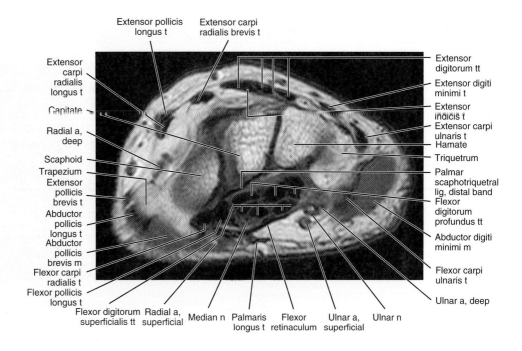

Extensor pollicis
longus t

Extensor carpi
radialis brevis t

Extensor
carpi
radialis
longus t

Capitate

Radial a,
deep

Scaphoid

Trapezium

Extensor
pollicis
brevis t

Abductor
pollicis
longus t

Abductor
pollicis
brevis m

Flexor carpi
radialis t

Flexor pollicis
longus t

Extensor
digitorum tt

Extensor digiti
minimi t

Extensor
indicis t

Extensor carpi
ulnaris t

Hamate

Triquetrum

Palmar
scaphotriquetral
lig, distal band

Flexor
digitorum
profundus tt

Abductor digiti
minimi m

Flexor carpi
ulnaris t

Ulnar a, deep

Flexor digitorum
superficialis tt

Radial a,
superficial

Median n

Palmaris
longus t

Flexor
retinaculum

Ulnar a,
superficial

Ulnar n

Figure 7.1.13

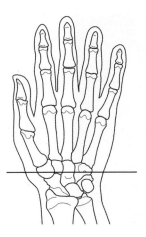

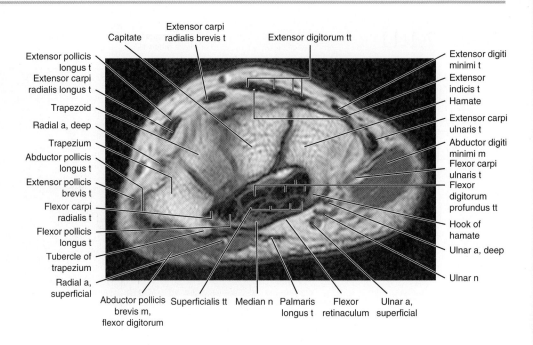

Capitate

Extensor carpi radialis brevis t

Extensor digitorum tt

Extensor pollicis longus t
Extensor carpi radialis longus t
Trapezoid
Radial a, deep
Trapezium
Abductor pollicis longus t
Extensor pollicis brevis t
Flexor carpi radialis t
Flexor pollicis longus t
Tubercle of trapezium
Radial a, superficial

Extensor digiti minimi t
Extensor indicis t
Hamate
Extensor carpi ulnaris t
Abductor digiti minimi m
Flexor carpi ulnaris t
Flexor digitorum profundus tt
Hook of hamate
Ulnar a, deep
Ulnar n

Abductor pollicis brevis m, flexor digitorum
Superficialis tt
Median n
Palmaris longus t
Flexor retinaculum
Ulnar a, superficial

Figure 7.1.14

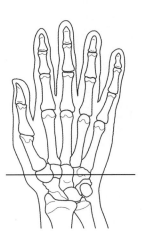

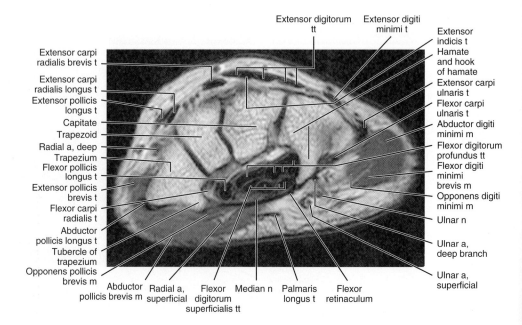

Extensor digitorum tt
Extensor digiti minimi t

Extensor carpi radialis brevis t
Extensor carpi radialis longus t
Extensor pollicis longus t
Capitate
Trapezoid
Radial a, deep
Trapezium
Flexor pollicis longus t
Extensor pollicis brevis t
Flexor carpi radialis t
Abductor pollicis longus t
Tubercle of trapezium
Opponens pollicis brevis m

Extensor indicis t
Hamate and hook of hamate
Extensor carpi ulnaris t
Flexor carpi ulnaris t
Abductor digiti minimi m
Flexor digitorum profundus tt
Flexor digiti minimi brevis m
Opponens digiti minimi m
Ulnar n
Ulnar a, deep branch
Ulnar a, superficial

Abductor pollicis brevis m
Radial a, superficial
Flexor digitorum superficialis tt
Median n
Palmaris longus t
Flexor retinaculum

Figure 7.1.15

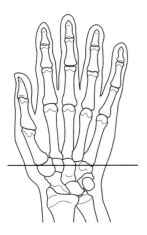

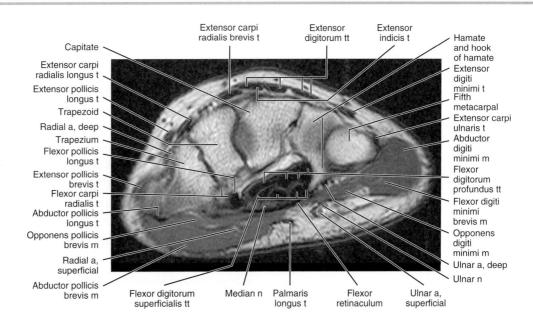

Capitate

Extensor carpi radialis longus t

Extensor pollicis longus t

Trapezoid

Radial a, deep

Trapezium

Flexor pollicis longus t

Extensor pollicis brevis t

Flexor carpi radialis t

Abductor pollicis longus t

Opponens pollicis brevis m

Radial a, superficial

Abductor pollicis brevis m

Extensor carpi radialis brevis t

Extensor digitorum tt

Extensor indicis t

Hamate and hook of hamate

Extensor digiti minimi t

Fifth metacarpal

Extensor carpi ulnaris t

Abductor digiti minimi m

Flexor digitorum profundus tt

Flexor digiti minimi brevis m

Opponens digiti minimi m

Ulnar a, deep

Ulnar n

Flexor digitorum superficialis tt

Median n

Palmaris longus t

Flexor retinaculum

Ulnar a, superficial

Figure 7.1.16

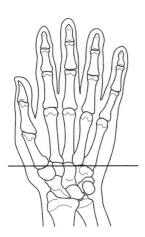

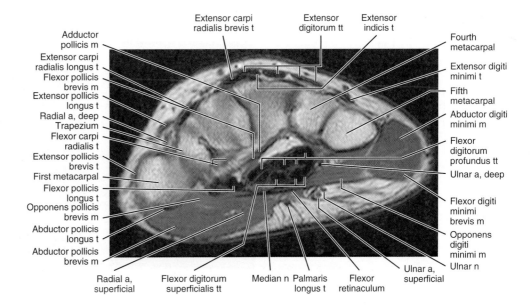

Adductor pollicis m

Extensor carpi radialis longus t

Flexor pollicis brevis m

Extensor pollicis longus t

Radial a, deep

Trapezium

Flexor carpi radialis t

Extensor pollicis brevis t

First metacarpal

Flexor pollicis longus t

Opponens pollicis brevis m

Abductor pollicis longus t

Abductor pollicis brevis m

Extensor carpi radialis brevis t

Extensor digitorum tt

Extensor indicis t

Fourth metacarpal

Extensor digiti minimi t

Fifth metacarpal

Abductor digiti minimi m

Flexor digitorum profundus tt

Ulnar a, deep

Flexor digiti minimi brevis m

Opponens digiti minimi m

Ulnar n

Radial a, superficial

Flexor digitorum superficialis tt

Median n

Palmaris longus t

Flexor retinaculum

Ulnar a, superficial

Figure 7.1.17

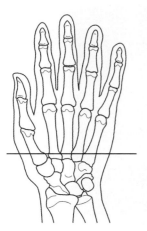

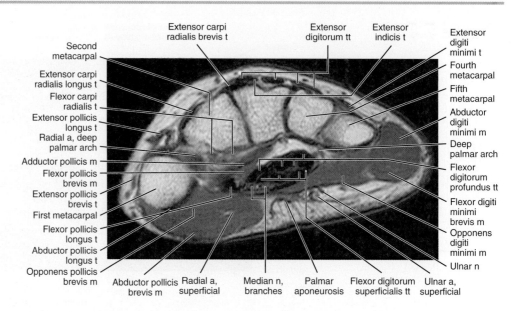

Extensor carpi radialis brevis t

Extensor digitorum tt

Extensor indicis t

Extensor digiti minimi t

Second metacarpal

Extensor carpi radialis longus t

Flexor carpi radialis t

Extensor pollicis longus t

Radial a, deep palmar arch

Adductor pollicis m

Flexor pollicis brevis m

Extensor pollicis brevis t

First metacarpal

Flexor pollicis longus t

Abductor pollicis longus t

Opponens pollicis brevis m

Fourth metacarpal

Fifth metacarpal

Abductor digiti minimi m

Deep palmar arch

Flexor digitorum profundus tt

Flexor digiti minimi brevis m

Opponens digiti minimi m

Ulnar n

Abductor pollicis brevis m

Radial a, superficial

Median n, branches

Palmar aponeurosis

Flexor digitorum superficialis tt

Ulnar a, superficial

Figure 7.1.18

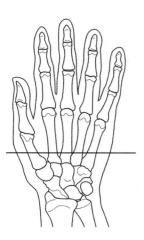

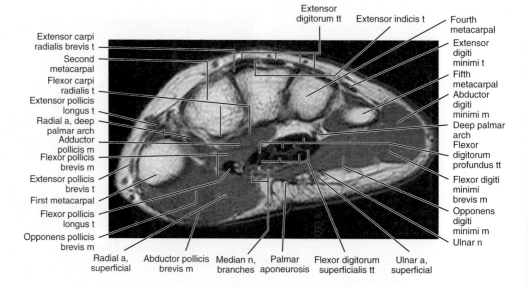

Extensor digitorum tt

Extensor indicis t

Fourth metacarpal

Extensor carpi radialis brevis t

Second metacarpal

Flexor carpi radialis t

Extensor pollicis longus t

Radial a, deep palmar arch

Adductor pollicis m

Flexor pollicis brevis m

Extensor pollicis brevis t

First metacarpal

Flexor pollicis longus t

Opponens pollicis brevis m

Extensor digiti minimi t

Fifth metacarpal

Abductor digiti minimi m

Deep palmar arch

Flexor digitorum profundus tt

Flexor digiti minimi brevis m

Opponens digiti minimi m

Ulnar n

Radial a, superficial

Abductor pollicis brevis m

Median n, branches

Palmar aponeurosis

Flexor digitorum superficialis tt

Ulnar a, superficial

SAGITTAL
Figure 7.2.1

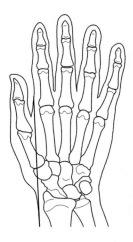

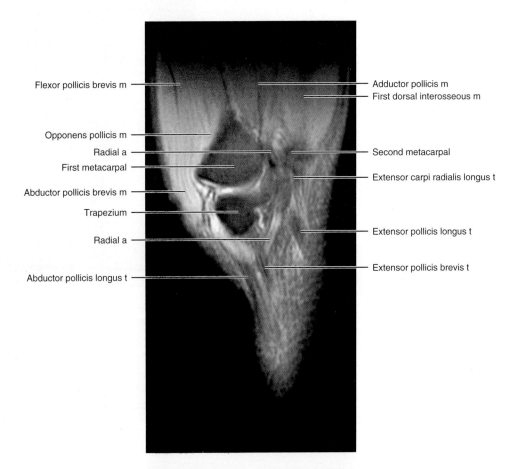

Flexor pollicis brevis m

Opponens pollicis m
Radial a
First metacarpal
Abductor pollicis brevis m
Trapezium
Radial a

Abductor pollicis longus t

Adductor pollicis m
First dorsal interosseous m

Second metacarpal

Extensor carpi radialis longus t

Extensor pollicis longus t

Extensor pollicis brevis t

Figure 7.2.2

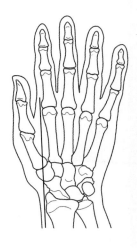

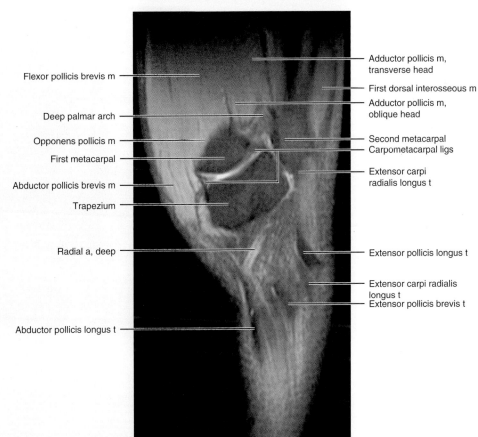

Flexor pollicis brevis m

Deep palmar arch

Opponens pollicis m
First metacarpal

Abductor pollicis brevis m
Trapezium

Radial a, deep

Abductor pollicis longus t

Adductor pollicis m, transverse head

First dorsal interosseous m
Adductor pollicis m, oblique head

Second metacarpal
Carpometacarpal ligs

Extensor carpi radialis longus t

Extensor pollicis longus t

Extensor carpi radialis longus t
Extensor pollicis brevis t

Figure 7.2.3

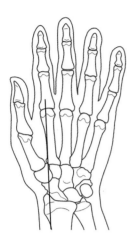

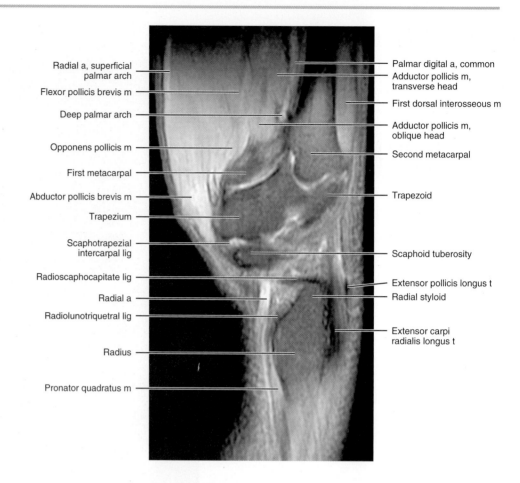

Radial a, superficial palmar arch
Flexor pollicis brevis m
Deep palmar arch
Opponens pollicis m
First metacarpal
Abductor pollicis brevis m
Trapezium
Scaphotrapezial intercarpal lig
Radioscaphocapitate lig
Radial a
Radiolunotriquetral lig
Radius
Pronator quadratus m

Palmar digital a, common
Adductor pollicis m, transverse head
First dorsal interosseous m
Adductor pollicis m, oblique head
Second metacarpal
Trapezoid
Scaphoid tuberosity
Extensor pollicis longus t
Radial styloid
Extensor carpi radialis longus t

Figure 7.2.4

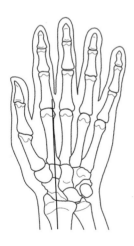

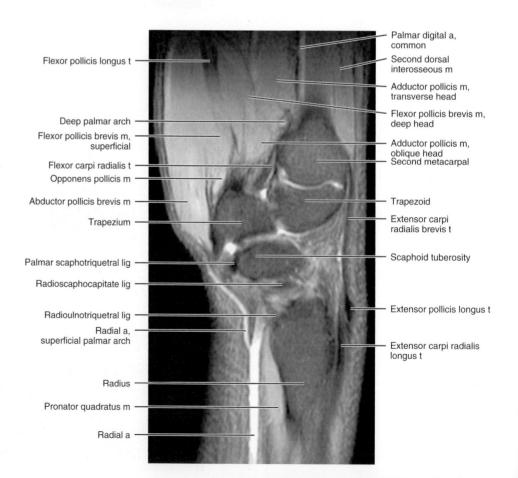

Flexor pollicis longus t
Deep palmar arch
Flexor pollicis brevis m, superficial
Flexor carpi radialis t
Opponens pollicis m
Abductor pollicis brevis m
Trapezium
Palmar scaphotriquetral lig
Radioscaphocapitate lig
Radioulnotriquetral lig
Radial a, superficial palmar arch
Radius
Pronator quadratus m
Radial a

Palmar digital a, common
Second dorsal interosseous m
Adductor pollicis m, transverse head
Flexor pollicis brevis m, deep head
Adductor pollicis m, oblique head
Second metacarpal
Trapezoid
Extensor carpi radialis brevis t
Scaphoid tuberosity
Extensor pollicis longus t
Extensor carpi radialis longus t

Figure 7.2.5

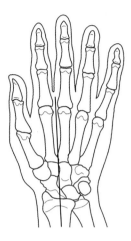

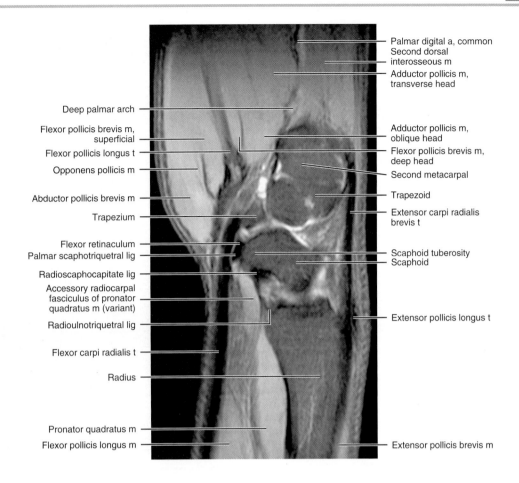

Deep palmar arch
Flexor pollicis brevis m, superficial
Flexor pollicis longus t
Opponens pollicis m

Abductor pollicis brevis m
Trapezium

Flexor retinaculum
Palmar scaphotriquetral lig
Radioscaphocapitate lig
Accessory radiocarpal fasciculus of pronator quadratus m (variant)
Radioulnotriquetral lig

Flexor carpi radialis t

Radius

Pronator quadratus m
Flexor pollicis longus m

Palmar digital a, common
Second dorsal interosseous m
Adductor pollicis m, transverse head

Adductor pollicis m, oblique head
Flexor pollicis brevis m, deep head
Second metacarpal

Trapezoid
Extensor carpi radialis brevis t

Scaphoid tuberosity
Scaphoid

Extensor pollicis longus t

Extensor pollicis brevis m

Figure 7.2.6

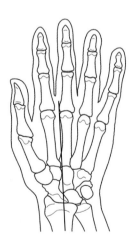

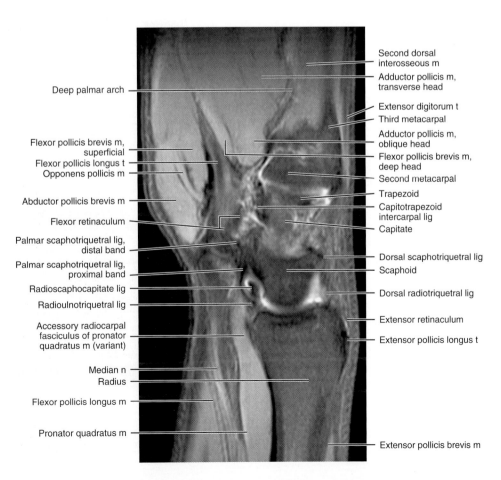

Deep palmar arch

Flexor pollicis brevis m, superficial
Flexor pollicis longus t
Opponens pollicis m

Abductor pollicis brevis m

Flexor retinaculum
Palmar scaphotriquetral lig, distal band
Palmar scaphotriquetral lig, proximal band
Radioscaphocapitate lig
Radioulnotriquetral lig

Accessory radiocarpal fasciculus of pronator quadratus m (variant)

Median n
Radius

Flexor pollicis longus m

Pronator quadratus m

Second dorsal interosseous m
Adductor pollicis m, transverse head

Extensor digitorum t
Third metacarpal
Adductor pollicis m, oblique head
Flexor pollicis brevis m, deep head
Second metacarpal
Trapezoid
Capitotrapezoid intercarpal lig
Capitate

Dorsal scaphotriquetral lig
Scaphoid

Dorsal radiotriquetral lig

Extensor retinaculum

Extensor pollicis longus t

Extensor pollicis brevis m

Figure 7.2.7

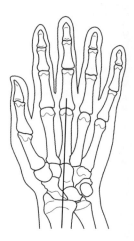

Second lumbrical m

Deep palmar arch

Ulnar n, branch

Flexor digitorum profundus t

Flexor pollicis brevis m, superficial

Opponens pollicis m

Palmar aponeurosis

Abductor pollicis brevis m

Flexor retinaculum

Palmar scaphotriquetral lig, distal band

Radioscaphocapitate lig

Palmar scaphotriquetral lig, proximal band

Median n

Radiolunotriquetral lig

Flexor pollicis longus t

Radioscapholunate lig

Radius

Flexor digitorum profundus t

Flexor digitorum superficialis m and t

Palmaris longus t

Pronator quadratus m

Second dorsal interosseous m

Extensor digitorum t

Palmar v

Third metacarpal

Adductor pollicis m, transverse head

Adductor pollicis m, oblique head

Flexor pollicis brevis m, deep head

Capitate

Extensor digitorum t

Dorsal scaphotriquetral lig

Scaphoid

Dorsal radiotriquetral lig

Extensor retinaculum

Extensor pollicis longus t

Figure 7.2.8

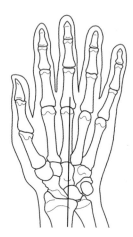

Second lumbrical m

Deep palmar arch

Flexor digitorum profundus t

Median n, branch

Flexor pollicis brevis m

Palmar aponeurosis

Opponens pollicis m

Abductor pollicis brevis m

Palmar scaphotriquetral lig, distal band

Flexor retinaculum

Median n

Radioscaphocapitate lig

Palmar scaphotriquetral lig, distal band

Palmaris longus t

Radiolunotriquetral lig

Scapholunate intercarpal lig

Radius

Flexor digitorum profundus t

Flexor digitorum superficialis m and t

Pronator quadratus m

Second dorsal interosseous m

Third metacarpal

Adductor pollicis m, transverse head

Extensor digitorum t

Adductor pollicis m, oblique head

Carpometacarpal lig

Capitate

Extensor indicis t

Dorsal scaphotriquetral lig

Scaphoid

Dorsal radiotriquetral lig

Extensor retinaculum

Lister's tubercle

Extensor pollicis longus m

Figure 7.2.9

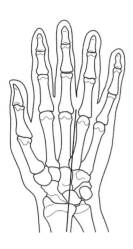

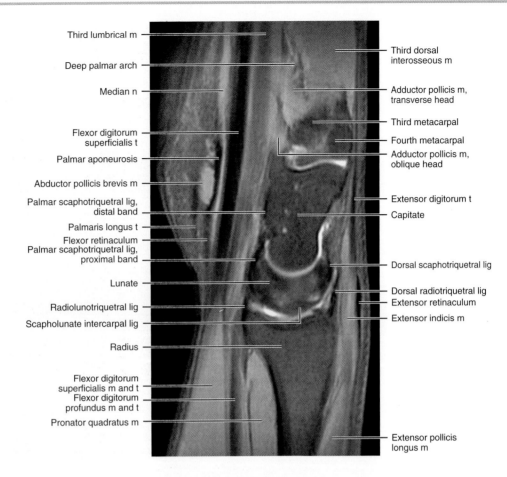

Third lumbrical m

Deep palmar arch

Median n

Flexor digitorum superficialis t

Palmar aponeurosis

Abductor pollicis brevis m

Palmar scaphotriquetral lig, distal band

Palmaris longus t

Flexor retinaculum
Palmar scaphotriquetral lig, proximal band

Lunate

Radiolunotriquetral lig

Scapholunate intercarpal lig

Radius

Flexor digitorum superficialis m and t
Flexor digitorum profundus m and t

Pronator quadratus m

Third dorsal interosseous m

Adductor pollicis m, transverse head

Third metacarpal

Fourth metacarpal
Adductor pollicis m, oblique head

Extensor digitorum t

Capitate

Dorsal scaphotriquetral lig

Dorsal radiotriquetral lig
Extensor retinaculum
Extensor indicis m

Extensor pollicis longus m

Figure 7.2.10

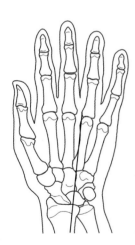

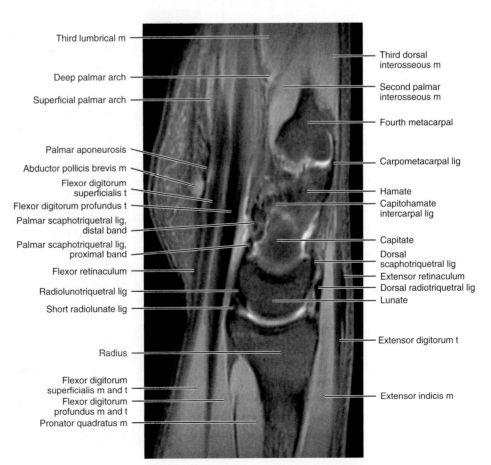

Third lumbrical m

Deep palmar arch

Superficial palmar arch

Palmar aponeurosis

Abductor pollicis brevis m

Flexor digitorum superficialis t

Flexor digitorum profundus t

Palmar scaphotriquetral lig, distal band

Palmar scaphotriquetral lig, proximal band

Flexor retinaculum

Radiolunotriquetral lig

Short radiolunate lig

Radius

Flexor digitorum superficialis m and t
Flexor digitorum profundus m and t
Pronator quadratus m

Third dorsal interosseous m

Second palmar interosseous m

Fourth metacarpal

Carpometacarpal lig

Hamate

Capitohamate intercarpal lig

Capitate

Dorsal scaphotriquetral lig

Extensor retinaculum
Dorsal radiotriquetral lig

Lunate

Extensor digitorum t

Extensor indicis m

Figure 7.2.11

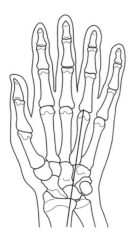

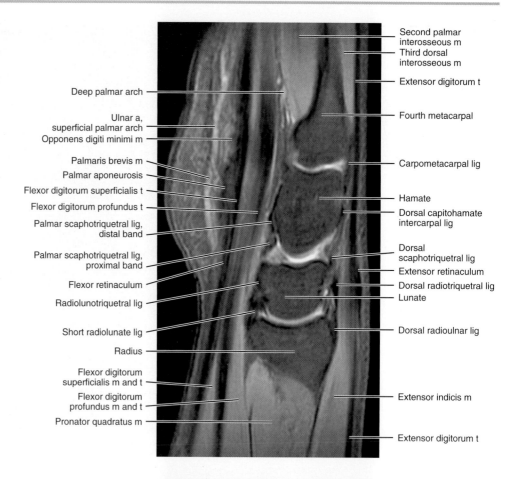

Deep palmar arch

Ulnar a, superficial palmar arch
Opponens digiti minimi m

Palmaris brevis m
Palmar aponeurosis
Flexor digitorum superficialis t
Flexor digitorum profundus t
Palmar scaphotriquetral lig, distal band

Palmar scaphotriquetral lig, proximal band

Flexor retinaculum

Radiolunotriquetral lig

Short radiolunate lig

Radius

Flexor digitorum superficialis m and t
Flexor digitorum profundus m and t
Pronator quadratus m

Second palmar interosseous m
Third dorsal interosseous m
Extensor digitorum t

Fourth metacarpal

Carpometacarpal lig

Hamate
Dorsal capitohamate intercarpal lig

Dorsal scaphotriquetral lig
Extensor retinaculum
Dorsal radiotriquetral lig
Lunate

Dorsal radioulnar lig

Extensor indicis m

Extensor digitorum t

Figure 7.2.12

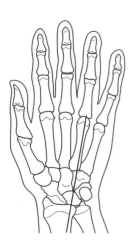

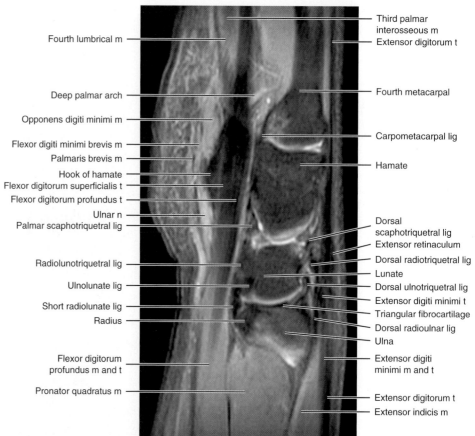

Fourth lumbrical m

Deep palmar arch

Opponens digiti minimi m

Flexor digiti minimi brevis m
Palmaris brevis m
Hook of hamate
Flexor digitorum superficialis t
Flexor digitorum profundus t
Ulnar n
Palmar scaphotriquetral lig

Radiolunotriquetral lig

Ulnolunate lig

Short radiolunate lig
Radius

Flexor digitorum profundus m and t

Pronator quadratus m

Third palmar interosseous m
Extensor digitorum t

Fourth metacarpal

Carpometacarpal lig

Hamate

Dorsal scaphotriquetral lig
Extensor retinaculum
Dorsal radiotriquetral lig
Lunate
Dorsal ulnotriquetral lig
Extensor digiti minimi t
Triangular fibrocartilage
Dorsal radioulnar lig
Ulna
Extensor digiti minimi m and t

Extensor digitorum t
Extensor indicis m

Figure 7.2.13

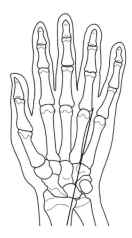

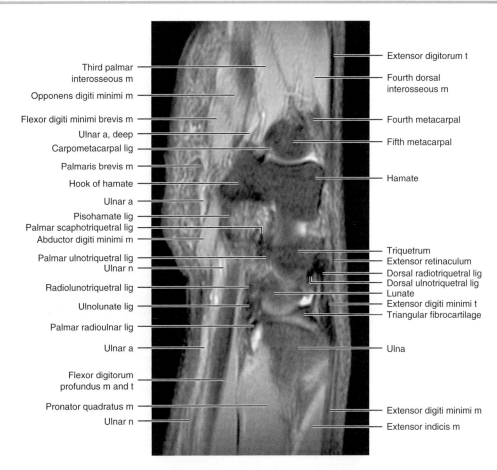

Third palmar interosseous m
Opponens digiti minimi m
Flexor digiti minimi brevis m
Ulnar a, deep
Carpometacarpal lig
Palmaris brevis m
Hook of hamate
Ulnar a
Pisohamate lig
Palmar scaphotriquetral lig
Abductor digiti minimi m
Palmar ulnotriquetral lig
Ulnar n
Radiolunotriquetral lig
Ulnolunate lig
Palmar radioulnar lig
Ulnar a
Flexor digitorum profundus m and t
Pronator quadratus m
Ulnar n

Extensor digitorum t
Fourth dorsal interosseous m
Fourth metacarpal
Fifth metacarpal
Hamate
Triquetrum
Extensor retinaculum
Dorsal radiotriquetral lig
Dorsal ulnotriquetral lig
Lunate
Extensor digiti minimi t
Triangular fibrocartilage
Ulna
Extensor digiti minimi m
Extensor indicis m

Figure 7.2.14

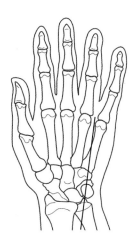

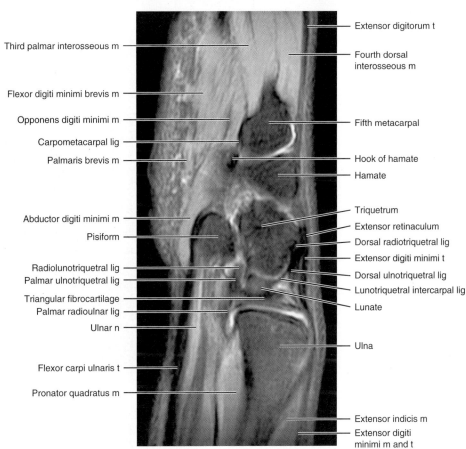

Third palmar interosseous m
Flexor digiti minimi brevis m
Opponens digiti minimi m
Carpometacarpal lig
Palmaris brevis m
Abductor digiti minimi m
Pisiform
Radiolunotriquetral lig
Palmar ulnotriquetral lig
Triangular fibrocartilage
Palmar radioulnar lig
Ulnar n
Flexor carpi ulnaris t
Pronator quadratus m

Extensor digitorum t
Fourth dorsal interosseous m
Fifth metacarpal
Hook of hamate
Hamate
Triquetrum
Extensor retinaculum
Dorsal radiotriquetral lig
Extensor digiti minimi t
Dorsal ulnotriquetral lig
Lunotriquetral intercarpal lig
Lunate
Ulna
Extensor indicis m
Extensor digiti minimi m and t

Figure 7.2.15

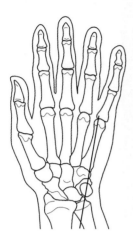

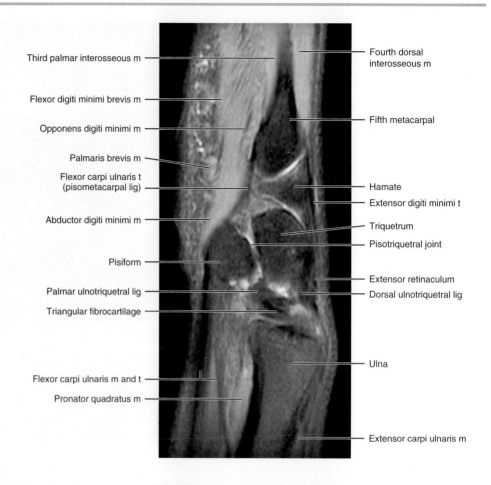

Third palmar interosseous m

Flexor digiti minimi brevis m

Opponens digiti minimi m

Palmaris brevis m

Flexor carpi ulnaris t
(pisometacarpal lig)

Abductor digiti minimi m

Pisiform

Palmar ulnotriquetral lig

Triangular fibrocartilage

Flexor carpi ulnaris m and t

Pronator quadratus m

Fourth dorsal
interosseous m

Fifth metacarpal

Hamate

Extensor digiti minimi t

Triquetrum

Pisotriquetral joint

Extensor retinaculum

Dorsal ulnotriquetral lig

Ulna

Extensor carpi ulnaris m

Figure 7.2.16

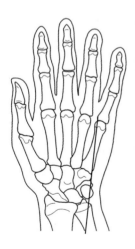

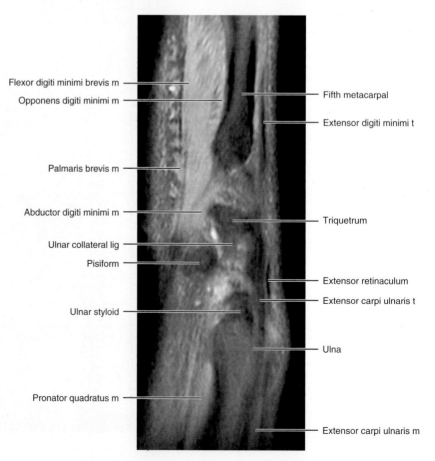

Flexor digiti minimi brevis m

Opponens digiti minimi m

Palmaris brevis m

Abductor digiti minimi m

Ulnar collateral lig

Pisiform

Ulnar styloid

Pronator quadratus m

Fifth metacarpal

Extensor digiti minimi t

Triquetrum

Extensor retinaculum

Extensor carpi ulnaris t

Ulna

Extensor carpi ulnaris m

Figure 7.2.17

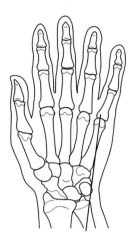

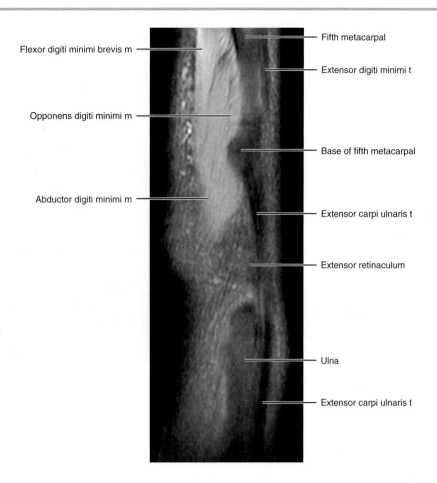

Flexor digiti minimi brevis m

Opponens digiti minimi m

Abductor digiti minimi m

Fifth metacarpal

Extensor digiti minimi t

Base of fifth metacarpal

Extensor carpi ulnaris t

Extensor retinaculum

Ulna

Extensor carpi ulnaris t

CORONAL

Figure 7.3.1

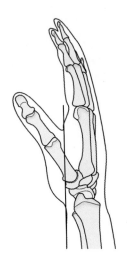

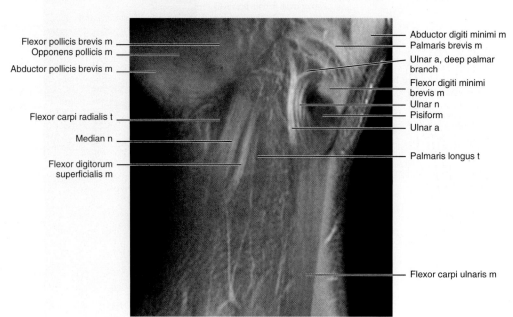

Flexor pollicis brevis m
Opponens pollicis m

Abductor pollicis brevis m

Flexor carpi radialis t

Median n

Flexor digitorum superficialis m

Abductor digiti minimi m
Palmaris brevis m
Ulnar a, deep palmar branch
Flexor digiti minimi brevis m
Ulnar n
Pisiform
Ulnar a

Palmaris longus t

Flexor carpi ulnaris m

Figure 7.3.2

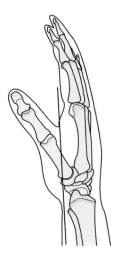

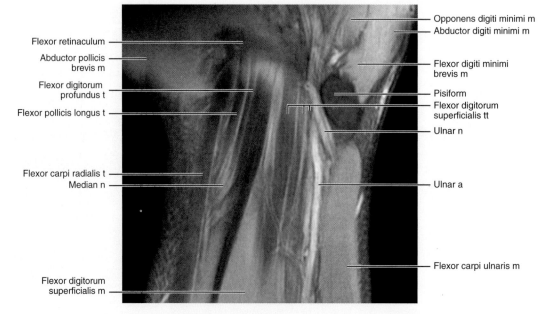

Flexor retinaculum

Abductor pollicis brevis m

Flexor digitorum profundus t

Flexor pollicis longus t

Flexor carpi radialis t
Median n

Flexor digitorum superficialis m

Opponens digiti minimi m
Abductor digiti minimi m

Flexor digiti minimi brevis m

Pisiform
Flexor digitorum superficialis tt

Ulnar n

Ulnar a

Flexor carpi ulnaris m

Figure 7.3.3

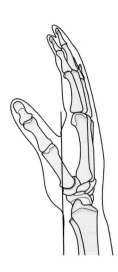

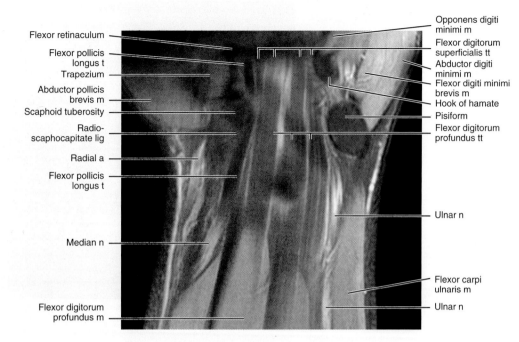

Flexor retinaculum

Flexor pollicis longus t

Trapezium

Abductor pollicis brevis m

Scaphoid tuberosity

Radio-scaphocapitate lig

Radial a

Flexor pollicis longus t

Median n

Flexor digitorum profundus m

Opponens digiti minimi m

Flexor digitorum superficialis tt

Abductor digiti minimi m

Flexor digiti minimi brevis m

Hook of hamate

Pisiform

Flexor digitorum profundus tt

Ulnar n

Flexor carpi ulnaris m

Ulnar n

Figure 7.3.4

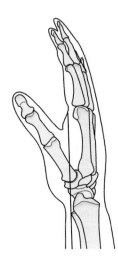

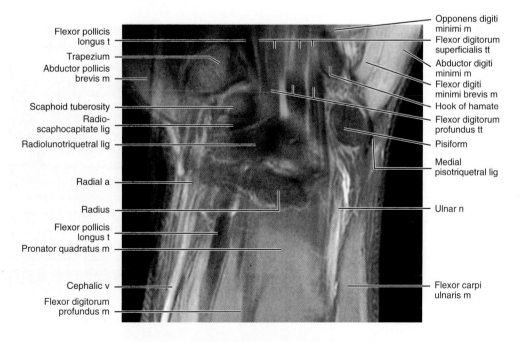

Flexor pollicis longus t

Trapezium

Abductor pollicis brevis m

Scaphoid tuberosity

Radio-scaphocapitate lig

Radiolunotriquetral lig

Radial a

Radius

Flexor pollicis longus t

Pronator quadratus m

Cephalic v

Flexor digitorum profundus m

Opponens digiti minimi m

Flexor digitorum superficialis tt

Abductor digiti minimi m

Flexor digiti minimi brevis m

Hook of hamate

Flexor digitorum profundus tt

Pisiform

Medial pisotriquetral lig

Ulnar n

Flexor carpi ulnaris m

Figure 7.3.5

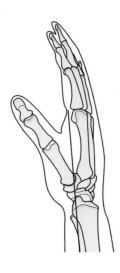

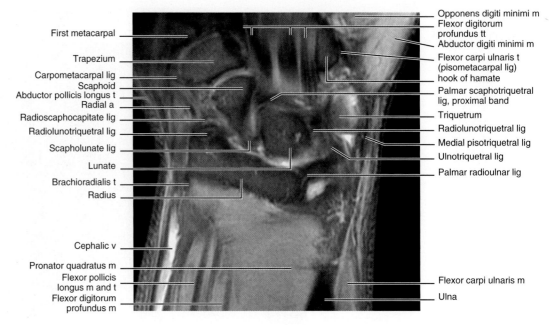

First metacarpal

Trapezium

Carpometacarpal lig
Scaphoid
Abductor pollicis longus t
Radial a
Radioscaphocapitate lig
Radiolunotriquetral lig
Scapholunate lig
Lunate
Brachioradialis t
Radius

Cephalic v

Pronator quadratus m
Flexor pollicis
longus m and t
Flexor digitorum
profundus m

Opponens digiti minimi m
Flexor digitorum
profundus tt
Abductor digiti minimi m
Flexor carpi ulnaris t
(pisometacarpal lig)
hook of hamate
Palmar scaphotriquetral
lig, proximal band
Triquetrum
Radiolunotriquetral lig
Medial pisotriquetral lig
Ulnotriquetral lig
Palmar radioulnar lig

Flexor carpi ulnaris m
Ulna

Figure 7.3.6

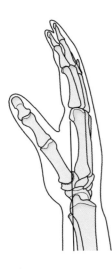

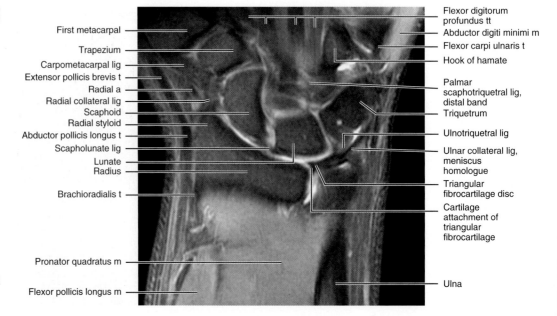

First metacarpal

Trapezium

Carpometacarpal lig
Extensor pollicis brevis t
Radial a
Radial collateral lig
Scaphoid
Radial styloid
Abductor pollicis longus t
Scapholunate lig
Lunate
Radius

Brachioradialis t

Pronator quadratus m

Flexor pollicis longus m

Flexor digitorum
profundus tt
Abductor digiti minimi m
Flexor carpi ulnaris t
Hook of hamate
Palmar
scaphotriquetral lig,
distal band
Triquetrum
Ulnotriquetral lig
Ulnar collateral lig,
meniscus
homologue
Triangular
fibrocartilage disc
Cartilage
attachment of
triangular
fibrocartilage
Ulna

Figure 7.3.7

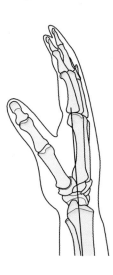

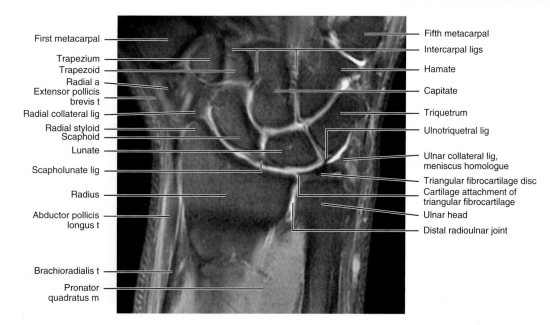

First metacarpal
Trapezium
Trapezoid
Radial a
Extensor pollicis brevis t
Radial collateral lig
Radial styloid
Scaphoid
Lunate
Scapholunate lig
Radius
Abductor pollicis longus t
Brachioradialis t
Pronator quadratus m

Fifth metacarpal
Intercarpal ligs
Hamate
Capitate
Triquetrum
Ulnotriquetral lig
Ulnar collateral lig, meniscus homologue
Triangular fibrocartilage disc
Cartilage attachment of triangular fibrocartilage
Ulnar head
Distal radioulnar joint

Figure 7.3.8

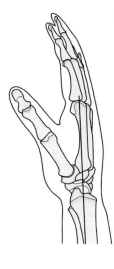

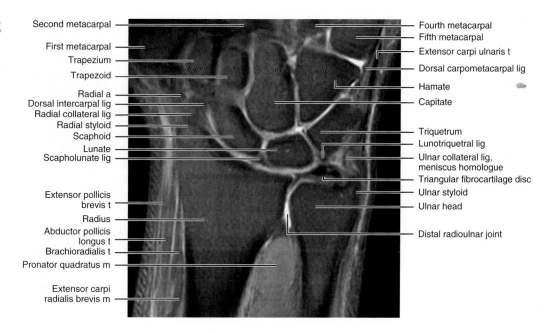

Second metacarpal
First metacarpal
Trapezium
Trapezoid
Radial a
Dorsal intercarpal lig
Radial collateral lig
Radial styloid
Scaphoid
Lunate
Scapholunate lig
Extensor pollicis brevis t
Radius
Abductor pollicis longus t
Brachioradialis t
Pronator quadratus m
Extensor carpi radialis brevis m

Fourth metacarpal
Fifth metacarpal
Extensor carpi ulnaris t
Dorsal carpometacarpal lig
Hamate
Capitate
Triquetrum
Lunotriquetral lig
Ulnar collateral lig, meniscus homologue
Triangular fibrocartilage disc
Ulnar styloid
Ulnar head
Distal radioulnar joint

Figure 7.3.9

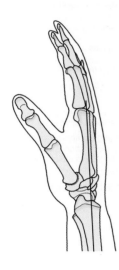

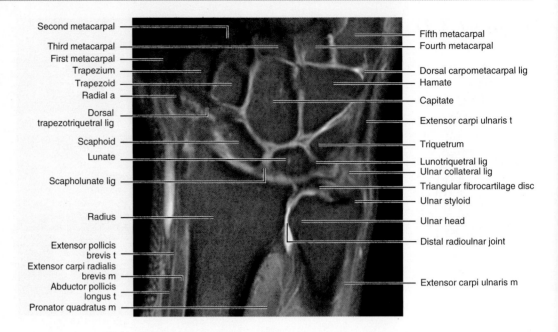

Second metacarpal
Third metacarpal
First metacarpal
Trapezium
Trapezoid
Radial a
Dorsal trapezotriquetral lig
Scaphoid
Lunate
Scapholunate lig
Radius
Extensor pollicis brevis t
Extensor carpi radialis brevis m
Abductor pollicis longus t
Pronator quadratus m

Fifth metacarpal
Fourth metacarpal
Dorsal carpometacarpal lig
Hamate
Capitate
Extensor carpi ulnaris t
Triquetrum
Lunotriquetral lig
Ulnar collateral lig
Triangular fibrocartilage disc
Ulnar styloid
Ulnar head
Distal radioulnar joint
Extensor carpi ulnaris m

Figure 7.3.10

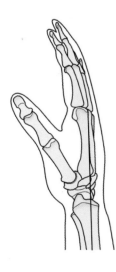

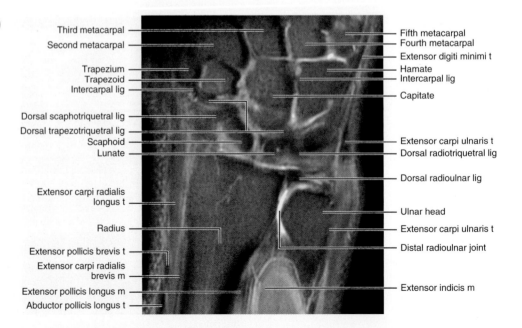

Third metacarpal
Second metacarpal
Trapezium
Trapezoid
Intercarpal lig
Dorsal scaphotriquetral lig
Dorsal trapezotriquetral lig
Scaphoid
Lunate
Extensor carpi radialis longus t
Radius
Extensor pollicis brevis t
Extensor carpi radialis brevis m
Extensor pollicis longus m
Abductor pollicis longus t

Fifth metacarpal
Fourth metacarpal
Extensor digiti minimi t
Hamate
Intercarpal lig
Capitate
Extensor carpi ulnaris t
Dorsal radiotriquetral lig
Dorsal radioulnar lig
Ulnar head
Extensor carpi ulnaris t
Distal radioulnar joint
Extensor indicis m

Figure 7.3.11

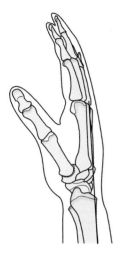

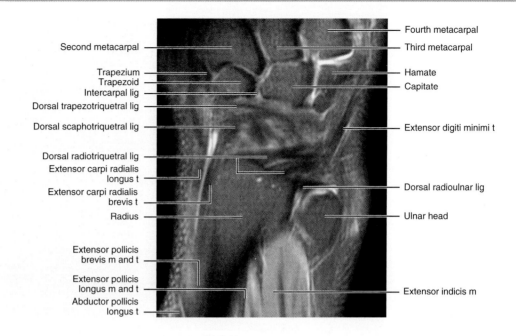

Second metacarpal

Trapezium
Trapezoid
Intercarpal lig
Dorsal trapezotriquetral lig

Dorsal scaphotriquetral lig

Dorsal radiotriquetral lig
Extensor carpi radialis
longus t
Extensor carpi radialis
brevis t
Radius

Extensor pollicis
brevis m and t

Extensor pollicis
longus m and t
Abductor pollicis
longus t

Fourth metacarpal
Third metacarpal

Hamate
Capitate

Extensor digiti minimi t

Dorsal radioulnar lig

Ulnar head

Extensor indicis m

Figure 7.3.12

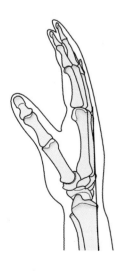

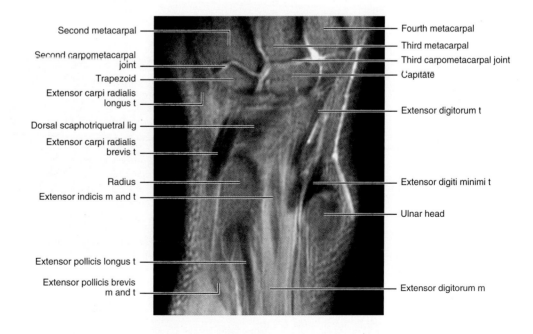

Second metacarpal

Second carpometacarpal
joint
Trapezoid
Extensor carpi radialis
longus t
Dorsal scaphotriquetral lig
Extensor carpi radialis
brevis t
Radius
Extensor indicis m and t

Extensor pollicis longus t

Extensor pollicis brevis
m and t

Fourth metacarpal
Third metacarpal
Third carpometacarpal joint
Capitate

Extensor digitorum t

Extensor digiti minimi t

Ulnar head

Extensor digitorum m

Figure 7.3.13

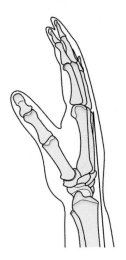

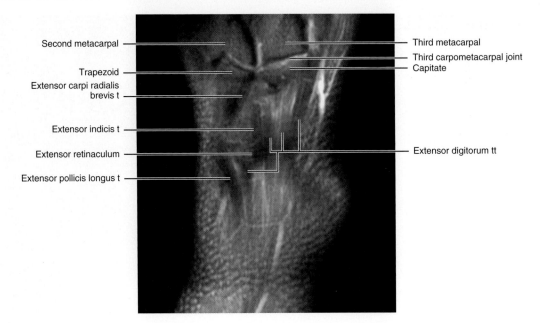

Second metacarpal

Trapezoid

Extensor carpi radialis
brevis t

Extensor indicis t

Extensor retinaculum

Extensor pollicis longus t

Third metacarpal

Third carpometacarpal joint
Capitate

Extensor digitorum tt

Chapter 8

MRI of the Hand

Table 4: Muscles of the Hand

MUSCLE	ORIGIN	INSERTION	NERVE SUPPLY
Palmaris brevis	Ulnar border of the palmar aponeurosis	Deep surface of the skin along the ulnar border of the palm	Superficial branch of ulnar (C8, T1)
Abductor pollicis brevis	Palmar surface of the flexor retinaculum, trapezium, and occasionally scaphoid	Radial side of the base of the proximal phalanx of the thumb	Recurrent branch of median (C8, T1)
Opponens pollicis	Palmar surface of the flexor retinaculum and tubercle of the trapezium	Lateral part of the palmar surface of the shaft of the first the metacarpal	Recurrent branch of median (C8, T1)
Flexor pollicis brevis	Superficial head: trapezium, adjacent part of the flexor retinaculum, and tendon sheath of the flexor carpi radialis; deep head: trapezoid and capitate	Superficial head: lateral side of the front of the base of the proximal phalanx; deep head: into a tendon of the superficial head	Recurrent branch of median and deep branch of ulnar (C8, T1)
Adductor pollicis brevis	Carpal head: flexor retinaculum, capitate, bases of the second and third metacarpals; metacarpal head: palmar ridges of the third metacarpal and capsules of the second, third, and fourth metacarpo-phalangeal articulations	Ulnar side of the front of the base of the proximal phalanx of the thumb	Recurrent branch of median (C8, T1)
Abductor digiti minimi	Distal half of the pisiform, pisihamate ligament, tendon of the flexor carpi ulnaris, and frequently the flexor retinaculum	Two tendons: (1) the ulnar side of the base of the proximal phalanx of the little finger and (2) the aponeurosis of the extensor tendon of the little finger	Deep palmar division of ulnar (C8, T1)
Flexor digiti minimi brevis	Hook of the hamate and adjacent parts of the flexor retinaculum	Ulnar side of the base of the proximal phalanx of the little finger	Superficial or deep palmar branch of ulnar (C8, T1)
Opponens digiti minimi	Distal border of the hook of the hamate and adjacent flexor retinaculum	Medial surface of the body and particularly onto the head of the fifth metacarpal	Deep palmar branch of ulnar (C8, T1)
Lumbrical	Two lateral lumbricals: radial and palmar sides of the first and second tendons of the flexor digitorum profundus Two medial lumbricals: adjacent side of the second and third tendons, and the third and fourth tendons of the flexor digitorum profundus	Into the radial border of the tendon of the extensor digitorum on the back of the proximal phalanx	Median, lateral two or three lumbricals; ulnar, deep palmar branch, medial one or two lumbricals (C8, T1)

Table 4: Muscles of the Hand—Cont'd

MUSCLE	ORIGIN	INSERTION	NERVE SUPPLY
Interosseous	Palmar interosseous: anterior border of the shaft of the first, second, fourth, and fifth metacarpals. The first arises near the base and the others arise from three fourths of the shaft of the bone. Dorsal interosseous: adjacent sides of the metacarpal bones in each metacarpal interspace	Into the expansion on the axial side of the corresponding digit. The first palmar interosseous is described frequently as a division of the flexor brevis or adductor pollicis. The first dorsal interosseous usually inserts onto the proximal phalanx. The other three insert into the extensor expansion and proximal phalanx	Deep palmar branch of ulnar (C8, T1)

AXIAL

Figure 8.1.1

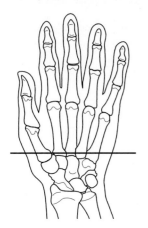

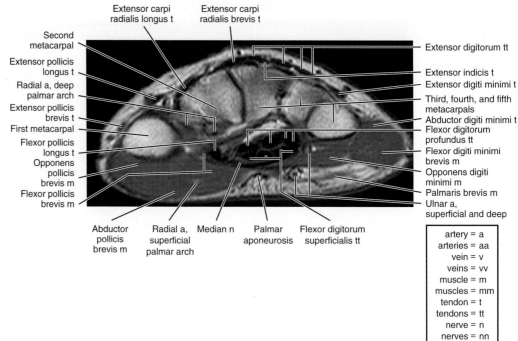

Extensor carpi radialis longus t
Extensor carpi radialis brevis t
Extensor digitorum tt
Extensor indicis t
Extensor digiti minimi t
Third, fourth, and fifth metacarpals
Abductor digiti minimi t
Flexor digitorum profundus tt
Flexor digiti minimi brevis m
Opponens digiti minimi m
Palmaris brevis m
Ulnar a, superficial and deep

Second metacarpal
Extensor pollicis longus t
Radial a, deep palmar arch
Extensor pollicis brevis t
First metacarpal
Flexor pollicis longus t
Opponens pollicis brevis m
Flexor pollicis brevis m

Abductor pollicis brevis m
Radial a, superficial palmar arch
Median n
Palmar aponeurosis
Flexor digitorum superficialis tt

artery = a
arteries = aa
vein = v
veins = vv
muscle = m
muscles = mm
tendon = t
tendons = tt
nerve = n
nerves = nn
ligament = lig
ligaments = ligs

Figure 8.1.2

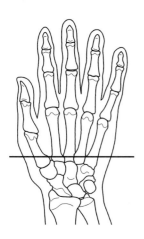

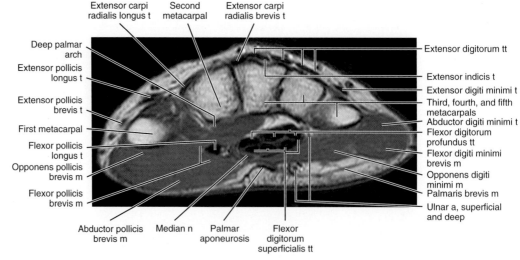

Extensor carpi radialis longus t
Second metacarpal
Extensor carpi radialis brevis t
Extensor digitorum tt

Deep palmar arch
Extensor pollicis longus t
Extensor pollicis brevis t
First metacarpal
Flexor pollicis longus t
Opponens pollicis brevis m
Flexor pollicis brevis m

Extensor indicis t
Extensor digiti minimi t
Third, fourth, and fifth metacarpals
Abductor digiti minimi t
Flexor digitorum profundus tt
Flexor digiti minimi brevis m
Opponens digiti minimi m
Palmaris brevis m
Ulnar a, superficial and deep

Abductor pollicis brevis m
Median n
Palmar aponeurosis
Flexor digitorum superficialis tt

Figure 8.1.3

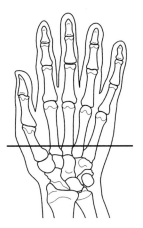

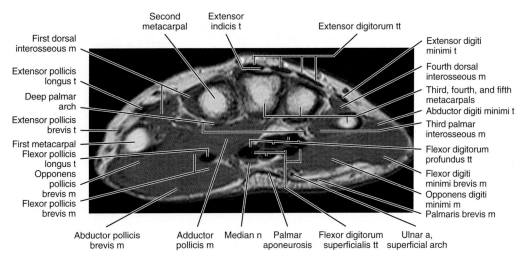

First dorsal interosseous m

Extensor pollicis longus t

Deep palmar arch

Extensor pollicis brevis t

First metacarpal
Flexor pollicis longus t
Opponens pollicis brevis m
Flexor pollicis brevis m

Second metacarpal

Extensor indicis t

Extensor digitorum tt

Extensor digiti minimi t

Fourth dorsal interosseous m

Third, fourth, and fifth metacarpals

Abductor digiti minimi t

Third palmar interosseous m

Flexor digitorum profundus tt

Flexor digiti minimi brevis m

Opponens digiti minimi m

Palmaris brevis m

Abductor pollicis brevis m

Adductor pollicis m

Median n

Palmar aponeurosis

Flexor digitorum superficialis tt

Ulnar a, superficial arch

Figure 8.1.4

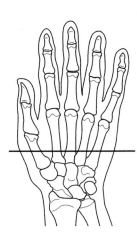

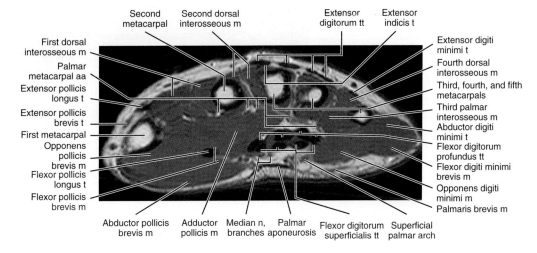

First dorsal interosseous m

Palmar metacarpal aa

Extensor pollicis longus t

Extensor pollicis brevis t

First metacarpal
Opponens pollicis brevis m
Flexor pollicis longus t
Flexor pollicis brevis m

Second metacarpal

Second dorsal interosseous m

Extensor digitorum tt

Extensor indicis t

Extensor digiti minimi t

Fourth dorsal interosseous m

Third, fourth, and fifth metacarpals

Third palmar interosseous m

Abductor digiti minimi t

Flexor digitorum profundus tt

Flexor digiti minimi brevis m

Opponens digiti minimi m

Palmaris brevis m

Abductor pollicis brevis m

Adductor pollicis m

Median n, branches

Palmar aponeurosis

Flexor digitorum superficialis tt

Superficial palmar arch

Figure 8.1.5

Figure 8.1.6

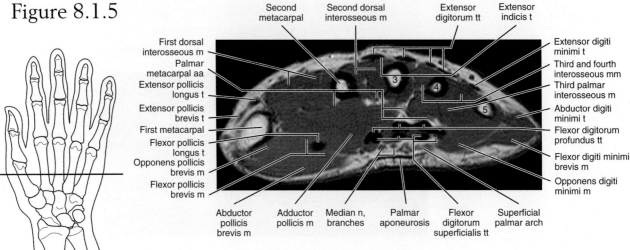

Figure 8.1.7

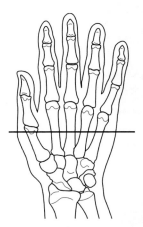

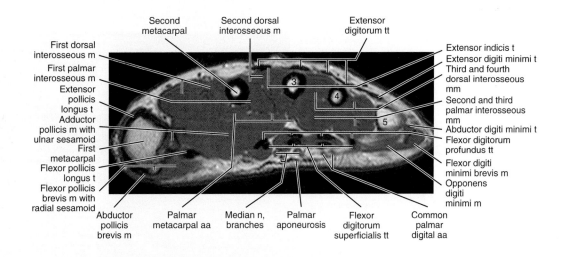

Second metacarpal

Second dorsal interosseous m

Extensor digitorum tt

First dorsal interosseous m

First palmar interosseous m

Extensor pollicis longus t

Adductor pollicis m with ulnar sesamoid

First metacarpal

Flexor pollicis longus t

Flexor pollicis brevis m with radial sesamoid

Extensor indicis t

Extensor digiti minimi t

Third and fourth dorsal interosseous mm

Second and third palmar interosseous mm

Abductor digiti minimi t

Flexor digitorum profundus tt

Flexor digiti minimi brevis m

Opponens digiti minimi m

Abductor pollicis brevis m

Palmar metacarpal aa

Median n, branches

Palmar aponeurosis

Flexor digitorum superficialis tt

Common palmar digital aa

Figure 8.1.8

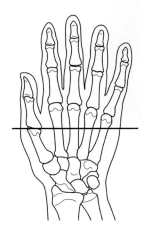

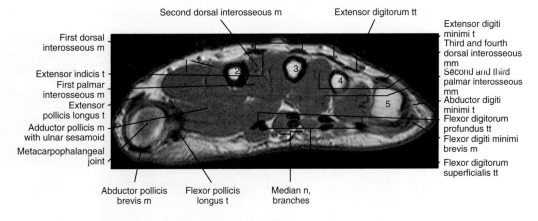

Second dorsal interosseous m

Extensor digitorum tt

First dorsal interosseous m

Extensor indicis t

First palmar interosseous m

Extensor pollicis longus t

Adductor pollicis m with ulnar sesamoid

Metacarpophalangeal joint

Extensor digiti minimi t

Third and fourth dorsal interosseous mm

Second and third palmar interosseous mm

Abductor digiti minimi t

Flexor digitorum profundus tt

Flexor digiti minimi brevis m

Flexor digitorum superficialis tt

Abductor pollicis brevis m

Flexor pollicis longus t

Median n, branches

Figure 8.1.9

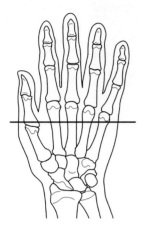

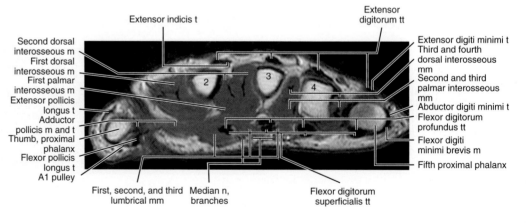

Extensor indicis t
Second dorsal
interosseous m
First dorsal
interosseous m
First palmar
interosseous m
Extensor pollicis
longus t
Adductor
pollicis m and t
Thumb, proximal
phalanx

Extensor digitorum tt
Extensor digiti minimi t
Third and fourth
dorsal interosseous mm
Second and third
palmar interosseous mm
Abductor digiti minimi t
Flexor digitorum
profundus tt
Flexor digiti minimi
brevis m

Flexor pollicis
longus t

Median n,
branches

Flexor digitorum
superficialis tt

Volar plate
sesamoid

Figure 8.1.10

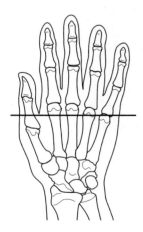

Extensor indicis t

Extensor
digitorum tt

Second dorsal
interosseous m
First dorsal
interosseous m
First palmar
interosseous m
Extensor pollicis
longus t
Adductor
pollicis m and t
Thumb, proximal
phalanx
Flexor pollicis
longus t
A1 pulley

Extensor digiti minimi t
Third and fourth
dorsal interosseous
mm
Second and third
palmar interosseous
mm
Abductor digiti minimi t
Flexor digitorum
profundus tt
Flexor digiti
minimi brevis m
Fifth proximal phalanx

First, second, and third
lumbrical mm

Median n,
branches

Flexor digitorum
superficialis tt

Figure 8.1.11

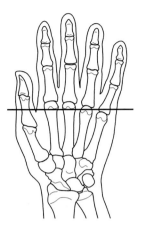

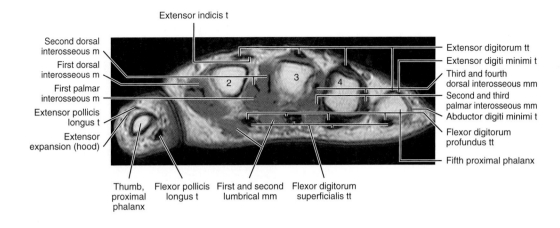

Extensor indicis t

Second dorsal interosseous m

First dorsal interosseous m

First palmar interosseous m

Extensor pollicis longus t

Extensor expansion (hood)

Extensor digitorum tt

Extensor digiti minimi t

Third and fourth dorsal interosseous mm

Second and third palmar interosseous mm

Abductor digiti minimi t

Flexor digitorum profundus tt

Fifth proximal phalanx

Thumb, proximal phalanx

Flexor pollicis longus t

First and second lumbrical mm

Flexor digitorum superficialis tt

Figure 8.1.12

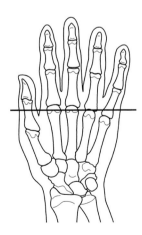

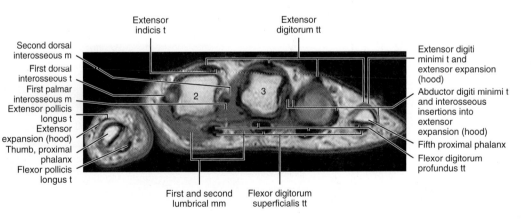

Extensor indicis t

Extensor digitorum tt

Second dorsal interosseous m

First dorsal interosseous t

First palmar interosseous m

Extensor pollicis longus t

Extensor expansion (hood)

Thumb, proximal phalanx

Flexor pollicis longus t

Extensor digiti minimi t and extensor expansion (hood)

Abductor digiti minimi t and interosseous insertions into extensor expansion (hood)

Fifth proximal phalanx

Flexor digitorum profundus tt

First and second lumbrical mm

Flexor digitorum superficialis tt

Figure 8.1.13

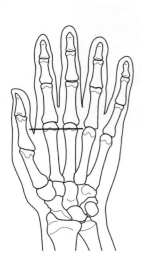

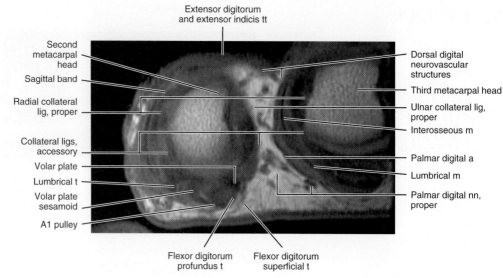

Extensor digitorum
and extensor indicis tt

Second
metacarpal
head

Sagittal band

Radial collateral
lig, proper

Collateral ligs,
accessory

Volar plate

Lumbrical t

Volar plate
sesamoid

A1 pulley

Dorsal digital
neurovascular
structures

Third metacarpal head

Ulnar collateral lig,
proper

Interosseous m

Palmar digital a

Lumbrical m

Palmar digital nn,
proper

Flexor digitorum
profundus t

Flexor digitorum
superficial t

Figure 8.1.14

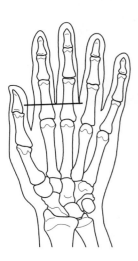

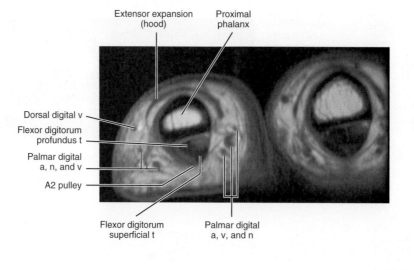

Extensor expansion
(hood)

Proximal
phalanx

Dorsal digital v

Flexor digitorum
profundus t

Palmar digital
a, n, and v

A2 pulley

Flexor digitorum
superficial t

Palmar digital
a, v, and n

SAGITTAL

Figure 8.2.1

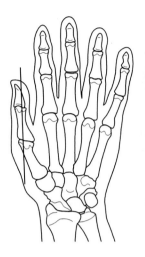

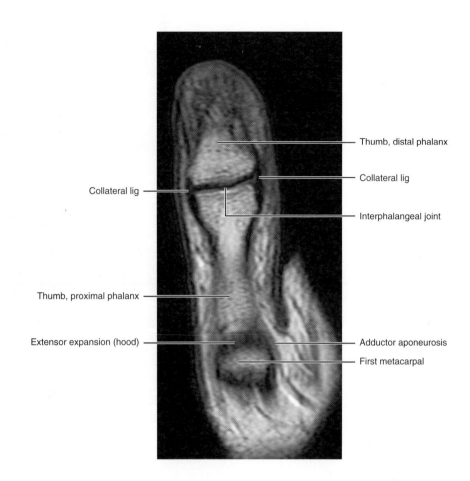

Collateral lig

Thumb, distal phalanx

Collateral lig

Interphalangeal joint

Thumb, proximal phalanx

Extensor expansion (hood)

Adductor aponeurosis

First metacarpal

Figure 8.2.2

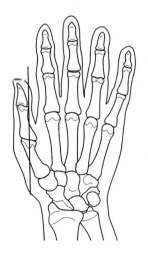

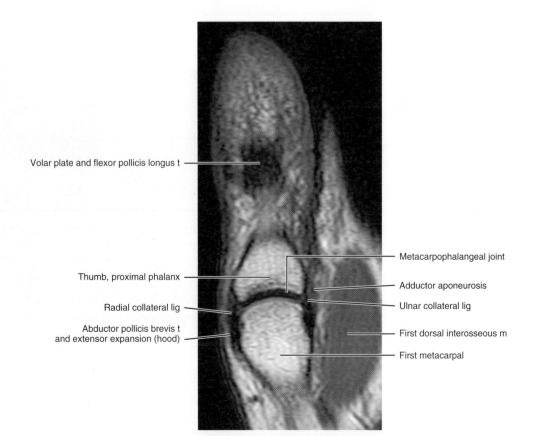

Volar plate and flexor pollicis longus t

Metacarpophalangeal joint

Thumb, proximal phalanx

Adductor aponeurosis

Radial collateral lig

Ulnar collateral lig

Abductor pollicis brevis t
and extensor expansion (hood)

First dorsal interosseous m

First metacarpal

Figure 8.2.3

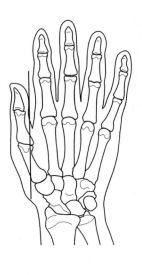

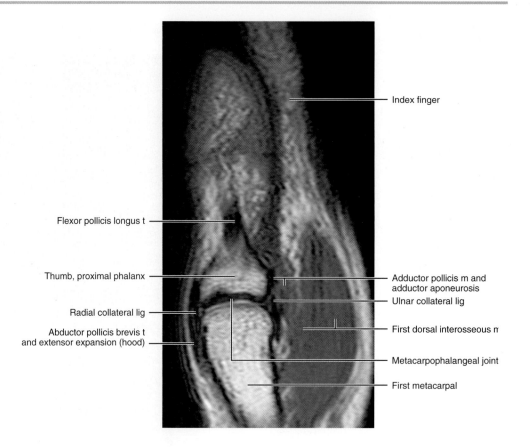

Index finger

Flexor pollicis longus t

Thumb, proximal phalanx

Adductor pollicis m and adductor aponeurosis

Ulnar collateral lig

Radial collateral lig

First dorsal interosseous m

Abductor pollicis brevis t and extensor expansion (hood)

Metacarpophalangeal joint

First metacarpal

Figure 8.2.4

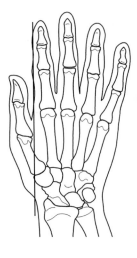

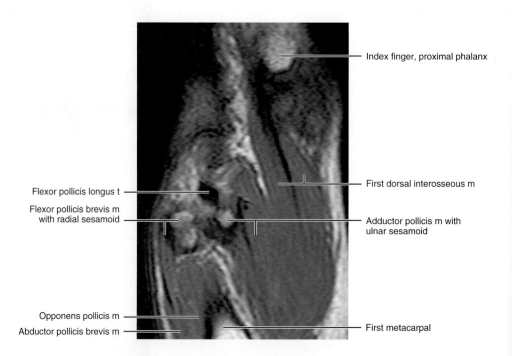

Index finger, proximal phalanx

Flexor pollicis longus t

First dorsal interosseous m

Flexor pollicis brevis m with radial sesamoid

Adductor pollicis m with ulnar sesamoid

Opponens pollicis m

Abductor pollicis brevis m

First metacarpal

Figure 8.2.5

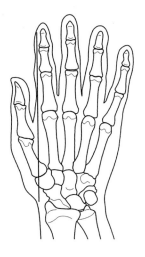

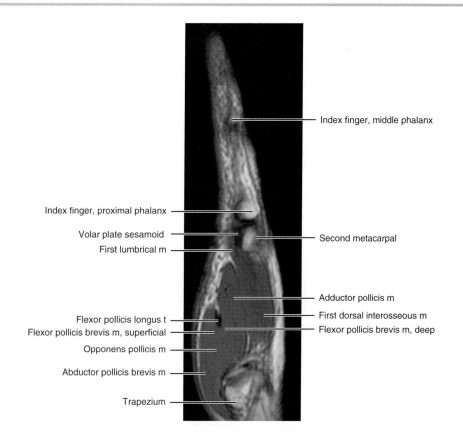

Index finger, middle phalanx

Index finger, proximal phalanx

Volar plate sesamoid

First lumbrical m

Second metacarpal

Adductor pollicis m

First dorsal interosseous m

Flexor pollicis longus t

Flexor pollicis brevis m, superficial

Flexor pollicis brevis m, deep

Opponens pollicis m

Abductor pollicis brevis m

Trapezium

Figure 8.2.6

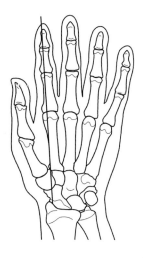

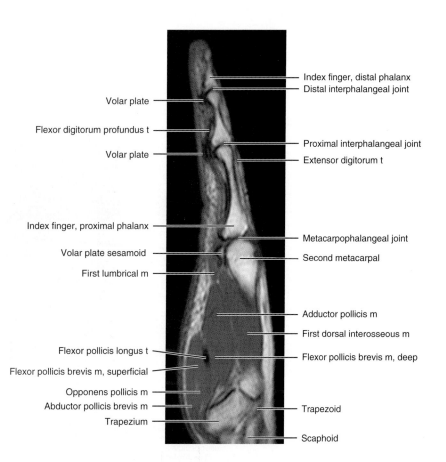

Index finger, distal phalanx

Distal interphalangeal joint

Volar plate

Flexor digitorum profundus t

Proximal interphalangeal joint

Volar plate

Extensor digitorum t

Index finger, proximal phalanx

Metacarpophalangeal joint

Volar plate sesamoid

Second metacarpal

First lumbrical m

Adductor pollicis m

First dorsal interosseous m

Flexor pollicis longus t

Flexor pollicis brevis m, deep

Flexor pollicis brevis m, superficial

Opponens pollicis m

Abductor pollicis brevis m

Trapezoid

Trapezium

Scaphoid

Figure 8.2.7

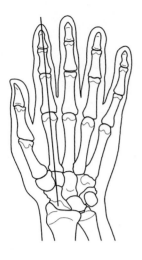

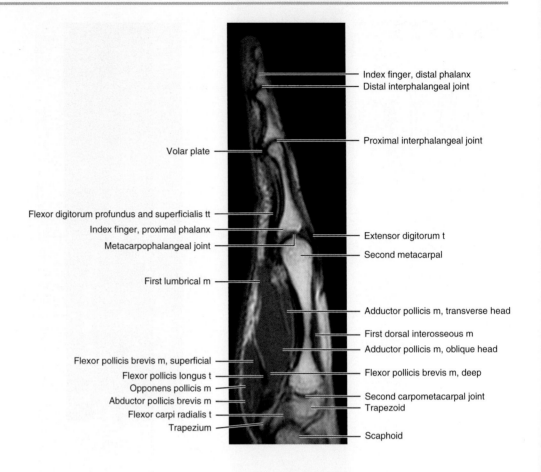

Index finger, distal phalanx
Distal interphalangeal joint

Proximal interphalangeal joint

Volar plate

Flexor digitorum profundus and superficialis tt
Index finger, proximal phalanx
Metacarpophalangeal joint

Extensor digitorum t
Second metacarpal

First lumbrical m

Adductor pollicis m, transverse head
First dorsal interosseous m
Adductor pollicis m, oblique head

Flexor pollicis brevis m, superficial
Flexor pollicis longus t
Opponens pollicis m
Abductor pollicis brevis m
Flexor carpi radialis t
Trapezium

Flexor pollicis brevis m, deep
Second carpometacarpal joint
Trapezoid
Scaphoid

Figure 8.2.8

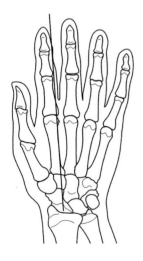

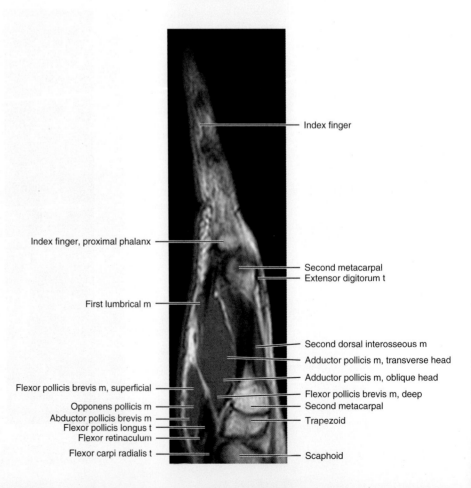

Index finger

Index finger, proximal phalanx

Second metacarpal
Extensor digitorum t

First lumbrical m

Second dorsal interosseous m
Adductor pollicis m, transverse head
Adductor pollicis m, oblique head

Flexor pollicis brevis m, superficial
Opponens pollicis m
Abductor pollicis brevis m
Flexor pollicis longus t
Flexor retinaculum
Flexor carpi radialis t

Flexor pollicis brevis m, deep
Second metacarpal
Trapezoid

Scaphoid

Figure 8.2.9

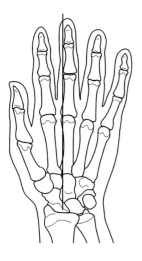

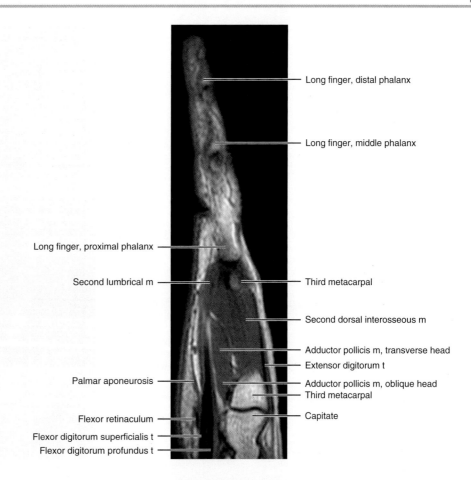

Long finger, distal phalanx

Long finger, middle phalanx

Long finger, proximal phalanx

Second lumbrical m

Third metacarpal

Second dorsal interosseous m

Adductor pollicis m, transverse head
Extensor digitorum t
Palmar aponeurosis
Adductor pollicis m, oblique head
Third metacarpal

Flexor retinaculum
Capitate
Flexor digitorum superficialis t
Flexor digitorum profundus t

Figure 8.2.10

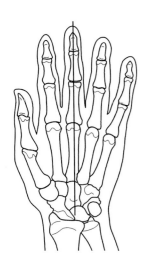

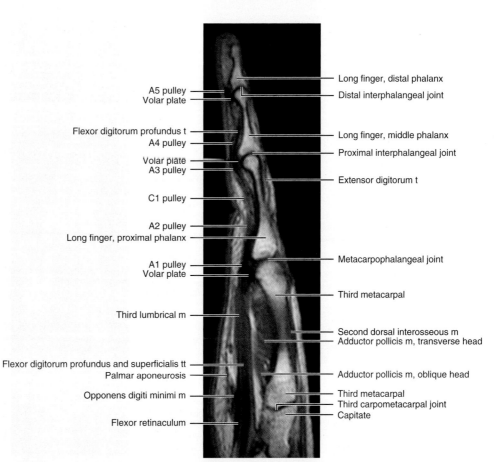

A5 pulley
Volar plate
Long finger, distal phalanx
Distal interphalangeal joint

Flexor digitorum profundus t
A4 pulley
Long finger, middle phalanx
Volar plate
Proximal interphalangeal joint
A3 pulley

C1 pulley
Extensor digitorum t

A2 pulley
Long finger, proximal phalanx

A1 pulley
Volar plate
Metacarpophalangeal joint

Third metacarpal

Third lumbrical m

Second dorsal interosseous m
Adductor pollicis m, transverse head

Flexor digitorum profundus and superficialis tt
Palmar aponeurosis
Adductor pollicis m, oblique head

Opponens digiti minimi m
Third metacarpal
Third carpometacarpal joint
Capitate

Flexor retinaculum

Figure 8.2.11

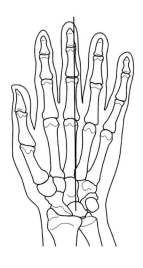

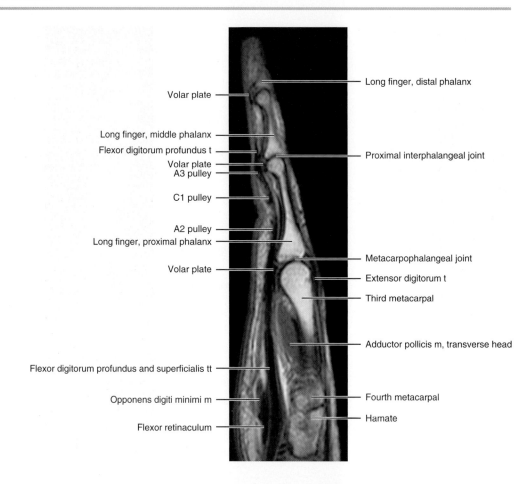

Volar plate — Long finger, distal phalanx

Long finger, middle phalanx
Flexor digitorum profundus t — Proximal interphalangeal joint
Volar plate
A3 pulley

C1 pulley

A2 pulley
Long finger, proximal phalanx — Metacarpophalangeal joint

Volar plate — Extensor digitorum t
— Third metacarpal

— Adductor pollicis m, transverse head

Flexor digitorum profundus and superficialis tt

Opponens digiti minimi m — Fourth metacarpal
— Hamate
Flexor retinaculum

Figure 8.2.12

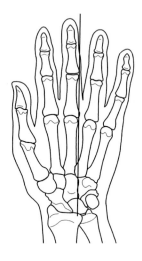

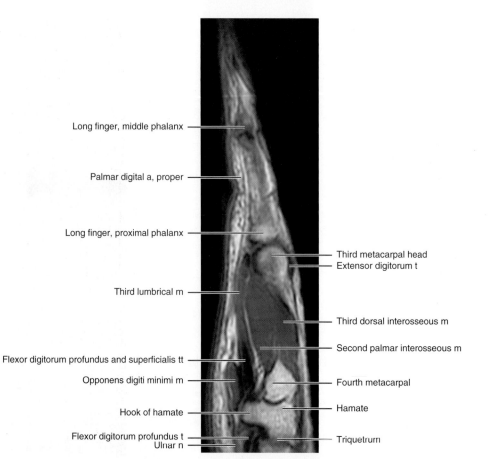

Long finger, middle phalanx

Palmar digital a, proper

Long finger, proximal phalanx — Third metacarpal head
— Extensor digitorum t

Third lumbrical m

— Third dorsal interosseous m

— Second palmar interosseous m

Flexor digitorum profundus and superficialis tt
Opponens digiti minimi m — Fourth metacarpal

Hook of hamate — Hamate

Flexor digitorum profundus t — Triquetrum
Ulnar n

Figure 8.2.13

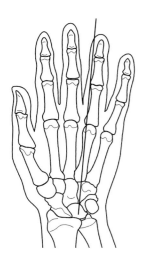

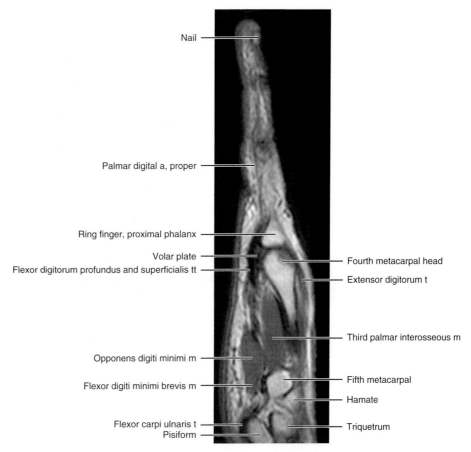

- Nail
- Palmar digital a, proper
- Ring finger, proximal phalanx
- Volar plate
- Flexor digitorum profundus and superficialis tt
- Fourth metacarpal head
- Extensor digitorum t
- Third palmar interosseous m
- Opponens digiti minimi m
- Flexor digiti minimi brevis m
- Fifth metacarpal
- Hamate
- Flexor carpi ulnaris t
- Pisiform
- Triquetrum

Figure 8.2.14

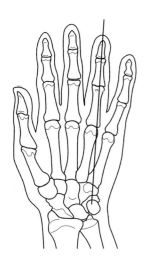

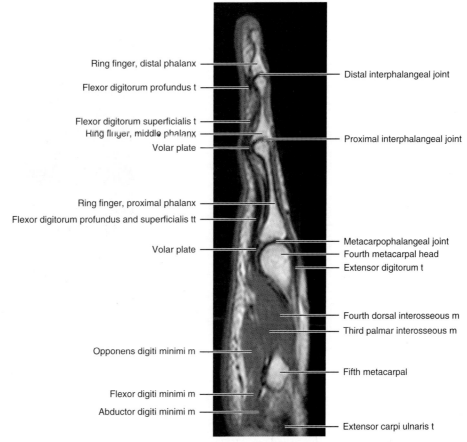

- Ring finger, distal phalanx
- Flexor digitorum profundus t
- Distal interphalangeal joint
- Flexor digitorum superficialis t
- Ring finger, middle phalanx
- Volar plate
- Proximal interphalangeal joint
- Ring finger, proximal phalanx
- Flexor digitorum profundus and superficialis tt
- Volar plate
- Metacarpophalangeal joint
- Fourth metacarpal head
- Extensor digitorum t
- Fourth dorsal interosseous m
- Third palmar interosseous m
- Opponens digiti minimi m
- Fifth metacarpal
- Flexor digiti minimi m
- Abductor digiti minimi m
- Extensor carpi ulnaris t

Figure 8.2.15

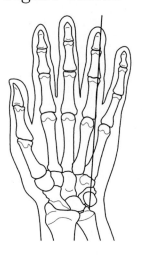

Ring finger, distal phalanx

Ring finger, middle phalanx
Flexor digitorum profundus and superficialis tt
Volar plate

Proximal interphalangeal joint

Ring finger, proximal phalanx

Fourth lumbrical m

Flexor digitorum profundus and superficialis tt

Fourth metacarpal head

Extensor digitorum and extensor digiti minimi tt

Third palmar interosseous m
Fourth dorsal interosseous m

Opponens digiti minimi m

Flexor digiti minimi m

Abductor digiti minimi m

Fifth metacarpal

Extensor carpi ulnaris t

Figure 8.2.16

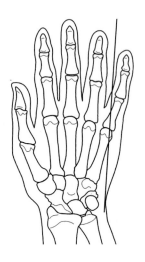
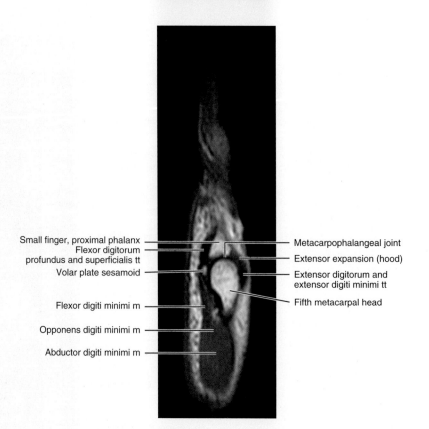

Small finger, proximal phalanx
Flexor digitorum profundus and superficialis tt
Volar plate sesamoid

Metacarpophalangeal joint
Extensor expansion (hood)
Extensor digitorum and extensor digiti minimi tt

Flexor digiti minimi m

Fifth metacarpal head

Opponens digiti minimi m

Abductor digiti minimi m

Figure 8.2.17

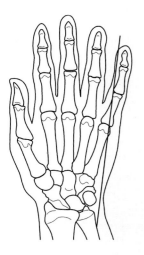

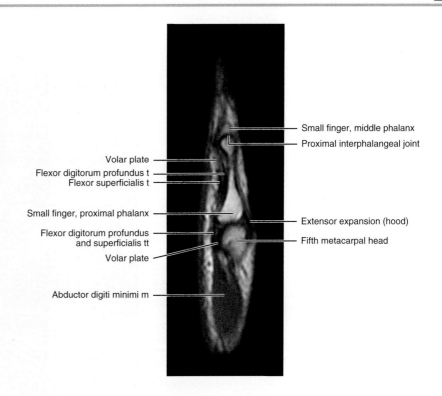

Small finger, middle phalanx
Proximal interphalangeal joint

Volar plate
Flexor digitorum profundus t
Flexor superficialis t

Small finger, proximal phalanx

Extensor expansion (hood)

Flexor digitorum profundus
and superficialis tt

Fifth metacarpal head

Volar plate

Abductor digiti minimi m

Figure 8.2.18

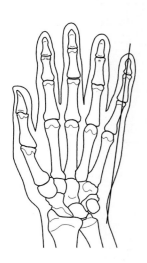

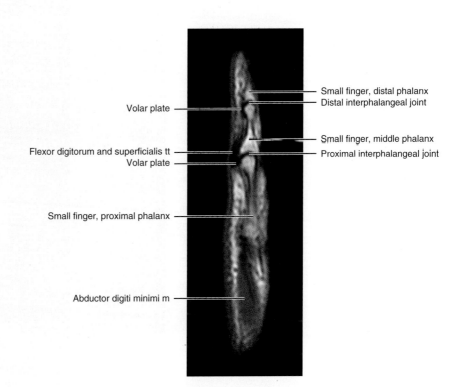

Volar plate

Small finger, distal phalanx
Distal interphalangeal joint

Small finger, middle phalanx
Proximal interphalangeal joint

Flexor digitorum and superficialis tt
Volar plate

Small finger, proximal phalanx

Abductor digiti minimi m

CORONAL
Figure 8.3.1

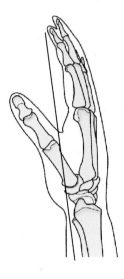

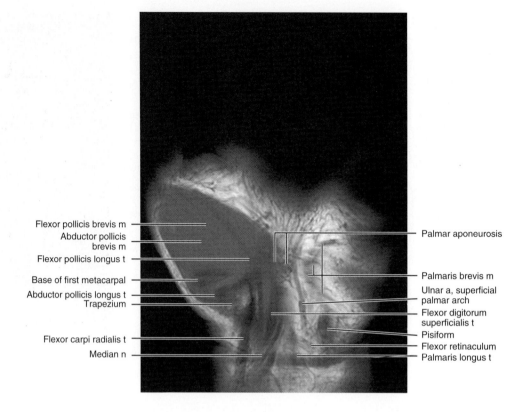

Flexor pollicis brevis m

Abductor pollicis brevis m

Flexor pollicis longus t

Base of first metacarpal

Abductor pollicis longus t

Trapezium

Flexor carpi radialis t

Median n

Palmar aponeurosis

Palmaris brevis m

Ulnar a, superficial palmar arch

Flexor digitorum superficialis t

Pisiform

Flexor retinaculum

Palmaris longus t

Figure 8.3.2

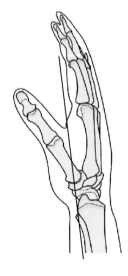

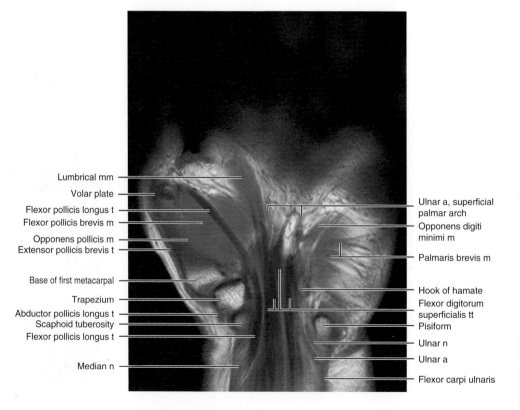

Lumbrical mm

Volar plate

Flexor pollicis longus t

Flexor pollicis brevis m

Opponens pollicis m

Extensor pollicis brevis t

Base of first metacarpal

Trapezium

Abductor pollicis longus t

Scaphoid tuberosity

Flexor pollicis longus t

Median n

Ulnar a, superficial palmar arch

Opponens digiti minimi m

Palmaris brevis m

Hook of hamate

Flexor digitorum superficialis tt

Pisiform

Ulnar n

Ulnar a

Flexor carpi ulnaris

Figure 8.3.3

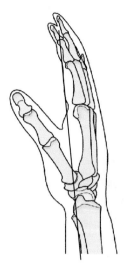

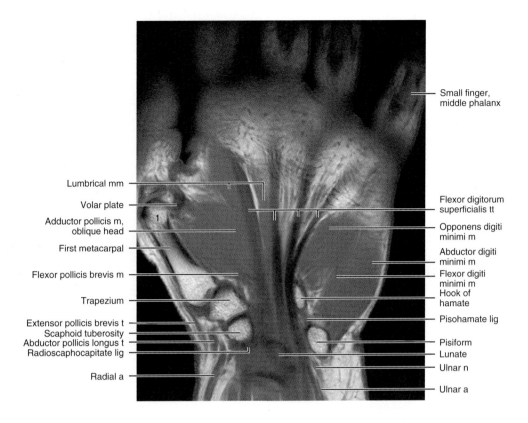

Lumbrical mm

Volar plate

Adductor pollicis m, oblique head

First metacarpal

Flexor pollicis brevis m

Trapezium

Extensor pollicis brevis t
Scaphoid tuberosity
Abductor pollicis longus t
Radioscaphocapitate lig

Radial a

Small finger, middle phalanx

Flexor digitorum superficialis tt

Opponens digiti minimi m

Abductor digiti minimi m

Flexor digiti minimi m

Hook of hamate

Pisohamate lig

Pisiform

Lunate

Ulnar n

Ulnar a

Figure 8.3.4

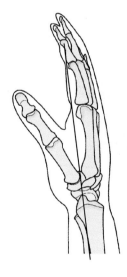

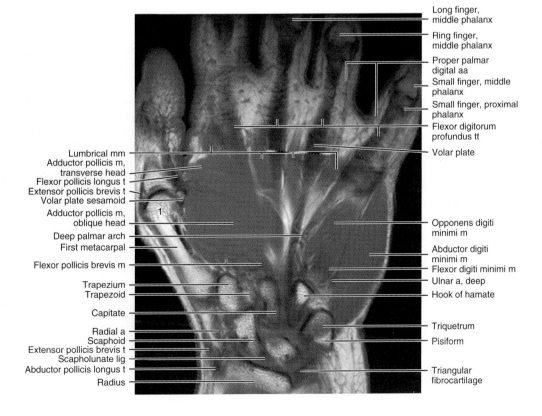

Lumbrical mm
Adductor pollicis m, transverse head
Flexor pollicis longus t
Extensor pollicis brevis t
Volar plate sesamoid
Adductor pollicis m, oblique head

Deep palmar arch
First metacarpal

Flexor pollicis brevis m

Trapezium
Trapezoid

Capitate

Radial a
Scaphoid
Extensor pollicis brevis t
Scapholunate lig
Abductor pollicis longus t

Radius

Long finger, middle phalanx

Ring finger, middle phalanx

Proper palmar digital aa

Small finger, middle phalanx

Small finger, proximal phalanx

Flexor digitorum profundus tt

Volar plate

Opponens digiti minimi m

Abductor digiti minimi m

Flexor digiti minimi m

Ulnar a, deep

Hook of hamate

Triquetrum

Pisiform

Triangular fibrocartilage

Figure 8.3.5

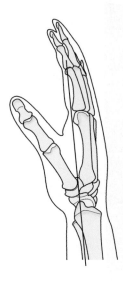

Palmar digital aa, proper
Index finger, proximal phalanx
Thumb, distal phalanx
Collateral ligs, accessory

Thumb, proximal phalanx
Interosseous tt
Adductor pollicis m, transverse head
Flexor pollicis longus t
Volar plate
Extensor pollicis brevis t
Adductor pollicis m, oblique head
First dorsal interosseous m
Deep palmar arch
Base of second, third, fourth, and fifth metacarpals
Trapezium
Trapezoid
Radial a
Intercarpal lig
Capitate
Scaphoid
Radial styloid
Scapholunate lig
Radius
Extensor pollicis brevis t

Long finger, proximal phalanx
Ring finger, proximal phalanx
Small finger, middle phalanx
Small finger, proximal phalanx
Part of extensor expansion (hood)
Collateral ligs, accessory
Fifth metacarpal head
Second palmar interosseous m
Fourth dorsal interosseous m
Third palmar interosseous m
Opponens digiti minimi m
Abductor digiti minimi m
Extensor carpi ulnaris t
Hamate
Triquetrum
Lunate
Triangular fibrocartilage, meniscus homologue

Figure 8.3.6

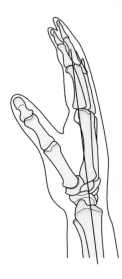

Index finger, proximal phalanx
Thumb, distal phalanx
Ulnar collateral ligs, accessory
Extensor pollicis longus t
Radial collateral ligs, accessory
First dorsal interosseous t
Joint capsule
Interosseous tt
Thumb, proximal phalanx
First palmar interosseous m
Second dorsal interosseous m
Deep palmar arch
First dorsal interosseous m
Extensor pollicis longus t
Base of second, third, fourth, and fifth metacarpals
Extensor carpi radialis longus t
Radial a
Trapezoid
Intercarpal lig
Capitate
Dorsal trapezotriquetral lig
Scaphoid
Radial styloid
Lunate
Radius
Extensor pollicis brevis t

Part of extensor expansion (hood)
Long finger, proximal phalanx
Ring finger, proximal phalanx
Radial and ulnar collateral ligs, proper
Radial and ulnar collateral ligs, proper
Third dorsal interosseous m
Fourth dorsal interosseous m
Hamate
Extensor carpi ulnaris t
Triquetrum
Triangular fibrocartilage
Ulnar styloid
Ulna

Figure 8.3.7

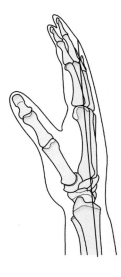

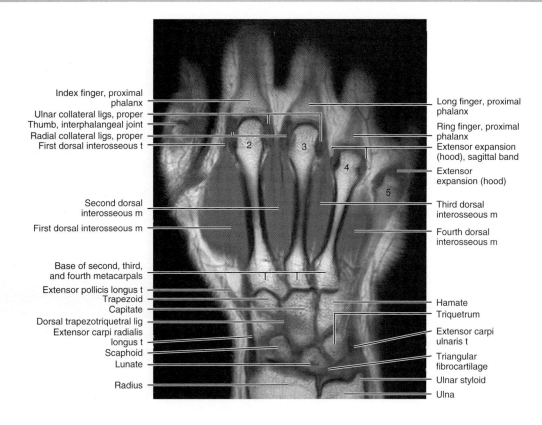

Index finger, proximal phalanx
Ulnar collateral ligs, proper
Thumb, interphalangeal joint
Radial collateral ligs, proper
First dorsal interosseous t

Long finger, proximal phalanx
Ring finger, proximal phalanx
Extensor expansion (hood), sagittal band
Extensor expansion (hood)

Second dorsal interosseous m
First dorsal interosseous m

Third dorsal interosseous m
Fourth dorsal interosseous m

Base of second, third, and fourth metacarpals
Extensor pollicis longus t
Trapezoid
Capitate
Dorsal trapezotriquetral lig
Extensor carpi radialis longus t
Scaphoid
Lunate
Radius

Hamate
Triquetrum
Extensor carpi ulnaris t
Triangular fibrocartilage
Ulnar styloid
Ulna

Figure 8.3.8

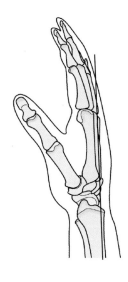

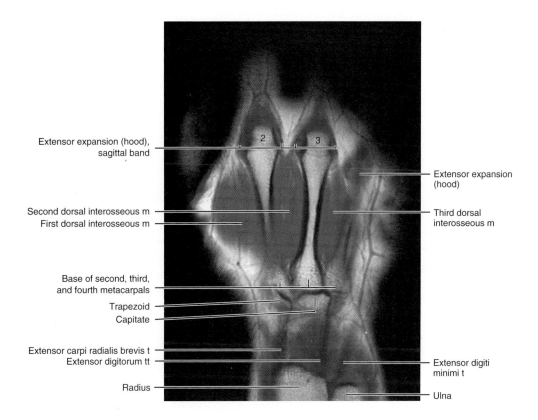

Extensor expansion (hood), sagittal band

Extensor expansion (hood)

Second dorsal interosseous m
First dorsal interosseous m

Third dorsal interosseous m

Base of second, third, and fourth metacarpals
Trapezoid
Capitate

Extensor carpi radialis brevis t
Extensor digitorum tt
Radius

Extensor digiti minimi t
Ulna

Figure 8.3.9

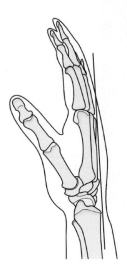

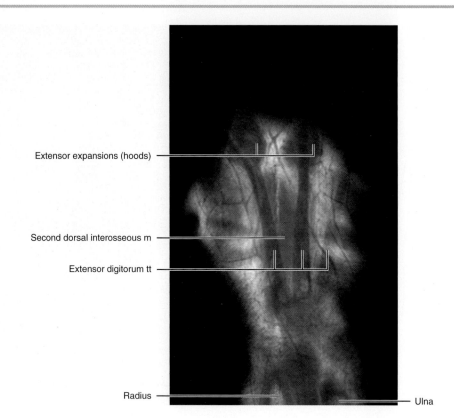

Extensor expansions (hoods) —

Second dorsal interosseous m —

Extensor digitorum tt —

Radius —

Ulna

Lower Extremity

Chapter 9

MRI of the Hip

Table 5: Muscles of the Hip

MUSCLE	ORIGIN	INSERTION	NERVE SUPPLY
Obturator internus	Pelvic surface of the pubic rami near the obturator foramen, pelvic surface of the ischium between the foramen and the greater sciatic notch, deep surface of the obturator internus fascia, fibrous arch that surrounds the foramen for obturator vessels and nerve, most of the pelvic surface of the obturator membrane except the lower part	Medial side of the greater trochanter in front of the trochanteric fossa of the femur	Nerve to the obturator internus, from the lumbosacral trunk, and first and second sacral
Obturator externus	Lateral surface of the pubic and ischial rami, where they surround the obturator membrane, lateral surface of the obturator membrane	Trochanteric fossa	Obturator
Gemellus superior	Outer surface of the ischial spine and edge of the lesser sciatic notch	After union with the tendon of the obturator internus, inserts into the medial side of the greater trochanter in front of the trochanteric fossa	By a small nerve, branch of the to the obturator nerve internus or branch of the nerve to the quadratus femoris
Gemellus inferior	Upper part of the inner border of the tuberosity of the ischium, sacrotuberous ligament, and edge of the lesser sciatic notch	By union with the tendon of the obturator internus or with the tendon onto the greater trochanter below the obturator internus muscle	By a small nerve, branch of the nerve to the quadratus femoris
Quadratus femoris	Upper part of the outer border of the tuberosity of the ischium	Onto the inferior dorsal angle of the greater trochanter	Lumbosacral trunk and first sacral
Psoas major	By a series of thick fasciculi from the intervertebral discs and bodies between T12 and L5, from the bodies of L1 to L4, and from slender fascicles from the ventral surfaces of the transverse processes of the lumbar vertebrae	Inserts onto the lesser trochanter of the femur	Branches from L1 (often), L2, L3, and L4
Iliacus	Iliac crest, iliolumbar ligament, iliac fossa, anterior sacroiliac ligaments, often from the ala of the sacrum, and from the ventral border of the ilium between the two anterior spines	Lateral surface of the psoas tendon (above the inguinal ligament) onto the femur immediately distal to the lesser trochanter; the lateral portion arises from the ventral border of the ilium and is attached to the tendon of the rectus femoris and the capsule of the hip joint	Femoral and L1 to L4

Table 5: Muscles of the Hip—Cont'd

MUSCLE	ORIGIN	INSERTION	NERVE SUPPLY
Tensor fasciae latae	Anterior superior iliac spine and anterior part of the external lip of the iliac crest	Muscle fibers pass distally in parallel array, unite with the tendon, and join the iliotibial tract about one third of the way down the thigh	Superior gluteal
Gluteus medius	Ventral three fourths of the iliac crest, outer surface of the ilium between the anterior and posterior gluteal lines, and from the investing fascia	Onto the posterosuperior angle and the external surface of the greater trochanter	Superior gluteal (L4, L5, S1)
Piriformis	Lateral part of the ventral surface of S2, S3, and S4, posterior border of the greater sciatic notch, from the sacrotuberous ligament near the sacrum	Onto the anterior and inner parts of the upper border of the greater trochanter	S1 or S2 or from a loop between S1 and S2
Gluteus maximus	Dorsal fifth of the outer lip of the iliac crest, ilium dorsal to the posterior gluteal line, thoracolumbar fascia between the posterior superior spine of the ilium and the side of the sacrum, lateral parts of S4, S5, and coccygeal vertebrae, and from the back of the sacrotuberous ligament	Into the iliotibial tract, gluteal tuberosity of the femur, adjacent part of the tendinous origin of the vastus lateralis	Inferior gluteal by two branches from the sacral plexus (separately or as a united nerve)
Gluteus minimus	Outer surface of the ilium between the anterior and inferior gluteal lines, from the septum between the gluteus minimus and the gluteus medius near the anterior superior, iliac spine and the capsule of the hip joint	Onto the anterior border of the greater trochanter of the femur	Superior gluteal from a branch that supplies the tensor fasciae latae
Biceps femoris, long head	Medial facet on the posterior surface of the ischial tuberosity and sacrotuberous ligament	By a tendon that extends to the lateral condyle of the femur	Tibial part of the sciatic
Semitendinosus	Distal margin of the ischial tuberosity and from the tendon common to it and the long head of the biceps femoris	By a triangular tendinous expansion into the proximal part of the medial surface of the tibia behind and distal to the insertion of the gracilis	Sciatic or directly from the lumbosacral plexus by two nerves: from S1 and S2 and from L5 and S1
Semimembranosus	Lateral facet on the posterior surface of the ischial tuberosity	Posterior aspect of the medial tibial condyle	Sciatic branch (also supplies the adductor magnus)

AXIAL

Figure 9.1.1

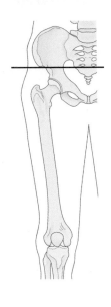

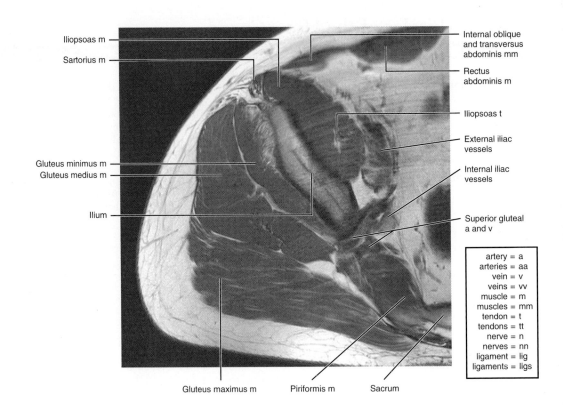

Iliopsoas m

Sartorius m

Internal oblique and transversus abdominis mm

Rectus abdominis m

Iliopsoas t

External iliac vessels

Internal iliac vessels

Gluteus minimus m

Gluteus medius m

Ilium

Superior gluteal a and v

artery	= a
arteries	= aa
vein	= v
veins	= vv
muscle	= m
muscles	= mm
tendon	= t
tendons	= tt
nerve	= n
nerves	= nn
ligament	= lig
ligaments	= ligs

Gluteus maximus m

Piriformis m

Sacrum

Figure 9.1.2

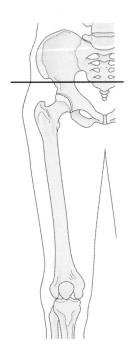

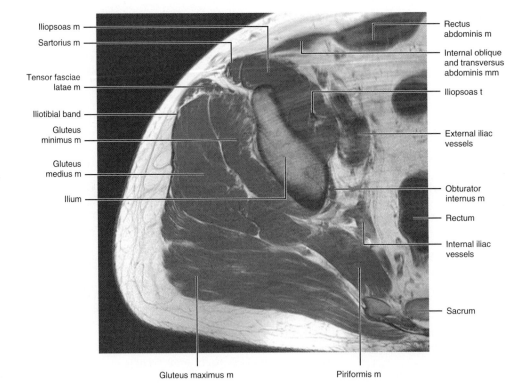

Iliopsoas m

Sartorius m

Tensor fasciae latae m

Iliotibial band

Gluteus minimus m

Gluteus medius m

Ilium

Rectus abdominis m

Internal oblique and transversus abdominis mm

Iliopsoas t

External iliac vessels

Obturator internus m

Rectum

Internal iliac vessels

Sacrum

Gluteus maximus m

Piriformis m

Figure 9.1.3

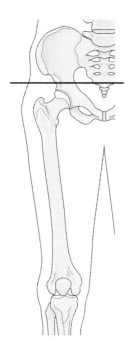

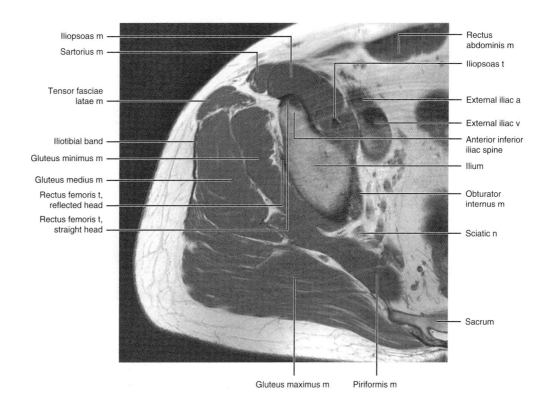

Iliopsoas m
Sartorius m
Tensor fasciae latae m
Iliotibial band
Gluteus minimus m
Gluteus medius m
Rectus femoris t, reflected head
Rectus femoris t, straight head

Rectus abdominis m
Iliopsoas t
External iliac a
External iliac v
Anterior inferior iliac spine
Ilium
Obturator internus m
Sciatic n
Sacrum

Gluteus maximus m   Piriformis m

Figure 9.1.4

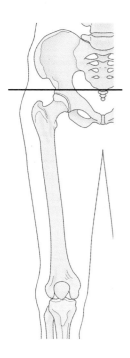

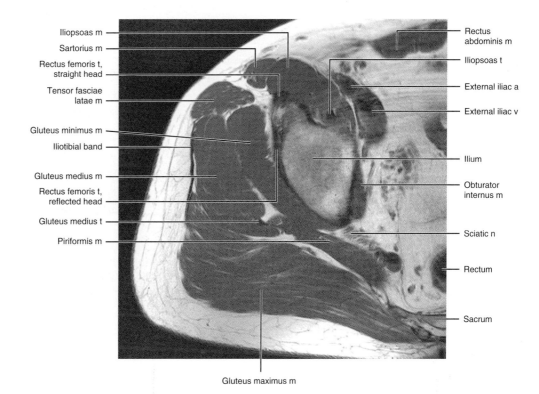

Iliopsoas m
Sartorius m
Rectus femoris t, straight head
Tensor fasciae latae m
Gluteus minimus m
Iliotibial band
Gluteus medius m
Rectus femoris t, reflected head
Gluteus medius t
Piriformis m

Rectus abdominis m
Iliopsoas t
External iliac a
External iliac v
Ilium
Obturator internus m
Sciatic n
Rectum
Sacrum

Gluteus maximus m

Figure 9.1.5

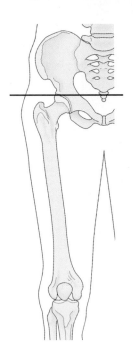

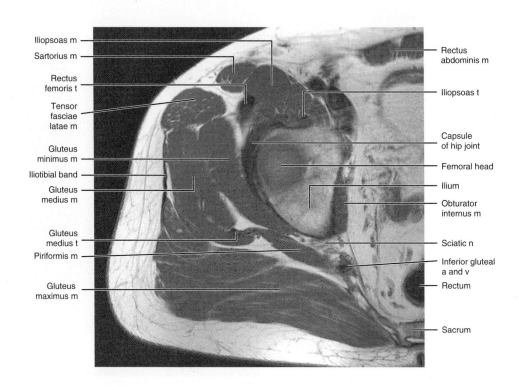

Iliopsoas m
Sartorius m
Rectus femoris t
Tensor fasciae latae m
Gluteus minimus m
Iliotibial band
Gluteus medius m
Gluteus medius t
Piriformis m
Gluteus maximus m

Rectus abdominis m
Iliopsoas t
Capsule of hip joint
Femoral head
Ilium
Obturator internus m
Sciatic n
Inferior gluteal a and v
Rectum
Sacrum

Figure 9.1.6

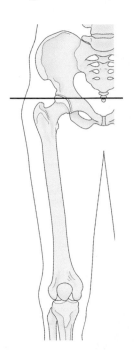

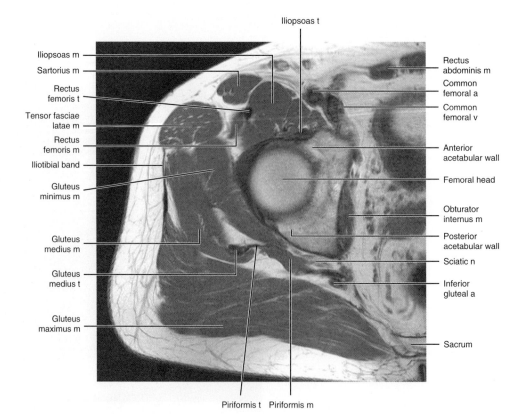

Iliopsoas t

Iliopsoas m
Sartorius m
Rectus femoris t
Tensor fasciae latae m
Rectus femoris m
Iliotibial band
Gluteus minimus m
Gluteus medius m
Gluteus medius t
Gluteus maximus m

Rectus abdominis m
Common femoral a
Common femoral v
Anterior acetabular wall
Femoral head
Obturator internus m
Posterior acetabular wall
Sciatic n
Inferior gluteal a
Sacrum

Piriformis t   Piriformis m

Figure 9.1.7

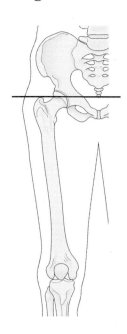

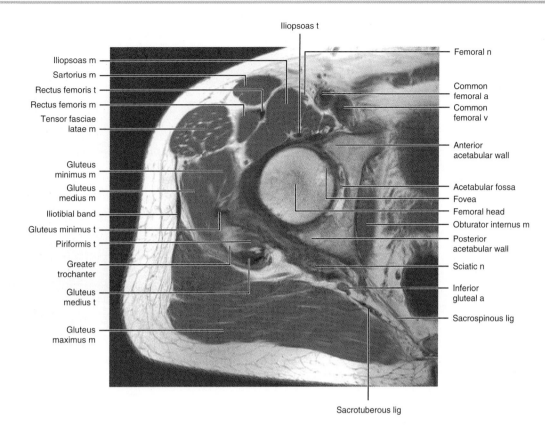

Iliopsoas t

Iliopsoas m
Sartorius m
Rectus femoris t
Rectus femoris m
Tensor fasciae latae m

Gluteus minimus m
Gluteus medius m
Iliotibial band
Gluteus minimus t
Piriformis t
Greater trochanter
Gluteus medius t
Gluteus maximus m

Femoral n
Common femoral a
Common femoral v
Anterior acetabular wall
Acetabular fossa
Fovea
Femoral head
Obturator internus m
Posterior acetabular wall
Sciatic n
Inferior gluteal a
Sacrospinous lig

Sacrotuberous lig

Figure 9.1.8

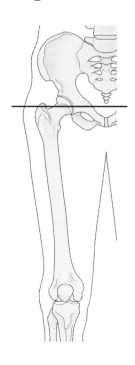

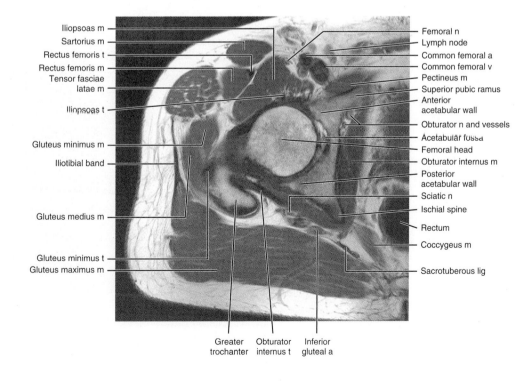

Iliopsoas m
Sartorius m
Rectus femoris t
Rectus femoris m
Tensor fasciae latae m
Iliopsoas t

Gluteus minimus m
Iliotibial band

Gluteus medius m

Gluteus minimus t
Gluteus maximus m

Femoral n
Lymph node
Common femoral a
Common femoral v
Pectineus m
Superior pubic ramus
Anterior acetabular wall
Obturator n and vessels
Acetabular fossa
Femoral head
Obturator internus m
Posterior acetabular wall
Sciatic n
Ischial spine
Rectum
Coccygeus m
Sacrotuberous lig

Greater trochanter　Obturator internus t　Inferior gluteal a

Figure 9.1.9

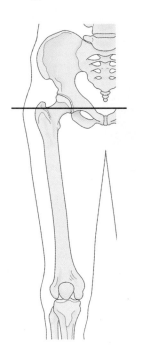

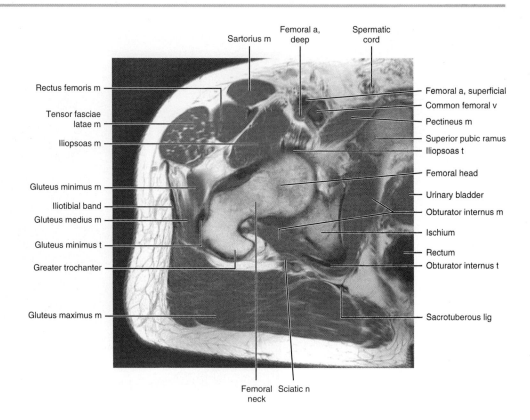

Sartorius m

Femoral a, deep

Spermatic cord

Rectus femoris m

Tensor fasciae latae m

Iliopsoas m

Gluteus minimus m

Iliotibial band

Gluteus medius m

Gluteus minimus t

Greater trochanter

Gluteus maximus m

Femoral a, superficial

Common femoral v

Pectineus m

Superior pubic ramus

Iliopsoas t

Femoral head

Urinary bladder

Obturator internus m

Ischium

Rectum

Obturator internus t

Sacrotuberous lig

Femoral neck

Sciatic n

Figure 9.1.10

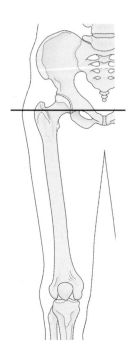

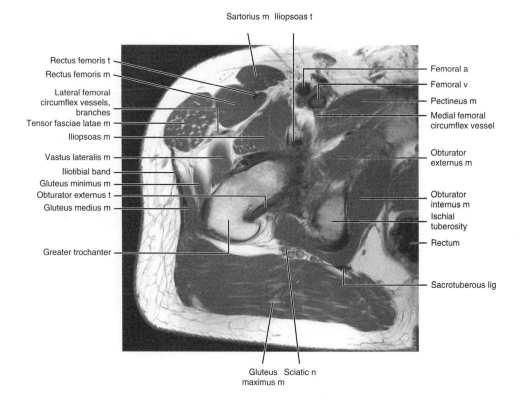

Sartorius m   Iliopsoas t

Rectus femoris t

Rectus femoris m

Lateral femoral circumflex vessels, branches

Tensor fasciae latae m

Iliopsoas m

Vastus lateralis m

Iliotibial band

Gluteus minimus m

Obturator externus t

Gluteus medius m

Greater trochanter

Femoral a

Femoral v

Pectineus m

Medial femoral circumflex vessel

Obturator externus m

Obturator internus m

Ischial tuberosity

Rectum

Sacrotuberous lig

Gluteus maximus m   Sciatic n

Figure 9.1.11

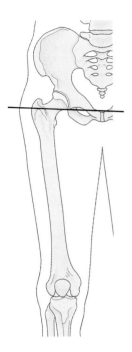

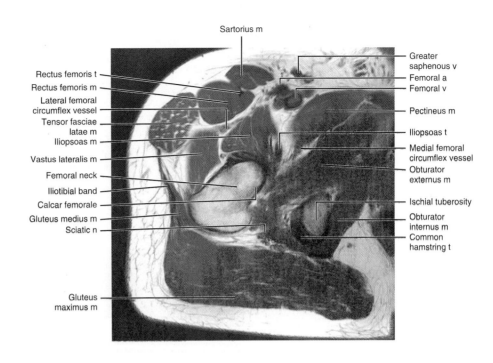

Sartorius m

Rectus femoris t
Rectus femoris m
Lateral femoral circumflex vessel
Tensor fasciae latae m
Iliopsoas m
Vastus lateralis m
Femoral neck
Iliotibial band
Calcar femorale
Gluteus medius m
Sciatic n

Gluteus maximus m

Greater saphenous v
Femoral a
Femoral v
Pectineus m
Iliopsoas t
Medial femoral circumflex vessel
Obturator externus m
Ischial tuberosity
Obturator internus m
Common hamstring t

Figure 9.1.12

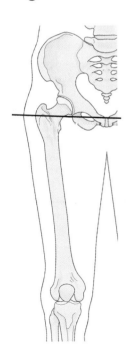

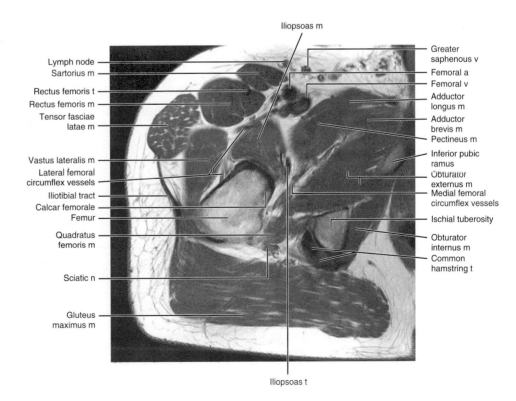

Iliopsoas m

Lymph node
Sartorius m
Rectus femoris t
Rectus femoris m
Tensor fasciae latae m
Vastus lateralis m
Lateral femoral circumflex vessels
Iliotibial tract
Calcar femorale
Femur
Quadratus femoris m
Sciatic n
Gluteus maximus m

Greater saphenous v
Femoral a
Femoral v
Adductor longus m
Adductor brevis m
Pectineus m
Inferior pubic ramus
Obturator externus m
Medial femoral circumflex vessels
Ischial tuberosity
Obturator internus m
Common hamstring t

Iliopsoas t

Figure 9.1.13

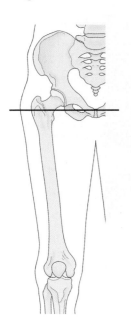

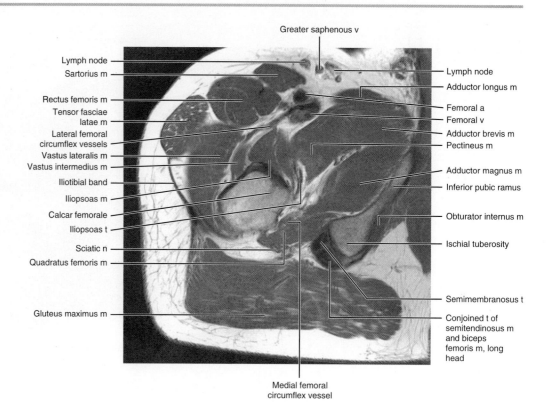

Greater saphenous v

Lymph node
Sartorius m

Rectus femoris m
Tensor fasciae latae m
Lateral femoral circumflex vessels
Vastus lateralis m
Vastus intermedius m
Iliotibial band
Iliopsoas m
Calcar femorale
Iliopsoas t
Sciatic n
Quadratus femoris m

Gluteus maximus m

Lymph node
Adductor longus m
Femoral a
Femoral v
Adductor brevis m
Pectineus m
Adductor magnus m
Inferior pubic ramus
Obturator internus m
Ischial tuberosity

Semimembranosus t
Conjoined t of semitendinosus m and biceps femoris m, long head

Medial femoral circumflex vessel

Figure 9.1.14

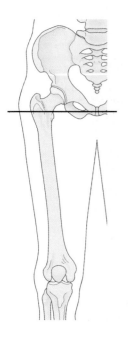

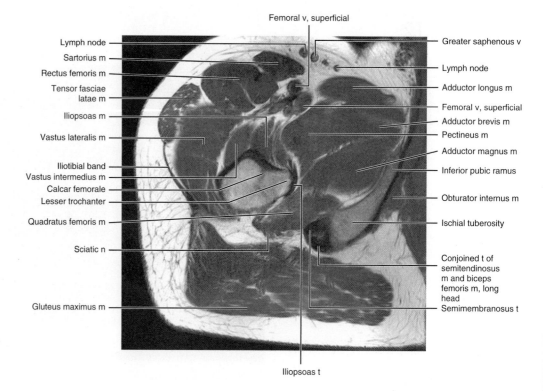

Femoral v, superficial

Lymph node
Sartorius m
Rectus femoris m
Tensor fasciae latae m
Iliopsoas m
Vastus lateralis m
Iliotibial band
Vastus intermedius m
Calcar femorale
Lesser trochanter
Quadratus femoris m
Sciatic n

Gluteus maximus m

Greater saphenous v
Lymph node
Adductor longus m
Femoral v, superficial
Adductor brevis m
Pectineus m
Adductor magnus m
Inferior pubic ramus
Obturator internus m
Ischial tuberosity
Conjoined t of semitendinosus m and biceps femoris m, long head
Semimembranosus t

Iliopsoas t

Figure 9.1.15

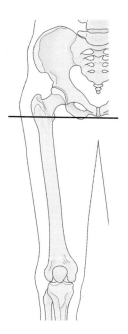

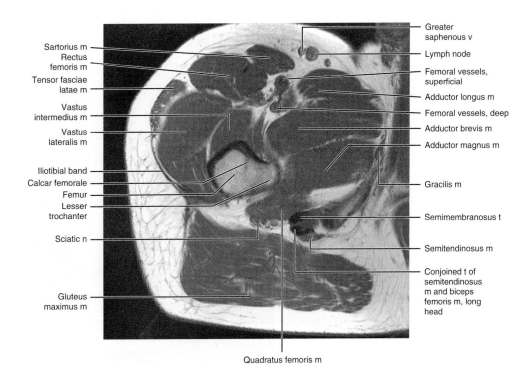

Sartorius m
Rectus femoris m
Tensor fasciae latae m
Vastus intermedius m
Vastus lateralis m
Iliotibial band
Calcar femorale
Femur
Lesser trochanter
Sciatic n
Gluteus maximus m

Greater saphenous v
Lymph node
Femoral vessels, superficial
Adductor longus m
Femoral vessels, deep
Adductor brevis m
Adductor magnus m
Gracilis m
Semimembranosus t
Semitendinosus m
Conjoined t of semitendinosus m and biceps femoris m, long head

Quadratus femoris m

Figure 9.1.16

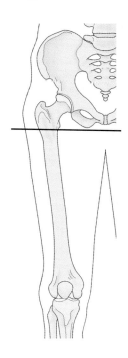

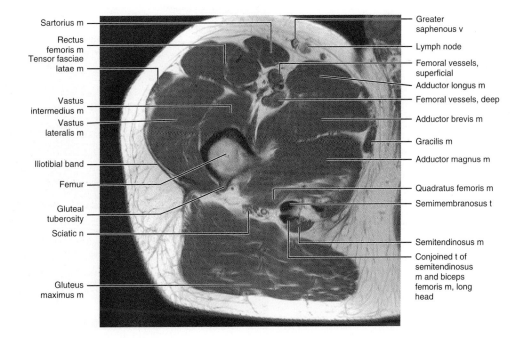

Sartorius m
Rectus femoris m
Tensor fasciae latae m
Vastus intermedius m
Vastus lateralis m
Iliotibial band
Femur
Gluteal tuberosity
Sciatic n
Gluteus maximus m

Greater saphenous v
Lymph node
Femoral vessels, superficial
Adductor longus m
Femoral vessels, deep
Adductor brevis m
Gracilis m
Adductor magnus m
Quadratus femoris m
Semimembranosus t
Semitendinosus m
Conjoined t of semitendinosus m and biceps femoris m, long head

Figure 9.1.17

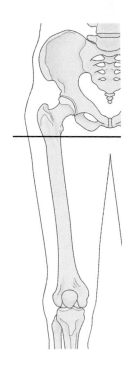

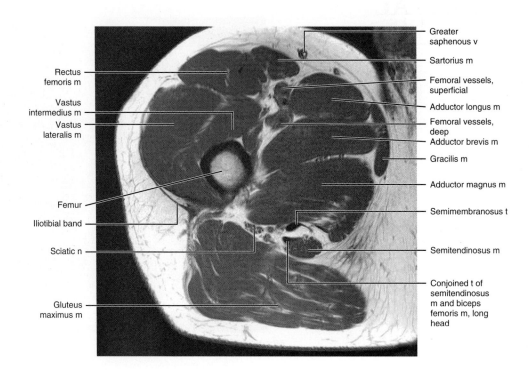

Rectus femoris m
Vastus intermedius m
Vastus lateralis m
Femur
Iliotibial band
Sciatic n
Gluteus maximus m

Greater saphenous v
Sartorius m
Femoral vessels, superficial
Adductor longus m
Femoral vessels, deep
Adductor brevis m
Gracilis m
Adductor magnus m
Semimembranosus t
Semitendinosus m
Conjoined t of semitendinosus m and biceps femoris m, long head

Figure 9.1.18

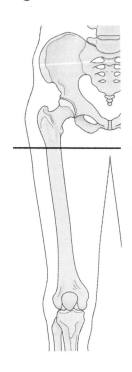

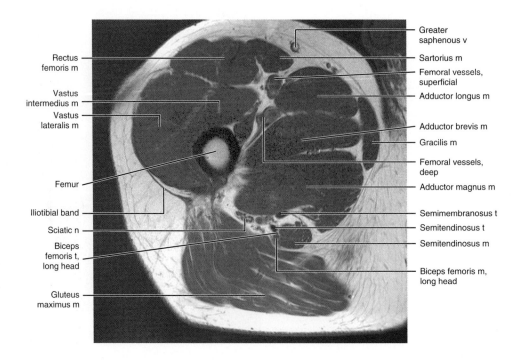

Rectus femoris m
Vastus intermedius m
Vastus lateralis m
Femur
Iliotibial band
Sciatic n
Biceps femoris t, long head
Gluteus maximus m

Greater saphenous v
Sartorius m
Femoral vessels, superficial
Adductor longus m
Adductor brevis m
Gracilis m
Femoral vessels, deep
Adductor magnus m
Semimembranosus t
Semitendinosus t
Semitendinosus m
Biceps femoris m, long head

SAGITTAL

Figure 9.2.1

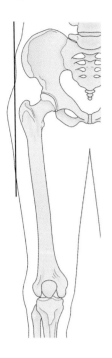

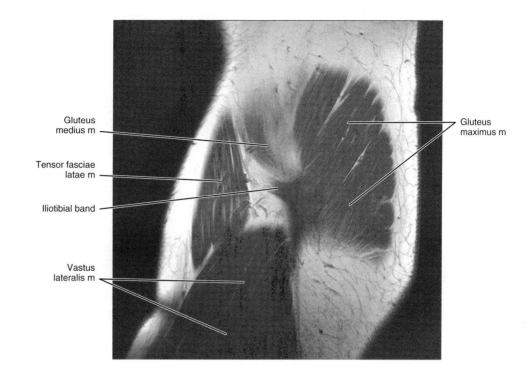

Gluteus medius m

Tensor fasciae latae m

Iliotibial band

Vastus lateralis m

Gluteus maximus m

Figure 9.2.2

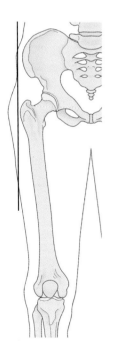

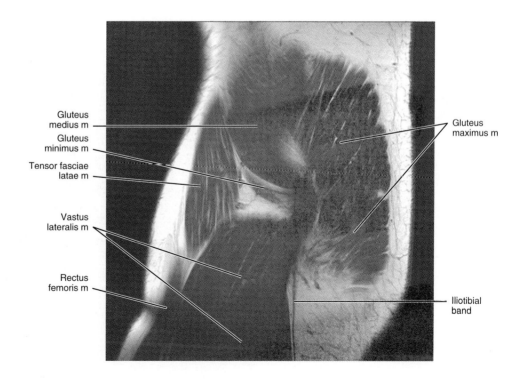

Gluteus medius m

Gluteus minimus m

Tensor fasciae latae m

Vastus lateralis m

Rectus femoris m

Gluteus maximus m

Iliotibial band

Figure 9.2.3

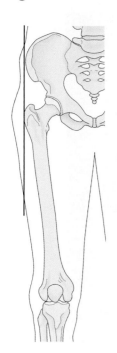

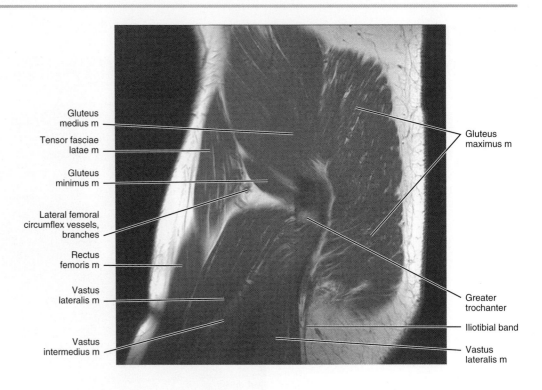

Gluteus medius m

Tensor fasciae latae m

Gluteus minimus m

Lateral femoral circumflex vessels, branches

Rectus femoris m

Vastus lateralis m

Vastus intermedius m

Gluteus maximus m

Greater trochanter

Iliotibial band

Vastus lateralis m

Figure 9.2.4

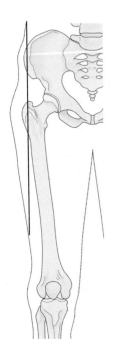

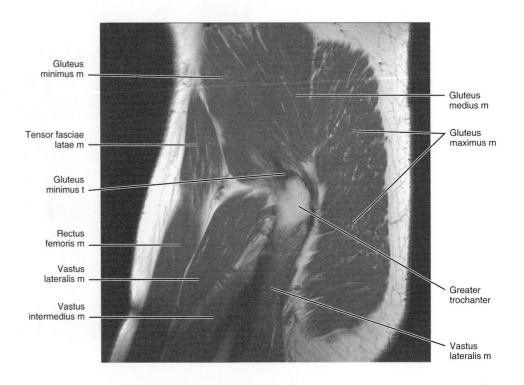

Gluteus minimus m

Tensor fasciae latae m

Gluteus minimus t

Rectus femoris m

Vastus lateralis m

Vastus intermedius m

Gluteus medius m

Gluteus maximus m

Greater trochanter

Vastus lateralis m

Figure 9.2.5

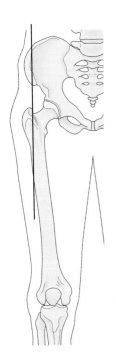

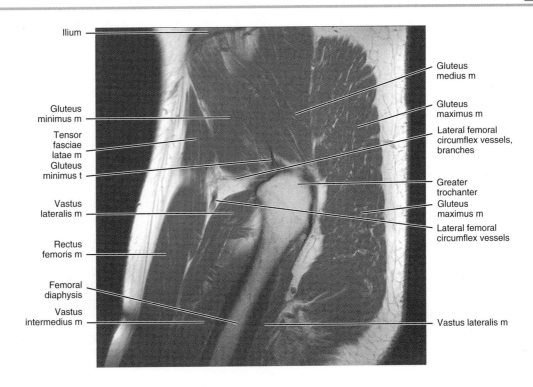

Ilium

Gluteus minimus m

Tensor fasciae latae m

Gluteus minimus t

Vastus lateralis m

Rectus femoris m

Femoral diaphysis

Vastus intermedius m

Gluteus medius m

Gluteus maximus m

Lateral femoral circumflex vessels, branches

Greater trochanter

Gluteus maximus m

Lateral femoral circumflex vessels

Vastus lateralis m

Figure 9.2.6

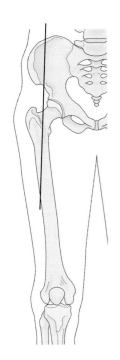

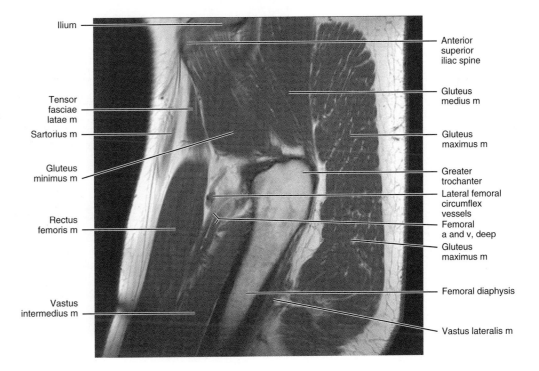

Ilium

Tensor fasciae latae m

Sartorius m

Gluteus minimus m

Rectus femoris m

Vastus intermedius m

Anterior superior iliac spine

Gluteus medius m

Gluteus maximus m

Greater trochanter

Lateral femoral circumflex vessels

Femoral a and v, deep

Gluteus maximus m

Femoral diaphysis

Vastus lateralis m

Figure 9.2.7

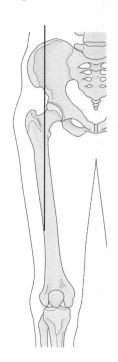

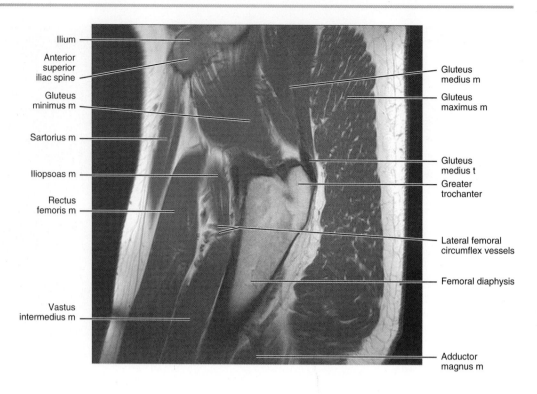

Ilium

Anterior superior iliac spine

Gluteus minimus m

Sartorius m

Iliopsoas m

Rectus femoris m

Vastus intermedius m

Gluteus medius m

Gluteus maximus m

Gluteus medius t

Greater trochanter

Lateral femoral circumflex vessels

Femoral diaphysis

Adductor magnus m

Figure 9.2.8

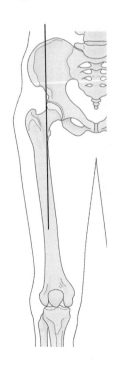

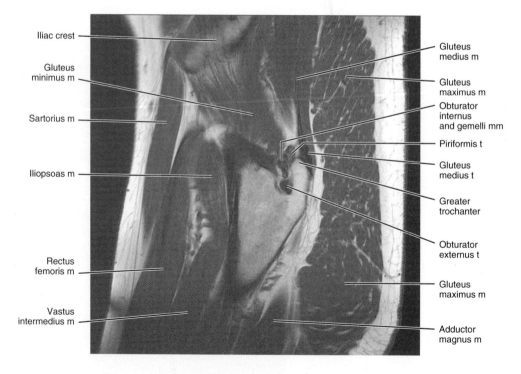

Iliac crest

Gluteus minimus m

Sartorius m

Iliopsoas m

Rectus femoris m

Vastus intermedius m

Gluteus medius m

Gluteus maximus m

Obturator internus and gemelli mm

Piriformis t

Gluteus medius t

Greater trochanter

Obturator externus t

Gluteus maximus m

Adductor magnus m

Figure 9.2.9

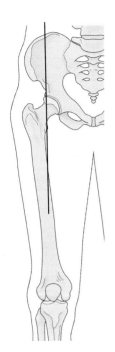

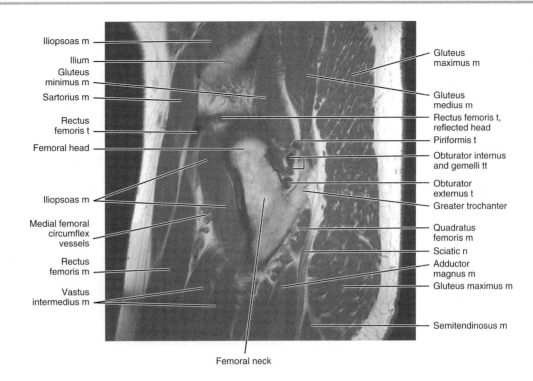

Iliopsoas m
Ilium
Gluteus minimus m
Sartorius m
Rectus femoris t
Femoral head
Iliopsoas m
Medial femoral circumflex vessels
Rectus femoris m
Vastus intermedius m

Gluteus maximus m
Gluteus medius m
Rectus femoris t, reflected head
Piriformis t
Obturator internus and gemelli tt
Obturator externus t
Greater trochanter
Quadratus femoris m
Sciatic n
Adductor magnus m
Gluteus maximus m
Semitendinosus m

Femoral neck

Figure 9.2.10

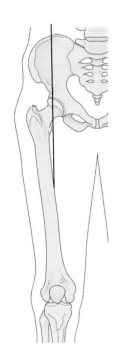

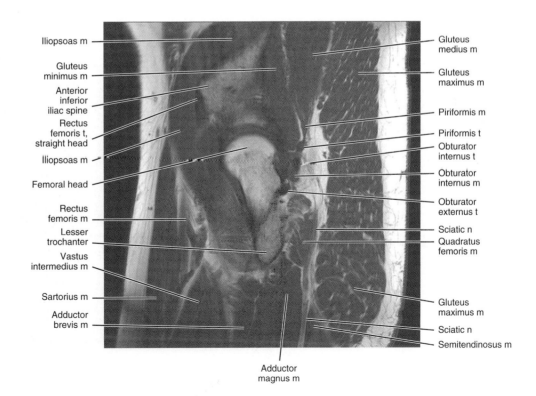

Iliopsoas m
Gluteus minimus m
Anterior inferior iliac spine
Rectus femoris t, straight head
Iliopsoas m
Femoral head
Rectus femoris m
Lesser trochanter
Vastus intermedius m
Sartorius m
Adductor brevis m

Gluteus medius m
Gluteus maximus m
Piriformis m
Piriformis t
Obturator internus t
Obturator internus m
Obturator externus t
Sciatic n
Quadratus femoris m
Gluteus maximus m
Sciatic n
Semitendinosus m

Adductor magnus m

Figure 9.2.11

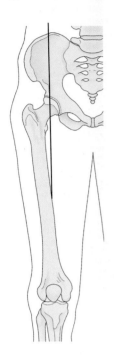

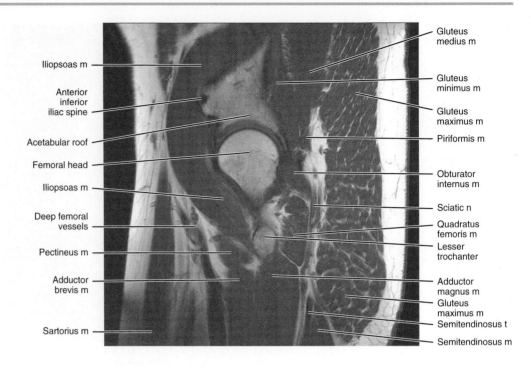

Iliopsoas m

Anterior inferior iliac spine

Acetabular roof

Femoral head

Iliopsoas m

Deep femoral vessels

Pectineus m

Adductor brevis m

Sartorius m

Gluteus medius m

Gluteus minimus m

Gluteus maximus m

Piriformis m

Obturator internus m

Sciatic n

Quadratus femoris m

Lesser trochanter

Adductor magnus m

Gluteus maximus m

Semitendinosus t

Semitendinosus m

Figure 9.2.12

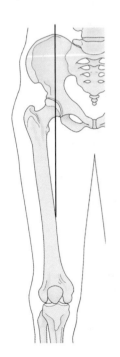

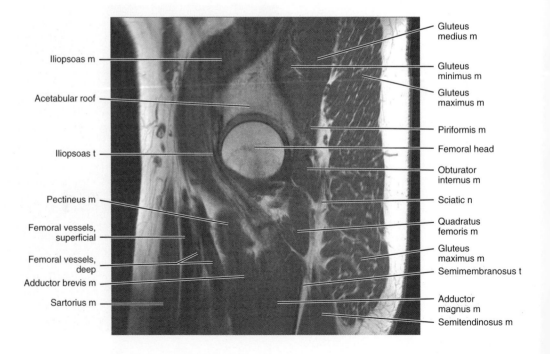

Iliopsoas m

Acetabular roof

Iliopsoas t

Pectineus m

Femoral vessels, superficial

Femoral vessels, deep

Adductor brevis m

Sartorius m

Gluteus medius m

Gluteus minimus m

Gluteus maximus m

Piriformis m

Femoral head

Obturator internus m

Sciatic n

Quadratus femoris m

Gluteus maximus m

Semimembranosus t

Adductor magnus m

Semitendinosus m

Figure 9.2.13

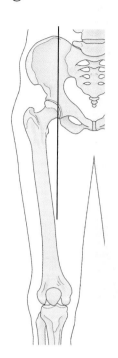

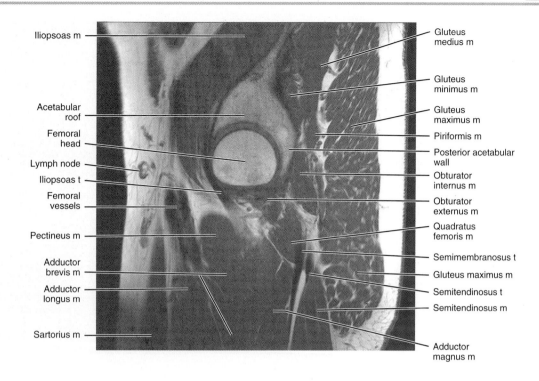

Iliopsoas m

Acetabular roof

Femoral head

Lymph node

Iliopsoas t

Femoral vessels

Pectineus m

Adductor brevis m

Adductor longus m

Sartorius m

Gluteus medius m

Gluteus minimus m

Gluteus maximus m

Piriformis m

Posterior acetabular wall

Obturator internus m

Obturator externus m

Quadratus femoris m

Semimembranosus t

Gluteus maximus m

Semitendinosus t

Semitendinosus m

Adductor magnus m

Figure 9.2.14

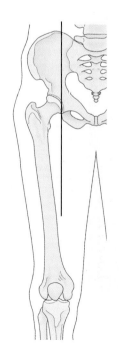

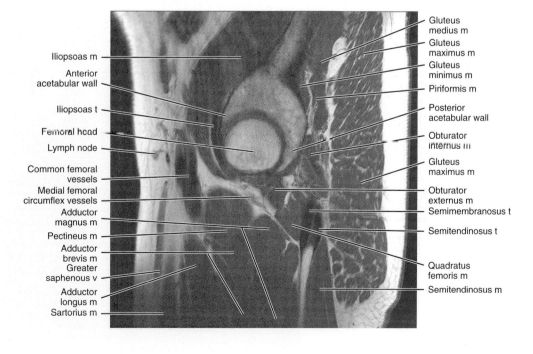

Iliopsoas m

Anterior acetabular wall

Iliopsoas t

Femoral head

Lymph node

Common femoral vessels

Medial femoral circumflex vessels

Adductor magnus m

Pectineus m

Adductor brevis m

Greater saphenous v

Adductor longus m

Sartorius m

Gluteus medius m

Gluteus maximus m

Gluteus minimus m

Piriformis m

Posterior acetabular wall

Obturator internus m

Gluteus maximus m

Obturator externus m

Semimembranosus t

Semitendinosus t

Quadratus femoris m

Semitendinosus m

Figure 9.2.15

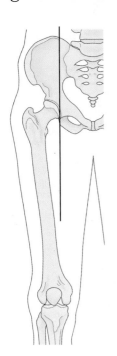

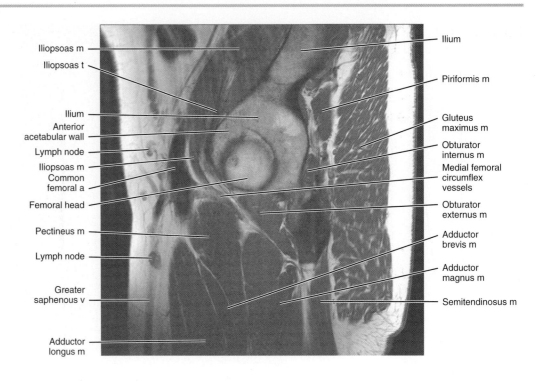

Iliopsoas m

Iliopsoas t

Ilium

Anterior acetabular wall

Lymph node

Iliopsoas m
Common femoral a

Femoral head

Pectineus m

Lymph node

Greater saphenous v

Adductor longus m

Ilium

Piriformis m

Gluteus maximus m

Obturator internus m

Medial femoral circumflex vessels

Obturator externus m

Adductor brevis m

Adductor magnus m

Semitendinosus m

Figure 9.2.16

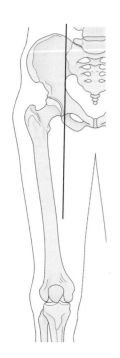

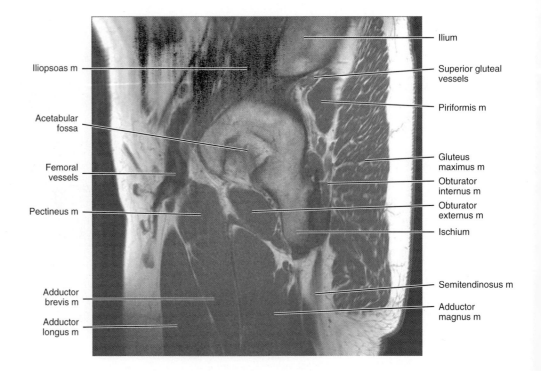

Iliopsoas m

Acetabular fossa

Femoral vessels

Pectineus m

Adductor brevis m

Adductor longus m

Ilium

Superior gluteal vessels

Piriformis m

Gluteus maximus m

Obturator internus m

Obturator externus m

Ischium

Semitendinosus m

Adductor magnus m

Figure 9.2.17

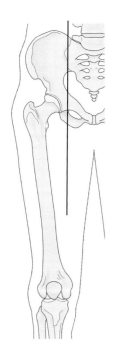

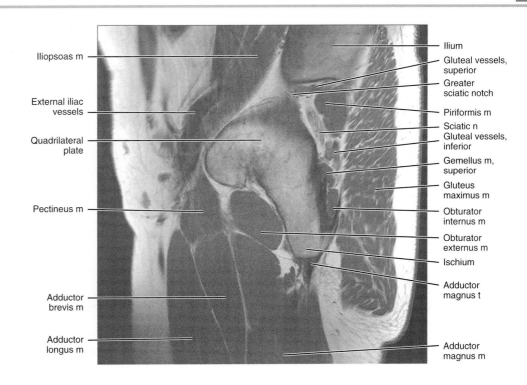

Iliopsoas m

External iliac vessels

Quadrilateral plate

Pectineus m

Adductor brevis m

Adductor longus m

Ilium

Gluteal vessels, superior

Greater sciatic notch

Piriformis m

Sciatic n

Gluteal vessels, inferior

Gemellus m, superior

Gluteus maximus m

Obturator internus m

Obturator externus m

Ischium

Adductor magnus t

Adductor magnus m

Figure 9.2.18

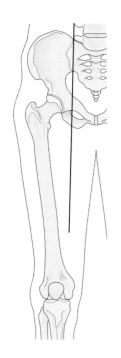

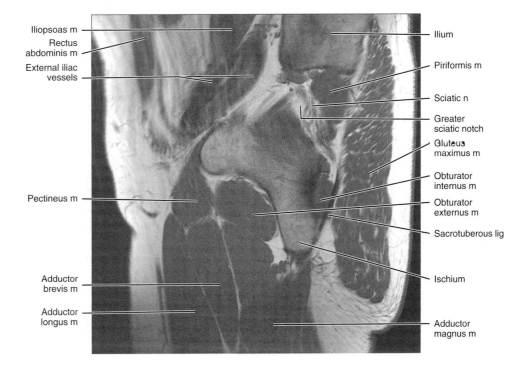

Iliopsoas m

Rectus abdominis m

External iliac vessels

Pectineus m

Adductor brevis m

Adductor longus m

Ilium

Piriformis m

Sciatic n

Greater sciatic notch

Gluteus maximus m

Obturator internus m

Obturator externus m

Sacrotuberous lig

Ischium

Adductor magnus m

Figure 9.2.19

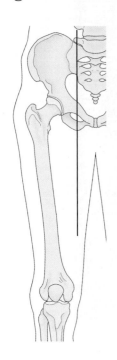

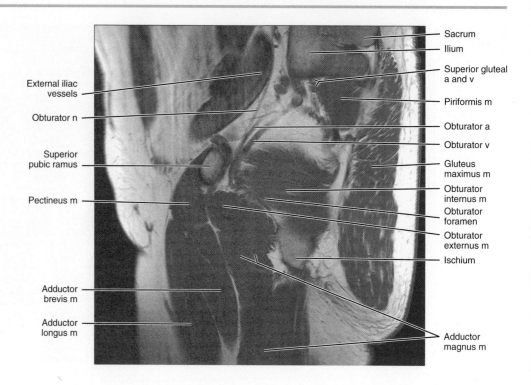

External iliac vessels

Obturator n

Superior pubic ramus

Pectineus m

Adductor brevis m

Adductor longus m

Sacrum

Ilium

Superior gluteal a and v

Piriformis m

Obturator a

Obturator v

Gluteus maximus m

Obturator internus m

Obturator foramen

Obturator externus m

Ischium

Adductor magnus m

CORONAL
Figure 9.3.1

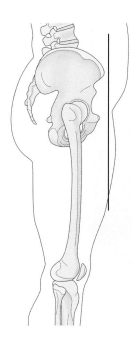

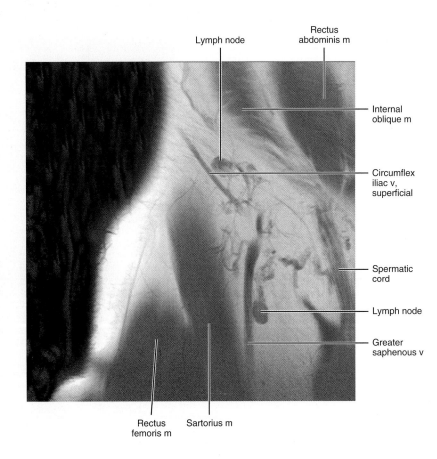

Lymph node

Rectus abdominis m

Internal oblique m

Circumflex iliac v, superficial

Spermatic cord

Lymph node

Greater saphenous v

Rectus femoris m

Sartorius m

Figure 9.3.2

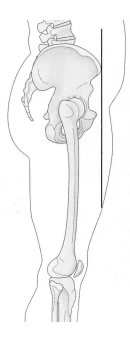

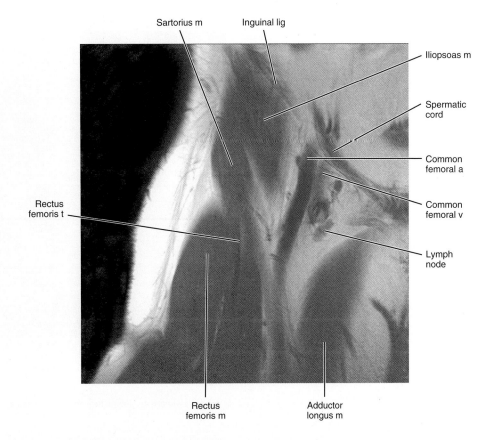

Sartorius m

Inguinal lig

Iliopsoas m

Spermatic cord

Common femoral a

Common femoral v

Lymph node

Rectus femoris t

Rectus femoris m

Adductor longus m

Figure 9.3.3

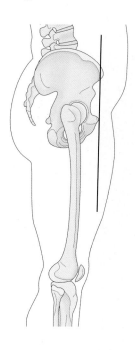

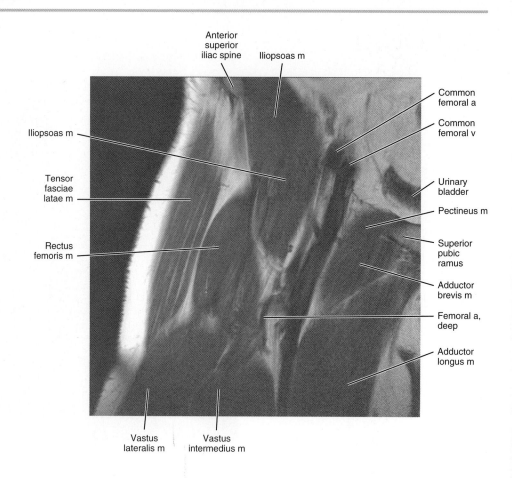

Anterior superior iliac spine

Iliopsoas m

Iliopsoas m

Tensor fasciae latae m

Rectus femoris m

Common femoral a

Common femoral v

Urinary bladder

Pectineus m

Superior pubic ramus

Adductor brevis m

Femoral a, deep

Adductor longus m

Vastus lateralis m

Vastus intermedius m

Figure 9.3.4

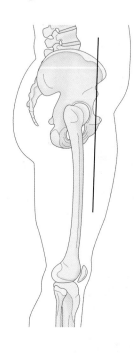

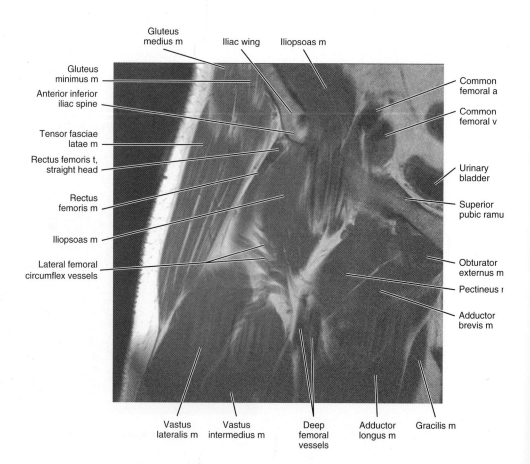

Gluteus medius m

Iliac wing

Iliopsoas m

Gluteus minimus m

Anterior inferior iliac spine

Tensor fasciae latae m

Rectus femoris t, straight head

Rectus femoris m

Iliopsoas m

Lateral femoral circumflex vessels

Common femoral a

Common femoral v

Urinary bladder

Superior pubic ramu

Obturator externus m

Pectineus r

Adductor brevis m

Vastus lateralis m

Vastus intermedius m

Deep femoral vessels

Adductor longus m

Gracilis m

Figure 9.3.5

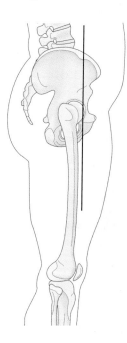

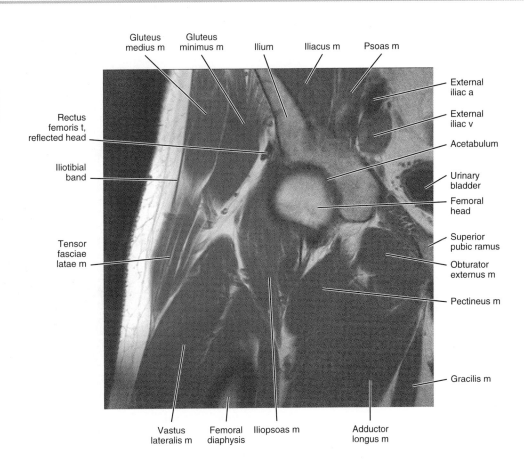

Gluteus medius m

Gluteus minimus m

Ilium

Iliacus m

Psoas m

External iliac a

External iliac v

Acetabulum

Urinary bladder

Femoral head

Superior pubic ramus

Obturator externus m

Pectineus m

Gracilis m

Rectus femoris t, reflected head

Iliotibial band

Tensor fasciae latae m

Vastus lateralis m

Femoral diaphysis

Iliopsoas m

Adductor longus m

Figure 9.3.6

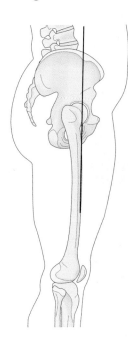

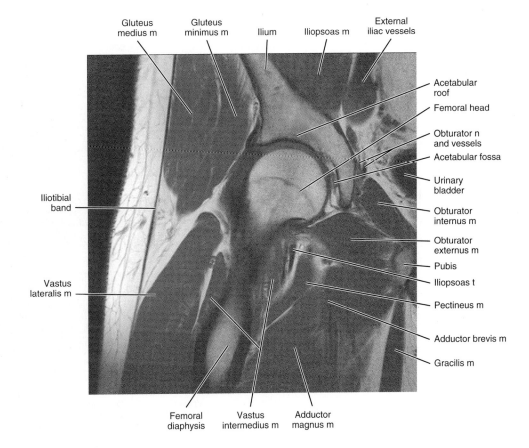

Gluteus medius m

Gluteus minimus m

Ilium

Iliopsoas m

External iliac vessels

Acetabular roof

Femoral head

Obturator n and vessels

Acetabular fossa

Urinary bladder

Obturator internus m

Obturator externus m

Pubis

Iliopsoas t

Pectineus m

Adductor brevis m

Gracilis m

Iliotibial band

Vastus lateralis m

Femoral diaphysis

Vastus intermedius m

Adductor magnus m

Figure 9.3.7

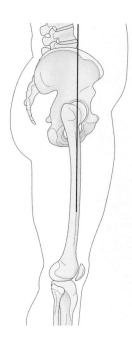

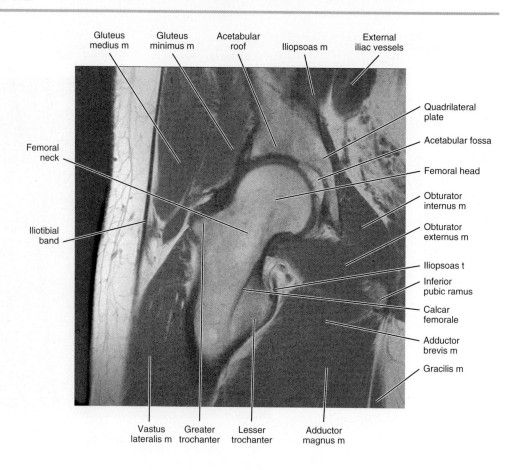

Gluteus medius m

Gluteus minimus m

Acetabular roof

Iliopsoas m

External iliac vessels

Femoral neck

Iliotibial band

Quadrilateral plate

Acetabular fossa

Femoral head

Obturator internus m

Obturator externus m

Iliopsoas t

Inferior pubic ramus

Calcar femorale

Adductor brevis m

Gracilis m

Vastus lateralis m

Greater trochanter

Lesser trochanter

Adductor magnus m

Figure 9.3.8

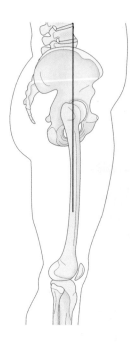

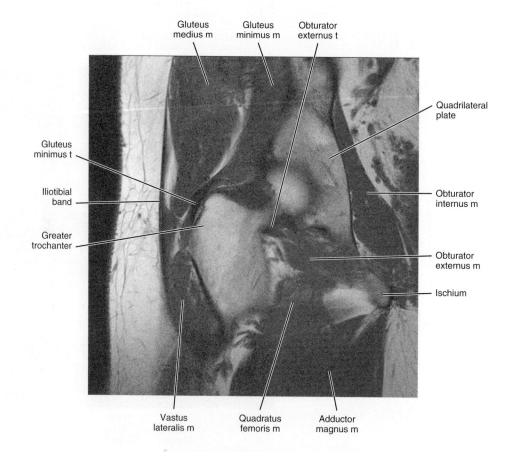

Gluteus medius m

Gluteus minimus m

Obturator externus t

Gluteus minimus t

Iliotibial band

Greater trochanter

Quadrilateral plate

Obturator internus m

Obturator externus m

Ischium

Vastus lateralis m

Quadratus femoris m

Adductor magnus m

Figure 9.3.9

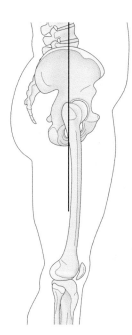

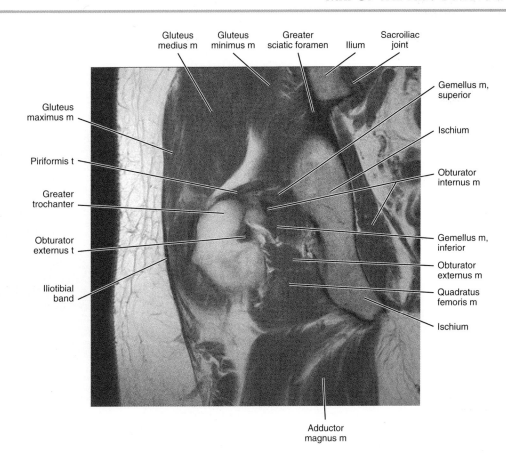

Gluteus medius m

Gluteus minimus m

Greater sciatic foramen

Ilium

Sacroiliac joint

Gluteus maximus m

Piriformis t

Greater trochanter

Obturator externus t

Iliotibial band

Gemellus m, superior

Ischium

Obturator internus m

Gemellus m, inferior

Obturator externus m

Quadratus femoris m

Ischium

Adductor magnus m

Figure 9.3.10

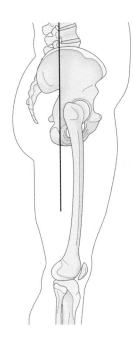

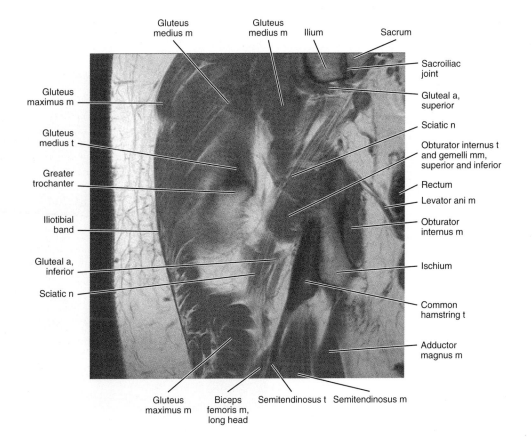

Gluteus medius m

Gluteus medius m

Ilium

Sacrum

Gluteus maximus m

Gluteus medius t

Greater trochanter

Iliotibial band

Gluteal a, inferior

Sciatic n

Sacroiliac joint

Gluteal a, superior

Sciatic n

Obturator internus t and gemelli mm, superior and inferior

Rectum

Levator ani m

Obturator internus m

Ischium

Common hamstring t

Adductor magnus m

Gluteus maximus m

Biceps femoris m, long head

Semitendinosus t

Semitendinosus m

Figure 9.3.11

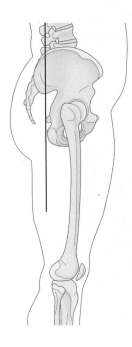

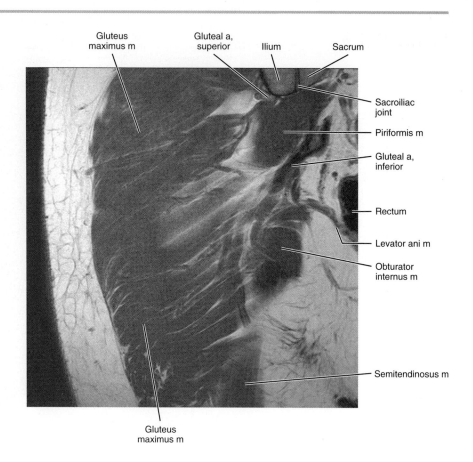

Gluteus maximus m

Gluteal a, superior

Ilium

Sacrum

Sacroiliac joint

Piriformis m

Gluteal a, inferior

Rectum

Levator ani m

Obturator internus m

Semitendinosus m

Gluteus maximus m

Figure 9.3.12

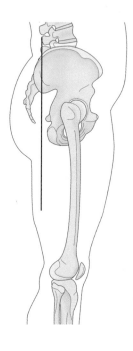

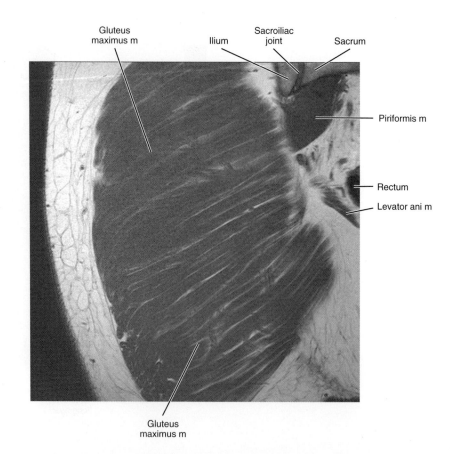

Gluteus maximus m

Ilium

Sacroiliac joint

Sacrum

Piriformis m

Rectum

Levator ani m

Gluteus maximus m

Figure 9.3.13

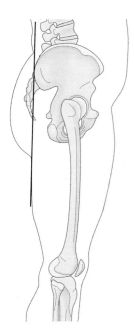

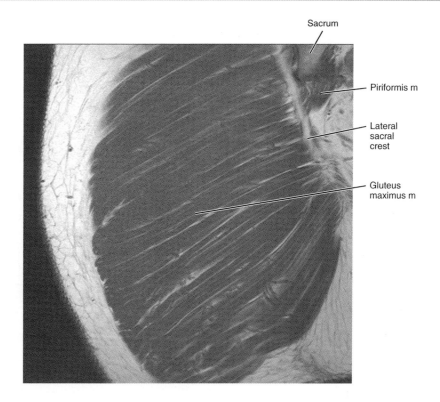

Sacrum

Piriformis m

Lateral
sacral
crest

Gluteus
maximus m

Chapter 10

MR Arthrography of the Hip

AXIAL

Figure 10.1.1

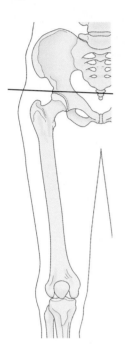

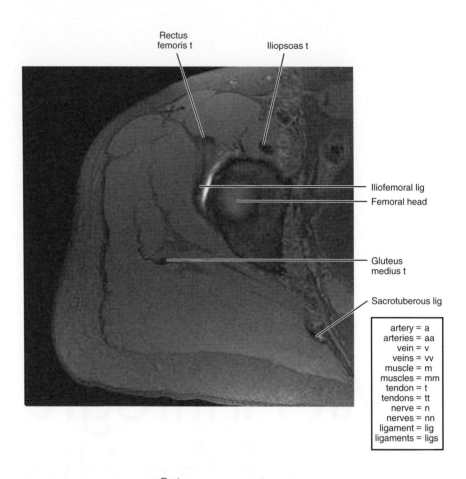

Rectus femoris t

Iliopsoas t

Iliofemoral lig

Femoral head

Gluteus medius t

Sacrotuberous lig

artery = a
arteries = aa
vein = v
veins = vv
muscle = m
muscles = mm
tendon = t
tendons = tt
nerve = n
nerves = nn
ligament = lig
ligaments = ligs

Figure 10.1.2

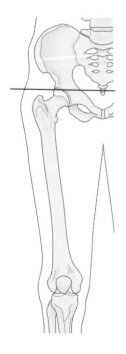

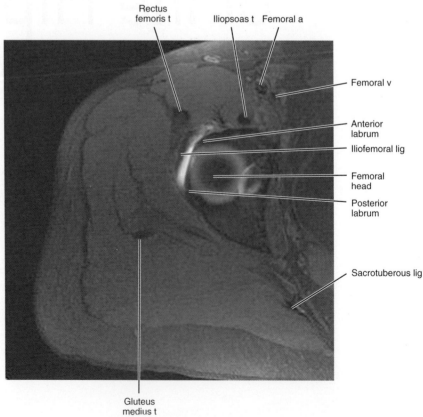

Rectus femoris t

Iliopsoas t   Femoral a

Femoral v

Anterior labrum

Iliofemoral lig

Femoral head

Posterior labrum

Sacrotuberous lig

Gluteus medius t

Figure 10.1.3

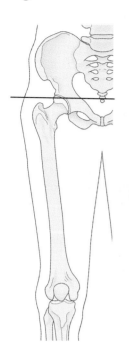

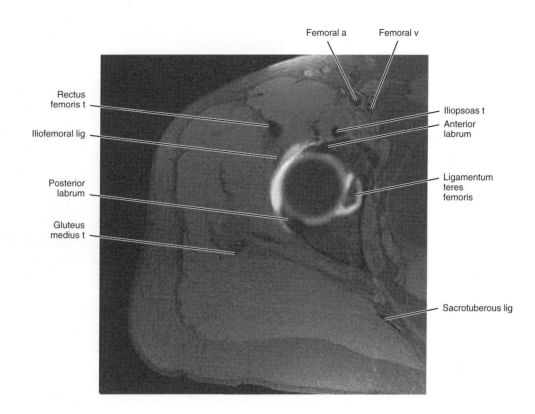

Femoral a   Femoral v

Rectus
femoris t

Iliofemoral lig

Posterior
labrum

Gluteus
medius t

Iliopsoas t

Anterior
labrum

Ligamentum
teres
femoris

Sacrotuberous lig

Figure 10.1.4

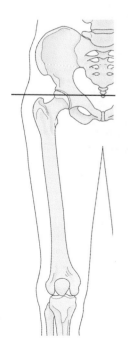

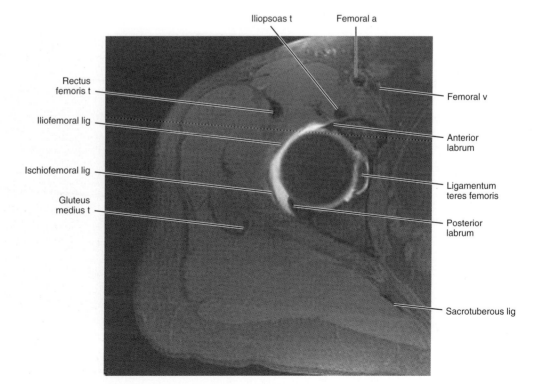

Iliopsoas t   Femoral a

Rectus
femoris t

Iliofemoral lig

Ischiofemoral lig

Gluteus
medius t

Femoral v

Anterior
labrum

Ligamentum
teres femoris

Posterior
labrum

Sacrotuberous lig

Figure 10.1.5

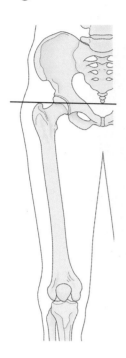

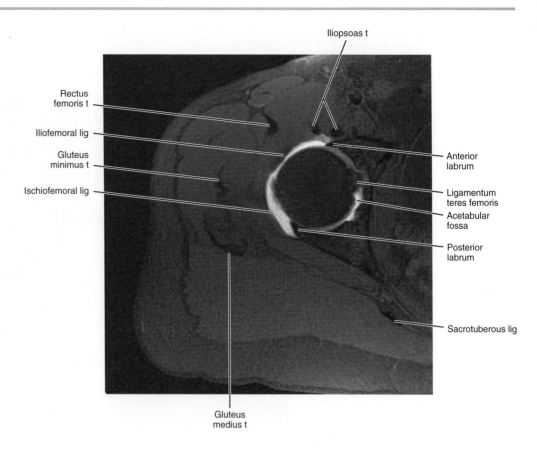

Iliopsoas t

Rectus femoris t

Iliofemoral lig

Gluteus minimus t

Ischiofemoral lig

Anterior labrum

Ligamentum teres femoris

Acetabular fossa

Posterior labrum

Sacrotuberous lig

Gluteus medius t

Figure 10.1.6

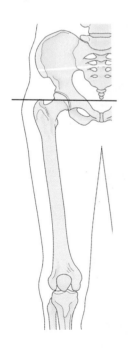

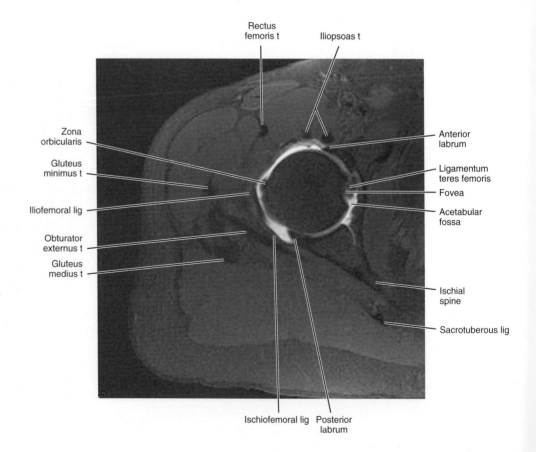

Rectus femoris t

Iliopsoas t

Zona orbicularis

Gluteus minimus t

Iliofemoral lig

Obturator externus t

Gluteus medius t

Anterior labrum

Ligamentum teres femoris

Fovea

Acetabular fossa

Ischial spine

Sacrotuberous lig

Ischiofemoral lig   Posterior labrum

Figure 10.1.7

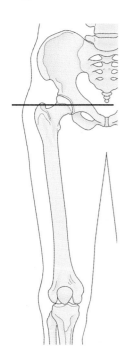

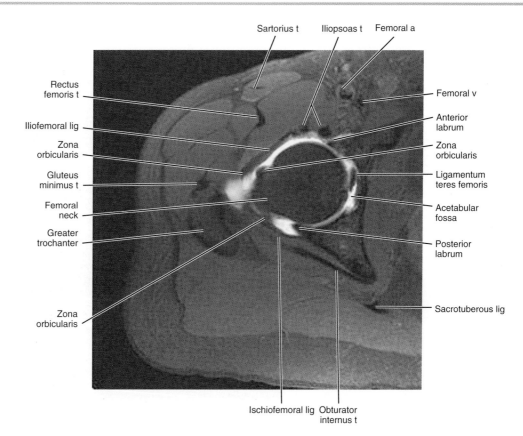

Sartorius t   Iliopsoas t   Femoral a

Rectus
femoris t

Iliofemoral lig

Zona
orbicularis

Gluteus
minimus t

Femoral
neck

Greater
trochanter

Zona
orbicularis

Femoral v

Anterior
labrum

Zona
orbicularis

Ligamentum
teres femoris

Acetabular
fossa

Posterior
labrum

Sacrotuberous lig

Ischiofemoral lig   Obturator
internus t

Figure 10.1.8

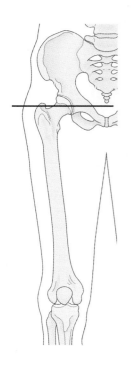

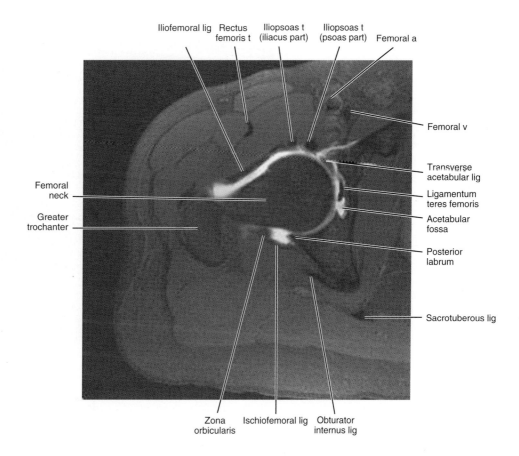

Iliofemoral lig   Rectus   Iliopsoas t   Iliopsoas t
                  femoris t   (iliacus part)   (psoas part)   Femoral a

Femoral v

Transverse
acetabular lig

Ligamentum
teres femoris

Acetabular
fossa

Posterior
labrum

Sacrotuberous lig

Femoral
neck

Greater
trochanter

Zona   Ischiofemoral lig   Obturator
orbicularis   internus lig

Figure 10.1.9

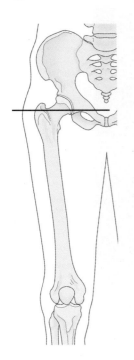

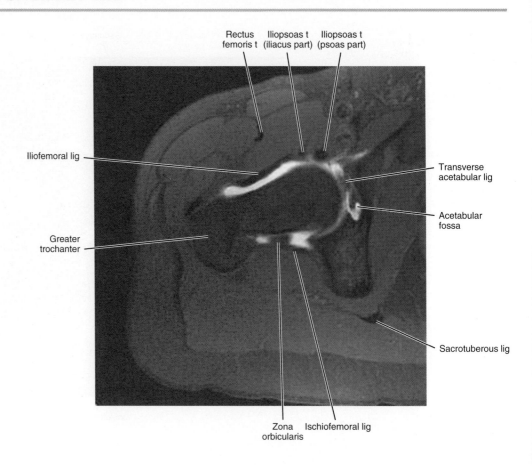

Rectus femoris t

Iliopsoas t (iliacus part)

Iliopsoas t (psoas part)

Iliofemoral lig

Transverse acetabular lig

Acetabular fossa

Greater trochanter

Sacrotuberous lig

Zona orbicularis

Ischiofemoral lig

Figure 10.1.10

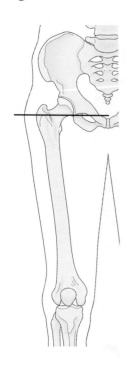

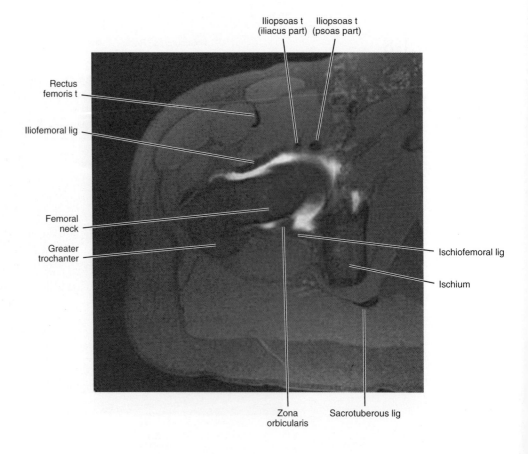

Iliopsoas t (iliacus part)

Iliopsoas t (psoas part)

Rectus femoris t

Iliofemoral lig

Femoral neck

Greater trochanter

Ischiofemoral lig

Ischium

Zona orbicularis

Sacrotuberous lig

Figure 10.1.11

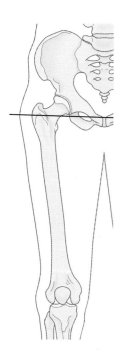

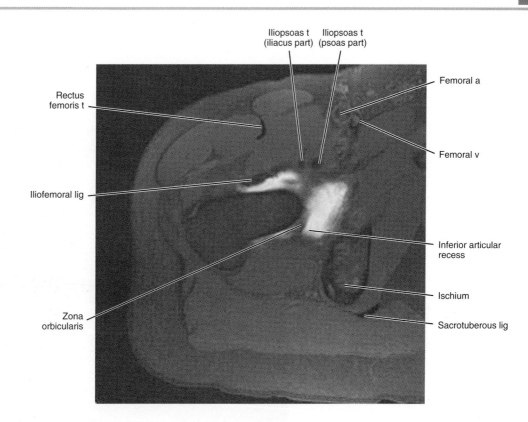

Iliopsoas t (iliacus part)   Iliopsoas t (psoas part)

Rectus femoris t

Femoral a

Femoral v

Iliofemoral lig

Inferior articular recess

Ischium

Sacrotuberous lig

Zona orbicularis

Figure 10.1.12

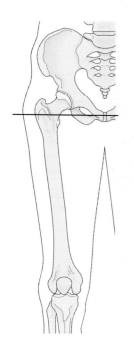

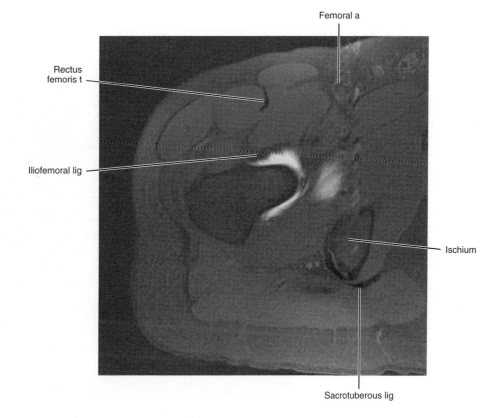

Femoral a

Rectus femoris t

Iliofemoral lig

Ischium

Sacrotuberous lig

SAGITTAL

Figure 10.2.1

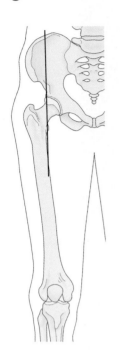

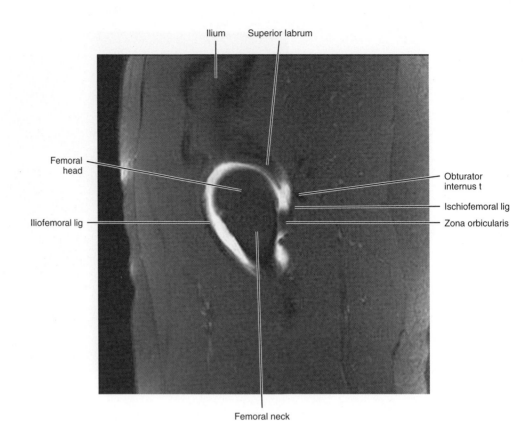

Ilium

Superior labrum

Femoral head

Obturator internus t

Ischiofemoral lig

Iliofemoral lig

Zona orbicularis

Femoral neck

Figure 10.2.2

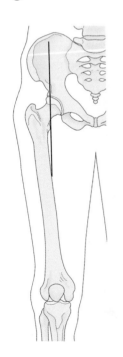

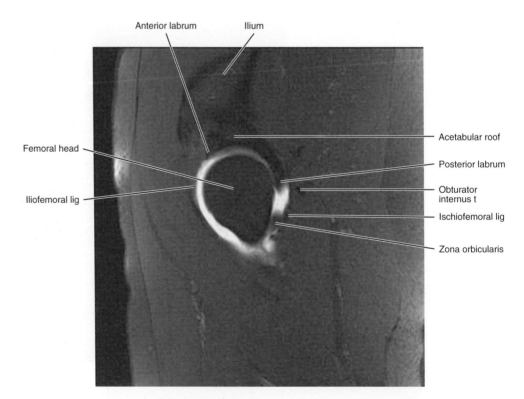

Anterior labrum

Ilium

Femoral head

Acetabular roof

Posterior labrum

Iliofemoral lig

Obturator internus t

Ischiofemoral lig

Zona orbicularis

Figure 10.2.3

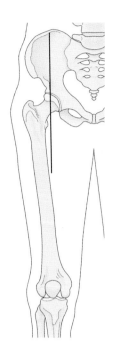

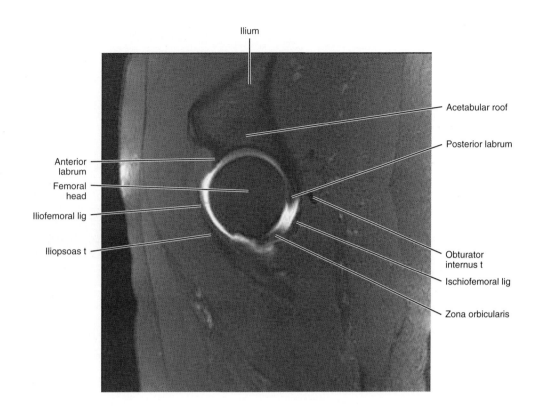

Ilium

Acetabular roof

Posterior labrum

Anterior labrum

Femoral head

Iliofemoral lig

Iliopsoas t

Obturator internus t

Ischiofemoral lig

Zona orbicularis

Figure 10.2.4

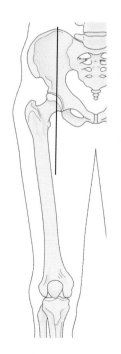

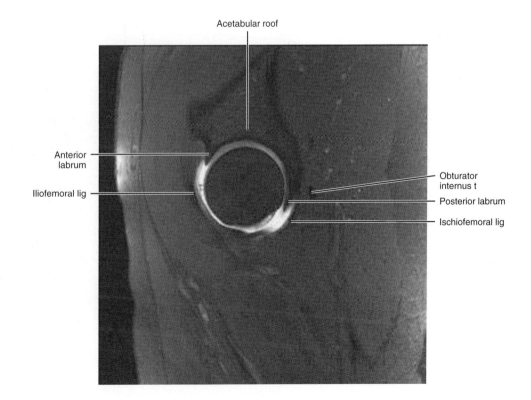

Acetabular roof

Anterior labrum

Iliofemoral lig

Obturator internus t

Posterior labrum

Ischiofemoral lig

Figure 10.2.5

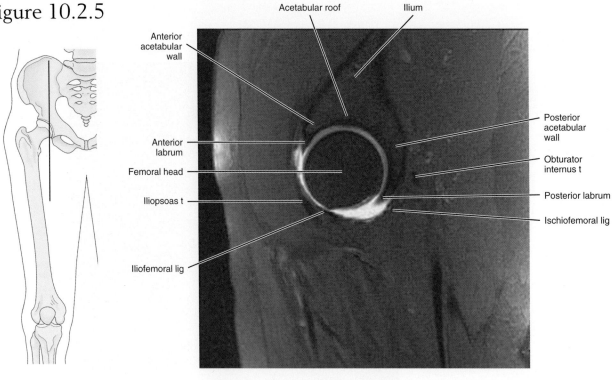

Acetabular roof
Ilium
Anterior acetabular wall
Posterior acetabular wall
Anterior labrum
Obturator internus t
Femoral head
Posterior labrum
Iliopsoas t
Ischiofemoral lig
Iliofemoral lig

Figure 10.2.6

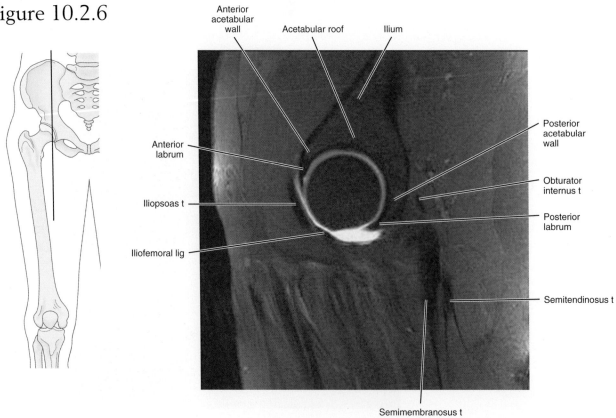

Anterior acetabular wall
Acetabular roof
Ilium
Posterior acetabular wall
Anterior labrum
Obturator internus t
Iliopsoas t
Posterior labrum
Iliofemoral lig
Semitendinosus t
Semimembranosus t

Figure 10.2.7

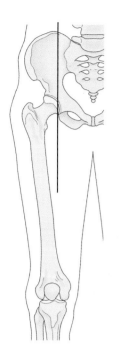

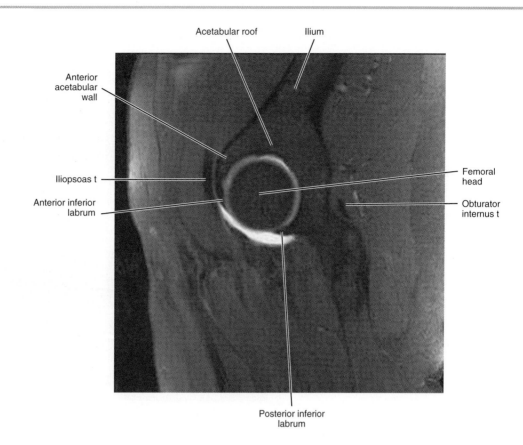

Acetabular roof

Ilium

Anterior acetabular wall

Iliopsoas t

Anterior inferior labrum

Femoral head

Obturator internus t

Posterior inferior labrum

Figure 10.2.8

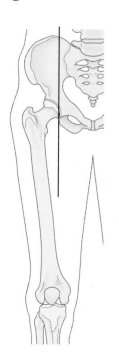

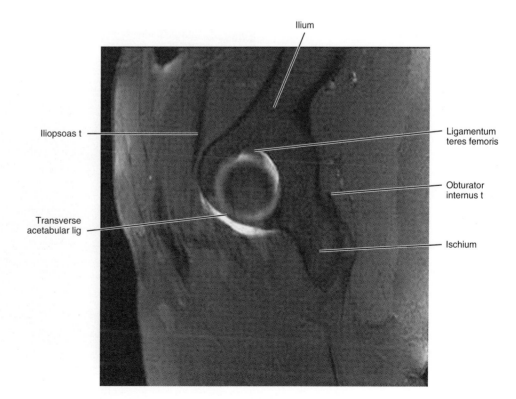

Ilium

Iliopsoas t

Ligamentum teres femoris

Obturator internus t

Transverse acetabular lig

Ischium

Figure 10.2.9

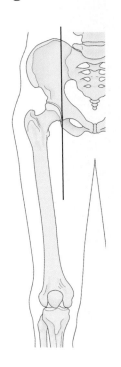

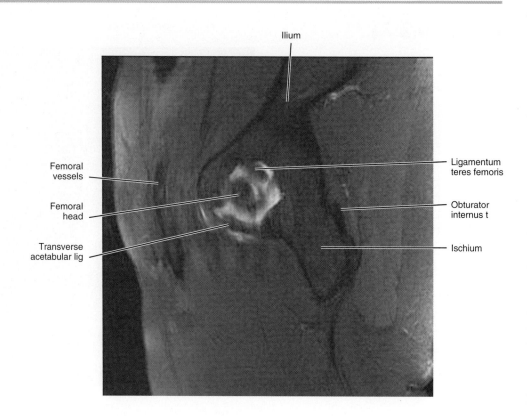

Ilium

Femoral
vessels

Femoral
head

Transverse
acetabular lig

Ligamentum
teres femoris

Obturator
internus t

Ischium

Figure 10.2.10

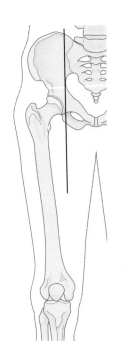

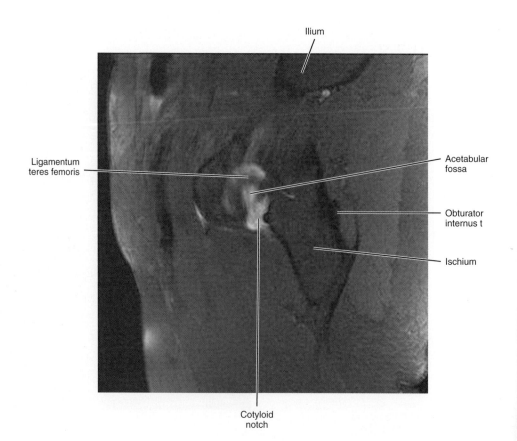

Ilium

Ligamentum
teres femoris

Acetabular
fossa

Obturator
internus t

Ischium

Cotyloid
notch

CORONAL
Figure 10.3.1

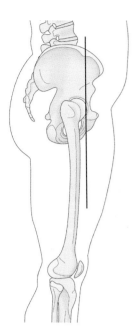

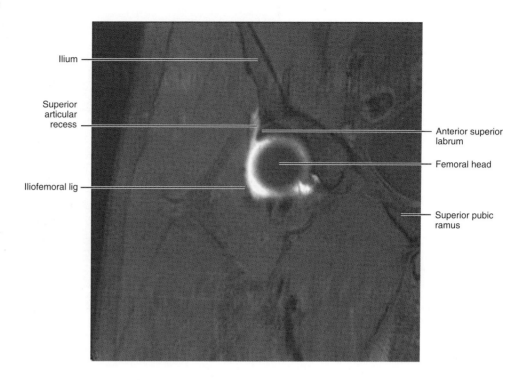

Ilium

Superior articular recess

Iliofemoral lig

Anterior superior labrum

Femoral head

Superior pubic ramus

Figure 10.3.2

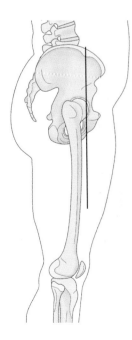

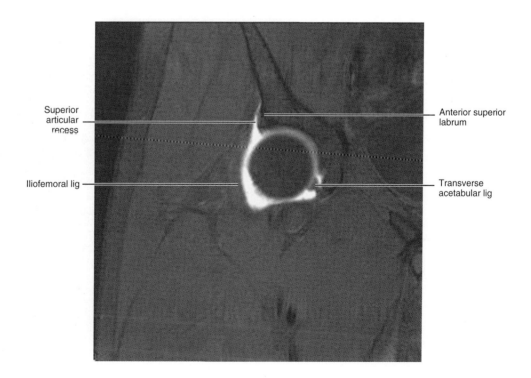

Superior articular recess

Iliofemoral lig

Anterior superior labrum

Transverse acetabular lig

Figure 10.3.3

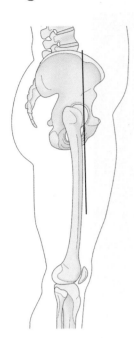

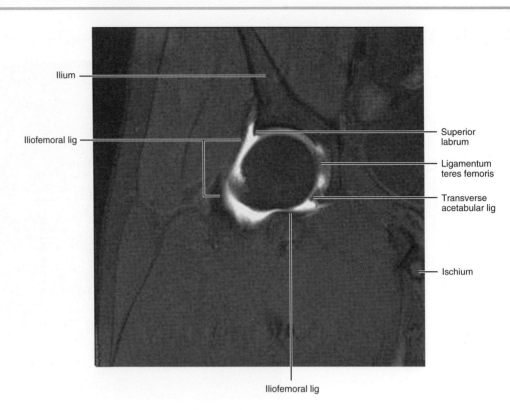

Ilium

Iliofemoral lig

Superior labrum

Ligamentum teres femoris

Transverse acetabular lig

Ischium

Iliofemoral lig

Figure 10.3.4

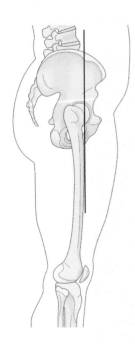

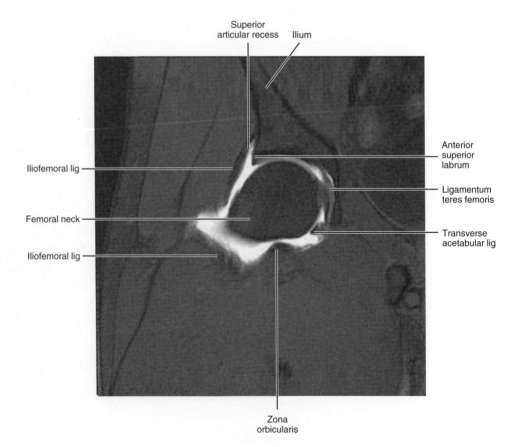

Superior articular recess

Ilium

Iliofemoral lig

Femoral neck

Iliofemoral lig

Anterior superior labrum

Ligamentum teres femoris

Transverse acetabular lig

Zona orbicularis

Figure 10.3.5

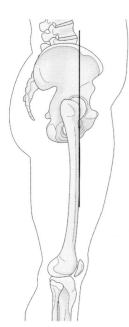

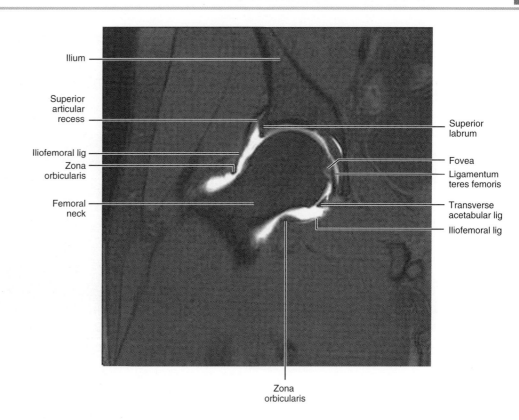

Ilium

Superior articular recess

Iliofemoral lig

Zona orbicularis

Femoral neck

Superior labrum

Fovea

Ligamentum teres femoris

Transverse acetabular lig

Iliofemoral lig

Zona orbicularis

Figure 10.3.6

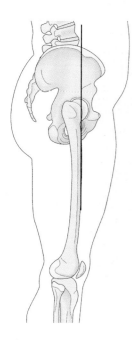

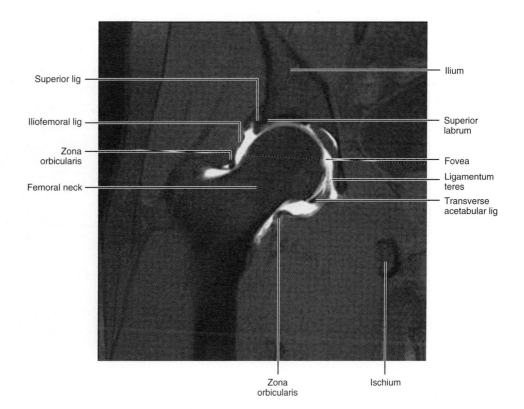

Superior lig

Iliofemoral lig

Zona orbicularis

Femoral neck

Ilium

Superior labrum

Fovea

Ligamentum teres

Transverse acetabular lig

Zona orbicularis

Ischium

Figure 10.3.7

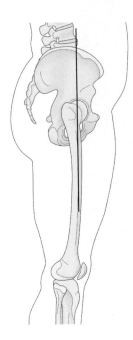

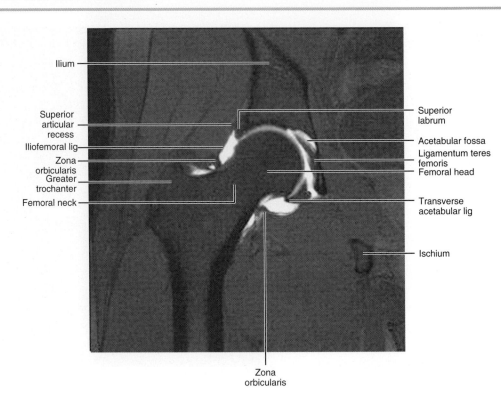

Ilium

Superior articular recess
Iliofemoral lig
Zona orbicularis
Greater trochanter
Femoral neck

Superior labrum
Acetabular fossa
Ligamentum teres femoris
Femoral head
Transverse acetabular lig

Ischium

Zona orbicularis

Figure 10.3.8

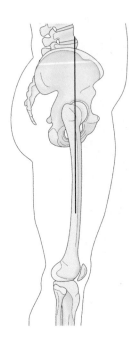

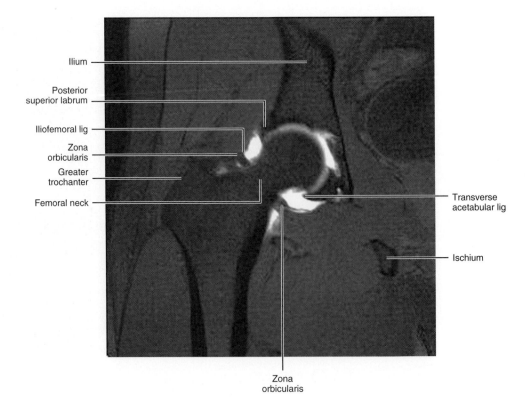

Ilium

Posterior superior labrum
Iliofemoral lig
Zona orbicularis
Greater trochanter
Femoral neck

Transverse acetabular lig

Ischium

Zona orbicularis

Figure 10.3.9

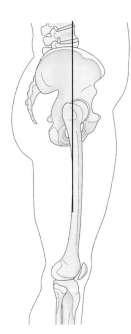

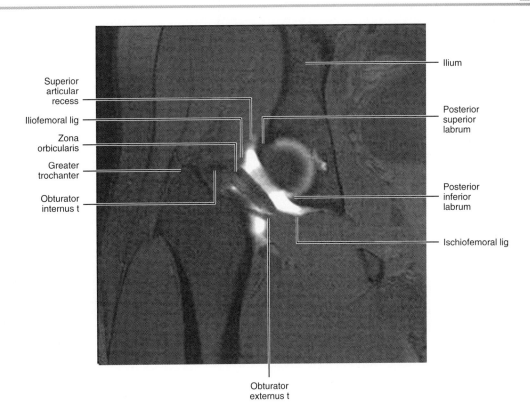

Superior articular recess
Iliofemoral lig
Zona orbicularis
Greater trochanter
Obturator internus t

Ilium
Posterior superior labrum
Posterior inferior labrum
Ischiofemoral lig

Obturator externus t

Figure 10.3.10

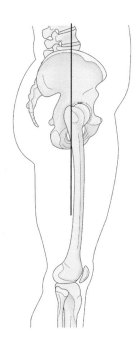

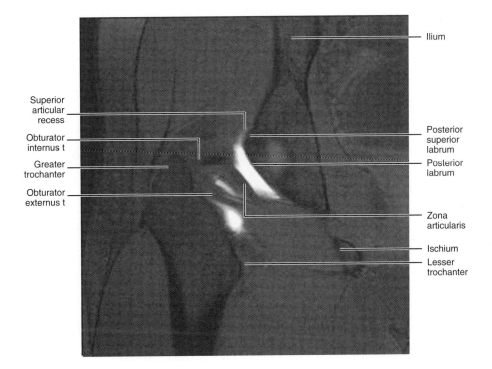

Superior articular recess
Obturator internus t
Greater trochanter
Obturator externus t

Ilium
Posterior superior labrum
Posterior labrum
Zona articularis
Ischium
Lesser trochanter

Chapter 11

MRI of the Thigh

Table 6: Muscles of the Thigh

MUSCLE	ORIGIN	INSERTION	NERVE SUPPLY
Sartorius	Anterior superior iliac spine and adjacent area below	Medial surface of the tibia; near the tuberosity and neighboring fascia	Femoral
Rectus femoris	Straight head: anterior inferior iliac spine; reflected head: posterosuperior surface of the rim of the acetabulum	Through the patellar ligament to the tibial tuberosity	Femoral
Vastus lateralis	Shaft of the femur along the anteroinferior margin of the greater trochanter, above the gluteal tuberosity, and the upper half of the linea aspera	Proximal border of the patella, front of the lateral condyle of the tibia and fascia of the leg	Femoral
Vastus medialis	Medial lip of the linea aspera and the distal half of the intertrochanteric line, and the aponeurosis of the tendons of insertion of the adductor muscles	Upper two thirds of the medial margin and proximal margin of the patella, medial condyle of the tibia, and investing deep fascia of the leg with the tendons of vastus intermedius, lateralis, and rectus, and through the patellar ligament onto the front of the tibial tuberosity	Femoral
Vastus intermedius	Distal half of the lateral margin of the linea aspera and its lateral bifurcation and from the anterolateral part of the shaft of the femur	Proximal margin and deep surface of the patella, aponeurosis of the vastus lateralis, medially and laterally to the tendons of vastus medialis and lateralis, to the patellar ligament and onto the tibial tuberosity	Femoral
Gracilis	Medial margin of inferior ramus of the pubis and the pubic end of the inferior ramus of the ischium	By an expanded tendinous process onto the tibia below the medial condyle	Anterior division of the obturator
Pectineus	Pectineal line, pectineal fascia, and anterior margin of the obturator sulcus, and from the pubofemoral ligament	Upper half of the pectineal line behind lesser trochanter	Femoral, also from the accessory obturator and/or obturator
Adductor longus	Pubic tubercle to symphysis pubis	Middle third of the linea aspera	Anterior division of the obturator, also occasionally, branch from the femoral
Adductor brevis	Medial part of the outer surface of the inferior ramus of the pubis	Distal two thirds of the pectineal line and the upper one third of the linea aspera	Anterior (or posterior) branch of the obturator

Table 6: Muscles of the Thigh—Cont'd

MUSCLE	ORIGIN	INSERTION	NERVE SUPPLY
Adductor magnus	Inferior ramus of the pubis	Medial side of the gluteal ridge and the superior part of the linea aspera by a tendon from the distal three fourths of the linea aspera and the adductor tubercle at the distal end of the medial supracondylar ridge	Posterior branch of the obturator and a branch from the sciatic
Biceps femoris	From the lateral lip of the linea aspera of the femur, from the middle of the shaft to the bifurcation of the linea aspera, proximal two thirds of the supracondylar ridge, and lateral intermuscular septum	Head of the fibula in front of the apex, partially onto the lateral condyle of the tibia, and into the fascia of the leg	Peroneal part of the sciatic

AXIAL

Figure 11.1.1

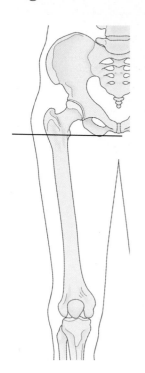

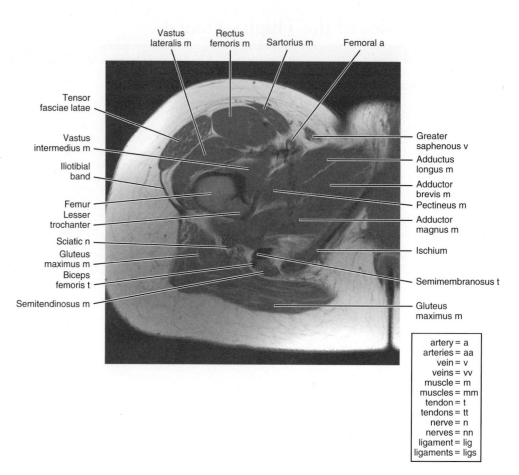

Vastus lateralis m
Rectus femoris m
Sartorius m
Femoral a

Tensor fasciae latae

Vastus intermedius m

Iliotibial band

Femur

Lesser trochanter

Sciatic n

Gluteus maximus m

Biceps femoris t

Semitendinosus m

Greater saphenous v

Adductus longus m

Adductor brevis m

Pectineus m

Adductor magnus m

Ischium

Semimembranosus t

Gluteus maximus m

artery = a
arteries = aa
vein = v
veins = vv
muscle = m
muscles = mm
tendon = t
tendons = tt
nerve = n
nerves = nn
ligament = lig
ligaments = ligs

Figure 11.1.2

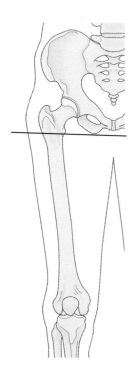

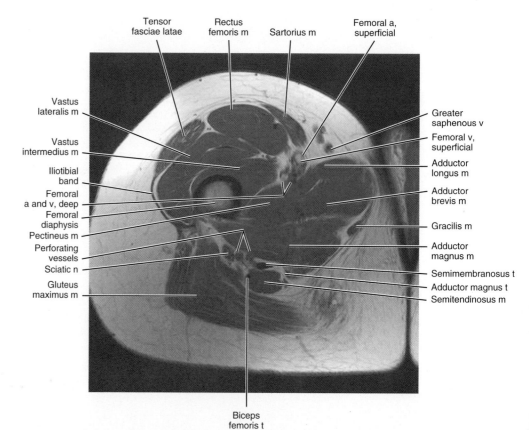

Tensor fasciae latae
Rectus femoris m
Sartorius m
Femoral a, superficial

Vastus lateralis m

Vastus intermedius m

Iliotibial band

Femoral a and v, deep

Femoral diaphysis

Pectineus m

Perforating vessels

Sciatic n

Gluteus maximus m

Greater saphenous v

Femoral v, superficial

Adductor longus m

Adductor brevis m

Gracilis m

Adductor magnus m

Semimembranosus t

Adductor magnus t

Semitendinosus m

Biceps femoris t

Figure 11.1.3

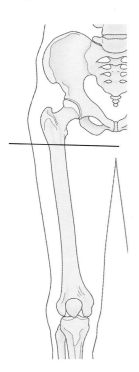

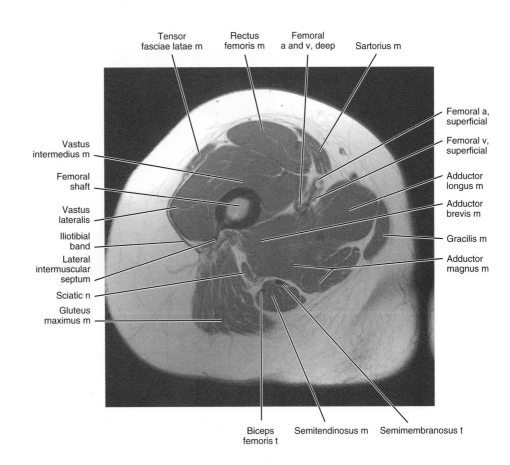

Tensor fasciae latae m · Rectus femoris m · Femoral a and v, deep · Sartorius m

Vastus intermedius m
Femoral shaft
Vastus lateralis
Iliotibial band
Lateral intermuscular septum
Sciatic n
Gluteus maximus m

Femoral a, superficial
Femoral v, superficial
Adductor longus m
Adductor brevis m
Gracilis m
Adductor magnus m

Biceps femoris t · Semitendinosus m · Semimembranosus t

Figure 11.1.4

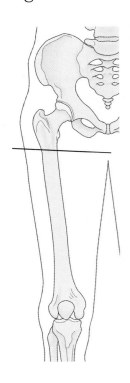

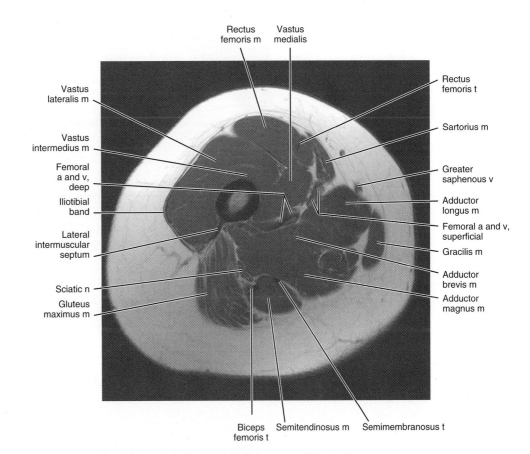

Rectus femoris m · Vastus medialis

Vastus lateralis m
Vastus intermedius m
Femoral a and v, deep
Iliotibial band
Lateral intermuscular septum
Sciatic n
Gluteus maximus m

Rectus femoris t
Sartorius m
Greater saphenous v
Adductor longus m
Femoral a and v, superficial
Gracilis m
Adductor brevis m
Adductor magnus m

Biceps femoris t · Semitendinosus m · Semimembranosus t

Figure 11.1.5

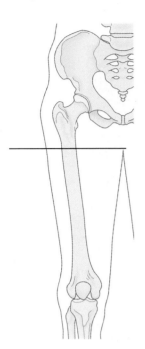

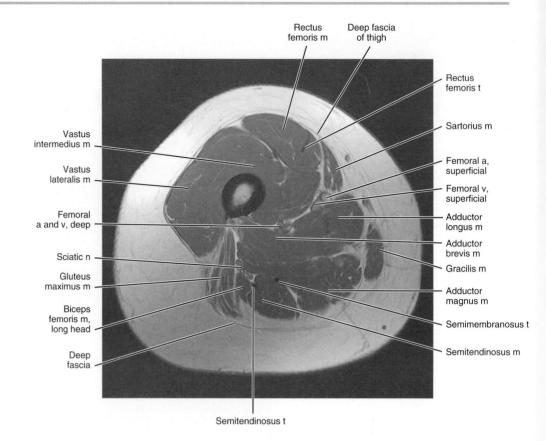

Rectus femoris m

Deep fascia of thigh

Vastus intermedius m

Vastus lateralis m

Femoral a and v, deep

Sciatic n

Gluteus maximus m

Biceps femoris m, long head

Deep fascia

Rectus femoris t

Sartorius m

Femoral a, superficial

Femoral v, superficial

Adductor longus m

Adductor brevis m

Gracilis m

Adductor magnus m

Semimembranosus t

Semitendinosus m

Semitendinosus t

Figure 11.1.6

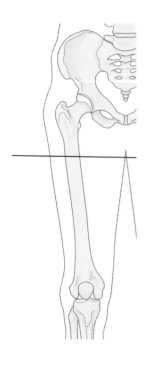

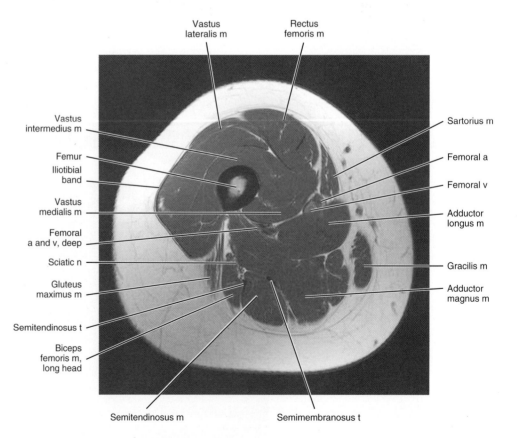

Vastus lateralis m

Rectus femoris m

Vastus intermedius m

Femur

Iliotibial band

Vastus medialis m

Femoral a and v, deep

Sciatic n

Gluteus maximus m

Semitendinosus t

Biceps femoris m, long head

Sartorius m

Femoral a

Femoral v

Adductor longus m

Gracilis m

Adductor magnus m

Semitendinosus m

Semimembranosus t

Figure 11.1.7

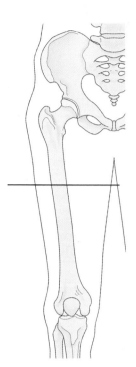

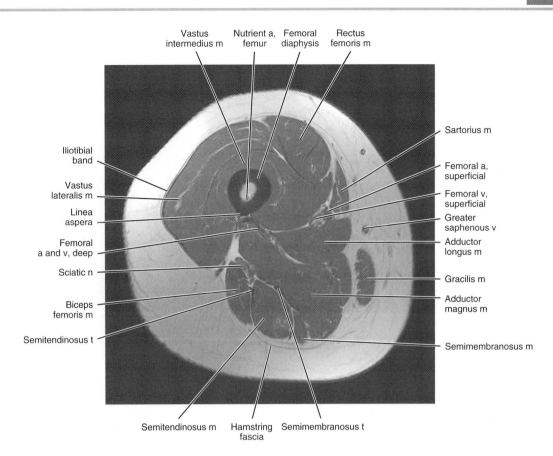

Vastus intermedius m
Nutrient a, femur
Femoral diaphysis
Rectus femoris m

Iliotibial band
Vastus lateralis m
Linea aspera
Femoral a and v, deep
Sciatic n
Biceps femoris m
Semitendinosus t

Sartorius m
Femoral a, superficial
Femoral v, superficial
Greater saphenous v
Adductor longus m
Gracilis m
Adductor magnus m
Semimembranosus m

Semitendinosus m
Hamstring fascia
Semimembranosus t

Figure 11.1.8

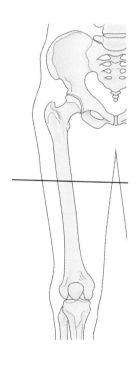

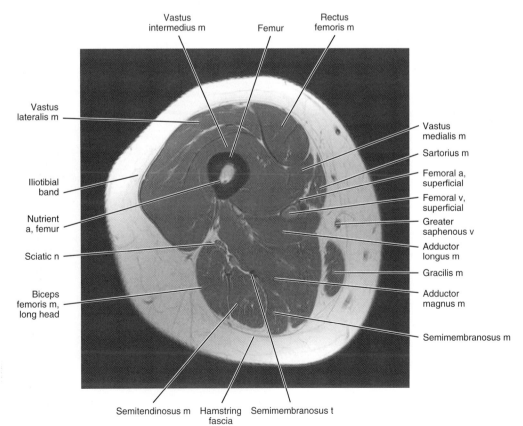

Vastus intermedius m
Femur
Rectus femoris m

Vastus lateralis m
Iliotibial band
Nutrient a, femur
Sciatic n
Biceps femoris m, long head

Vastus medialis m
Sartorius m
Femoral a, superficial
Femoral v, superficial
Greater saphenous v
Adductor longus m
Gracilis m
Adductor magnus m
Semimembranosus m

Semitendinosus m
Hamstring fascia
Semimembranosus t

Figure 11.1.9

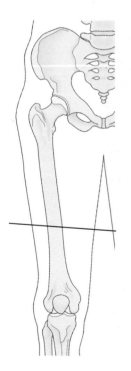

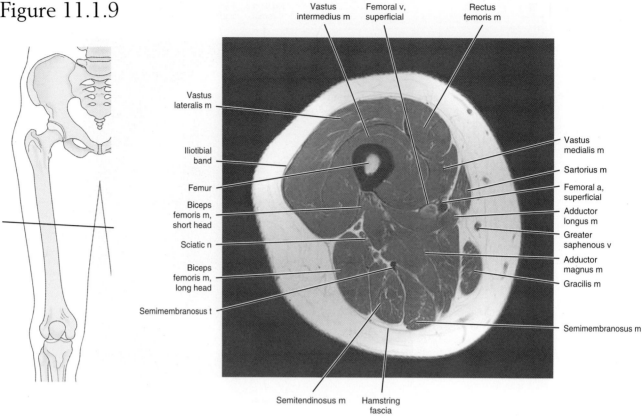

Vastus intermedius m

Femoral v, superficial

Rectus femoris m

Vastus lateralis m

Iliotibial band

Femur

Biceps femoris m, short head

Sciatic n

Biceps femoris m, long head

Semimembranosus t

Vastus medialis m

Sartorius m

Femoral a, superficial

Adductor longus m

Greater saphenous v

Adductor magnus m

Gracilis m

Semimembranosus m

Semitendinosus m

Hamstring fascia

Figure 11.1.10

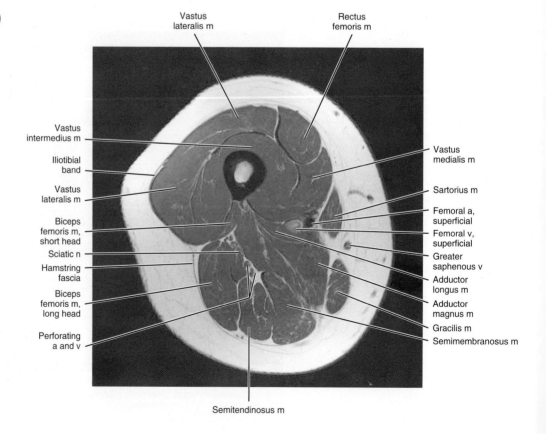

Vastus lateralis m

Rectus femoris m

Vastus intermedius m

Iliotibial band

Vastus lateralis m

Biceps femoris m, short head

Sciatic n

Hamstring fascia

Biceps femoris m, long head

Perforating a and v

Vastus medialis m

Sartorius m

Femoral a, superficial

Femoral v, superficial

Greater saphenous v

Adductor longus m

Adductor magnus m

Gracilis m

Semimembranosus m

Semitendinosus m

Figure 11.1.11

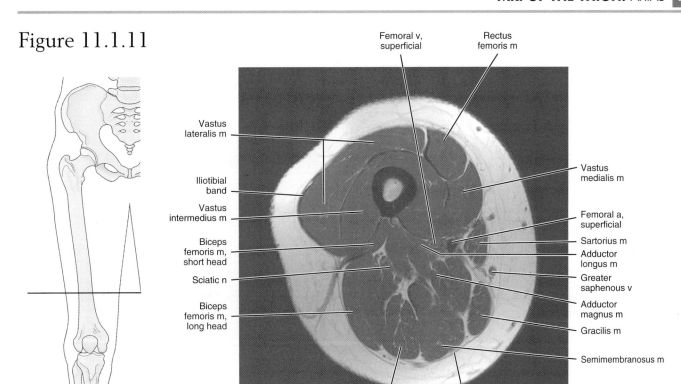

Femoral v, superficial
Rectus femoris m
Vastus lateralis m
Iliotibial band
Vastus intermedius m
Biceps femoris m, short head
Sciatic n
Biceps femoris m, long head
Vastus medialis m
Femoral a, superficial
Sartorius m
Adductor longus m
Greater saphenous v
Adductor magnus m
Gracilis m
Semimembranosus m
Semitendinosus m
Deep fascia

Figure 11.1.12

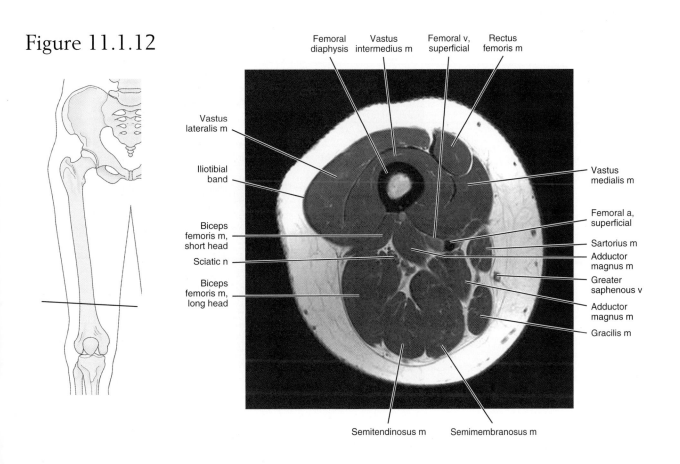

Femoral diaphysis
Vastus intermedius m
Femoral v, superficial
Rectus femoris m
Vastus lateralis m
Iliotibial band
Biceps femoris m, short head
Sciatic n
Biceps femoris m, long head
Vastus medialis m
Femoral a, superficial
Sartorius m
Adductor magnus m
Greater saphenous v
Adductor magnus m
Gracilis m
Semitendinosus m
Semimembranosus m

Figure 11.1.13

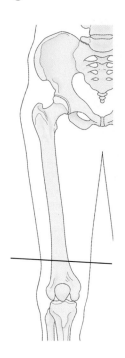

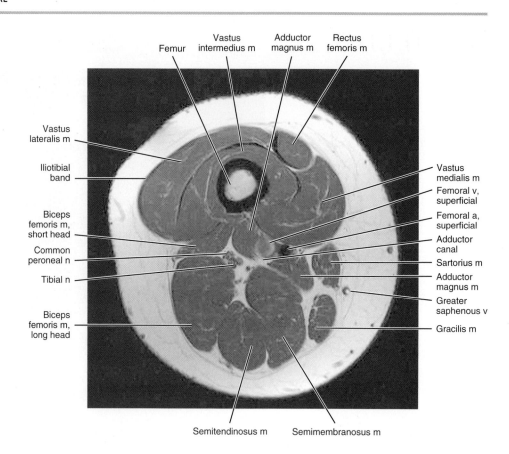

Femur

Vastus intermedius m

Adductor magnus m

Rectus femoris m

Vastus lateralis m

Iliotibial band

Biceps femoris m, short head

Common peroneal n

Tibial n

Biceps femoris m, long head

Vastus medialis m

Femoral v, superficial

Femoral a, superficial

Adductor canal

Sartorius m

Adductor magnus m

Greater saphenous v

Gracilis m

Semitendinosus m

Semimembranosus m

Figure 11.1.14

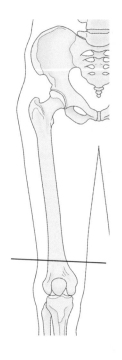

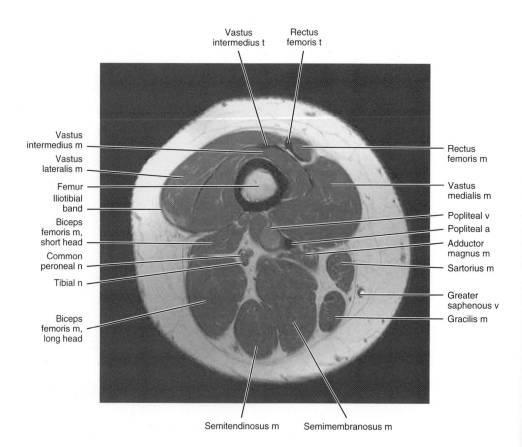

Vastus intermedius t

Rectus femoris t

Vastus intermedius m

Vastus lateralis m

Femur

Iliotibial band

Biceps femoris m, short head

Common peroneal n

Tibial n

Biceps femoris m, long head

Rectus femoris m

Vastus medialis m

Popliteal v

Popliteal a

Adductor magnus m

Sartorius m

Greater saphenous v

Gracilis m

Semitendinosus m

Semimembranosus m

Figure 11.1.15

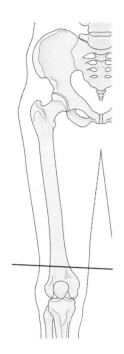

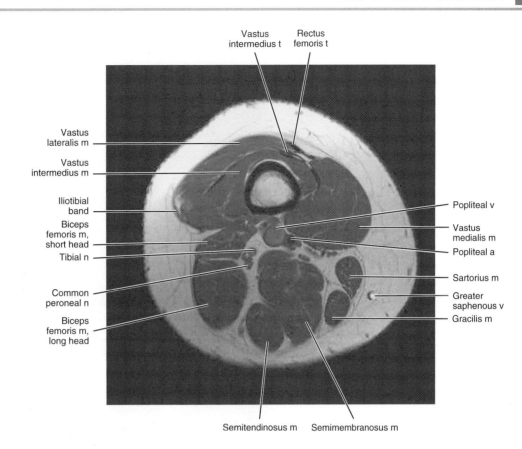

Vastus intermedius t
Rectus femoris t

Vastus lateralis m

Vastus intermedius m

Iliotibial band

Biceps femoris m, short head

Tibial n

Common peroneal n

Biceps femoris m, long head

Popliteal v

Vastus medialis m

Popliteal a

Sartorius m

Greater saphenous v

Gracilis m

Semitendinosus m   Semimembranosus m

Figure 11.1.16

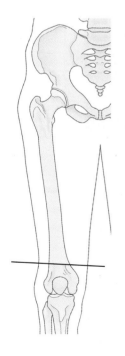

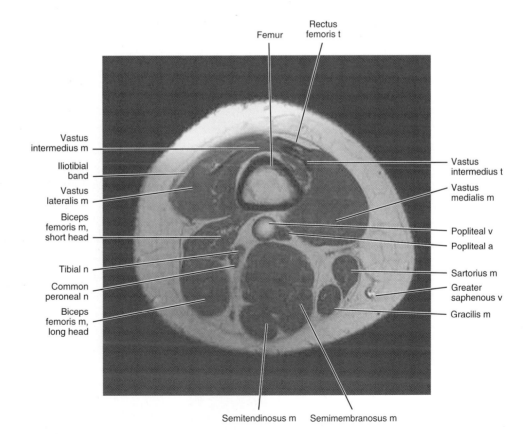

Femur
Rectus femoris t

Vastus intermedius m

Iliotibial band

Vastus lateralis m

Biceps femoris m, short head

Tibial n

Common peroneal n

Biceps femoris m, long head

Vastus intermedius t

Vastus medialis m

Popliteal v

Popliteal a

Sartorius m

Greater saphenous v

Gracilis m

Semitendinosus m   Semimembranosus m

SAGITTAL

Figure 11.2.1

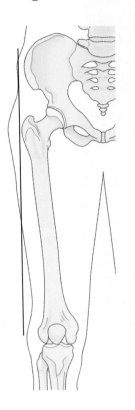

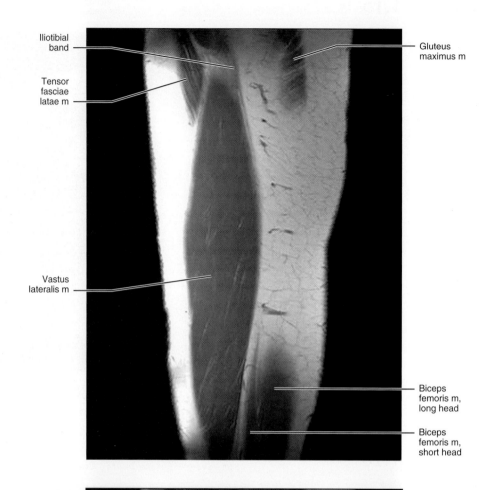

Iliotibial band

Tensor fasciae latae m

Gluteus maximus m

Vastus lateralis m

Biceps femoris m, long head

Biceps femoris m, short head

Figure 11.2.2

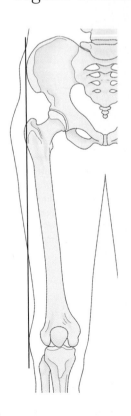

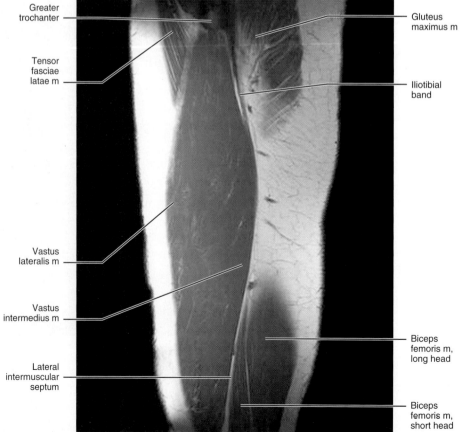

Greater trochanter

Tensor fasciae latae m

Gluteus maximus m

Iliotibial band

Vastus lateralis m

Vastus intermedius m

Lateral intermuscular septum

Biceps femoris m, long head

Biceps femoris m, short head

Figure 11.2.3

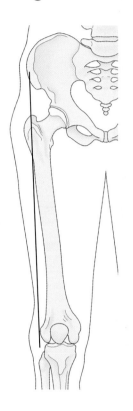

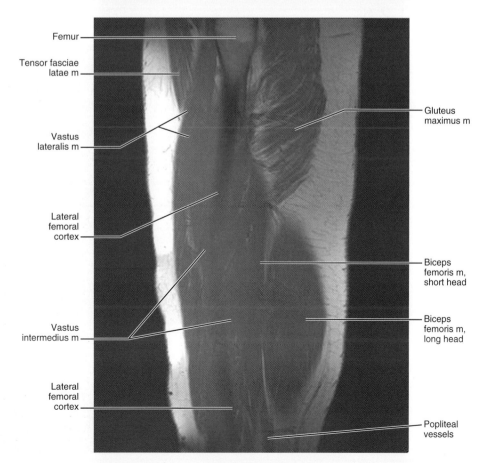

Greater trochanter

Tensor fasciae latae m

Vastus intermedius m

Vastus lateralis m

Vastus intermedius m

Lateral intermuscular septum

Gluteus maximus m

Biceps femoris m, long head

Biceps femoris m, short head

Figure 11.2.4

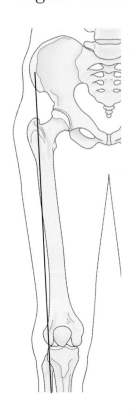

Femur

Tensor fasciae latae m

Vastus lateralis m

Lateral femoral cortex

Vastus intermedius m

Lateral femoral cortex

Gluteus maximus m

Biceps femoris m, short head

Biceps femoris m, long head

Popliteal vessels

Figure 11.2.5

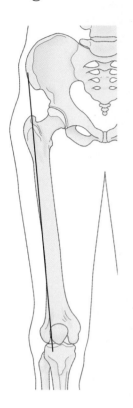

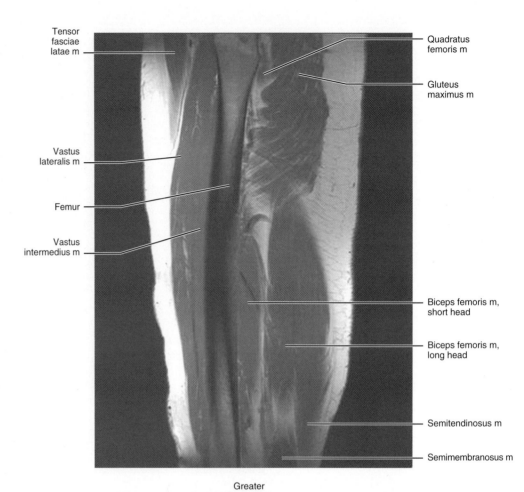

Tensor fasciae latae m

Vastus lateralis m

Femur

Vastus intermedius m

Quadratus femoris m

Gluteus maximus m

Biceps femoris m, short head

Biceps femoris m, long head

Semitendinosus m

Semimembranosus m

Figure 11.2.6

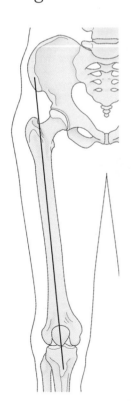

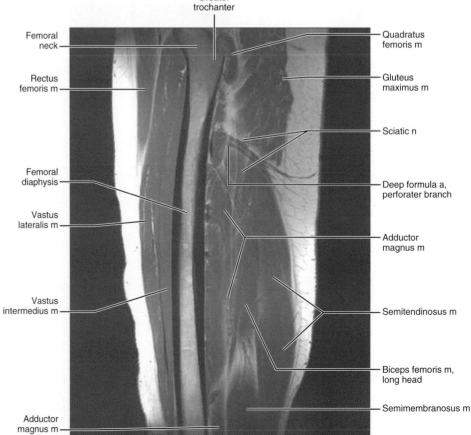

Greater trochanter

Femoral neck

Rectus femoris m

Femoral diaphysis

Vastus lateralis m

Vastus intermedius m

Adductor magnus m

Quadratus femoris m

Gluteus maximus m

Sciatic n

Deep formula a, perforater branch

Adductor magnus m

Semitendinosus m

Biceps femoris m, long head

Semimembranosus m

Figure 11.2.7

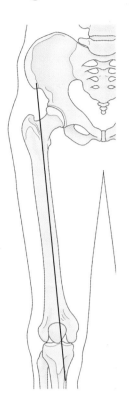

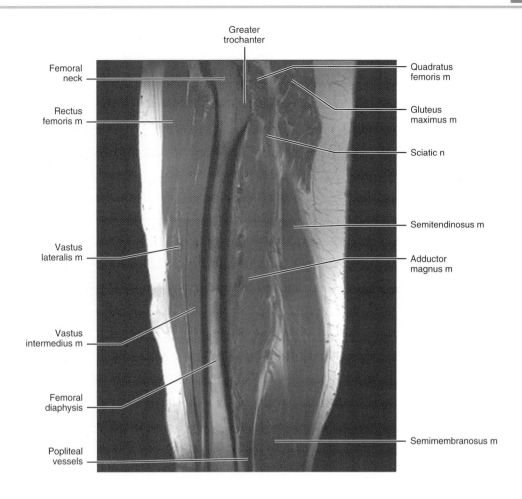

Greater trochanter

Femoral neck

Rectus femoris m

Vastus lateralis m

Vastus intermedius m

Femoral diaphysis

Popliteal vessels

Quadratus femoris m

Gluteus maximus m

Sciatic n

Semitendinosus m

Adductor magnus m

Semimembranosus m

Figure 11.2.8

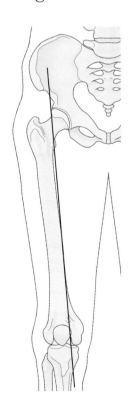

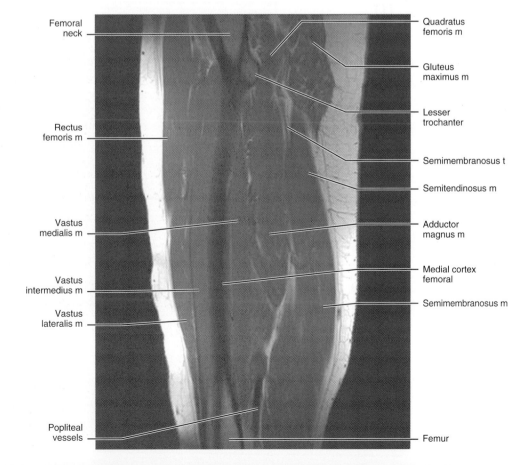

Femoral neck

Rectus femoris m

Vastus medialis m

Vastus intermedius m

Vastus lateralis m

Popliteal vessels

Quadratus femoris m

Gluteus maximus m

Lesser trochanter

Semimembranosus t

Semitendinosus m

Adductor magnus m

Medial cortex femoral

Semimembranosus m

Femur

Figure 11.2.9

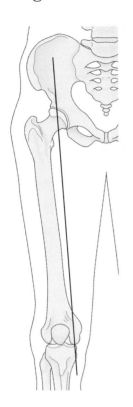

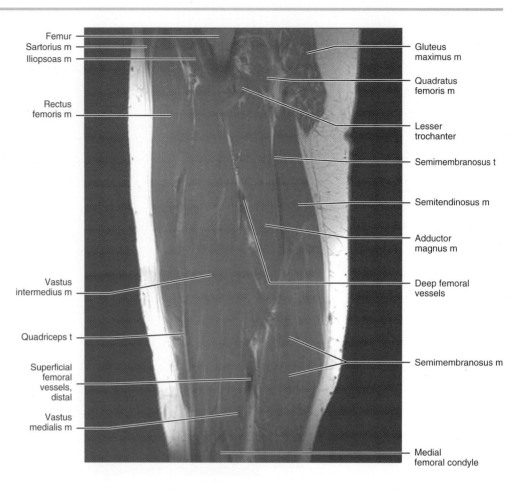

Femur
Sartorius m
Iliopsoas m

Rectus femoris m

Gluteus maximus m

Quadratus femoris m

Lesser trochanter

Semimembranosus t

Semitendinosus m

Adductor magnus m

Deep femoral vessels

Vastus intermedius m

Quadriceps t

Superficial femoral vessels, distal

Vastus medialis m

Semimembranosus m

Medial femoral condyle

Figure 11.2.10

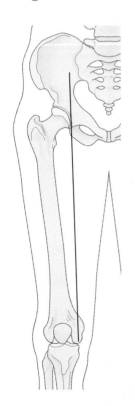

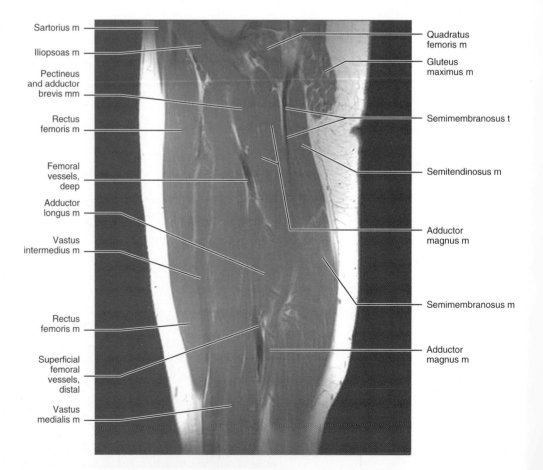

Sartorius m

Iliopsoas m

Pectineus and adductor brevis mm

Rectus femoris m

Femoral vessels, deep

Adductor longus m

Vastus intermedius m

Rectus femoris m

Superficial femoral vessels, distal

Vastus medialis m

Quadratus femoris m

Gluteus maximus m

Semimembranosus t

Semitendinosus m

Adductor magnus m

Semimembranosus m

Adductor magnus m

Figure 11.2.11

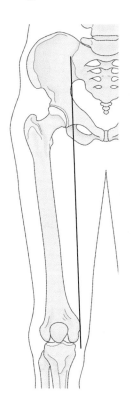

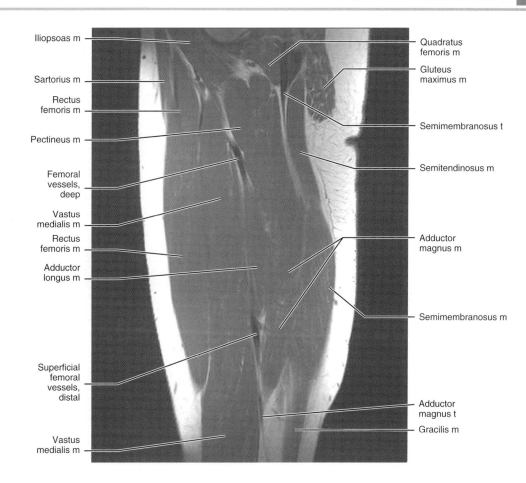

Iliopsoas m

Sartorius m

Rectus femoris m

Pectineus m

Femoral vessels, deep

Vastus medialis m

Rectus femoris m

Adductor longus m

Superficial femoral vessels, distal

Vastus medialis m

Quadratus femoris m

Gluteus maximus m

Semimembranosus t

Semitendinosus m

Adductor magnus m

Semimembranosus m

Adductor magnus t

Gracilis m

Figure 11.2.12

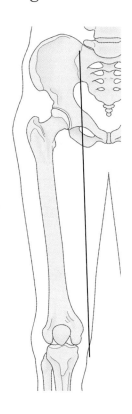

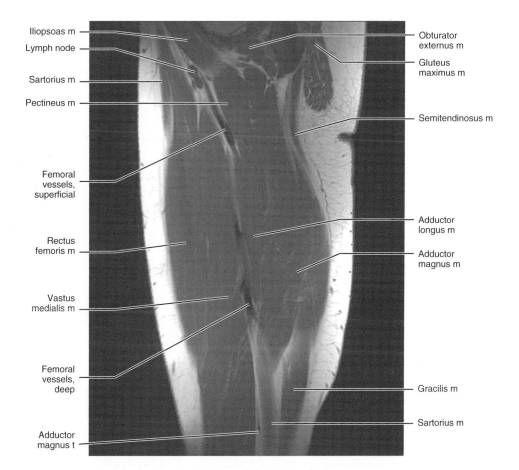

Iliopsoas m

Lymph node

Sartorius m

Pectineus m

Femoral vessels, superficial

Rectus femoris m

Vastus medialis m

Femoral vessels, deep

Adductor magnus t

Obturator externus m

Gluteus maximus m

Semitendinosus m

Adductor longus m

Adductor magnus m

Gracilis m

Sartorius m

Figure 11.2.13

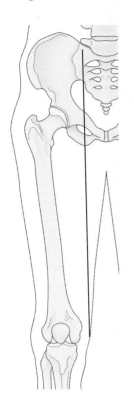

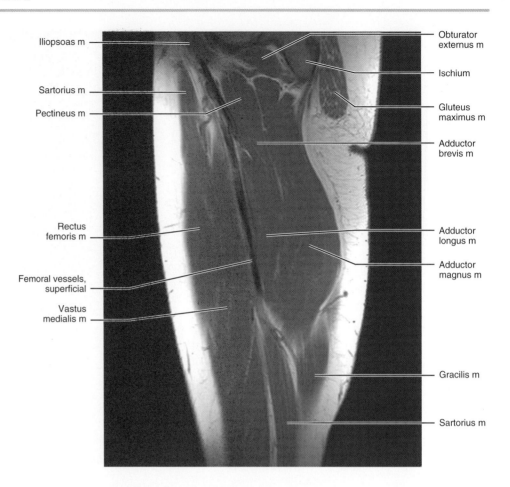

Iliopsoas m

Sartorius m

Pectineus m

Rectus femoris m

Femoral vessels, superficial

Vastus medialis m

Obturator externus m

Ischium

Gluteus maximus m

Adductor brevis m

Adductor longus m

Adductor magnus m

Gracilis m

Sartorius m

Figure 11.2.14

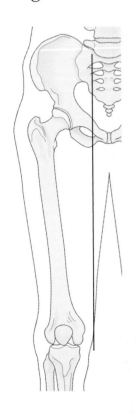

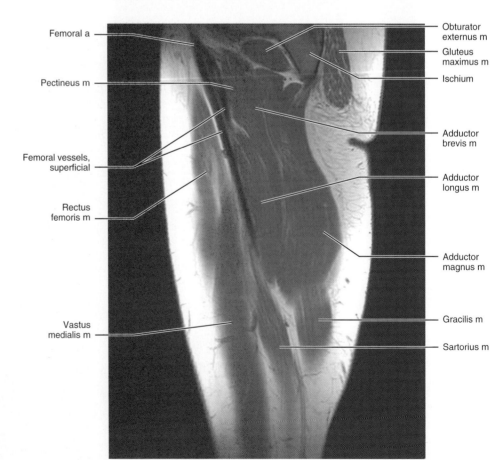

Femoral a

Pectineus m

Femoral vessels, superficial

Rectus femoris m

Vastus medialis m

Obturator externus m

Gluteus maximus m

Ischium

Adductor brevis m

Adductor longus m

Adductor magnus m

Gracilis m

Sartorius m

Figure 11.2.15

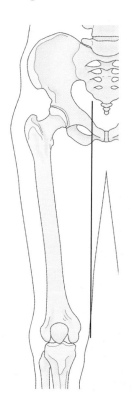

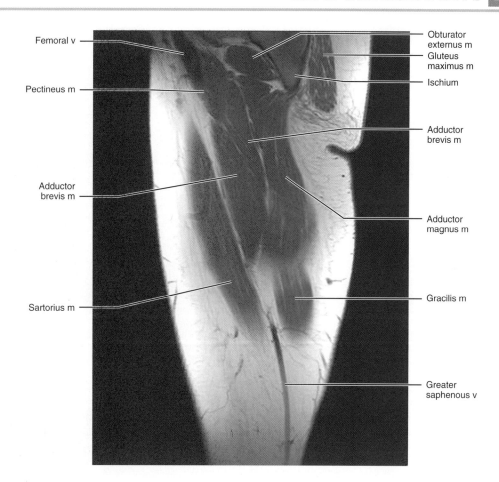

Femoral v — Obturator externus m

Pectineus m — Gluteus maximus m

— Ischium

— Adductor brevis m

Adductor brevis m — Adductor magnus m

Sartorius m — Gracilis m

— Greater saphenous v

Figure 11.2.16

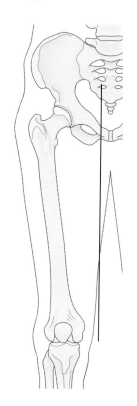

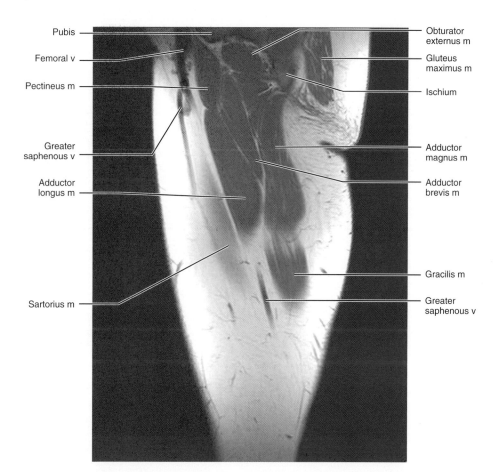

Pubis — Obturator externus m

Femoral v — Gluteus maximus m

Pectineus m — Ischium

Greater saphenous v — Adductor magnus m

Adductor longus m — Adductor brevis m

Sartorius m — Gracilis m

— Greater saphenous v

Figure 11.2.17

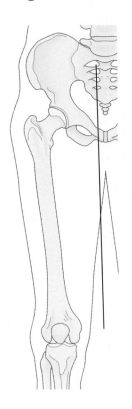

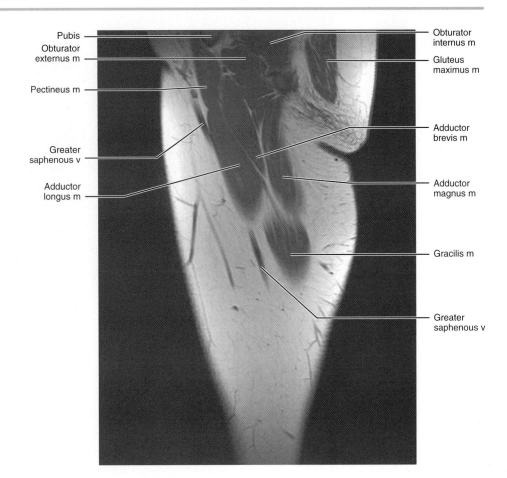

Pubis

Obturator
externus m

Pectineus m

Greater
saphenous v

Adductor
longus m

Obturator
internus m

Gluteus
maximus m

Adductor
brevis m

Adductor
magnus m

Gracilis m

Greater
saphenous v

CORONAL
Figure 11.3.1

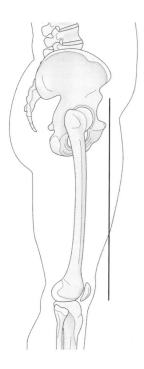

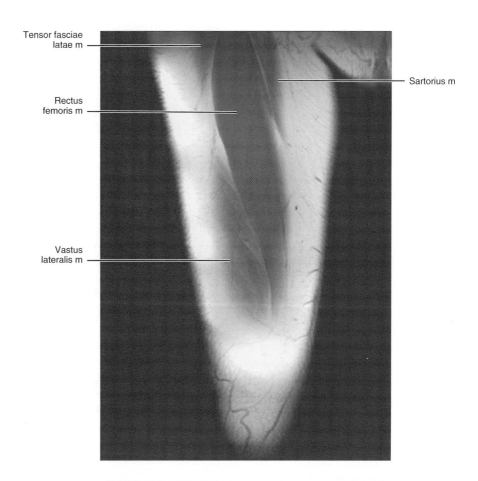

Tensor fasciae latae m

Rectus femoris m

Vastus lateralis m

Sartorius m

Figure 11.3.2

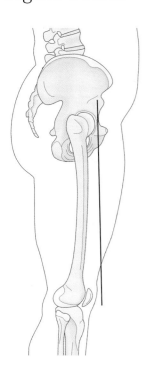

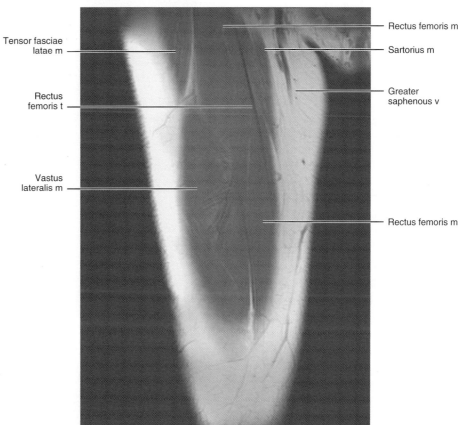

Tensor fasciae latae m

Rectus femoris t

Vastus lateralis m

Rectus femoris m

Sartorius m

Greater saphenous v

Rectus femoris m

Figure 11.3.3

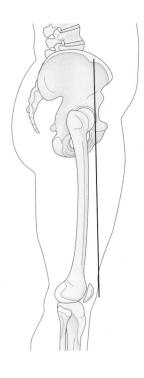

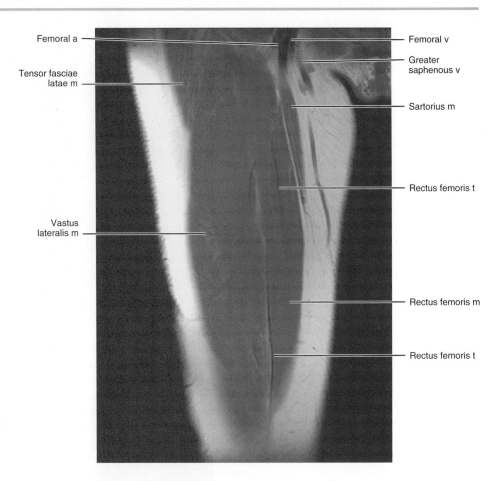

Femoral a — — Femoral v

— Greater saphenous v

Tensor fasciae latae m — — Sartorius m

— Rectus femoris t

Vastus lateralis m —

— Rectus femoris m

— Rectus femoris t

Figure 11.3.4

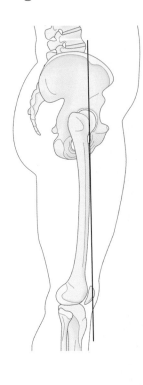

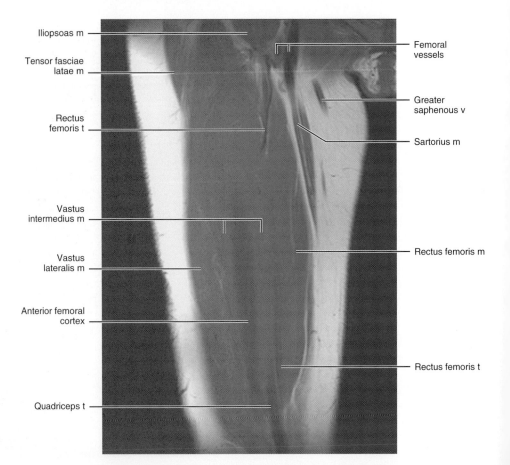

Iliopsoas m —

Tensor fasciae latae m — — Femoral vessels

Rectus femoris t — — Greater saphenous v

— Sartorius m

Vastus intermedius m —

Vastus lateralis m — — Rectus femoris m

Anterior femoral cortex —

— Rectus femoris t

Quadriceps t —

Figure 11.3.5

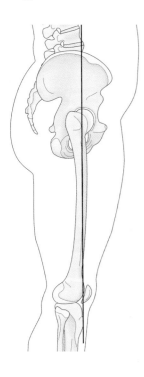

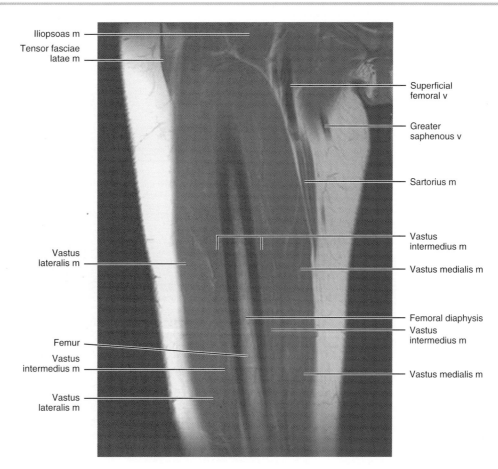

Iliopsoas m

Tensor fasciae latae m

Superficial femoral v

Greater saphenous v

Sartorius m

Vastus lateralis m

Vastus intermedius m

Vastus medialis m

Femoral diaphysis

Vastus intermedius m

Femur

Vastus intermedius m

Vastus medialis m

Vastus lateralis m

Figure 11.3.6

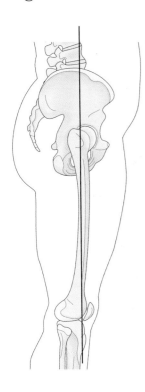

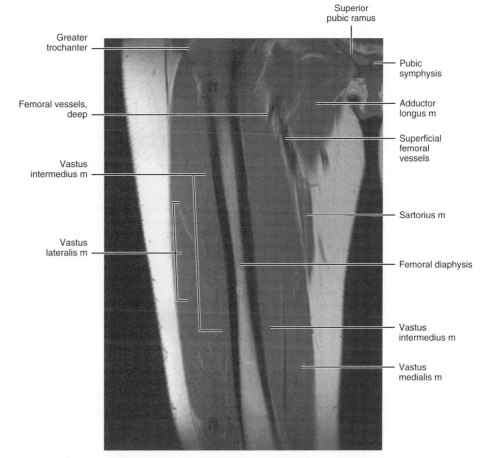

Superior pubic ramus

Greater trochanter

Pubic symphysis

Femoral vessels, deep

Adductor longus m

Superficial femoral vessels

Vastus intermedius m

Vastus lateralis m

Sartorius m

Femoral diaphysis

Vastus intermedius m

Vastus medialis m

Figure 11.3.7

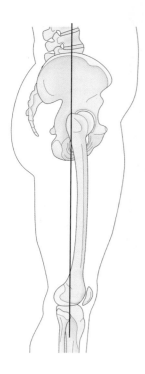

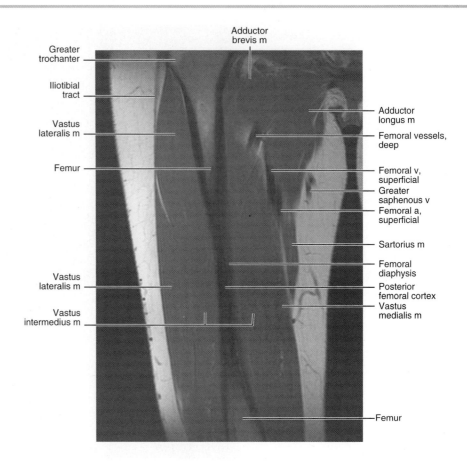

Greater trochanter

Iliotibial tract

Vastus lateralis m

Femur

Vastus lateralis m

Vastus intermedius m

Adductor brevis m

Adductor longus m

Femoral vessels, deep

Femoral v, superficial

Greater saphenous v

Femoral a, superficial

Sartorius m

Femoral diaphysis

Posterior femoral cortex

Vastus medialis m

Femur

Figure 11.3.8

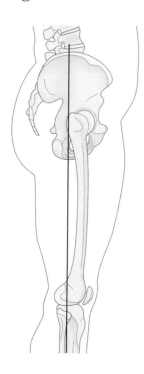

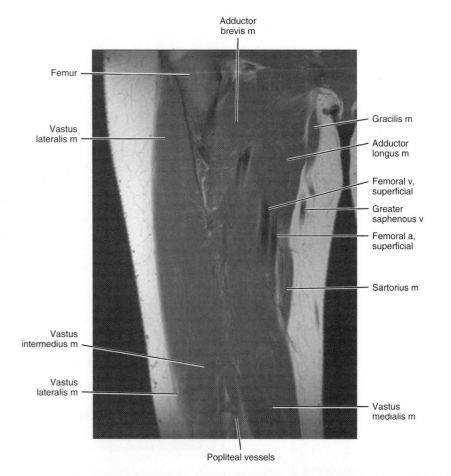

Femur

Vastus lateralis m

Vastus intermedius m

Vastus lateralis m

Adductor brevis m

Gracilis m

Adductor longus m

Femoral v, superficial

Greater saphenous v

Femoral a, superficial

Sartorius m

Vastus medialis m

Popliteal vessels

Figure 11.3.9

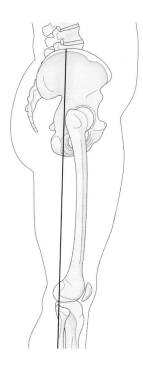

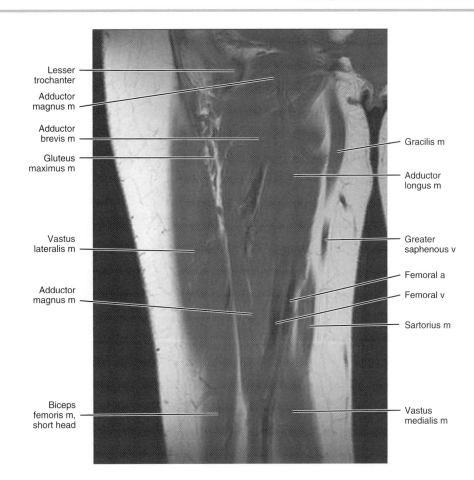

Lesser trochanter
Adductor magnus m
Adductor brevis m
Gluteus maximus m
Vastus lateralis m
Adductor magnus m
Biceps femoris m, short head

Gracilis m
Adductor longus m
Greater saphenous v
Femoral a
Femoral v
Sartorius m
Vastus medialis m

Figure 11.3.10

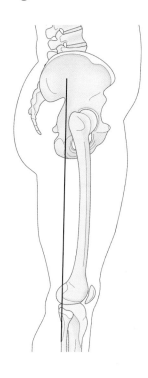

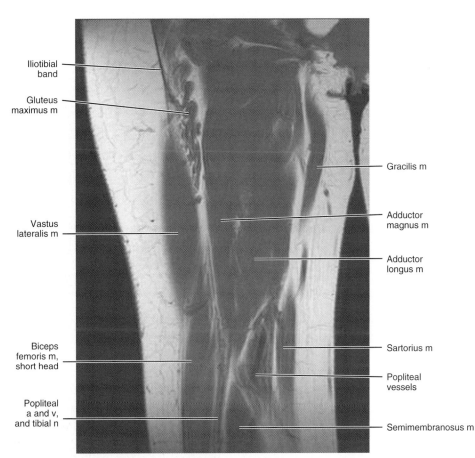

Iliotibial band
Gluteus maximus m
Vastus lateralis m
Biceps femoris m, short head
Popliteal a and v, and tibial n

Gracilis m
Adductor magnus m
Adductor longus m
Sartorius m
Popliteal vessels
Semimembranosus m

Figure 11.3.11

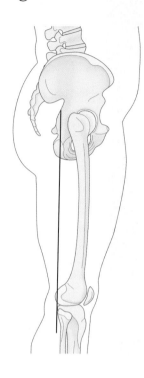

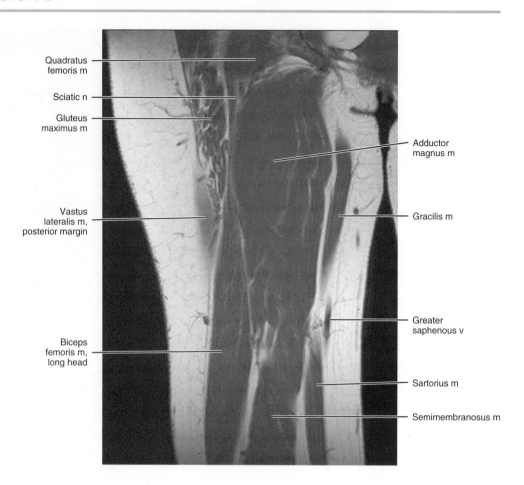

Quadratus femoris m

Sciatic n

Gluteus maximus m

Adductor magnus m

Gracilis m

Vastus lateralis m, posterior margin

Greater saphenous v

Sartorius m

Biceps femoris m, long head

Semimembranosus m

Figure 11.3.12

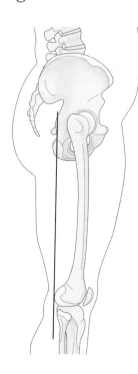

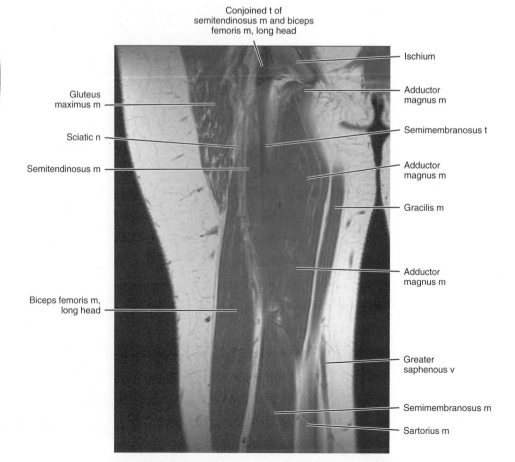

Conjoined t of semitendinosus m and biceps femoris m, long head

Ischium

Gluteus maximus m

Adductor magnus m

Sciatic n

Semimembranosus t

Semitendinosus m

Adductor magnus m

Gracilis m

Adductor magnus m

Biceps femoris m, long head

Greater saphenous v

Semimembranosus m

Sartorius m

Figure 11.3.13

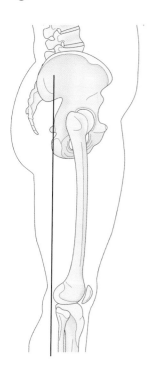

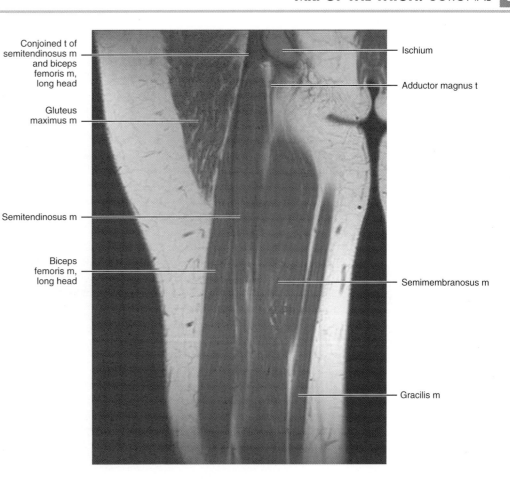

Conjoined t of semitendinosus m and biceps femoris m, long head

Gluteus maximus m

Semitendinosus m

Biceps femoris m, long head

Ischium

Adductor magnus t

Semimembranosus m

Gracilis m

Figure 11.3.14

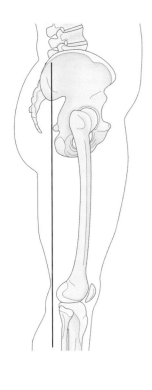

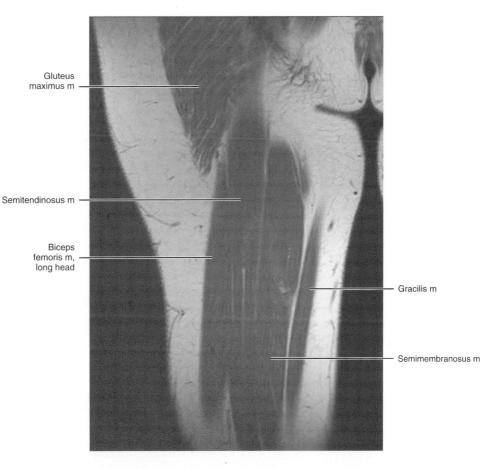

Gluteus maximus m

Semitendinosus m

Biceps femoris m, long head

Gracilis m

Semimembranosus m

Figure 11.3.15

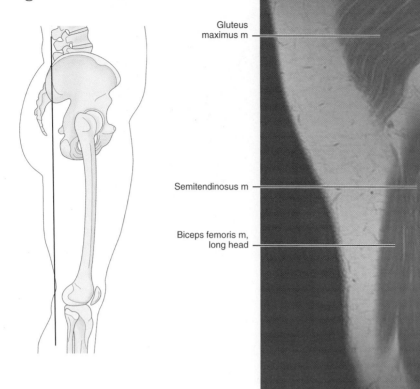

Gluteus maximus m

Semimembranosus m

Semitendinosus m

Biceps femoris m, long head

Gracilis m

Chapter 12

MRI of the Knee

AXIAL

Figure 12.1.1

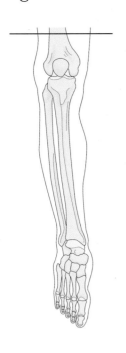

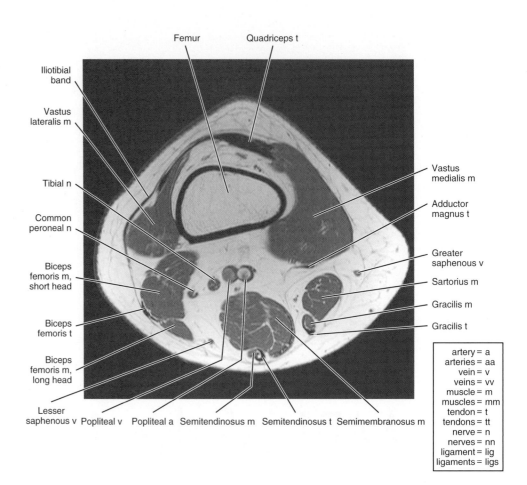

Femur

Quadriceps t

Iliotibial band

Vastus lateralis m

Vastus medialis m

Adductor magnus t

Tibial n

Common peroneal n

Greater saphenous v

Sartorius m

Biceps femoris m, short head

Gracilis m

Biceps femoris t

Gracilis t

Biceps femoris m, long head

Lesser saphenous v   Popliteal v   Popliteal a   Semitendinosus m   Semitendinosus t   Semimembranosus m

artery = a
arteries = aa
vein = v
veins = vv
muscle = m
muscles = mm
tendon = t
tendons = tt
nerve = n
nerves = nn
ligament = lig
ligaments = ligs

Figure 12.1.2

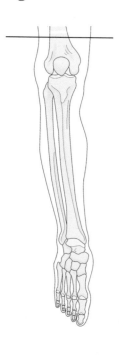

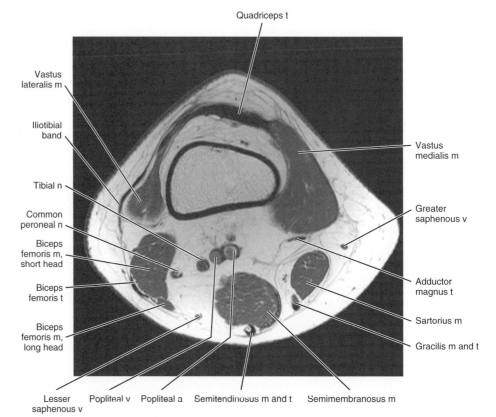

Quadriceps t

Vastus lateralis m

Iliotibial band

Vastus medialis m

Tibial n

Common peroneal n

Greater saphenous v

Biceps femoris m, short head

Biceps femoris t

Adductor magnus t

Biceps femoris m, long head

Sartorius m

Gracilis m and t

Lesser saphenous v   Popliteal v   Popliteal a   Semitendinosus m and t   Semimembranosus m

Figure 12.1.3

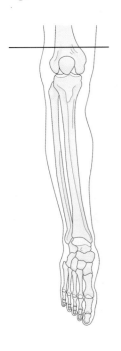

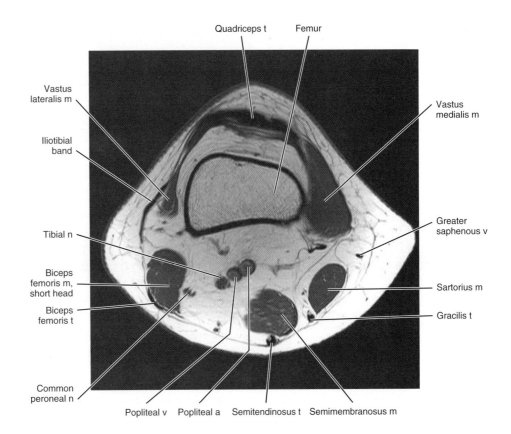

Quadriceps t   Femur

Vastus lateralis m

Iliotibial band

Vastus medialis m

Greater saphenous v

Tibial n

Biceps femoris m, short head

Biceps femoris t

Sartorius m

Gracilis t

Common peroneal n

Popliteal v   Popliteal a   Semitendinosus t   Semimembranosus m

Figure 12.1.4

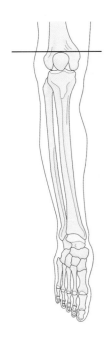

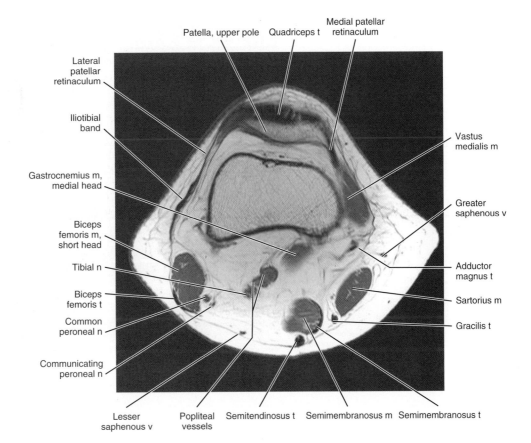

Patella, upper pole   Quadriceps t   Medial patellar retinaculum

Lateral patellar retinaculum

Iliotibial band

Gastrocnemius m, medial head

Biceps femoris m, short head

Tibial n

Biceps femoris t

Common peroneal n

Communicating peroneal n

Vastus medialis m

Greater saphenous v

Adductor magnus t

Sartorius m

Gracilis t

Lesser saphenous v   Popliteal vessels   Semitendinosus t   Semimembranosus m   Semimembranosus t

Figure 12.1.5

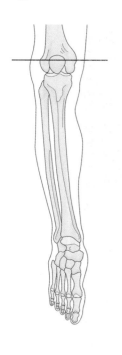

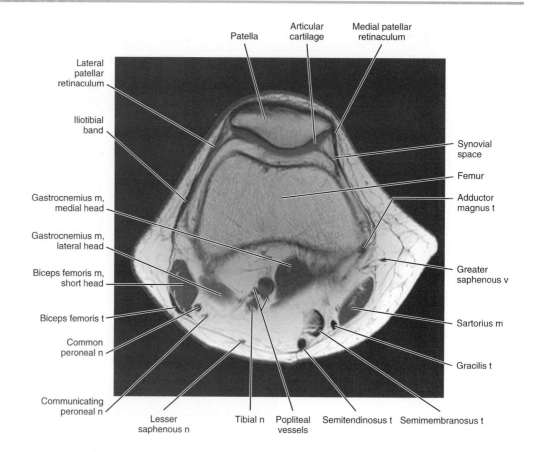

Lateral patellar retinaculum
Patella
Articular cartilage
Medial patellar retinaculum
Iliotibial band
Synovial space
Femur
Adductor magnus t
Gastrocnemius m, medial head
Gastrocnemius m, lateral head
Biceps femoris m, short head
Greater saphenous v
Biceps femoris t
Sartorius m
Common peroneal n
Gracilis t
Communicating peroneal n
Lesser saphenous n
Tibial n
Popliteal vessels
Semitendinosus t
Semimembranosus t

Figure 12.1.6

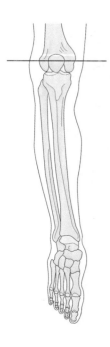

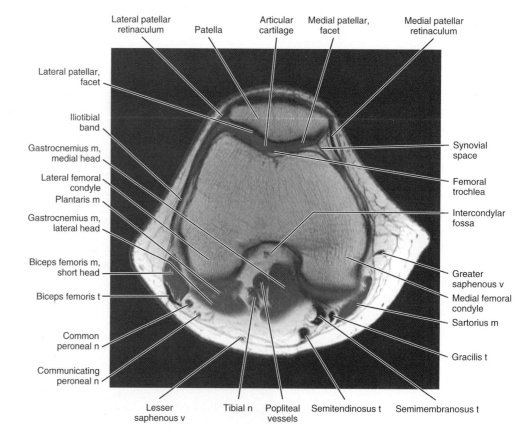

Lateral patellar retinaculum
Patella
Articular cartilage
Medial patellar, facet
Medial patellar retinaculum
Lateral patellar, facet
Iliotibial band
Synovial space
Gastrocnemius m, medial head
Femoral trochlea
Lateral femoral condyle
Plantaris m
Intercondylar fossa
Gastrocnemius m, lateral head
Biceps femoris m, short head
Greater saphenous v
Biceps femoris t
Medial femoral condyle
Sartorius m
Common peroneal n
Gracilis t
Communicating peroneal n
Lesser saphenous v
Tibial n
Popliteal vessels
Semitendinosus t
Semimembranosus t

Figure 12.1.7

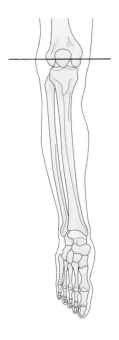

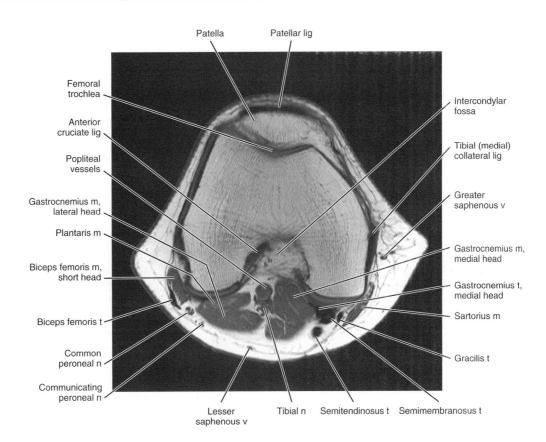

Patella
Patellar lig
Femoral trochlea
Anterior cruciate lig
Popliteal vessels
Gastrocnemius m, lateral head
Plantaris m
Biceps femoris m, short head
Biceps femoris t
Common peroneal n
Communicating peroneal n
Intercondylar fossa
Tibial (medial) collateral lig
Greater saphenous v
Gastrocnemius m, medial head
Gastrocnemius t, medial head
Sartorius m
Gracilis t
Lesser saphenous v
Tibial n
Semitendinosus t
Semimembranosus t

Figure 12.1.8

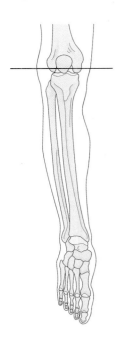

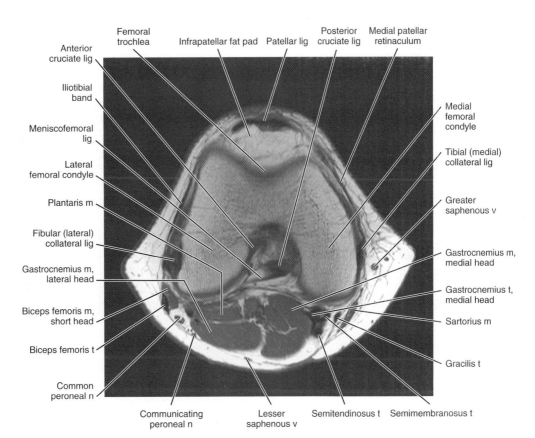

Femoral trochlea
Infrapatellar fat pad
Patellar lig
Posterior cruciate lig
Medial patellar retinaculum
Anterior cruciate lig
Iliotibial band
Meniscofemoral lig
Lateral femoral condyle
Plantaris m
Fibular (lateral) collateral lig
Gastrocnemius m, lateral head
Biceps femoris m, short head
Biceps femoris t
Common peroneal n
Medial femoral condyle
Tibial (medial) collateral lig
Greater saphenous v
Gastrocnemius m, medial head
Gastrocnemius t, medial head
Sartorius m
Gracilis t
Communicating peroneal n
Lesser saphenous v
Semitendinosus t
Semimembranosus t

Figure 12.1.9

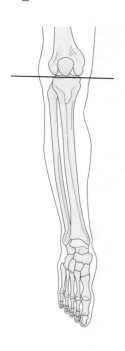

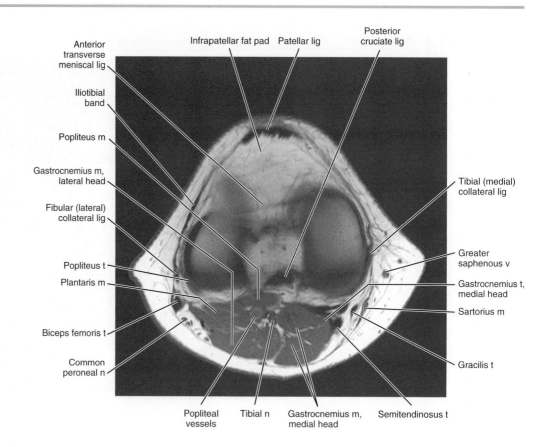

Anterior transverse meniscal lig

Iliotibial band

Popliteus m

Gastrocnemius m, lateral head

Fibular (lateral) collateral lig

Popliteus t

Plantaris m

Biceps femoris t

Common peroneal n

Infrapatellar fat pad

Patellar lig

Posterior cruciate lig

Tibial (medial) collateral lig

Greater saphenous v

Gastrocnemius t, medial head

Sartorius m

Gracilis t

Popliteal vessels

Tibial n

Gastrocnemius m, medial head

Semitendinosus t

Figure 12.1.10

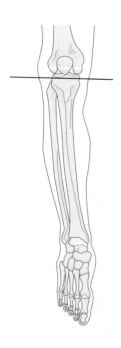

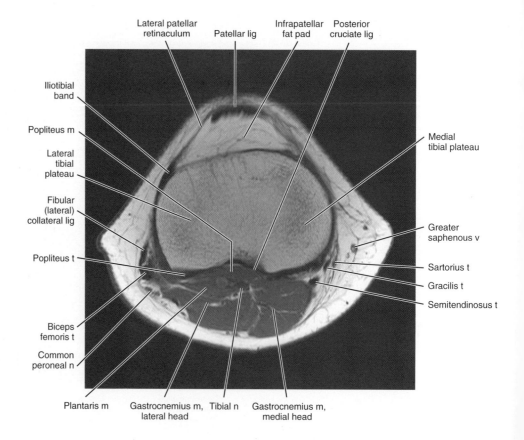

Lateral patellar retinaculum

Patellar lig

Infrapatellar fat pad

Posterior cruciate lig

Iliotibial band

Popliteus m

Lateral tibial plateau

Fibular (lateral) collateral lig

Popliteus t

Biceps femoris t

Common peroneal n

Medial tibial plateau

Greater saphenous v

Sartorius t

Gracilis t

Semitendinosus t

Plantaris m

Gastrocnemius m, lateral head

Tibial n

Gastrocnemius m, medial head

Figure 12.1.11

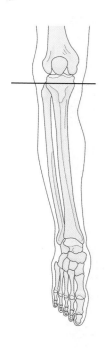
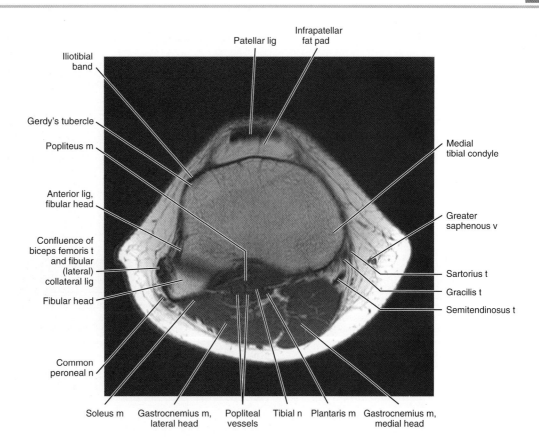

Figure 12.1.12

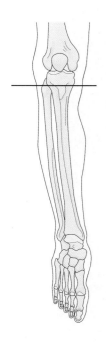
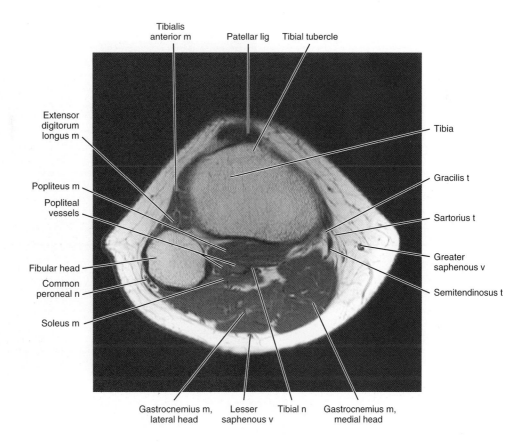

Figure 12.1.13

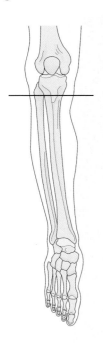

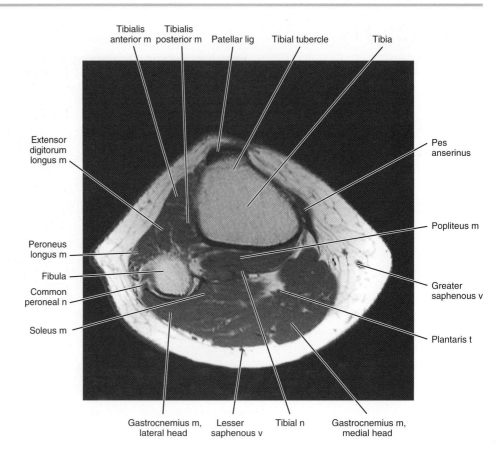

Tibialis anterior m | Tibialis posterior m | Patellar lig | Tibial tubercle | Tibia

Extensor digitorum longus m

Pes anserinus

Popliteus m

Peroneus longus m

Fibula

Common peroneal n

Soleus m

Greater saphenous v

Plantaris t

Gastrocnemius m, lateral head | Lesser saphenous v | Tibial n | Gastrocnemius m, medial head

Figure 12.1.14

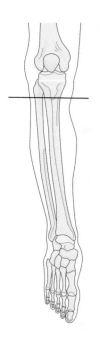

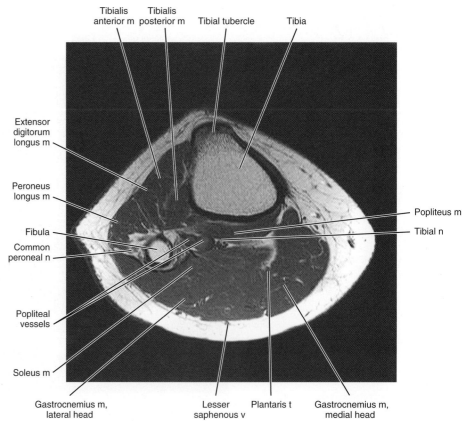

Tibialis anterior m | Tibialis posterior m | Tibial tubercle | Tibia

Extensor digitorum longus m

Peroneus longus m

Fibula

Common peroneal n

Popliteal vessels

Soleus m

Popliteus m

Tibial n

Gastrocnemius m, lateral head | Lesser saphenous v | Plantaris t | Gastrocnemius m, medial head

OBLIQUE SAGITTAL

Figure 12.2.1

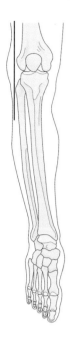

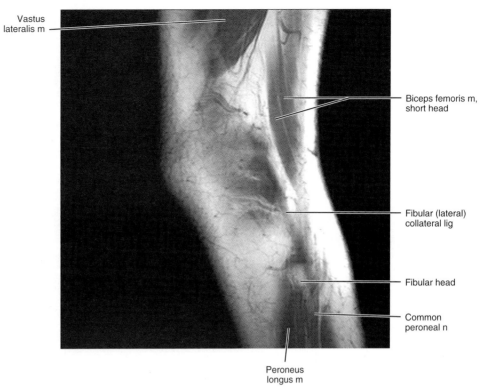

Vastus lateralis m

Biceps femoris m, short head

Fibular (lateral) collateral lig

Fibular head

Common peroneal n

Peroneus longus m

Figure 12.2.2

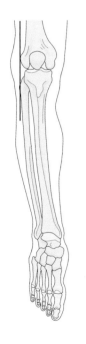

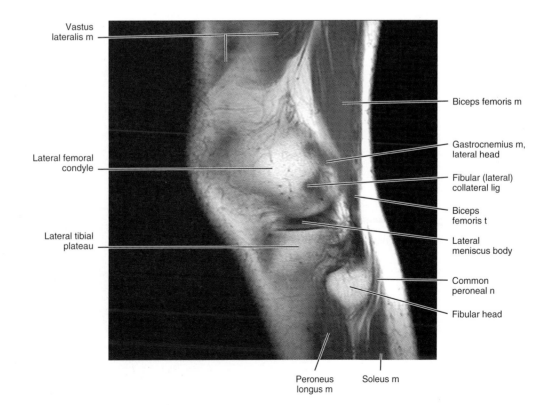

Vastus lateralis m

Lateral femoral condyle

Lateral tibial plateau

Biceps femoris m

Gastrocnemius m, lateral head

Fibular (lateral) collateral lig

Biceps femoris t

Lateral meniscus body

Common peroneal n

Fibular head

Peroneus longus m

Soleus m

Figure 12.2.3

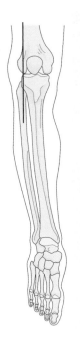

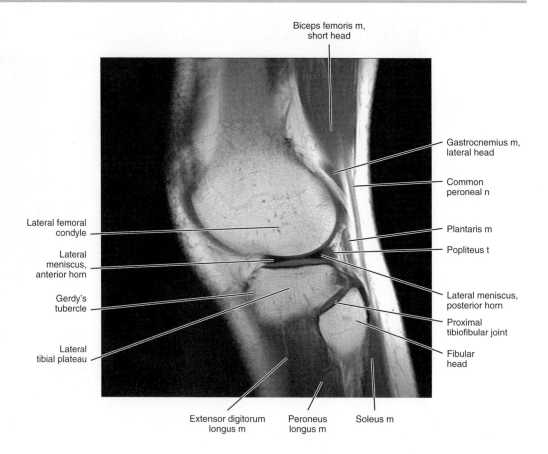

Biceps femoris m, short head

Gastrocnemius m, lateral head

Common peroneal n

Plantaris m

Popliteus t

Lateral meniscus, posterior horn

Proximal tibiofibular joint

Fibular head

Lateral femoral condyle

Lateral meniscus, anterior horn

Gerdy's tubercle

Lateral tibial plateau

Extensor digitorum longus m

Peroneus longus m

Soleus m

Figure 12.2.4

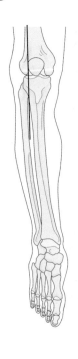

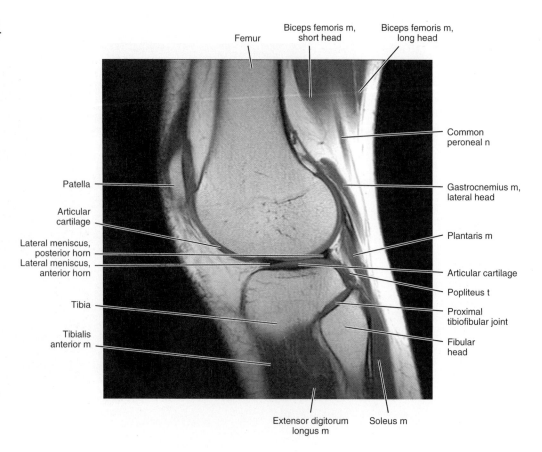

Femur

Biceps femoris m, short head

Biceps femoris m, long head

Common peroneal n

Gastrocnemius m, lateral head

Plantaris m

Articular cartilage

Popliteus t

Proximal tibiofibular joint

Fibular head

Patella

Articular cartilage

Lateral meniscus, posterior horn

Lateral meniscus, anterior horn

Tibia

Tibialis anterior m

Extensor digitorum longus m

Soleus m

Figure 12.2.5

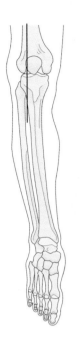

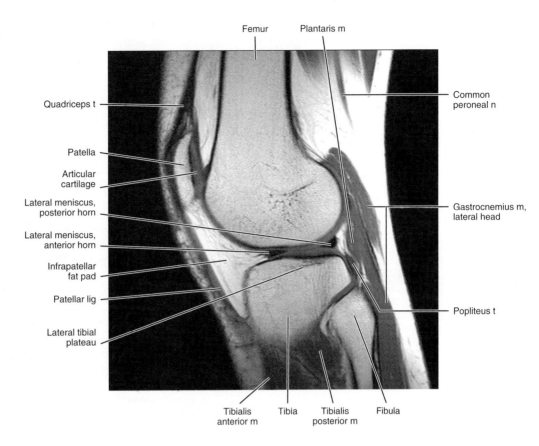

Femur
Plantaris m

Quadriceps t

Common peroneal n

Patella

Articular cartilage

Lateral meniscus, posterior horn

Gastrocnemius m, lateral head

Lateral meniscus, anterior horn

Infrapatellar fat pad

Patellar lig

Lateral tibial plateau

Popliteus t

Tibialis anterior m   Tibia   Tibialis posterior m   Fibula

Figure 12.2.6

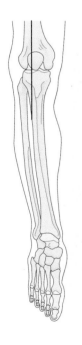

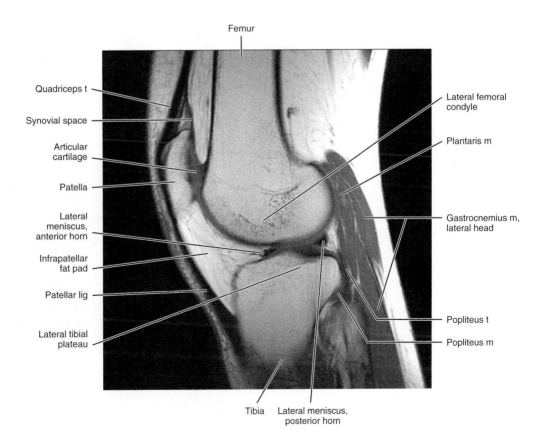

Femur

Quadriceps t

Lateral femoral condyle

Synovial space

Articular cartilage

Plantaris m

Patella

Lateral meniscus, anterior horn

Gastrocnemius m, lateral head

Infrapatellar fat pad

Patellar lig

Lateral tibial plateau

Popliteus t

Popliteus m

Tibia   Lateral meniscus, posterior horn

Figure 12.2.7

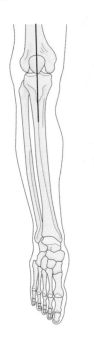

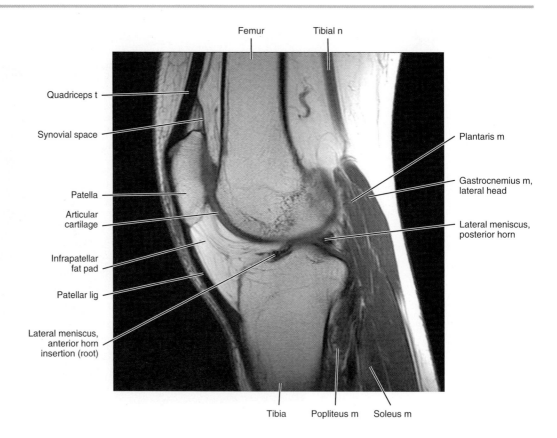

Femur   Tibial n

Quadriceps t

Synovial space

Patella

Articular cartilage

Infrapatellar fat pad

Patellar lig

Lateral meniscus, anterior horn insertion (root)

Plantaris m

Gastrocnemius m, lateral head

Lateral meniscus, posterior horn

Tibia   Popliteus m   Soleus m

Figure 12.2.8

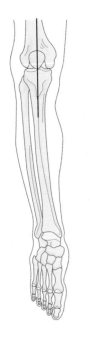

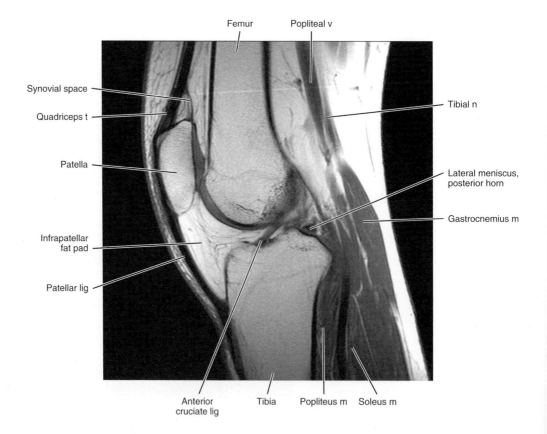

Femur   Popliteal v

Synovial space

Quadriceps t

Patella

Infrapatellar fat pad

Patellar lig

Tibial n

Lateral meniscus, posterior horn

Gastrocnemius m

Anterior cruciate lig   Tibia   Popliteus m   Soleus m

Figure 12.2.9

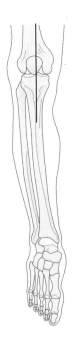

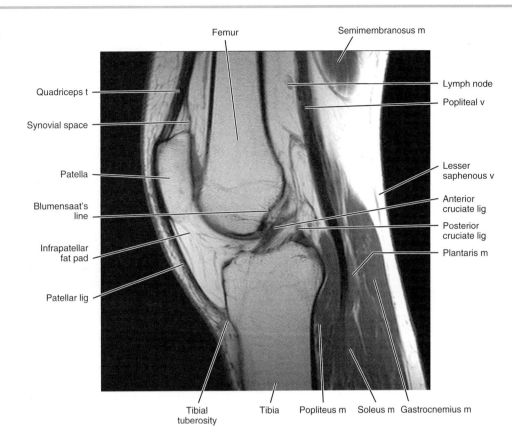

Femur
Semimembranosus m
Quadriceps t
Lymph node
Synovial space
Popliteal v
Patella
Lesser saphenous v
Blumensaat's line
Anterior cruciate lig
Infrapatellar fat pad
Posterior cruciate lig
Plantaris m
Patellar lig
Tibial tuberosity
Tibia
Popliteus m
Soleus m
Gastrocnemius m

Figure 12.2.10

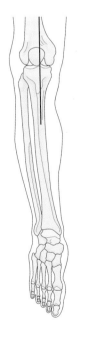

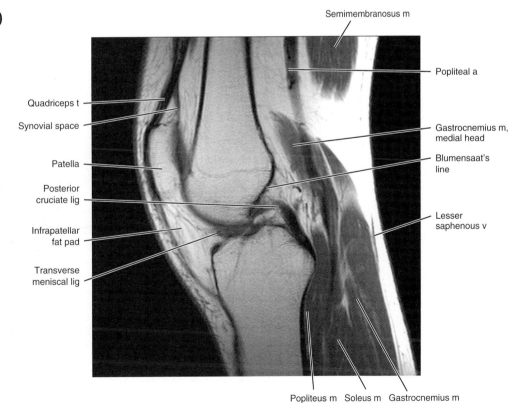

Semimembranosus m
Popliteal a
Quadriceps t
Synovial space
Gastrocnemius m, medial head
Patella
Blumensaat's line
Posterior cruciate lig
Infrapatellar fat pad
Lesser saphenous v
Transverse meniscal lig
Popliteus m
Soleus m
Gastrocnemius m

Figure 12.2.11

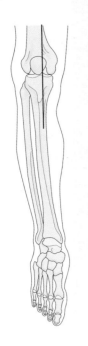

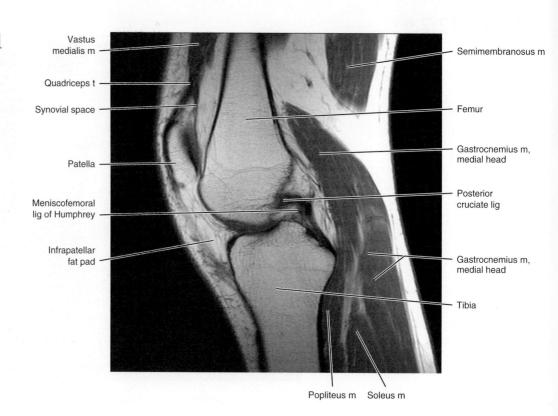

Vastus medialis m

Quadriceps t

Synovial space

Patella

Meniscofemoral lig of Humphrey

Infrapatellar fat pad

Semimembranosus m

Femur

Gastrocnemius m, medial head

Posterior cruciate lig

Gastrocnemius m, medial head

Tibia

Popliteus m   Soleus m

Figure 12.2.12

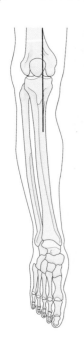

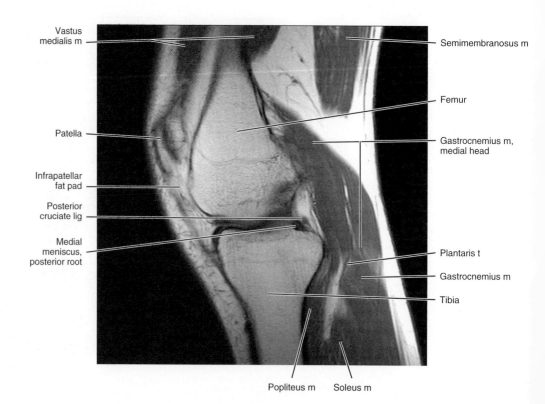

Vastus medialis m

Patella

Infrapatellar fat pad

Posterior cruciate lig

Medial meniscus, posterior root

Semimembranosus m

Femur

Gastrocnemius m, medial head

Plantaris t

Gastrocnemius m

Tibia

Popliteus m   Soleus m

Figure 12.2.13

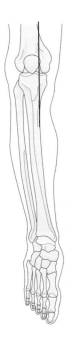

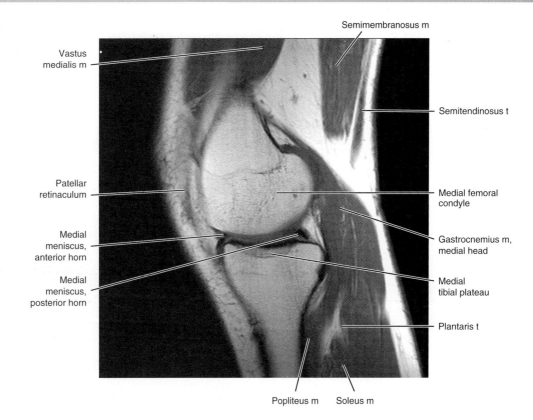

Semimembranosus m

Vastus medialis m

Semitendinosus t

Patellar retinaculum

Medial femoral condyle

Medial meniscus, anterior horn

Gastrocnemius m, medial head

Medial meniscus, posterior horn

Medial tibial plateau

Plantaris t

Popliteus m   Soleus m

Figure 12.2.14

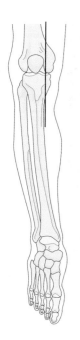

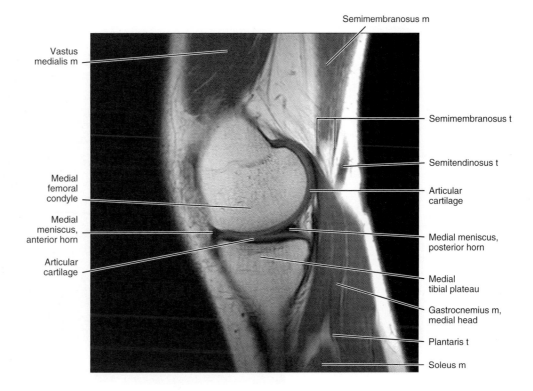

Semimembranosus m

Vastus medialis m

Semimembranosus t

Semitendinosus t

Medial femoral condyle

Articular cartilage

Medial meniscus, anterior horn

Medial meniscus, posterior horn

Articular cartilage

Medial tibial plateau

Gastrocnemius m, medial head

Plantaris t

Soleus m

Figure 12.2.15

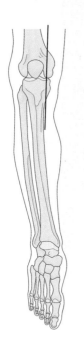

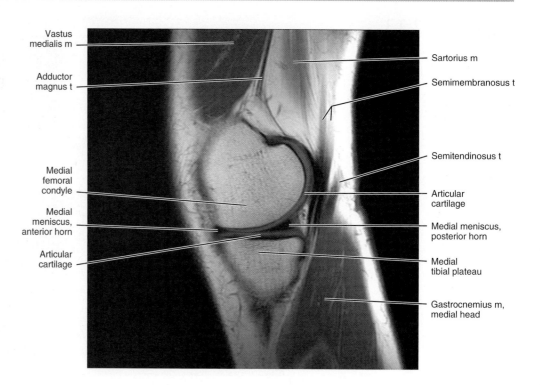

Vastus medialis m

Adductor magnus t

Medial femoral condyle

Medial meniscus, anterior horn

Articular cartilage

Sartorius m

Semimembranosus t

Semitendinosus t

Articular cartilage

Medial meniscus, posterior horn

Medial tibial plateau

Gastrocnemius m, medial head

Figure 12.2.16

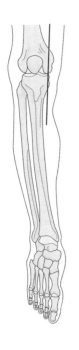

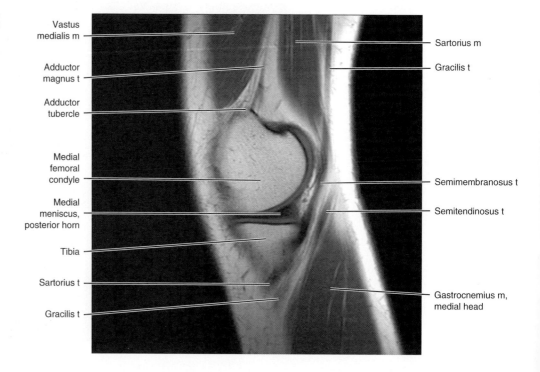

Vastus medialis m

Adductor magnus t

Adductor tubercle

Medial femoral condyle

Medial meniscus, posterior horn

Tibia

Sartorius t

Gracilis t

Sartorius m

Gracilis t

Semimembranosus t

Semitendinosus t

Gastrocnemius m, medial head

Figure 12.2.17

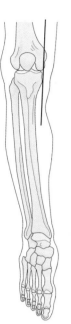

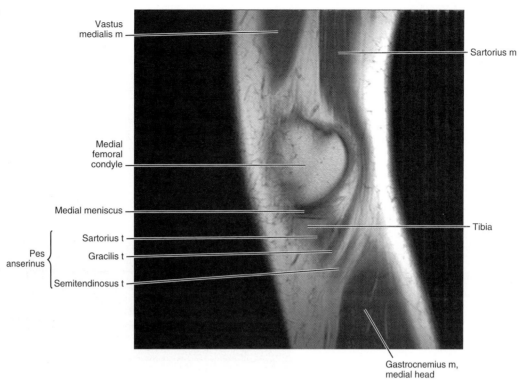

Vastus medialis m

Sartorius m

Medial femoral condyle

Medial meniscus

Tibia

Pes anserinus
- Sartorius t
- Gracilis t
- Semitendinosus t

Gastrocnemius m, medial head

CORONAL

Figure 12.3.1

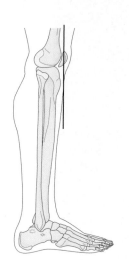

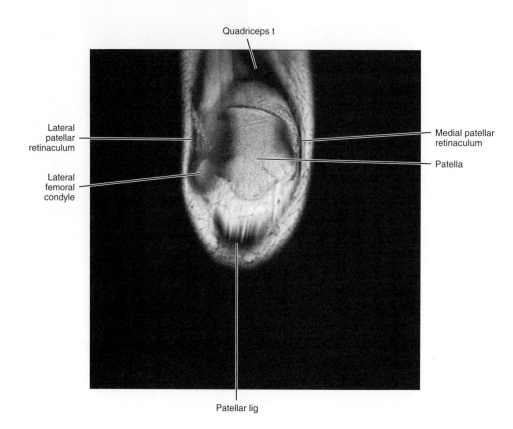

Quadriceps t

Lateral patellar retinaculum

Medial patellar retinaculum

Patella

Lateral femoral condyle

Patellar lig

Figure 12.3.2

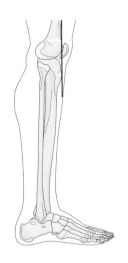

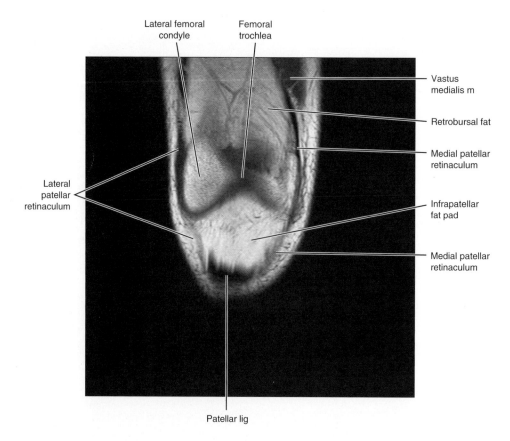

Lateral femoral condyle

Femoral trochlea

Vastus medialis m

Retrobursal fat

Medial patellar retinaculum

Lateral patellar retinaculum

Infrapatellar fat pad

Medial patellar retinaculum

Patellar lig

Figure 12.3.3

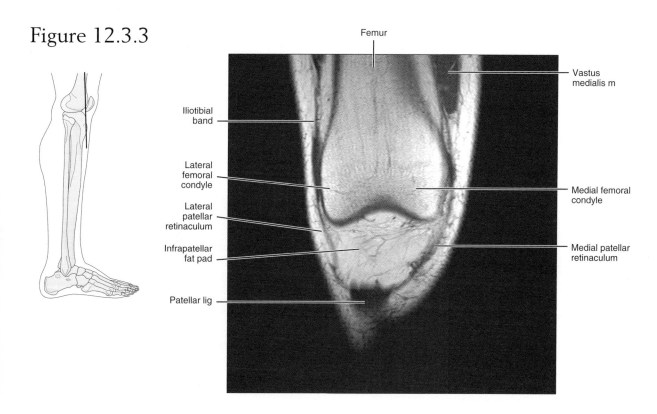

Femur

Vastus
medialis m

Iliotibial
band

Lateral
femoral
condyle

Medial femoral
condyle

Lateral
patellar
retinaculum

Infrapatellar
fat pad

Medial patellar
retinaculum

Patellar lig

Figure 12.3.4

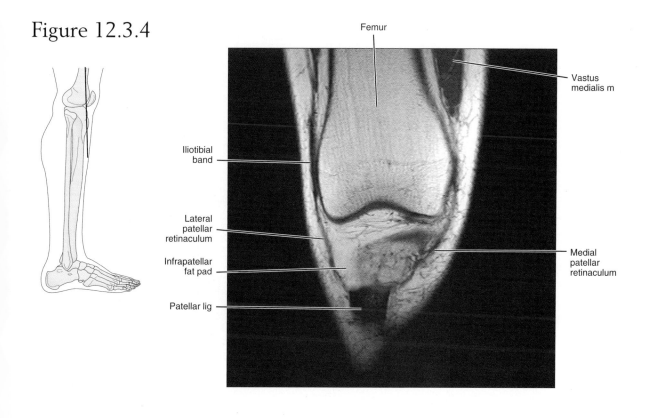

Femur

Vastus
medialis m

Iliotibial
band

Lateral
patellar
retinaculum

Infrapatellar
fat pad

Medial
patellar
retinaculum

Patellar lig

Figure 12.3.5

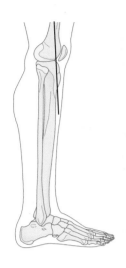

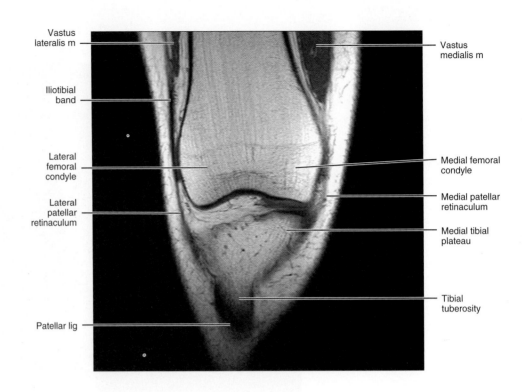

Vastus lateralis m

Vastus medialis m

Iliotibial band

Lateral femoral condyle

Medial femoral condyle

Lateral patellar retinaculum

Medial patellar retinaculum

Medial tibial plateau

Tibial tuberosity

Patellar lig

Figure 12.3.6

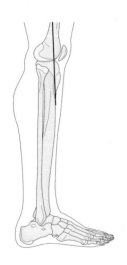

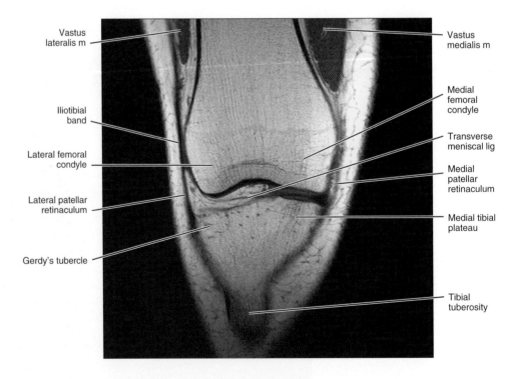

Vastus lateralis m

Vastus medialis m

Iliotibial band

Medial femoral condyle

Lateral femoral condyle

Transverse meniscal lig

Lateral patellar retinaculum

Medial patellar retinaculum

Medial tibial plateau

Gerdy's tubercle

Tibial tuberosity

Figure 12.3.7

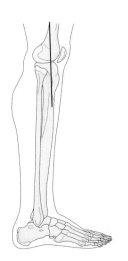

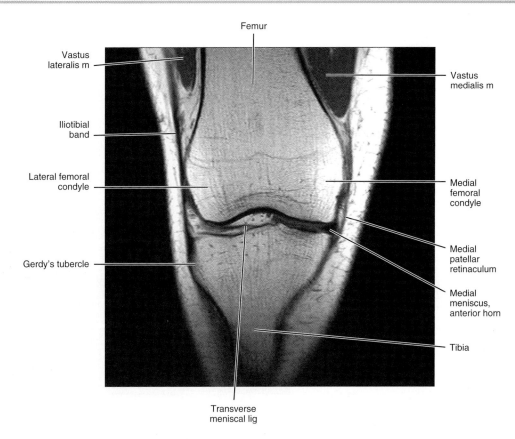

Vastus lateralis m

Iliotibial band

Lateral femoral condyle

Gerdy's tubercle

Femur

Vastus medialis m

Medial femoral condyle

Medial patellar retinaculum

Medial meniscus, anterior horn

Tibia

Transverse meniscal lig

Figure 12.3.8

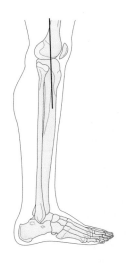

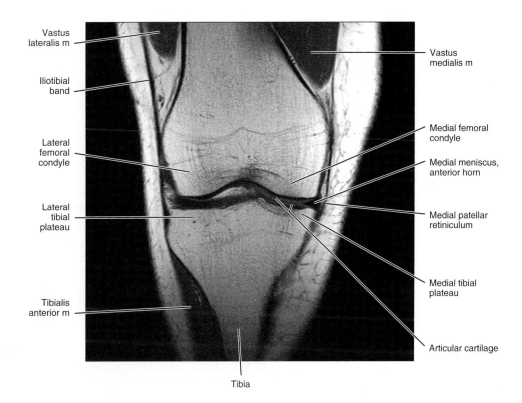

Vastus lateralis m

Iliotibial band

Lateral femoral condyle

Lateral tibial plateau

Tibialis anterior m

Vastus medialis m

Medial femoral condyle

Medial meniscus, anterior horn

Medial patellar retiniculum

Medial tibial plateau

Articular cartilage

Tibia

Figure 12.3.9

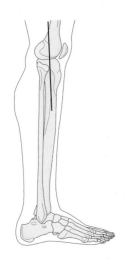

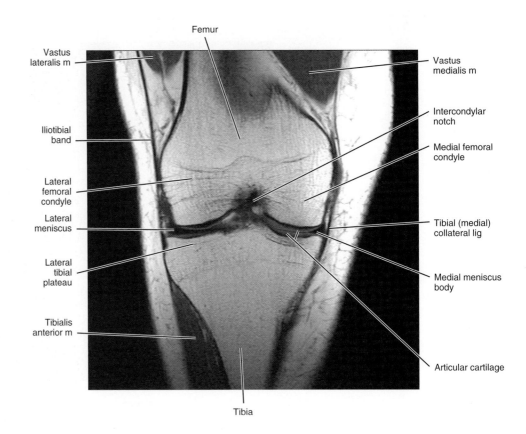

Femur

Vastus lateralis m

Vastus medialis m

Iliotibial band

Intercondylar notch

Lateral femoral condyle

Medial femoral condyle

Lateral meniscus

Tibial (medial) collateral lig

Lateral tibial plateau

Medial meniscus body

Tibialis anterior m

Articular cartilage

Tibia

Figure 12.3.10

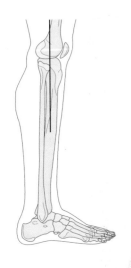

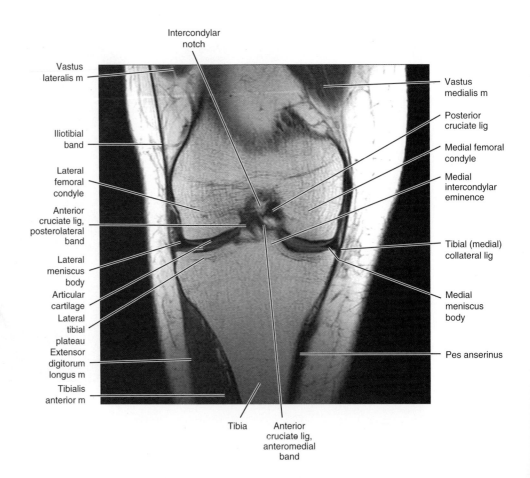

Intercondylar notch

Vastus lateralis m

Vastus medialis m

Iliotibial band

Posterior cruciate lig

Medial femoral condyle

Lateral femoral condyle

Medial intercondylar eminence

Anterior cruciate lig, posterolateral band

Lateral meniscus body

Tibial (medial) collateral lig

Articular cartilage

Medial meniscus body

Lateral tibial plateau

Pes anserinus

Extensor digitorum longus m

Tibialis anterior m

Tibia

Anterior cruciate lig, anteromedial band

Figure 12.3.11

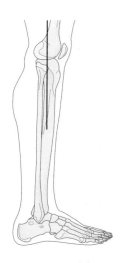

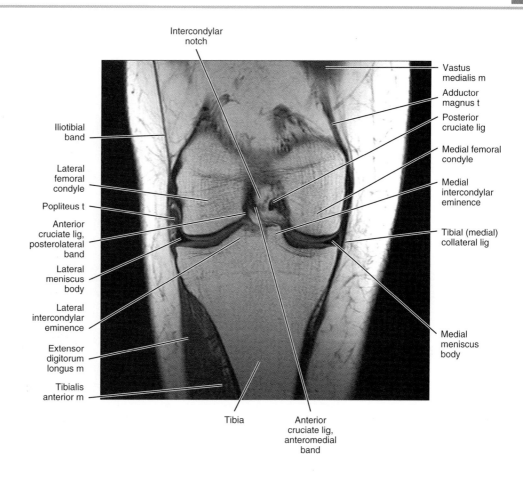

Intercondylar notch

Vastus medialis m

Adductor magnus t

Posterior cruciate lig

Medial femoral condyle

Medial intercondylar eminence

Tibial (medial) collateral lig

Medial meniscus body

Iliotibial band

Lateral femoral condyle

Popliteus t

Anterior cruciate lig, posterolateral band

Lateral meniscus body

Lateral intercondylar eminence

Extensor digitorum longus m

Tibialis anterior m

Tibia

Anterior cruciate lig, anteromedial band

Figure 12.3.12

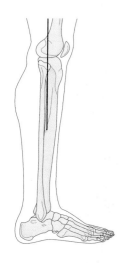

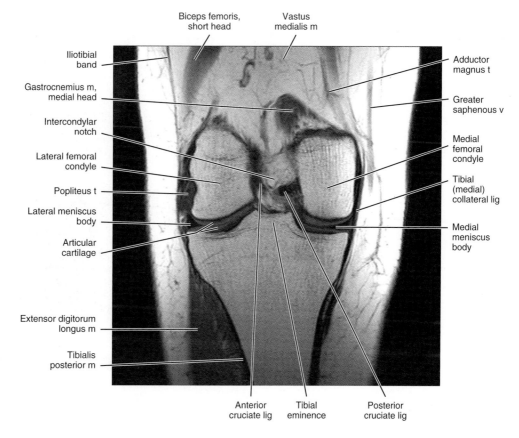

Biceps femoris, short head

Vastus medialis m

Iliotibial band

Gastrocnemius m, medial head

Intercondylar notch

Lateral femoral condyle

Popliteus t

Lateral meniscus body

Articular cartilage

Extensor digitorum longus m

Tibialis posterior m

Adductor magnus t

Greater saphenous v

Medial femoral condyle

Tibial (medial) collateral lig

Medial meniscus body

Anterior cruciate lig

Tibial eminence

Posterior cruciate lig

Figure 12.3.13

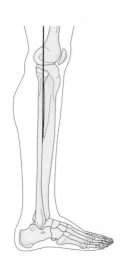

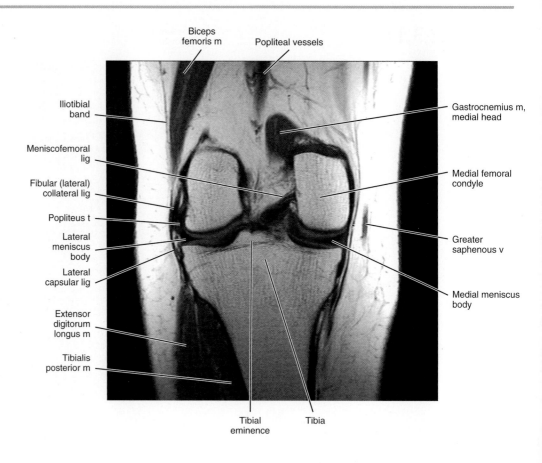

Biceps femoris m

Popliteal vessels

Iliotibial band

Meniscofemoral lig

Fibular (lateral) collateral lig

Popliteus t

Lateral meniscus body

Lateral capsular lig

Extensor digitorum longus m

Tibialis posterior m

Gastrocnemius m, medial head

Medial femoral condyle

Greater saphenous v

Medial meniscus body

Tibial eminence

Tibia

Figure 12.3.14

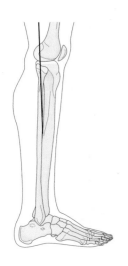

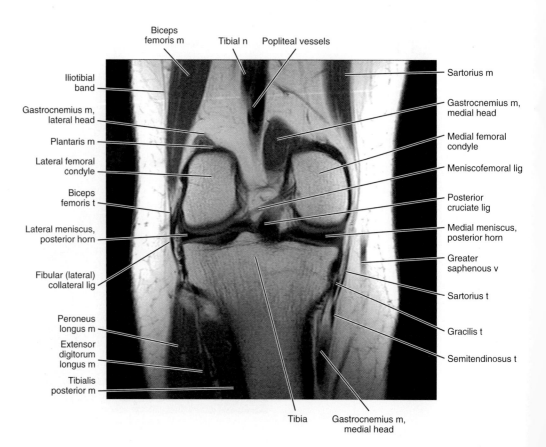

Biceps femoris m

Tibial n

Popliteal vessels

Iliotibial band

Gastrocnemius m, lateral head

Plantaris m

Lateral femoral condyle

Biceps femoris t

Lateral meniscus, posterior horn

Fibular (lateral) collateral lig

Peroneus longus m

Extensor digitorum longus m

Tibialis posterior m

Sartorius m

Gastrocnemius m, medial head

Medial femoral condyle

Meniscofemoral lig

Posterior cruciate lig

Medial meniscus, posterior horn

Greater saphenous v

Sartorius t

Gracilis t

Semitendinosus t

Tibia

Gastrocnemius m, medial head

Figure 12.3.15

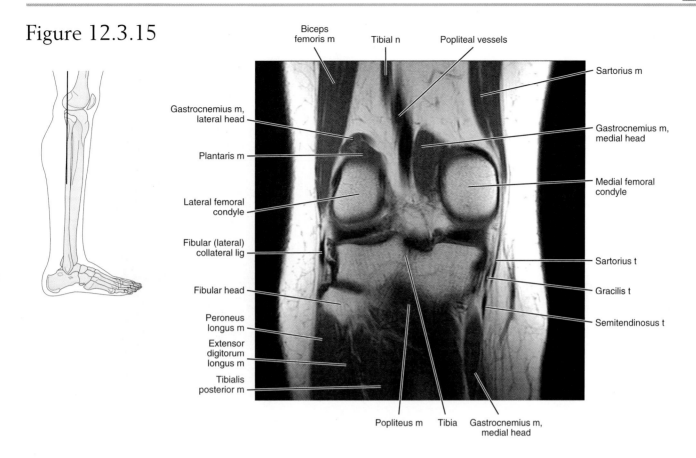

Biceps femoris m — Tibial n — Popliteal vessels — Sartorius m — Gastrocnemius m, lateral head — Gastrocnemius m, medial head — Plantaris m — Medial femoral condyle — Lateral femoral condyle — Fibular (lateral) collateral lig — Sartorius t — Fibular head — Gracilis t — Peroneus longus m — Semitendinosus t — Extensor digitorum longus m — Tibialis posterior m — Popliteus m — Tibia — Gastrocnemius m, medial head

Figure 12.3.16

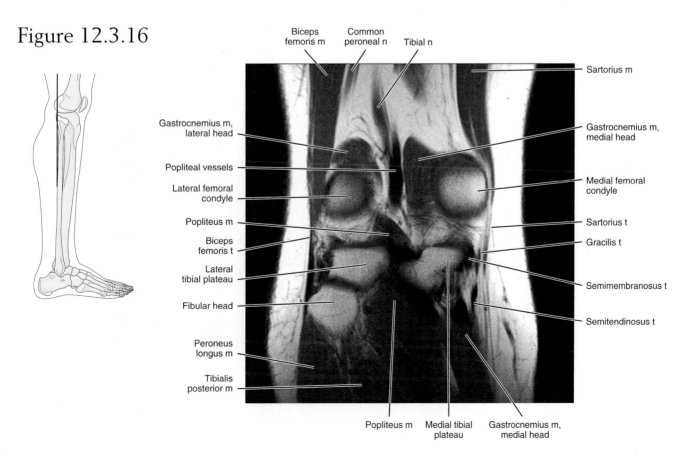

Biceps femoris m — Common peroneal n — Tibial n — Sartorius m — Gastrocnemius m, lateral head — Gastrocnemius m, medial head — Popliteal vessels — Medial femoral condyle — Lateral femoral condyle — Sartorius t — Popliteus m — Gracilis t — Biceps femoris t — Lateral tibial plateau — Semimembranosus t — Fibular head — Semitendinosus t — Peroneus longus m — Tibialis posterior m — Popliteus m — Medial tibial plateau — Gastrocnemius m, medial head

Figure 12.3.17

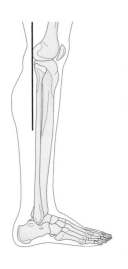

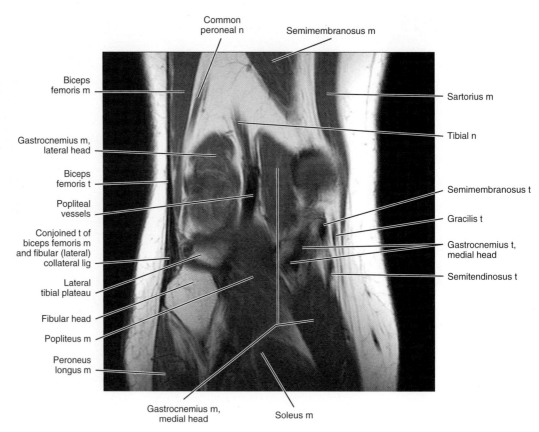

Common peroneal n

Semimembranosus m

Biceps femoris m

Sartorius m

Tibial n

Gastrocnemius m, lateral head

Biceps femoris t

Popliteal vessels

Semimembranosus t

Gracilis t

Conjoined t of biceps femoris m and fibular (lateral) collateral lig

Gastrocnemius t, medial head

Lateral tibial plateau

Semitendinosus t

Fibular head

Popliteus m

Peroneus longus m

Gastrocnemius m, medial head

Soleus m

Figure 12.3.18

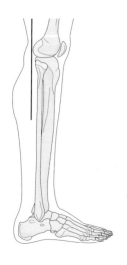

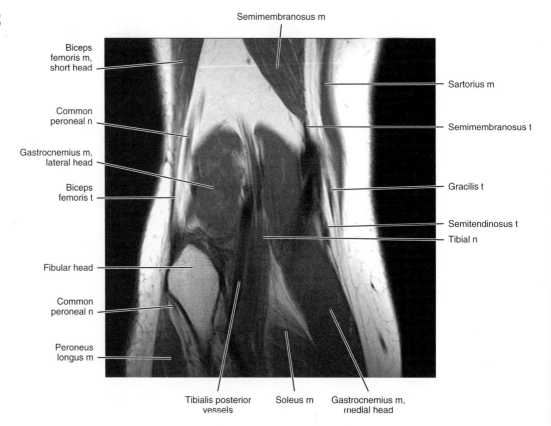

Semimembranosus m

Biceps femoris m, short head

Sartorius m

Common peroneal n

Semimembranosus t

Gastrocnemius m, lateral head

Biceps femoris t

Gracilis t

Semitendinosus t

Tibial n

Fibular head

Common peroneal n

Peroneus longus m

Tibialis posterior vessels

Soleus m

Gastrocnemius m, medial head

Figure 12.3.19

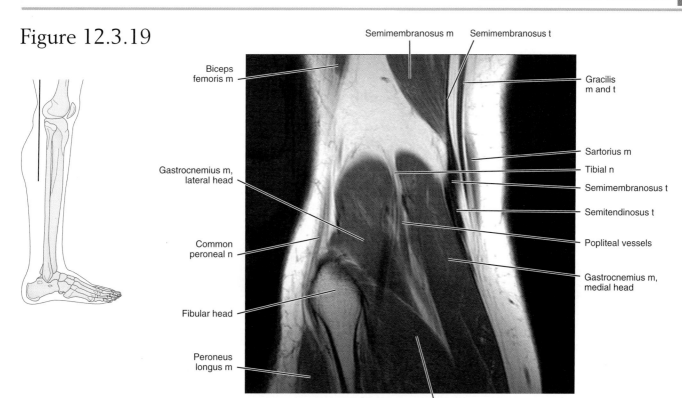

Biceps femoris m

Gastrocnemius m, lateral head

Common peroneal n

Fibular head

Peroneus longus m

Semimembranosus m

Semimembranosus t

Gracilis m and t

Sartorius m

Tibial n

Semimembranosus t

Semitendinosus t

Popliteal vessels

Gastrocnemius m, medial head

Soleus m

Chapter 13

MRI of the Leg

Table 7: Muscles of the Leg

MUSCLE	ORIGIN	INSERTION	NERVE SUPPLY
Tibialis anterior	Distal part of the lateral condyle of the tibia, lateral surface of the proximal half of the shaft of the tibia, adjacent interosseous membrane, overlying fascia near the condyle of the tibia, and intermuscular septum between it and the extensor digitorum longus	Medial surface of the first cuneiform and the base of the first metatarsal	Branch from the common peroneal and another from the deep peroneal
Extensor digitorum longus	Lateral condyle of the tibia, anterior crest of the fibula, intermuscular membrane between it and the tibialis anterior, lateral margin of the interosseous membrane, the septum between it and the peroneus longus, and fascia of the leg near the tibial origin	Each tendon, located on the dorsal surface of the toe to which it goes, divides into three fasciculi: the intermediate, attached to the dorsum of the base of the middle phalanx; and two lateral, which converge to the dorsum of the base on the distal phalanx. The margins of each tendon are bound to the sides of the back of the proximal phalanx	By two branches of the deep peroneal
Peroneus tertius	Distal one third of the anterior surface of the fibula, neighboring interosseous membrane, anterior intermuscular septum	Onto the base of the fifth metatarsal and often onto the base of the fourth	The more distal nerve to the extensor digitorum supplies this muscle (deep peroneal)
Extensor hallucis longus	Middle half of the anterior surface of the fibula near the interosseous crest, and distal half of the interosseous membrane	At the base of the dorsal aspect of the great toe	Deep peroneal
Peroneus longus	Proximal two thirds of the lateral surface of the fibula	Inferior surface of the first cuneiform and on the adjacent part of the inferolateral border and the base of the first metatarsal	Usually, the common peroneal, sometimes partially by superficial peroneal
Peroneus brevis	Middle one third of the lateral surface of the fibula, from the septum that separate it from the anterior and posterior groups of muscles	Dorsal aspect of the tuberosity of the fifth metatarsal	Superficial peroneal or a branch to peroneus longus

Table 7: Muscles of the Leg—Cont'd

MUSCLE	ORIGIN	INSERTION	NERVE SUPPLY
Popliteus	Facet at the anterior end of the groove on the lateral aspect of the femoral condyle	Proximal lip of the popliteal line of the tibia and the shaft of the tibia proximal to this line	Tibial: a branch that arises independently, or with the nerve to the posterior tibial muscle
Flexor digitorum longus	Popliteal line, medial side of the second quarter of the dorsal surface of the tibia, fibrous septum between the muscle and the tibialis fascia posterior, and the covering its proximal extremity	Onto the bases of the terminal phalanges of the second to fourth toes	Tibial: in company with nerves to other muscles of this group
Flexor hallucis longus	Distal two thirds of the posterior surface of the fibula, the septa between it and the tibialis posterior, and peroneal muscles	Onto the base of the terminal phalanx of the great toe	Tibial: often in company with the nerve to the flexor digitorum longus or other muscles of this group
Tibialis posterior	Lateral half of the popliteal line and lateral half of the middle one third of the posterior surface of the tibia, medial side of the head and part of the body of the fibula next to the interosseous membrane in the proximal two thirds, the entire proximal and lateral portion of the lateral part of the posterior surface of the interosseous membrane, and the septum between its proximal portion and the long flexor muscles	The tendon divides into two parts: the deep part becomes attached primarily to the tubercle of the navicular bone, and usually to the first cuneiform; the superficial part attaches to the third cuneiform and the base of the fourth metatarsal, and also, in part, to the second cuneiform, to the capsule of the naviculo-cuneiform joint, to the sulcus of the cuboid, and usually also to the origin of the short flexor of the big toe and base of the second metatarsal; slip may extend to other structures	Tibial: in company with nerves to other muscles of this group
Gastrocnemius	Medial head: posterior surface of the medial condyle of the femur above the articular surface; lateral head: a facet on the proximal part of the posterolateral surface of the lateral condyle of the femur	Via the Achilles tendon onto the posterior surface of the calcaneus	Sciatic, tibial part

Continued

Table 7: Muscles of the Leg—Cont'd

MUSCLE	ORIGIN	INSERTION	NERVE SUPPLY
Soleus	By a fibular head from the back of the head and the proximal one third of the posterior surface of the shaft of the fibula; intermuscular septum between it and the peroneus longus, by a tibial head from the popliteal line and the middle one third of the medial border of the tibia	Via the calcaneal tendon onto the posterior surface of the calcaneus	Sciatic, tibial part
Plantaris	Distal part of the lateral line of the bifurcation of the linea aspera, in close association with the lateral head of the gastrocnemius	Via a flat narrow tendon running along the medial edge of the Achilles tendon to the posterior surface of the calcaneus	Sciatic, tibial part

AXIAL
Figure 13.1.1

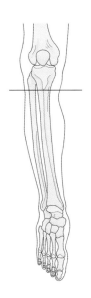

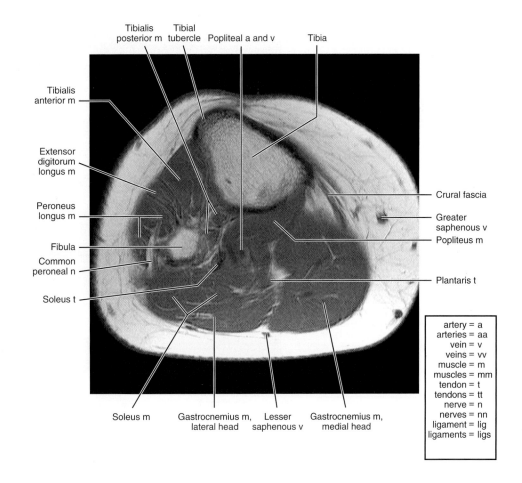

Tibialis posterior m — Tibial tubercle — Popliteal a and v — Tibia

Tibialis anterior m

Extensor digitorum longus m

Peroneus longus m

Fibula

Common peroneal n

Soleus t

Crural fascia

Greater saphenous v

Popliteus m

Plantaris t

Soleus m — Gastrocnemius m, lateral head — Lesser saphenous v — Gastrocnemius m, medial head

artery = a
arteries = aa
vein = v
veins = vv
muscle = m
muscles = mm
tendon = t
tendons = tt
nerve = n
nerves = nn
ligament = lig
ligaments = ligs

Figure 13.1.2

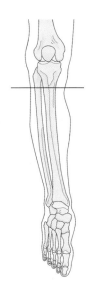

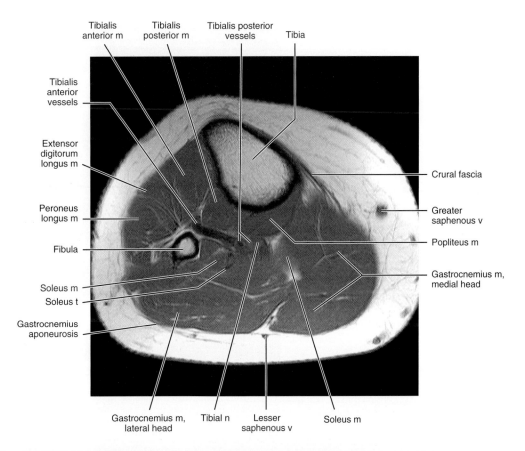

Tibialis anterior m — Tibialis posterior m — Tibialis posterior vessels — Tibia

Tibialis anterior vessels

Extensor digitorum longus m

Peroneus longus m

Fibula

Soleus m

Soleus t

Gastrocnemius aponeurosis

Crural fascia

Greater saphenous v

Popliteus m

Gastrocnemius m, medial head

Gastrocnemius m, lateral head — Tibial n — Lesser saphenous v — Soleus m

Figure 13.1.3

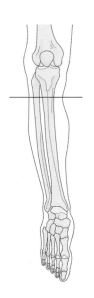

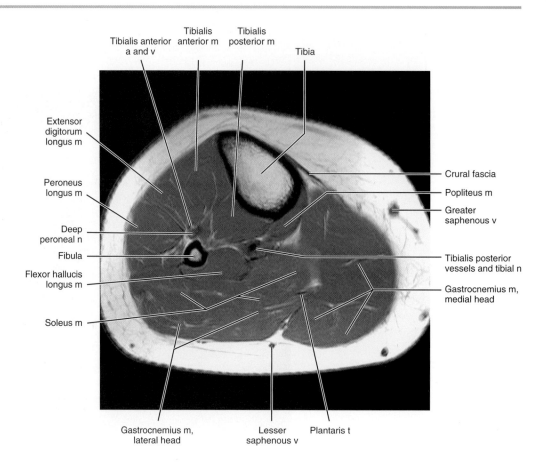

Figure 13.1.4

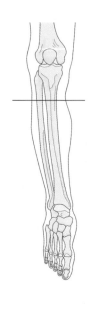

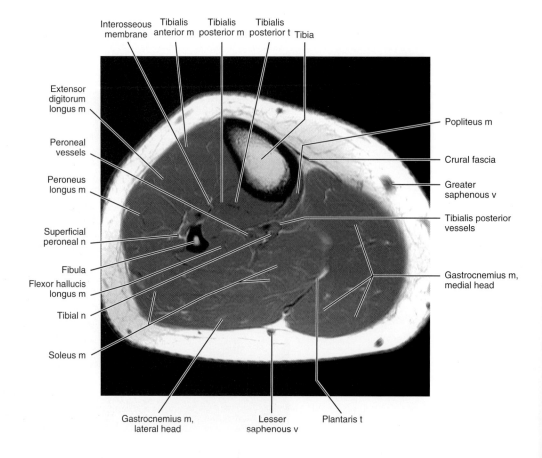

Figure 13.1.5

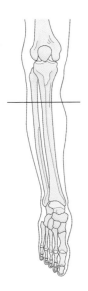

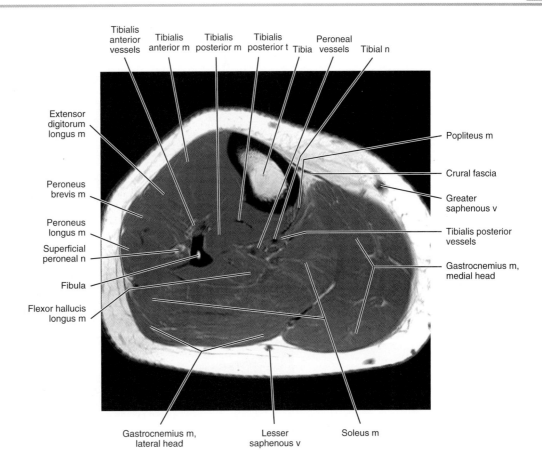

Tibialis anterior vessels · Tibialis anterior m · Tibialis posterior m · Tibialis posterior t · Tibia · Peroneal vessels · Tibial n

Extensor digitorum longus m

Peroneus brevis m

Peroneus longus m

Superficial peroneal n

Fibula

Flexor hallucis longus m

Popliteus m

Crural fascia

Greater saphenous v

Tibialis posterior vessels

Gastrocnemius m, medial head

Gastrocnemius m, lateral head · Lesser saphenous v · Soleus m

Figure 13.1.6

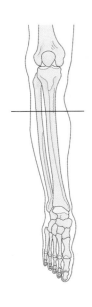

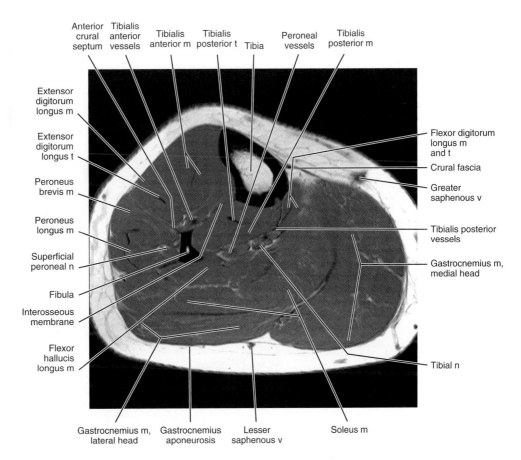

Anterior crural septum · Tibialis anterior vessels · Tibialis anterior m · Tibialis posterior t · Tibia · Peroneal vessels · Tibialis posterior m

Extensor digitorum longus m

Extensor digitorum longus t

Peroneus brevis m

Peroneus longus m

Superficial peroneal n

Fibula

Interosseous membrane

Flexor hallucis longus m

Flexor digitorum longus m and t

Crural fascia

Greater saphenous v

Tibialis posterior vessels

Gastrocnemius m, medial head

Tibial n

Gastrocnemius m, lateral head · Gastrocnemius aponeurosis · Lesser saphenous v · Soleus m

Figure 13.1.7

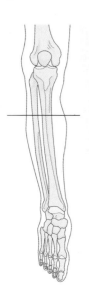

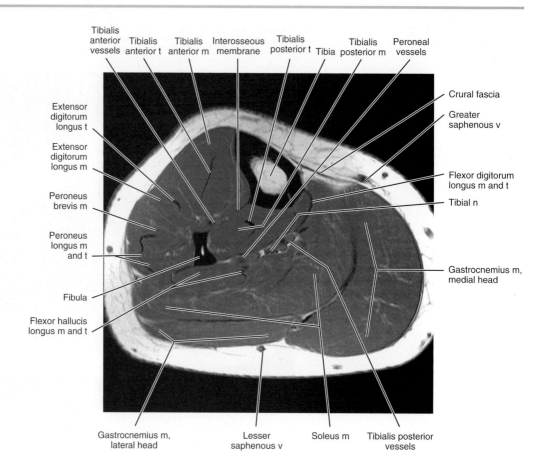

Tibialis anterior vessels
Tibialis anterior t
Tibialis anterior m
Interosseous membrane
Tibialis posterior t
Tibia
Tibialis posterior m
Peroneal vessels

Extensor digitorum longus t
Extensor digitorum longus m
Peroneus brevis m
Peroneus longus m and t
Fibula
Flexor hallucis longus m and t

Crural fascia
Greater saphenous v
Flexor digitorum longus m and t
Tibial n
Gastrocnemius m, medial head

Gastrocnemius m, lateral head
Lesser saphenous v
Soleus m
Tibialis posterior vessels

Figure 13.1.8

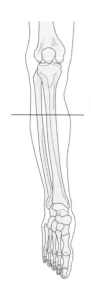

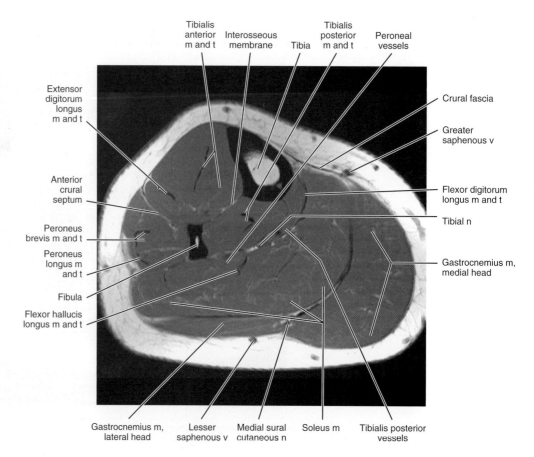

Tibialis anterior m and t
Interosseous membrane
Tibia
Tibialis posterior m and t
Peroneal vessels

Extensor digitorum longus m and t
Anterior crural septum
Peroneus brevis m and t
Peroneus longus m and t
Fibula
Flexor hallucis longus m and t

Crural fascia
Greater saphenous v
Flexor digitorum longus m and t
Tibial n
Gastrocnemius m, medial head

Gastrocnemius m, lateral head
Lesser saphenous v
Medial sural cutaneous n
Soleus m
Tibialis posterior vessels

Figure 13.1.9

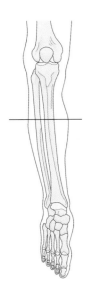

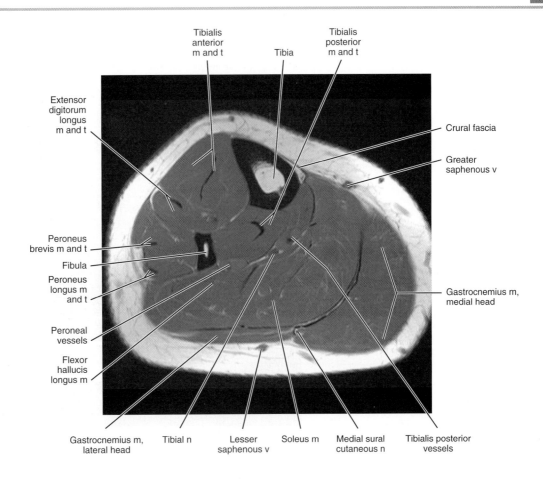

Extensor digitorum longus m and t

Tibialis anterior m and t

Tibia

Tibialis posterior m and t

Crural fascia

Greater saphenous v

Peroneus brevis m and t

Fibula

Peroneus longus m and t

Peroneal vessels

Flexor hallucis longus m

Gastrocnemius m, medial head

Gastrocnemius m, lateral head

Tibial n

Lesser saphenous v

Soleus m

Medial sural cutaneous n

Tibialis posterior vessels

Figure 13.1.10

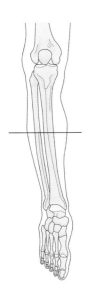

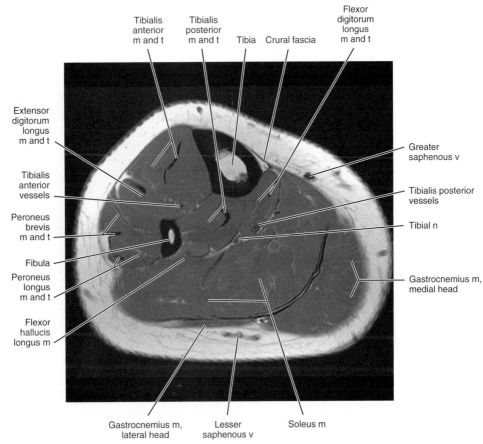

Tibialis anterior m and t

Tibialis posterior m and t

Tibia

Crural fascia

Flexor digitorum longus m and t

Extensor digitorum longus m and t

Tibialis anterior vessels

Peroneus brevis m and t

Fibula

Peroneus longus m and t

Flexor hallucis longus m

Greater saphenous v

Tibialis posterior vessels

Tibial n

Gastrocnemius m, medial head

Gastrocnemius m, lateral head

Lesser saphenous v

Soleus m

Figure 13.1.11

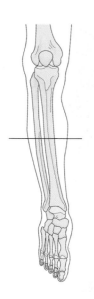

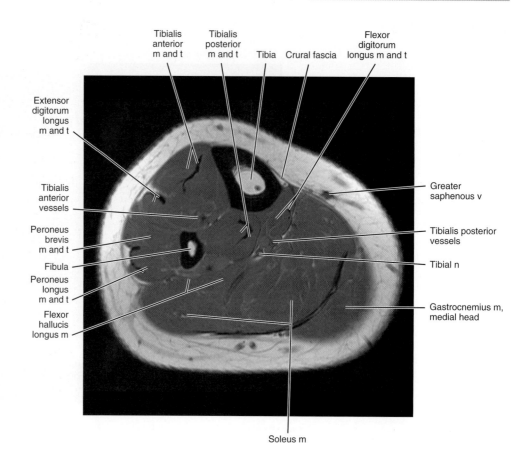

Extensor digitorum longus m and t

Tibialis anterior vessels

Peroneus brevis m and t

Fibula

Peroneus longus m and t

Flexor hallucis longus m

Tibialis anterior m and t

Tibialis posterior m and t

Tibia

Crural fascia

Flexor digitorum longus m and t

Greater saphenous v

Tibialis posterior vessels

Tibial n

Gastrocnemius m, medial head

Soleus m

Figure 13.1.12

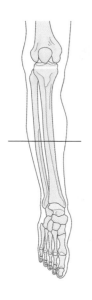

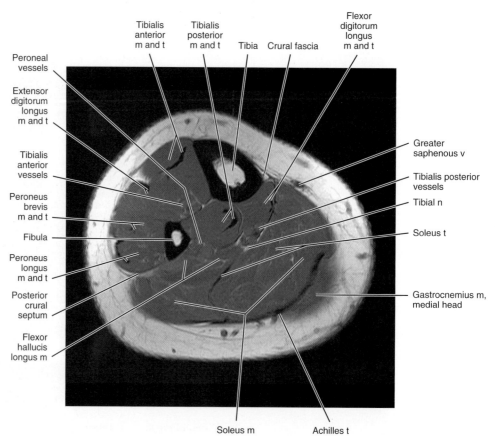

Peroneal vessels

Extensor digitorum longus m and t

Tibialis anterior vessels

Peroneus brevis m and t

Fibula

Peroneus longus m and t

Posterior crural septum

Flexor hallucis longus m

Tibialis anterior m and t

Tibialis posterior m and t

Tibia

Crural fascia

Flexor digitorum longus m and t

Greater saphenous v

Tibialis posterior vessels

Tibial n

Soleus t

Gastrocnemius m, medial head

Soleus m

Achilles t

Figure 13.1.13

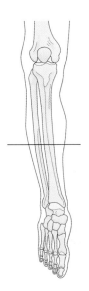

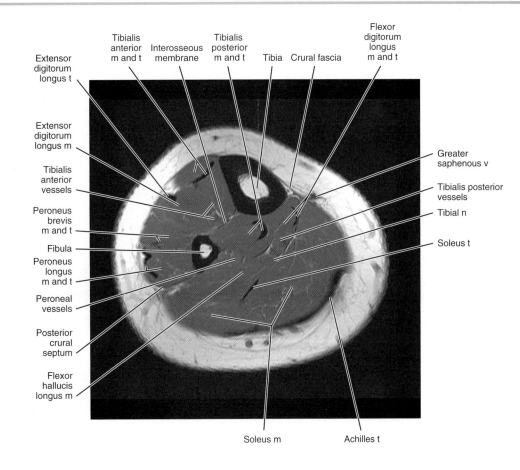

Extensor digitorum longus t

Extensor digitorum longus m

Tibialis anterior vessels

Peroneus brevis m and t

Fibula

Peroneus longus m and t

Peroneal vessels

Posterior crural septum

Flexor hallucis longus m

Tibialis anterior m and t

Interosseous membrane

Tibialis posterior m and t

Tibia

Crural fascia

Flexor digitorum longus m and t

Greater saphenous v

Tibialis posterior vessels

Tibial n

Soleus t

Soleus m

Achilles t

Figure 13.1.14

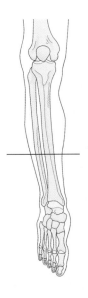

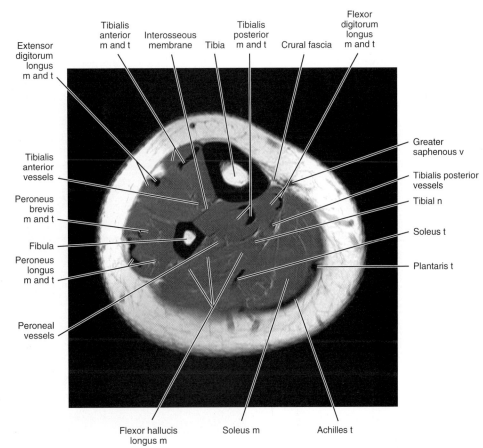

Extensor digitorum longus m and t

Tibialis anterior vessels

Peroneus brevis m and t

Fibula

Peroneus longus m and t

Peroneal vessels

Tibialis anterior m and t

Interosseous membrane

Tibia

Tibialis posterior m and t

Crural fascia

Flexor digitorum longus m and t

Greater saphenous v

Tibialis posterior vessels

Tibial n

Soleus t

Plantaris t

Flexor hallucis longus m

Soleus m

Achilles t

Figure 13.1.15

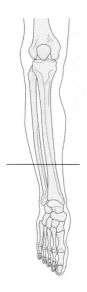

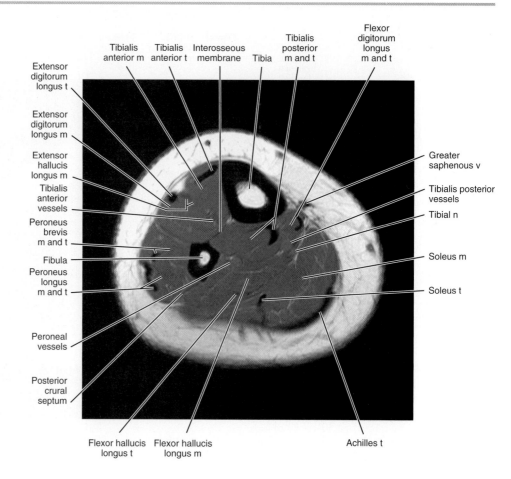

Extensor digitorum longus t

Extensor digitorum longus m

Extensor hallucis longus m

Tibialis anterior vessels

Peroneus brevis m and t

Fibula

Peroneus longus m and t

Peroneal vessels

Posterior crural septum

Tibialis anterior m

Tibialis anterior t

Interosseous membrane

Tibia

Tibialis posterior m and t

Flexor digitorum longus m and t

Greater saphenous v

Tibialis posterior vessels

Tibial n

Soleus m

Soleus t

Flexor hallucis longus t

Flexor hallucis longus m

Achilles t

Figure 13.1.16

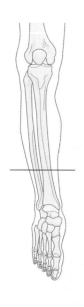

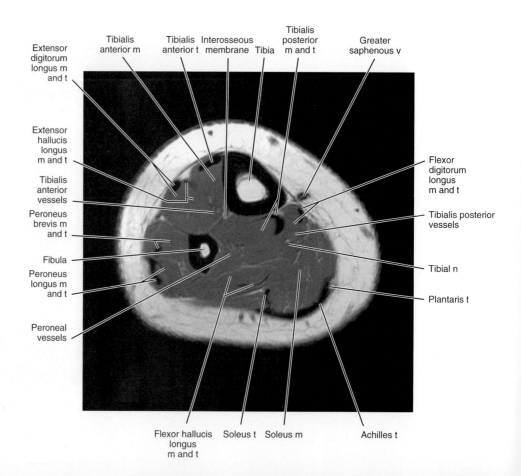

Extensor digitorum longus m and t

Extensor hallucis longus m and t

Tibialis anterior vessels

Peroneus brevis m and t

Fibula

Peroneus longus m and t

Peroneal vessels

Tibialis anterior m

Tibialis anterior t

Interosseous membrane

Tibia

Tibialis posterior m and t

Greater saphenous v

Flexor digitorum longus m and t

Tibialis posterior vessels

Tibial n

Plantaris t

Flexor hallucis longus m and t

Soleus t

Soleus m

Achilles t

Figure 13.1.17

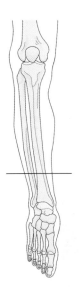

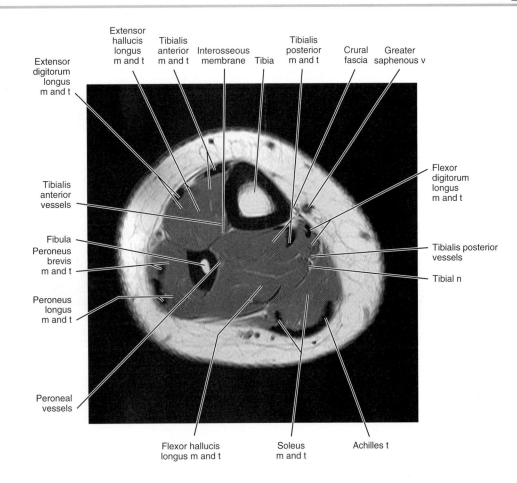

Extensor digitorum longus m and t

Extensor hallucis longus m and t

Tibialis anterior m and t

Interosseous membrane

Tibia

Tibialis posterior m and t

Crural fascia

Greater saphenous v

Tibialis anterior vessels

Flexor digitorum longus m and t

Fibula
Peroneus brevis m and t

Tibialis posterior vessels

Tibial n

Peroneus longus m and t

Peroneal vessels

Flexor hallucis longus m and t

Soleus m and t

Achilles t

Figure 13.1.18

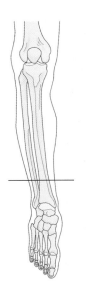

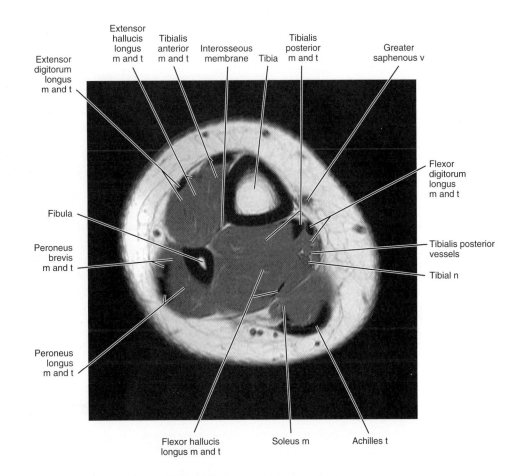

Extensor digitorum longus m and t

Extensor hallucis longus m and t

Tibialis anterior m and t

Interosseous membrane

Tibia

Tibialis posterior m and t

Greater saphenous v

Flexor digitorum longus m and t

Fibula

Peroneus brevis m and t

Tibialis posterior vessels

Tibial n

Peroneus longus m and t

Flexor hallucis longus m and t

Soleus m

Achilles t

Figure 13.1.19

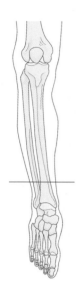

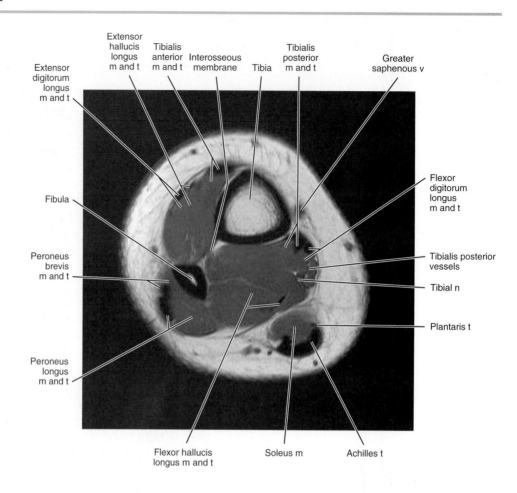

Extensor
digitorum
longus
m and t

Extensor
hallucis
longus
m and t

Tibialis
anterior
m and t

Interosseous
membrane

Tibia

Tibialis
posterior
m and t

Greater
saphenous v

Fibula

Flexor
digitorum
longus
m and t

Peroneus
brevis
m and t

Tibialis posterior
vessels

Tibial n

Plantaris t

Peroneus
longus
m and t

Flexor hallucis
longus m and t

Soleus m

Achilles t

Figure 13.1.20

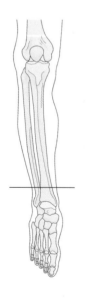

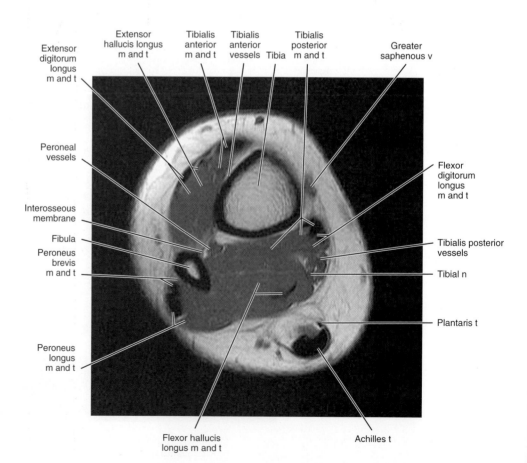

Extensor
digitorum
longus
m and t

Extensor
hallucis longus
m and t

Tibialis
anterior
m and t

Tibialis
anterior
vessels

Tibia

Tibialis
posterior
m and t

Greater
saphenous v

Peroneal
vessels

Flexor
digitorum
longus
m and t

Interosseous
membrane

Fibula

Peroneus
brevis
m and t

Tibialis posterior
vessels

Tibial n

Plantaris t

Peroneus
longus
m and t

Flexor hallucis
longus m and t

Achilles t

SAGITTAL

Figure 13.2.1

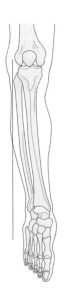

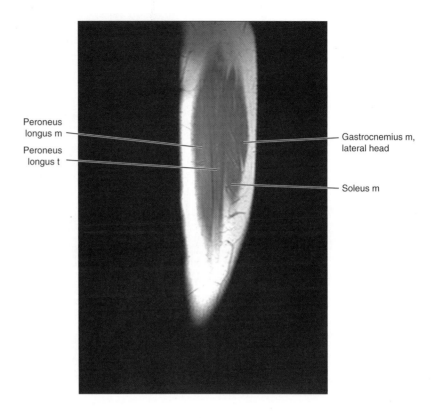

Peroneus longus m

Peroneus longus t

Gastrocnemius m, lateral head

Soleus m

Figure 13.2.2

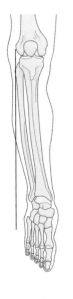

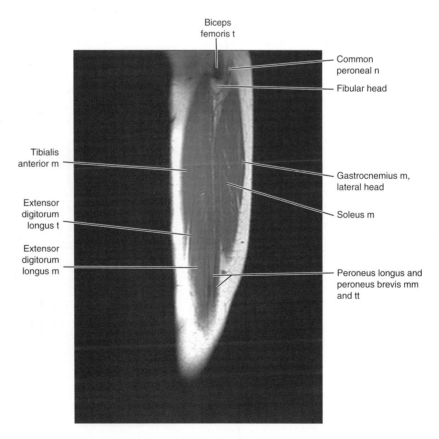

Biceps femoris t

Common peroneal n

Fibular head

Tibialis anterior m

Gastrocnemius m, lateral head

Soleus m

Extensor digitorum longus t

Extensor digitorum longus m

Peroneus longus and peroneus brevis mm and tt

Figure 13.2.3

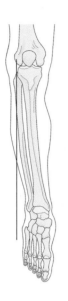

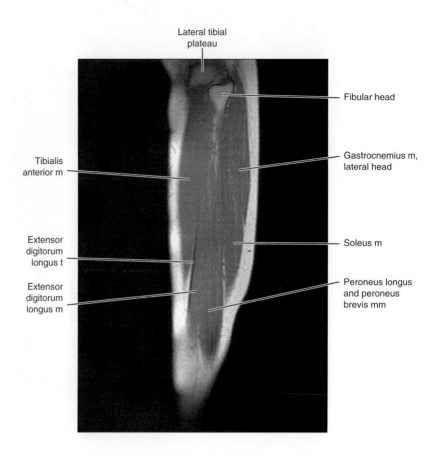

Lateral tibial plateau

Fibular head

Gastrocnemius m, lateral head

Tibialis anterior m

Soleus m

Extensor digitorum longus t

Peroneus longus and peroneus brevis mm

Extensor digitorum longus m

Figure 13.2.4

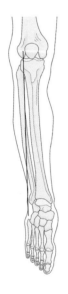

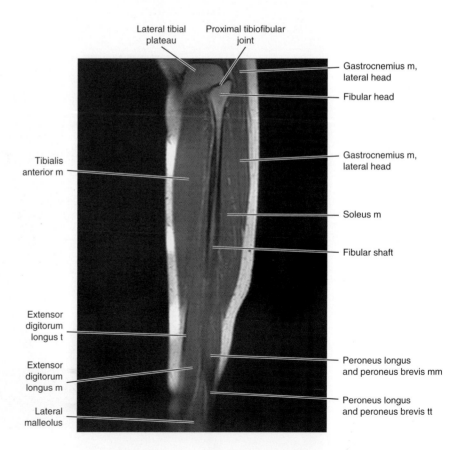

Lateral tibial plateau

Proximal tibiofibular joint

Gastrocnemius m, lateral head

Fibular head

Tibialis anterior m

Gastrocnemius m, lateral head

Soleus m

Fibular shaft

Extensor digitorum longus t

Extensor digitorum longus m

Peroneus longus and peroneus brevis mm

Lateral malleolus

Peroneus longus and peroneus brevis tt

Figure 13.2.5

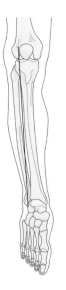

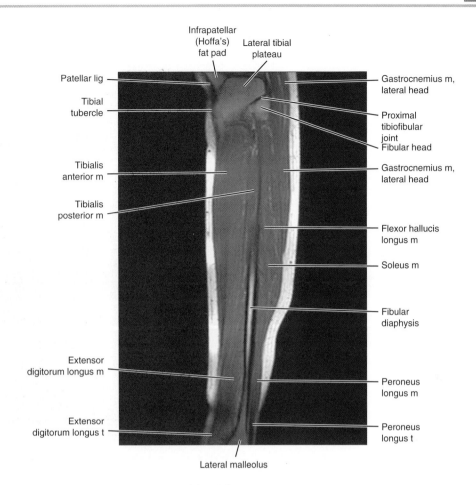

Infrapatellar
(Hoffa's)
fat pad

Lateral tibial
plateau

Patellar lig

Tibial
tubercle

Tibialis
anterior m

Tibialis
posterior m

Extensor
digitorum longus m

Extensor
digitorum longus t

Gastrocnemius m,
lateral head

Proximal
tibiofibular
joint
Fibular head

Gastrocnemius m,
lateral head

Flexor hallucis
longus m

Soleus m

Fibular
diaphysis

Peroneus
longus m

Peroneus
longus t

Lateral malleolus

Figure 13.2.6

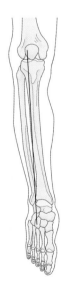

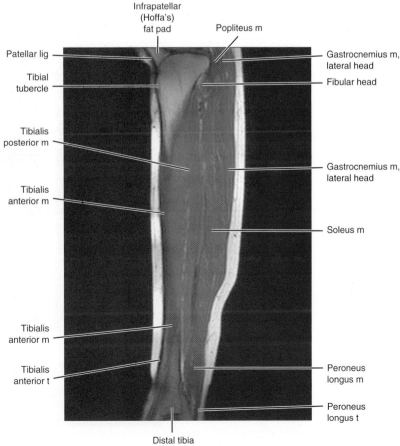

Infrapatellar
(Hoffa's)
fat pad

Popliteus m

Patellar lig

Tibial
tubercle

Tibialis
posterior m

Tibialis
anterior m

Tibialis
anterior m

Tibialis
anterior t

Gastrocnemius m,
lateral head

Fibular head

Gastrocnemius m,
lateral head

Soleus m

Peroneus
longus m

Peroneus
longus t

Distal tibia

Figure 13.2.7

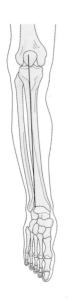

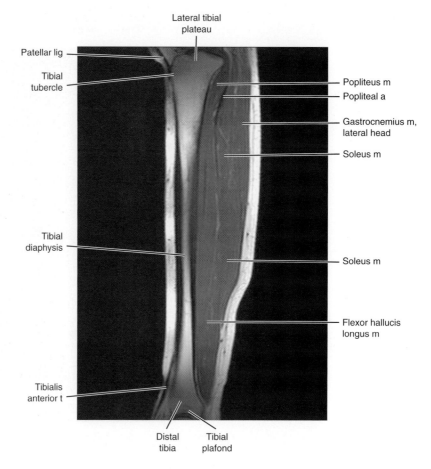

Lateral tibial plateau

Patellar lig

Tibial tubercle

Popliteus m

Popliteal a

Gastrocnemius m, lateral head

Soleus m

Tibial diaphysis

Soleus m

Flexor hallucis longus m

Tibialis anterior t

Distal tibia

Tibial plafond

Figure 13.2.8

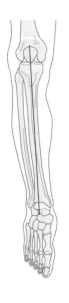

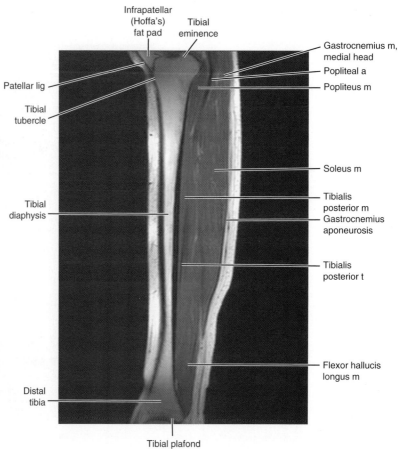

Infrapatellar (Hoffa's) fat pad

Tibial eminence

Gastrocnemius m, medial head

Popliteal a

Popliteus m

Patellar lig

Tibial tubercle

Soleus m

Tibialis posterior m

Tibial diaphysis

Gastrocnemius aponeurosis

Tibialis posterior t

Flexor hallucis longus m

Distal tibia

Tibial plafond

Figure 13.2.9

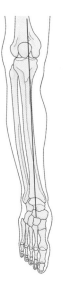
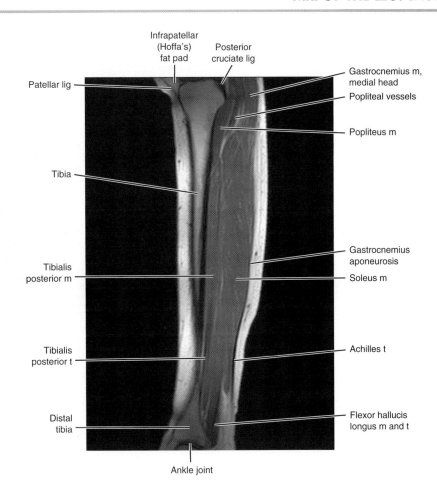

Infrapatellar (Hoffa's) fat pad
Posterior cruciate lig
Patellar lig
Gastrocnemius m, medial head
Popliteal vessels
Popliteus m
Tibia
Gastrocnemius aponeurosis
Tibialis posterior m
Soleus m
Tibialis posterior t
Achilles t
Distal tibia
Flexor hallucis longus m and t
Ankle joint

Figure 13.2.10

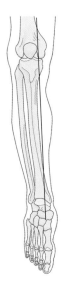
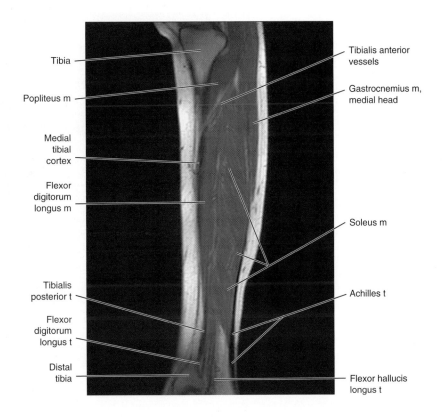

Tibia
Tibialis anterior vessels
Popliteus m
Gastrocnemius m, medial head
Medial tibial cortex
Flexor digitorum longus m
Soleus m
Tibialis posterior t
Achilles t
Flexor digitorum longus t
Distal tibia
Flexor hallucis longus t

Figure 13.2.11

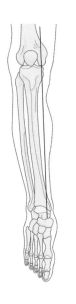

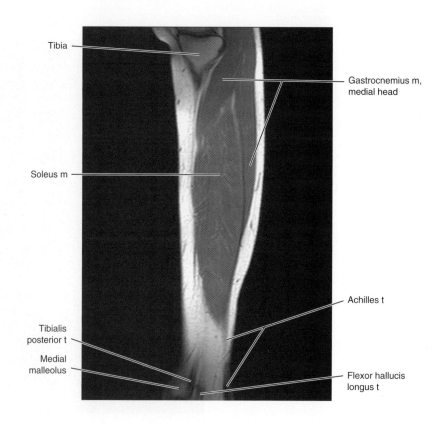

Tibia

Gastrocnemius m, medial head

Soleus m

Achilles t

Tibialis posterior t

Medial malleolus

Flexor hallucis longus t

Figure 13.2.12

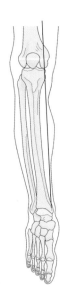

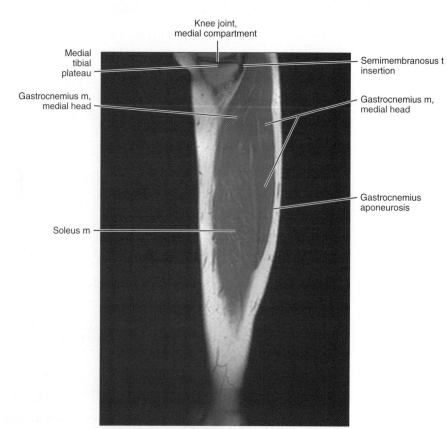

Knee joint, medial compartment

Medial tibial plateau

Semimembranosus t insertion

Gastrocnemius m, medial head

Gastrocnemius m, medial head

Gastrocnemius aponeurosis

Soleus m

Figure 13.2.13

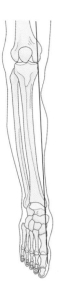

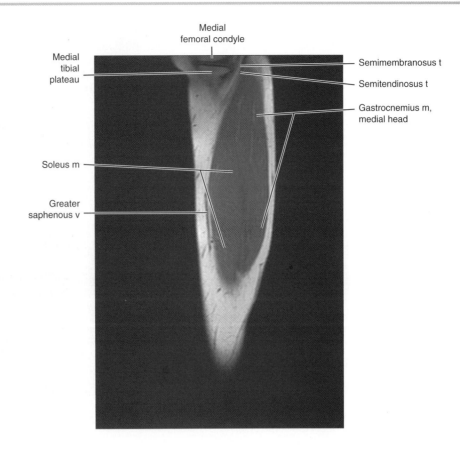

Medial femoral condyle

Medial tibial plateau

Semimembranosus t

Semitendinosus t

Gastrocnemius m, medial head

Soleus m

Greater saphenous v

Figure 13.2.14

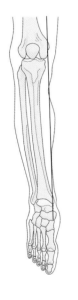

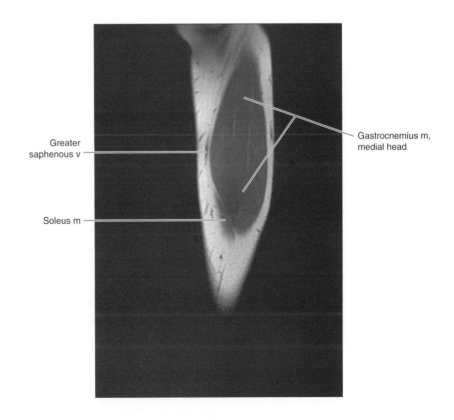

Greater saphenous v

Soleus m

Gastrocnemius m, medial head

Figure 13.2.15

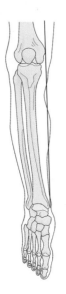

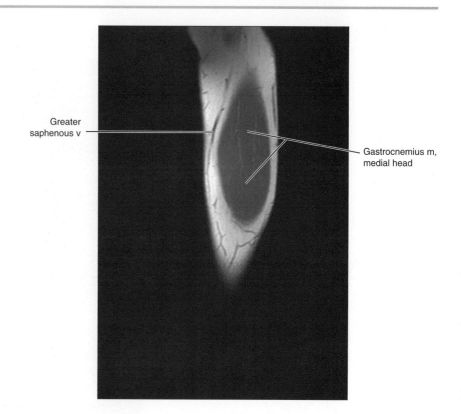

Greater
saphenous v

Gastrocnemius m,
medial head

CORONAL
Figure 13.3.1

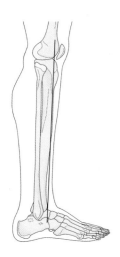

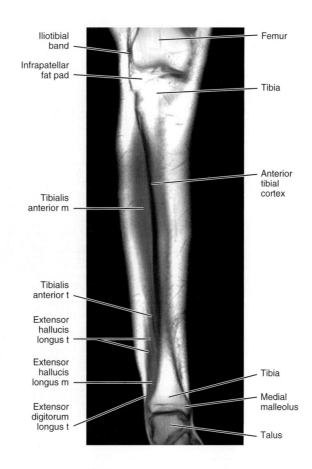

Iliotibial band

Infrapatellar fat pad

Tibialis anterior m

Tibialis anterior t

Extensor hallucis longus t

Extensor hallucis longus m

Extensor digitorum longus t

Femur

Tibia

Anterior tibial cortex

Tibia

Medial malleolus

Talus

Figure 13.3.2

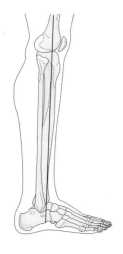

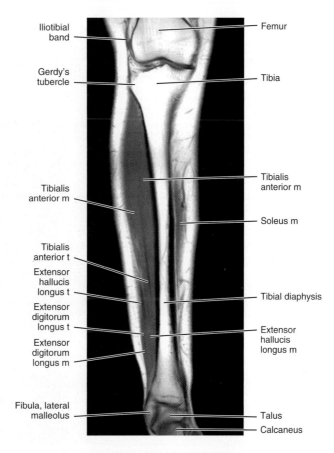

Iliotibial band

Gerdy's tubercle

Tibialis anterior m

Tibialis anterior t

Extensor hallucis longus t

Extensor digitorum longus t

Extensor digitorum longus m

Fibula, lateral malleolus

Femur

Tibia

Tibialis anterior m

Soleus m

Tibial diaphysis

Extensor hallucis longus m

Talus

Calcaneus

Figure 13.3.3

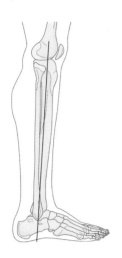

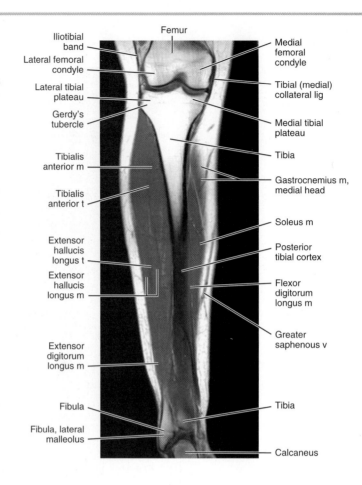

Iliotibial band
Lateral femoral condyle
Lateral tibial plateau
Gerdy's tubercle
Tibialis anterior m
Tibialis anterior t
Extensor hallucis longus t
Extensor hallucis longus m
Extensor digitorum longus m
Fibula
Fibula, lateral malleolus

Femur
Medial femoral condyle
Tibial (medial) collateral lig
Medial tibial plateau
Tibia
Gastrocnemius m, medial head
Soleus m
Posterior tibial cortex
Flexor digitorum longus m
Greater saphenous v
Tibia
Calcaneus

Figure 13.3.4

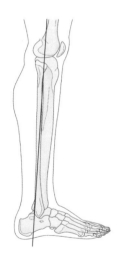

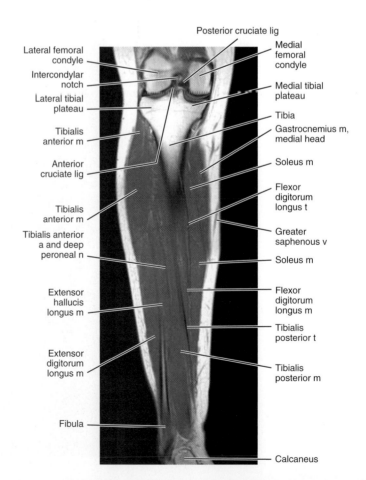

Lateral femoral condyle
Intercondylar notch
Lateral tibial plateau
Tibialis anterior m
Anterior cruciate lig
Tibialis anterior m
Tibialis anterior a and deep peroneal n
Extensor hallucis longus m
Extensor digitorum longus m
Fibula

Posterior cruciate lig
Medial femoral condyle
Medial tibial plateau
Tibia
Gastrocnemius m, medial head
Soleus m
Flexor digitorum longus t
Greater saphenous v
Soleus m
Flexor digitorum longus m
Tibialis posterior t
Tibialis posterior m
Calcaneus

Figure 13.3.5

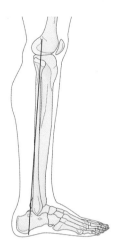

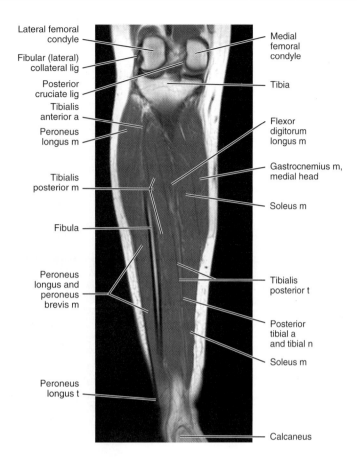

Lateral femoral condyle
Fibular (lateral) collateral lig
Posterior cruciate lig
Tibialis anterior a
Peroneus longus m
Tibialis posterior m
Fibula
Peroneus longus and peroneus brevis m
Peroneus longus t

Medial femoral condyle
Tibia
Flexor digitorum longus m
Gastrocnemius m, medial head
Soleus m
Tibialis posterior t
Posterior tibial a and tibial n
Soleus m
Calcaneus

Figure 13.3.6

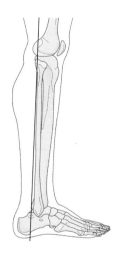

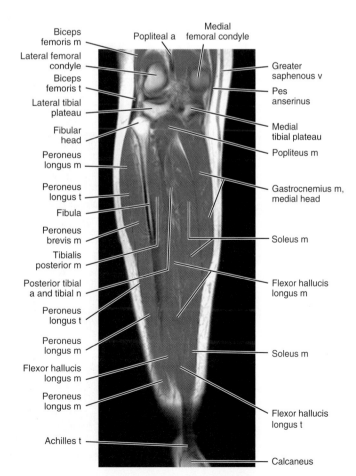

Biceps femoris m
Popliteal a
Medial femoral condyle
Lateral femoral condyle
Biceps femoris t
Lateral tibial plateau
Fibular head
Peroneus longus m
Peroneus longus t
Fibula
Peroneus brevis m
Tibialis posterior m
Posterior tibial a and tibial n
Peroneus longus t
Peroneus longus m
Flexor hallucis longus m
Peroneus longus m
Achilles t

Greater saphenous v
Pes anserinus
Medial tibial plateau
Popliteus m
Gastrocnemius m, medial head
Soleus m
Flexor hallucis longus m
Soleus m
Flexor hallucis longus t
Calcaneus

Figure 13.3.7

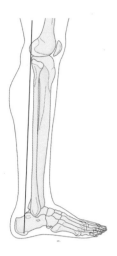

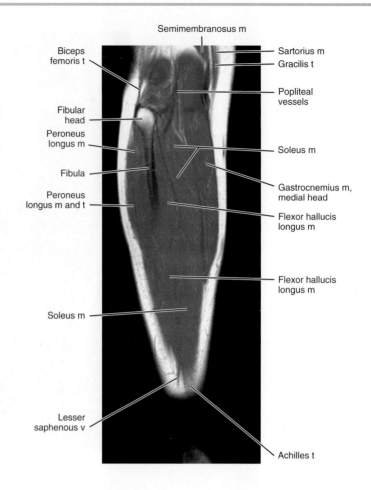

Semimembranosus m

Biceps femoris t

Sartorius m

Gracilis t

Popliteal vessels

Fibular head

Peroneus longus m

Soleus m

Fibula

Gastrocnemius m, medial head

Peroneus longus m and t

Flexor hallucis longus m

Flexor hallucis longus m

Soleus m

Lesser saphenous v

Achilles t

Figure 13.3.8

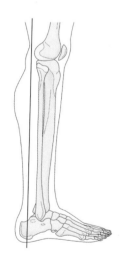

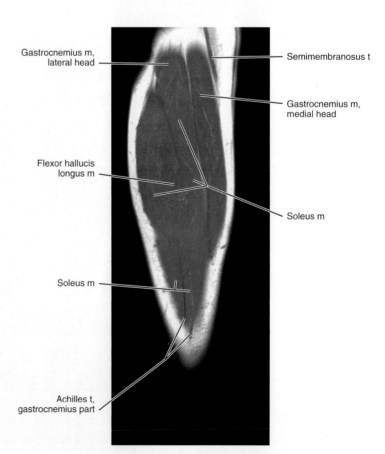

Gastrocnemius m, lateral head

Semimembranosus t

Gastrocnemius m, medial head

Flexor hallucis longus m

Soleus m

Soleus m

Achilles t, gastrocnemius part

Figure 13.3.9

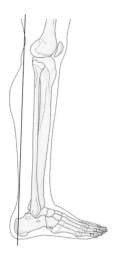

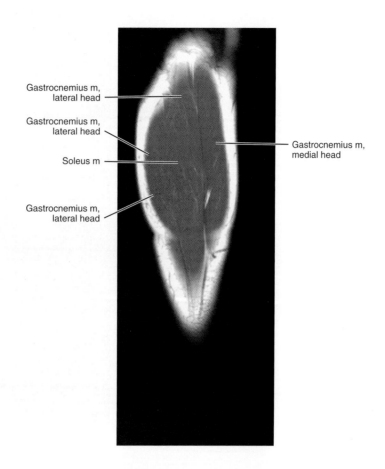

Gastrocnemius m, lateral head

Gastrocnemius m, lateral head

Soleus m

Gastrocnemius m, lateral head

Gastrocnemius m, medial head

Figure 13.3.10

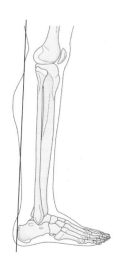

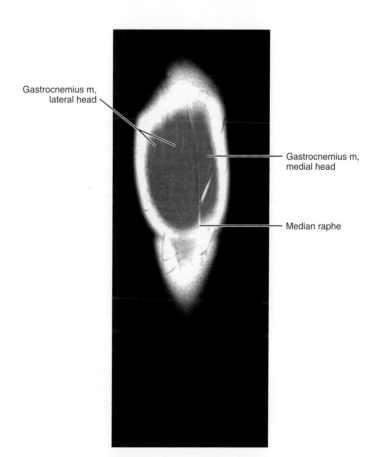

Gastrocnemius m, lateral head

Gastrocnemius m, medial head

Median raphe

Figure 13.3.11

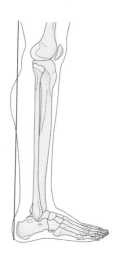

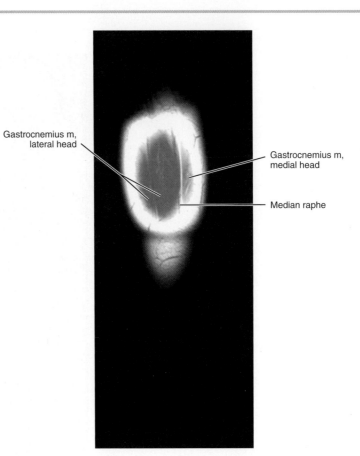

Gastrocnemius m, lateral head

Gastrocnemius m, medial head

Median raphe

Chapter 14

MRI of the Ankle

AXIAL

Figure 14.1.1

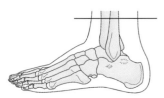

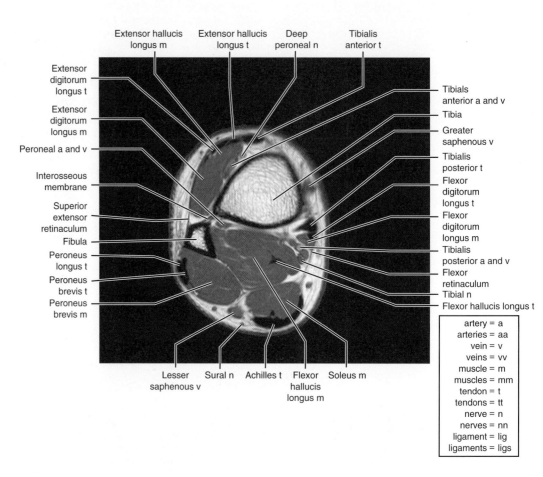

Extensor hallucis longus m

Extensor hallucis longus t

Deep peroneal n

Tibialis anterior t

Extensor digitorum longus t

Extensor digitorum longus m

Peroneal a and v

Interosseous membrane

Superior extensor retinaculum

Fibula

Peroneus longus t

Peroneus brevis t

Peroneus brevis m

Tibials anterior a and v

Tibia

Greater saphenous v

Tibialis posterior t

Flexor digitorum longus t

Flexor digitorum longus m

Tibialis posterior a and v

Flexor retinaculum

Tibial n

Flexor hallucis longus t

Lesser saphenous v

Sural n

Achilles t

Flexor hallucis longus m

Soleus m

artery = a
arteries = aa
vein = v
veins = vv
muscle = m
muscles = mm
tendon = t
tendons = tt
nerve = n
nerves = nn
ligament = lig
ligaments = ligs

Figure 14.1.2

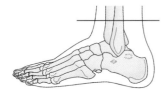

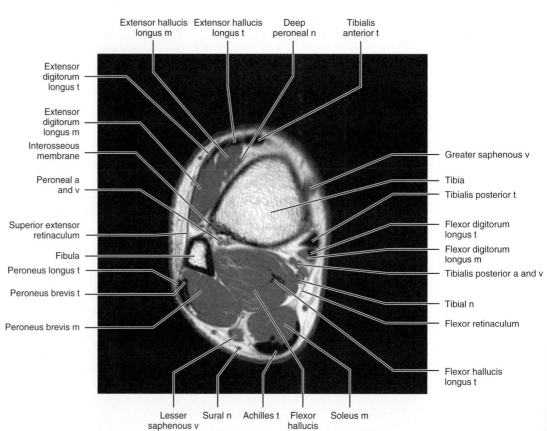

Extensor hallucis longus m

Extensor hallucis longus t

Deep peroneal n

Tibialis anterior t

Extensor digitorum longus t

Extensor digitorum longus m

Interosseous membrane

Peroneal a and v

Superior extensor retinaculum

Fibula

Peroneus longus t

Peroneus brevis t

Peroneus brevis m

Greater saphenous v

Tibia

Tibialis posterior t

Flexor digitorum longus t

Flexor digitorum longus m

Tibialis posterior a and v

Tibial n

Flexor retinaculum

Flexor hallucis longus t

Lesser saphenous v

Sural n

Achilles t

Flexor hallucis longus m

Soleus m

Figure 14.1.3

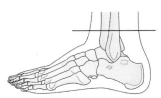

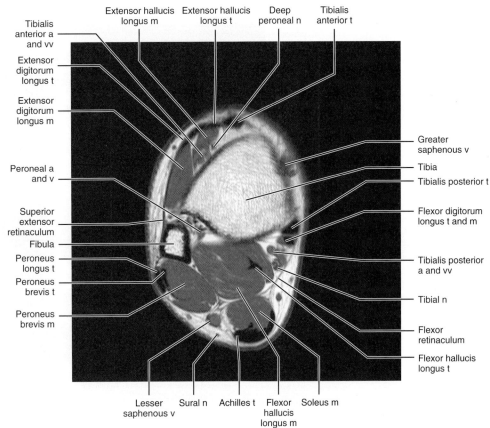

Tibialis anterior a and vv

Extensor digitorum longus t

Extensor digitorum longus m

Peroneal a and v

Superior extensor retinaculum

Fibula

Peroneus longus t

Peroneus brevis t

Peroneus brevis m

Extensor hallucis longus m

Extensor hallucis longus t

Deep peroneal n

Tibialis anterior t

Greater saphenous v

Tibia

Tibialis posterior t

Flexor digitorum longus t and m

Tibialis posterior a and vv

Tibial n

Flexor retinaculum

Flexor hallucis longus t

Lesser saphenous v

Sural n

Achilles t

Flexor hallucis longus m

Soleus m

Figure 14.1.4

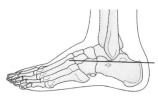

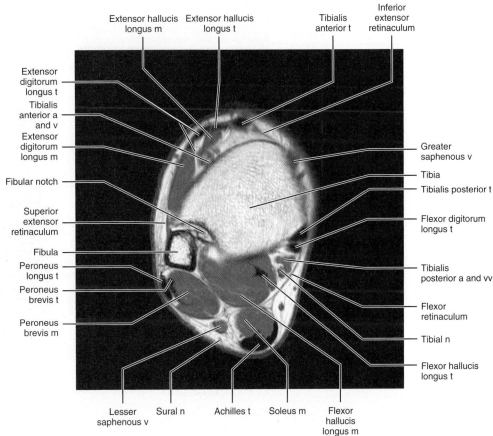

Extensor digitorum longus t

Tibialis anterior a and v

Extensor digitorum longus m

Fibular notch

Superior extensor retinaculum

Fibula

Peroneus longus t

Peroneus brevis t

Peroneus brevis m

Extensor hallucis longus m

Extensor hallucis longus t

Tibialis anterior t

Inferior extensor retinaculum

Greater saphenous v

Tibia

Tibialis posterior t

Flexor digitorum longus t

Tibialis posterior a and vv

Flexor retinaculum

Tibial n

Flexor hallucis longus t

Lesser saphenous v

Sural n

Achilles t

Soleus m

Flexor hallucis longus m

Figure 14.1.5

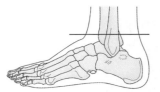

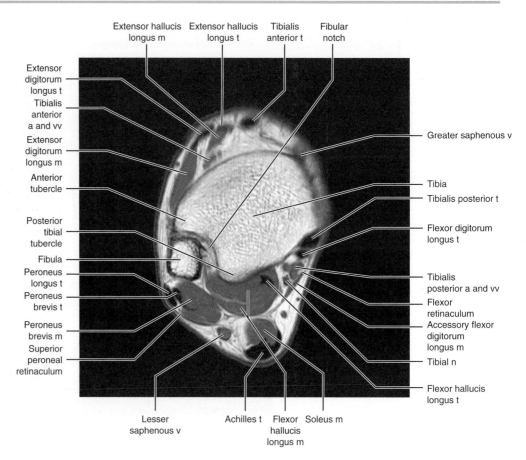

Extensor hallucis longus m
Extensor hallucis longus t
Tibialis anterior t
Fibular notch

Extensor digitorum longus t
Tibialis anterior a and vv
Extensor digitorum longus m
Anterior tubercle
Posterior tibial tubercle
Fibula
Peroneus longus t
Peroneus brevis t
Peroneus brevis m
Superior peroneal retinaculum

Greater saphenous v
Tibia
Tibialis posterior t
Flexor digitorum longus t
Tibialis posterior a and vv
Flexor retinaculum
Accessory flexor digitorum longus m
Tibial n
Flexor hallucis longus t

Lesser saphenous v
Achilles t
Flexor hallucis longus m
Soleus m

Figure 14.1.6

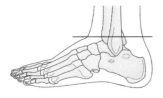

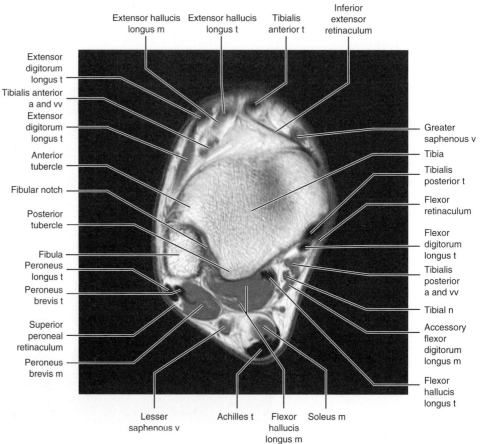

Extensor hallucis longus m
Extensor hallucis longus t
Tibialis anterior t
Inferior extensor retinaculum

Extensor digitorum longus t
Tibialis anterior a and vv
Extensor digitorum longus t
Anterior tubercle
Fibular notch
Posterior tubercle
Fibula
Peroneus longus t
Peroneus brevis t
Superior peroneal retinaculum
Peroneus brevis m

Greater saphenous v
Tibia
Tibialis posterior t
Flexor retinaculum
Flexor digitorum longus t
Tibialis posterior a and vv
Tibial n
Accessory flexor digitorum longus m
Flexor hallucis longus t

Lesser saphenous v
Achilles t
Flexor hallucis longus m
Soleus m

Figure 14.1.7

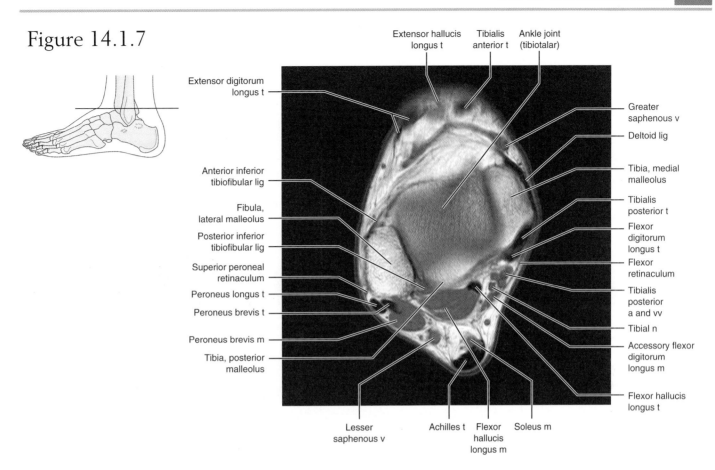

Extensor digitorum longus t

Extensor hallucis longus t

Tibialis anterior t

Ankle joint (tibiotalar)

Anterior inferior tibiofibular lig

Fibula, lateral malleolus

Posterior inferior tibiofibular lig

Superior peroneal retinaculum

Peroneus longus t

Peroneus brevis t

Peroneus brevis m

Tibia, posterior malleolus

Greater saphenous v

Deltoid lig

Tibia, medial malleolus

Tibialis posterior t

Flexor digitorum longus t

Flexor retinaculum

Tibialis posterior a and vv

Tibial n

Accessory flexor digitorum longus m

Flexor hallucis longus t

Lesser saphenous v

Achilles t

Flexor hallucis longus m

Soleus m

Figure 14.1.8

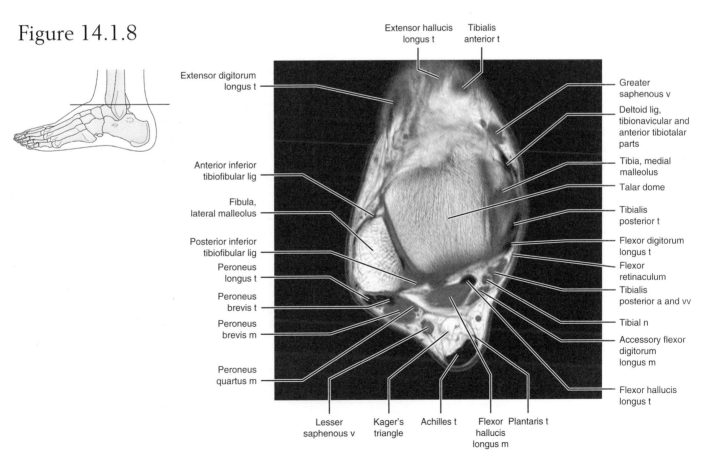

Extensor hallucis longus t

Tibialis anterior t

Extensor digitorum longus t

Anterior inferior tibiofibular lig

Fibula, lateral malleolus

Posterior inferior tibiofibular lig

Peroneus longus t

Peroneus brevis t

Peroneus brevis m

Peroneus quartus m

Greater saphenous v

Deltoid lig, tibionavicular and anterior tibiotalar parts

Tibia, medial malleolus

Talar dome

Tibialis posterior t

Flexor digitorum longus t

Flexor retinaculum

Tibialis posterior a and vv

Tibial n

Accessory flexor digitorum longus m

Flexor hallucis longus t

Lesser saphenous v

Kager's triangle

Achilles t

Flexor hallucis longus m

Plantaris t

Figure 14.1.9

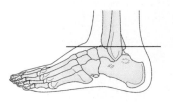

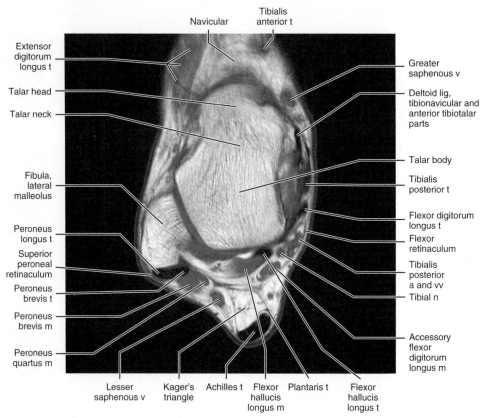

Extensor digitorum longus t
Talar head
Talar neck
Fibula, lateral malleolus
Peroneus longus t
Superior peroneal retinaculum
Peroneus brevis t
Peroneus brevis m
Peroneus quartus m

Navicular
Tibialis anterior t

Greater saphenous v
Deltoid lig, tibionavicular and anterior tibiotalar parts
Talar body
Tibialis posterior t
Flexor digitorum longus t
Flexor retinaculum
Tibialis posterior a and vv
Tibial n
Accessory flexor digitorum longus m

Lesser saphenous v
Kager's triangle
Achilles t
Flexor hallucis longus m
Plantaris t
Flexor hallucis longus t

Figure 14.1.10

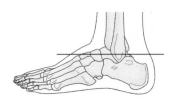

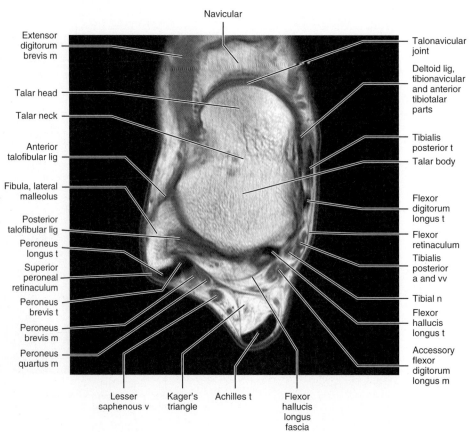

Extensor digitorum brevis m
Talar head
Talar neck
Anterior talofibular lig
Fibula, lateral malleolus
Posterior talofibular lig
Peroneus longus t
Superior peroneal retinaculum
Peroneus brevis t
Peroneus brevis m
Peroneus quartus m

Navicular

Talonavicular joint
Deltoid lig, tibionavicular and anterior tibiotalar parts
Tibialis posterior t
Talar body
Flexor digitorum longus t
Flexor retinaculum
Tibialis posterior a and vv
Tibial n
Flexor hallucis longus t
Accessory flexor digitorum longus m

Lesser saphenous v
Kager's triangle
Achilles t
Flexor hallucis longus fascia

Figure 14.1.11

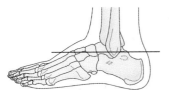

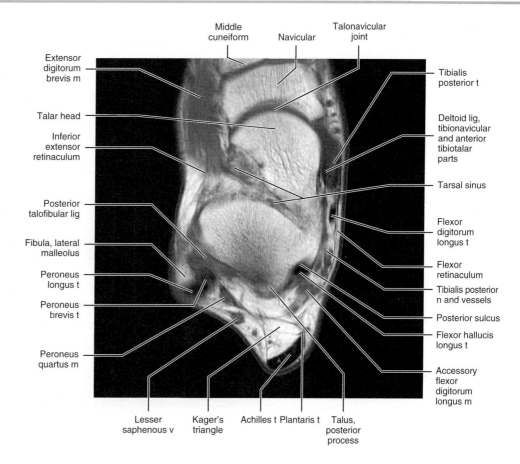

Middle cuneiform
Navicular
Talonavicular joint
Extensor digitorum brevis m
Tibialis posterior t
Talar head
Deltoid lig, tibionavicular and anterior tibiotalar parts
Inferior extensor retinaculum
Tarsal sinus
Posterior talofibular lig
Flexor digitorum longus t
Fibula, lateral malleolus
Flexor retinaculum
Peroneus longus t
Tibialis posterior n and vessels
Peroneus brevis t
Posterior sulcus
Flexor hallucis longus t
Peroneus quartus m
Accessory flexor digitorum longus m
Lesser saphenous v
Kager's triangle
Achilles t
Plantaris t
Talus, posterior process

Figure 14.1.12

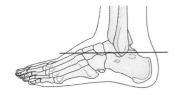

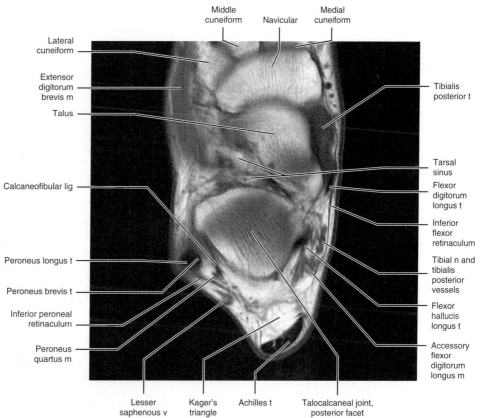

Middle cuneiform
Navicular
Medial cuneiform
Lateral cuneiform
Tibialis posterior t
Extensor digitorum brevis m
Talus
Tarsal sinus
Flexor digitorum longus t
Calcaneofibular lig
Inferior flexor retinaculum
Tibial n and tibialis posterior vessels
Peroneus longus t
Peroneus brevis t
Flexor hallucis longus t
Inferior peroneal retinaculum
Accessory flexor digitorum longus m
Peroneus quartus m
Lesser saphenous v
Kager's triangle
Achilles t
Talocalcaneal joint, posterior facet

Figure 14.1.13

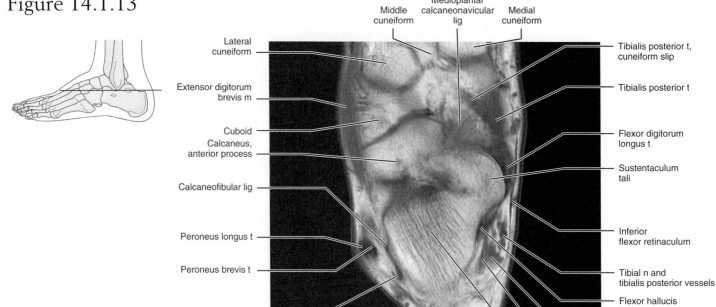

Middle cuneiform
Medioplantar calcaneonavicular lig
Medial cuneiform
Lateral cuneiform
Tibialis posterior t, cuneiform slip
Extensor digitorum brevis m
Tibialis posterior t
Cuboid
Flexor digitorum longus t
Calcaneus, anterior process
Sustentaculum tali
Calcaneofibular lig
Inferior flexor retinaculum
Peroneus longus t
Tibial n and tibialis posterior vessels
Peroneus brevis t
Flexor hallucis longus t
Accessory flexor digitorum longus m
Peroneus quartus t
Quadratus plantae m
Kager's triangle
Achilles t
Plantaris t
Calcaneus

Figure 14.1.14

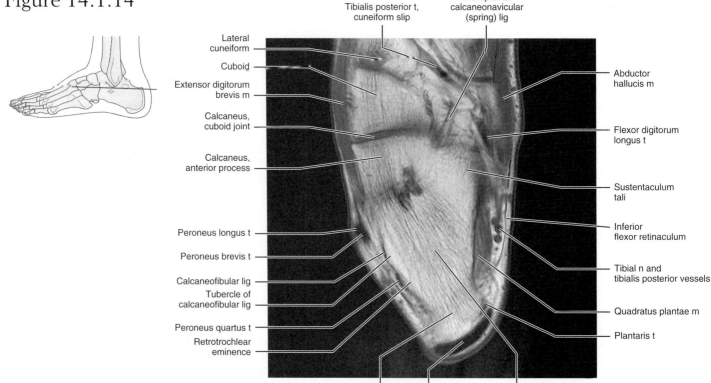

Tibialis posterior t, cuneiform slip
Inferoplantar calcaneonavicular (spring) lig
Lateral cuneiform
Cuboid
Abductor hallucis m
Extensor digitorum brevis m
Calcaneus, cuboid joint
Flexor digitorum longus t
Calcaneus, anterior process
Sustentaculum tali
Inferior flexor retinaculum
Peroneus longus t
Peroneus brevis t
Tibial n and tibialis posterior vessels
Calcaneofibular lig
Tubercle of calcaneofibular lig
Quadratus plantae m
Peroneus quartus t
Plantaris t
Retrotrochlear eminence
Calcaneal tuberosity
Achilles t
Calcaneus

Figure 14.1.15

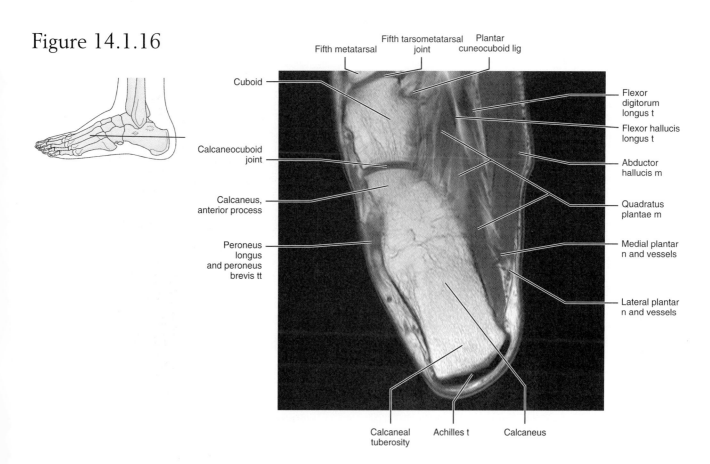

Plantar cuneocuboid lig

Cuboid

Extensor digitorum brevis m

Calcaneocuboid joint

Calcaneus, anterior process

Peroneal tubercle

Peroneus longus and peroneus brevis tt

Tubercle of calcaneofibular lig

Retrotrochlear eminence

Flexor digitorum longus t

Flexor hallucis longus t

Abductor hallucis m

Tibial n and tibialis posterior vessels

Quadratus plantae m

Calcaneal tuberosity

Achilles t

Calcaneus

Figure 14.1.16

Fifth tarsometatarsal joint

Plantar cuneocuboid lig

Fifth metatarsal

Cuboid

Calcaneocuboid joint

Calcaneus, anterior process

Peroneus longus and peroneus brevis tt

Flexor digitorum longus t

Flexor hallucis longus t

Abductor hallucis m

Quadratus plantae m

Medial plantar n and vessels

Lateral plantar n and vessels

Calcaneal tuberosity

Achilles t

Calcaneus

Figure 14.1.17

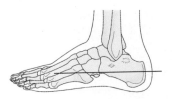

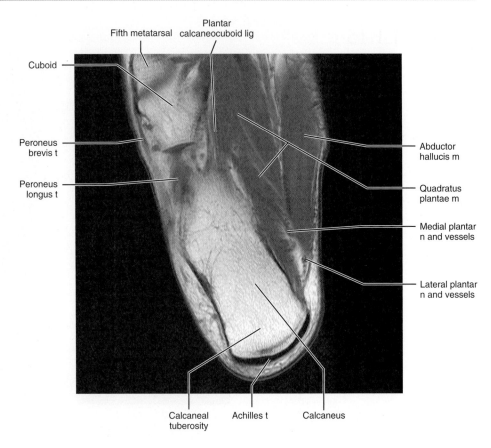

Fifth metatarsal

Plantar calcaneocuboid lig

Cuboid

Peroneus brevis t

Peroneus longus t

Abductor hallucis m

Quadratus plantae m

Medial plantar n and vessels

Lateral plantar n and vessels

Calcaneal tuberosity

Achilles t

Calcaneus

Figure 14.1.18

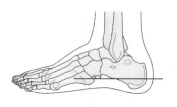

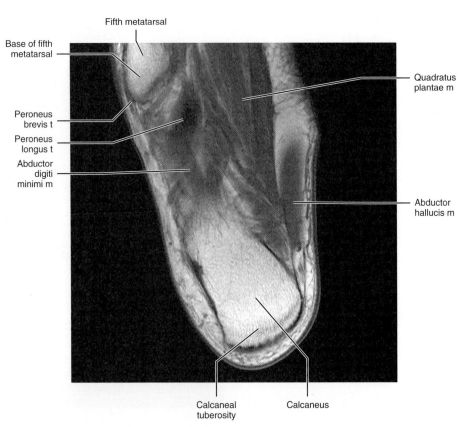

Fifth metatarsal

Base of fifth metatarsal

Peroneus brevis t

Peroneus longus t

Abductor digiti minimi m

Quadratus plantae m

Abductor hallucis m

Calcaneal tuberosity

Calcaneus

Figure 14.1.19

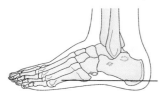

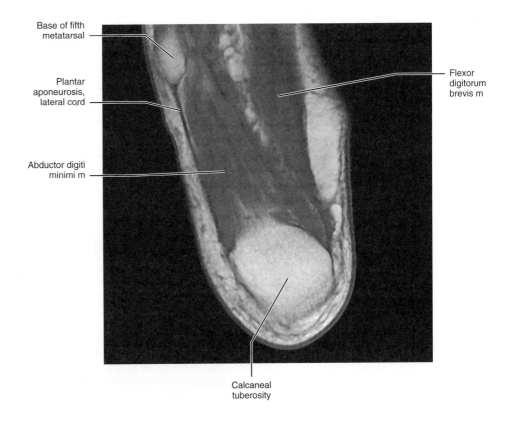

Base of fifth metatarsal

Plantar aponeurosis, lateral cord

Abductor digiti minimi m

Flexor digitorum brevis m

Calcaneal tuberosity

Figure 14.1.20

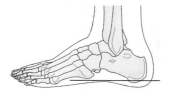

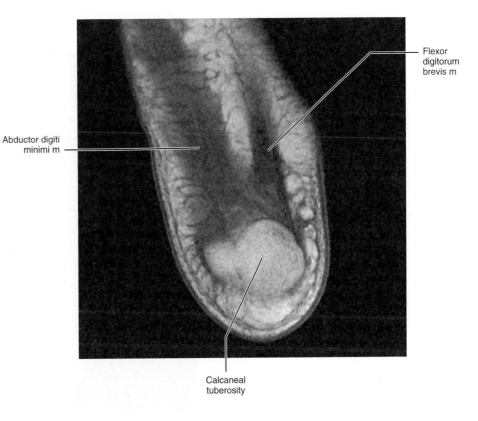

Flexor digitorum brevis m

Abductor digiti minimi m

Calcaneal tuberosity

OBLIQUE AXIAL

Figure 14.2.1

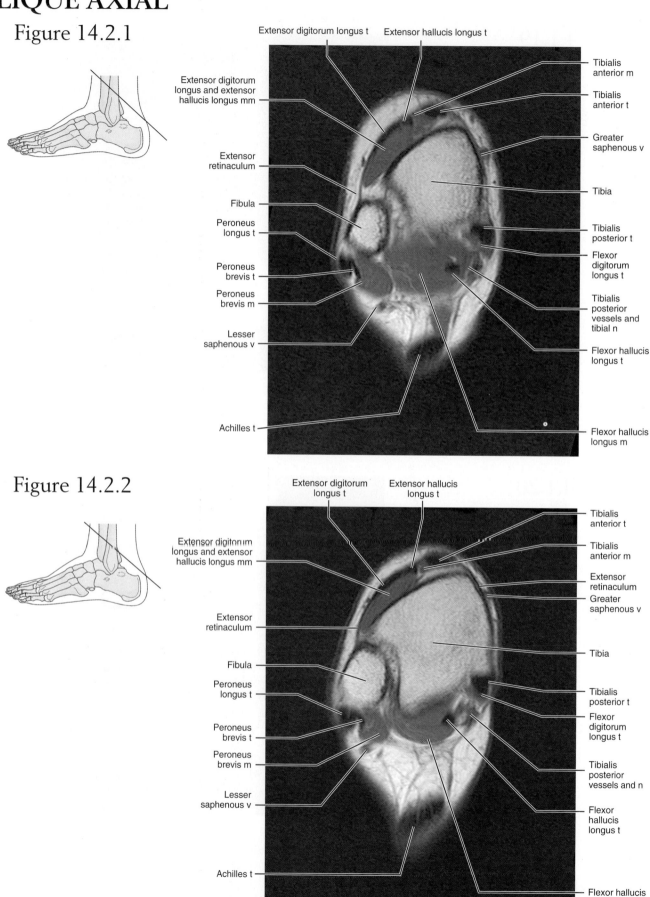

Extensor digitorum longus t
Extensor hallucis longus t
Extensor digitorum longus and extensor hallucis longus mm
Extensor retinaculum
Fibula
Peroneus longus t
Peroneus brevis t
Peroneus brevis m
Lesser saphenous v
Achilles t
Tibialis anterior m
Tibialis anterior t
Greater saphenous v
Tibia
Tibialis posterior t
Flexor digitorum longus t
Tibialis posterior vessels and tibial n
Flexor hallucis longus t
Flexor hallucis longus m

Figure 14.2.2

Extensor digitorum longus t
Extensor hallucis longus t
Extensor digitorum longus and extensor hallucis longus mm
Extensor retinaculum
Fibula
Peroneus longus t
Peroneus brevis t
Peroneus brevis m
Lesser saphenous v
Achilles t
Tibialis anterior t
Tibialis anterior m
Extensor retinaculum
Greater saphenous v
Tibia
Tibialis posterior t
Flexor digitorum longus t
Tibialis posterior vessels and n
Flexor hallucis longus t
Flexor hallucis longus m

Figure 14.2.3

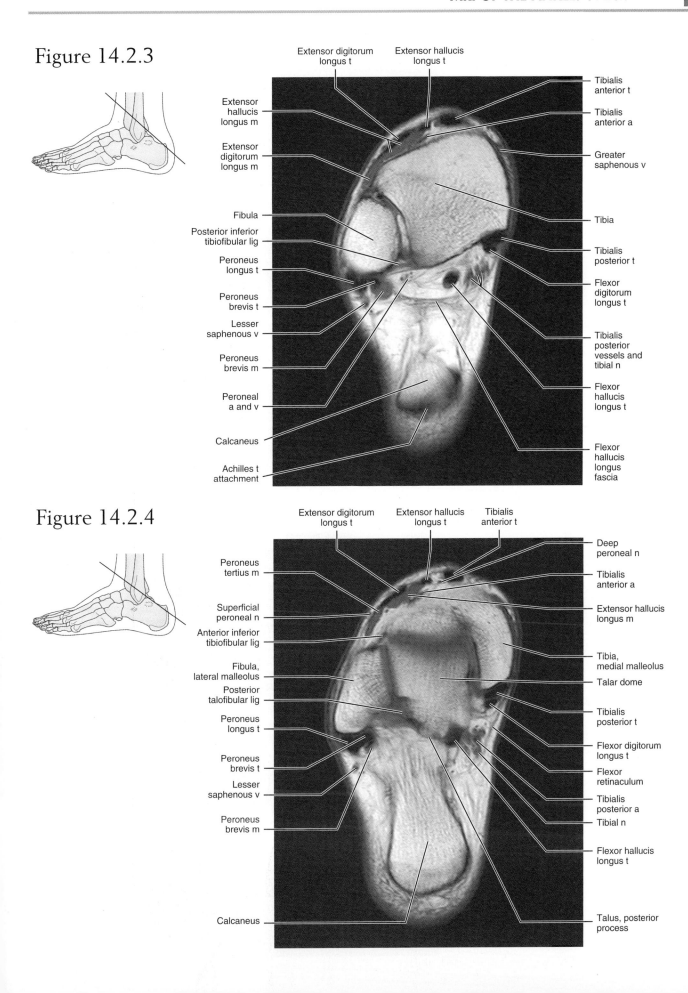

Extensor digitorum longus t

Extensor hallucis longus t

Extensor hallucis longus m

Extensor digitorum longus m

Fibula

Posterior inferior tibiofibular lig

Peroneus longus t

Peroneus brevis t

Lesser saphenous v

Peroneus brevis m

Peroneal a and v

Calcaneus

Achilles t attachment

Tibialis anterior t

Tibialis anterior a

Greater saphenous v

Tibia

Tibialis posterior t

Flexor digitorum longus t

Tibialis posterior vessels and tibial n

Flexor hallucis longus t

Flexor hallucis longus fascia

Figure 14.2.4

Extensor digitorum longus t

Extensor hallucis longus t

Tibialis anterior t

Peroneus tertius m

Superficial peroneal n

Anterior inferior tibiofibular lig

Fibula, lateral malleolus

Posterior talofibular lig

Peroneus longus t

Peroneus brevis t

Lesser saphenous v

Peroneus brevis m

Calcaneus

Deep peroneal n

Tibialis anterior a

Extensor hallucis longus m

Tibia, medial malleolus

Talar dome

Tibialis posterior t

Flexor digitorum longus t

Flexor retinaculum

Tibialis posterior a

Tibial n

Flexor hallucis longus t

Talus, posterior process

Figure 14.2.5

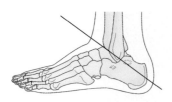

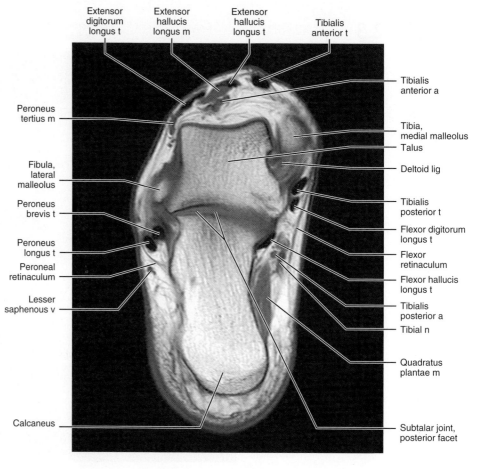

Extensor digitorum longus t
Extensor hallucis longus m
Extensor hallucis longus t
Tibialis anterior t

Peroneus tertius m

Fibula, lateral malleolus

Peroneus brevis t

Peroneus longus t

Peroneal retinaculum

Lesser saphenous v

Calcaneus

Tibialis anterior a

Tibia, medial malleolus

Talus

Deltoid lig

Tibialis posterior t

Flexor digitorum longus t

Flexor retinaculum

Flexor hallucis longus t

Tibialis posterior a

Tibial n

Quadratus plantae m

Subtalar joint, posterior facet

Figure 14.2.6

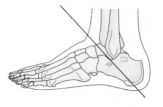

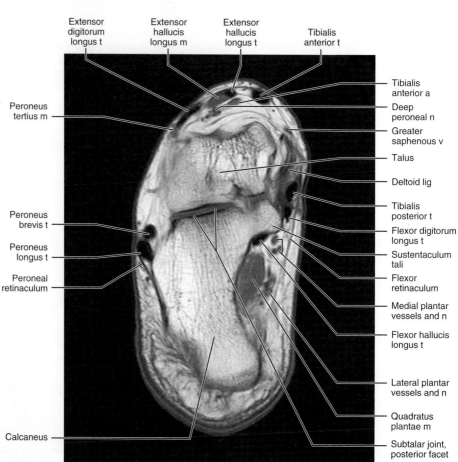

Extensor digitorum longus t
Extensor hallucis longus m
Extensor hallucis longus t
Tibialis anterior t

Peroneus tertius m

Peroneus brevis t

Peroneus longus t

Peroneal retinaculum

Calcaneus

Tibialis anterior a

Deep peroneal n

Greater saphenous v

Talus

Deltoid lig

Tibialis posterior t

Flexor digitorum longus t

Sustentaculum tali

Flexor retinaculum

Medial plantar vessels and n

Flexor hallucis longus t

Lateral plantar vessels and n

Quadratus plantae m

Subtalar joint, posterior facet

Figure 14.2.7

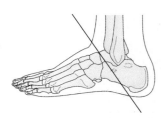

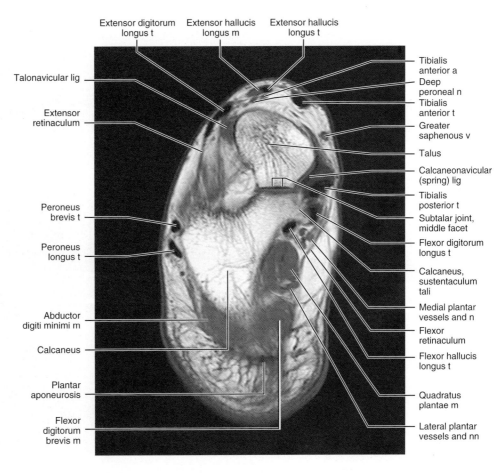

Extensor digitorum longus t
Extensor hallucis longus m
Extensor hallucis longus t
Talonavicular lig
Extensor retinaculum
Peroneus brevis t
Peroneus longus t
Abductor digiti minimi m
Calcaneus
Plantar aponeurosis
Flexor digitorum brevis m

Tibialis anterior a
Deep peroneal n
Tibialis anterior t
Greater saphenous v
Talus
Calcaneonavicular (spring) lig
Tibialis posterior t
Subtalar joint, middle facet
Flexor digitorum longus t
Calcaneus, sustentaculum tali
Medial plantar vessels and n
Flexor retinaculum
Flexor hallucis longus t
Quadratus plantae m
Lateral plantar vessels and nn

Figure 14.2.8

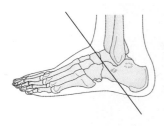

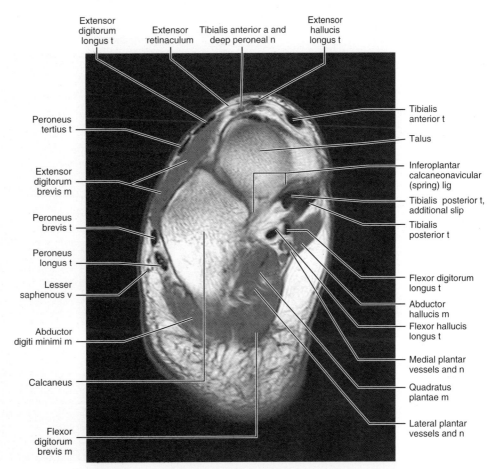

Extensor digitorum longus t
Extensor retinaculum
Tibialis anterior a and deep peroneal n
Extensor hallucis longus t
Peroneus tertius t
Extensor digitorum brevis m
Peroneus brevis t
Peroneus longus t
Lesser saphenous v
Abductor digiti minimi m
Calcaneus
Flexor digitorum brevis m

Tibialis anterior t
Talus
Inferoplantar calcaneonavicular (spring) lig
Tibialis posterior t, additional slip
Tibialis posterior t
Flexor digitorum longus t
Abductor hallucis m
Flexor hallucis longus t
Medial plantar vessels and n
Quadratus plantae m
Lateral plantar vessels and n

Figure 14.2.9

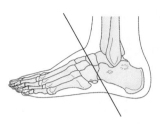

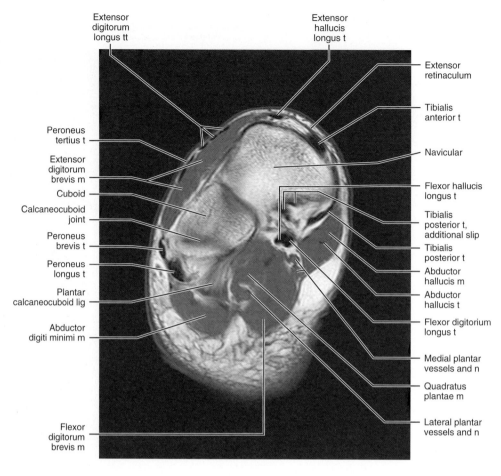

Extensor digitorum longus tt

Extensor hallucis longus t

Peroneus tertius t

Extensor digitorum brevis m

Cuboid

Calcaneocuboid joint

Peroneus brevis t

Peroneus longus t

Plantar calcaneocuboid lig

Abductor digiti minimi m

Flexor digitorum brevis m

Extensor retinaculum

Tibialis anterior t

Navicular

Flexor hallucis longus t

Tibialis posterior t, additional slip

Tibialis posterior t

Abductor hallucis m

Abductor hallucis t

Flexor digitorium longus t

Medial plantar vessels and n

Quadratus plantae m

Lateral plantar vessels and n

Figure 14.2.10

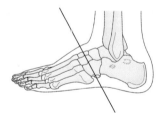

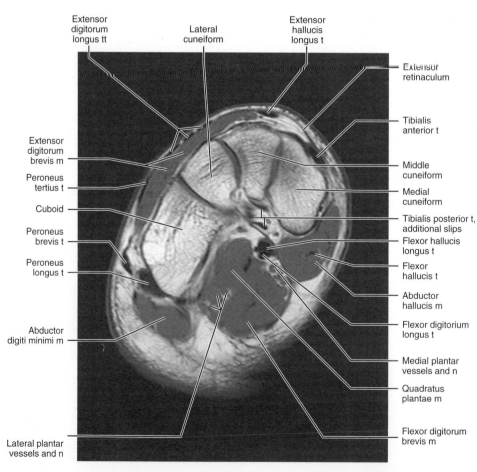

Extensor digitorum longus tt

Lateral cuneiform

Extensor hallucis longus t

Extensor digitorum brevis m

Peroneus tertius t

Cuboid

Peroneus brevis t

Peroneus longus t

Abductor digiti minimi m

Lateral plantar vessels and n

Extensor retinaculum

Tibialis anterior t

Middle cuneiform

Medial cuneiform

Tibialis posterior t, additional slips

Flexor hallucis longus t

Flexor hallucis t

Abductor hallucis m

Flexor digitorium longus t

Medial plantar vessels and n

Quadratus plantae m

Flexor digitorum brevis m

Figure 14.2.11

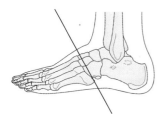

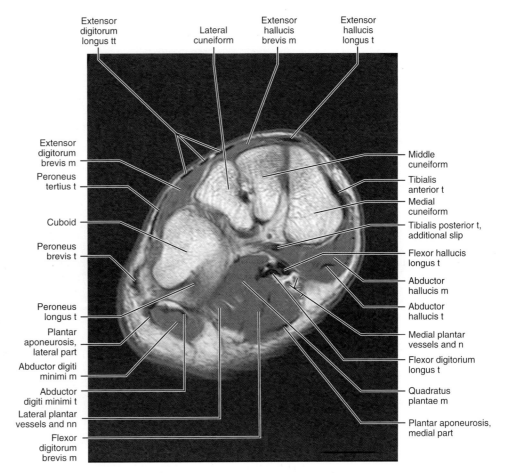

Extensor digitorum longus tt

Lateral cuneiform

Extensor hallucis brevis m

Extensor hallucis longus t

Extensor digitorum brevis m

Peroneus tertius t

Cuboid

Peroneus brevis t

Peroneus longus t

Plantar aponeurosis, lateral part

Abductor digiti minimi m

Abductor digiti minimi t

Lateral plantar vessels and nn

Flexor digitorum brevis m

Middle cuneiform

Tibialis anterior t

Medial cuneiform

Tibialis posterior t, additional slip

Flexor hallucis longus t

Abductor hallucis m

Abductor hallucis t

Medial plantar vessels and n

Flexor digitorium longus t

Quadratus plantae m

Plantar aponeurosis, medial part

SAGITTAL

Figure 14.3.1

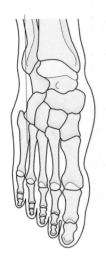

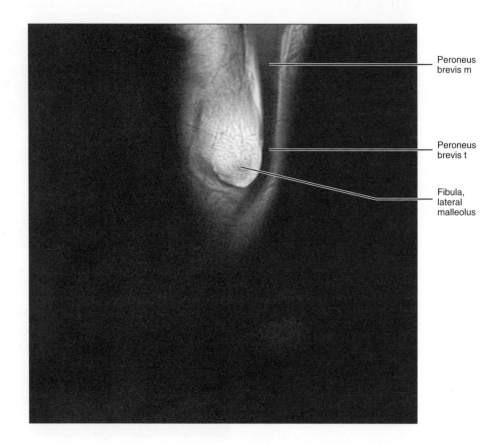

Peroneus brevis m

Peroneus brevis t

Fibula, lateral malleolus

Figure 14.3.2

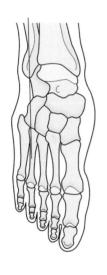

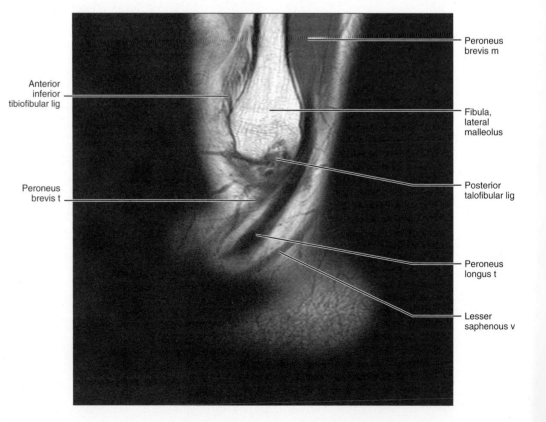

Anterior inferior tibiofibular lig

Peroneus brevis t

Peroneus brevis m

Fibula, lateral malleolus

Posterior talofibular lig

Peroneus longus t

Lesser saphenous v

Figure 14.3.3

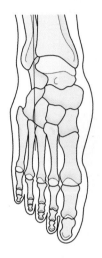

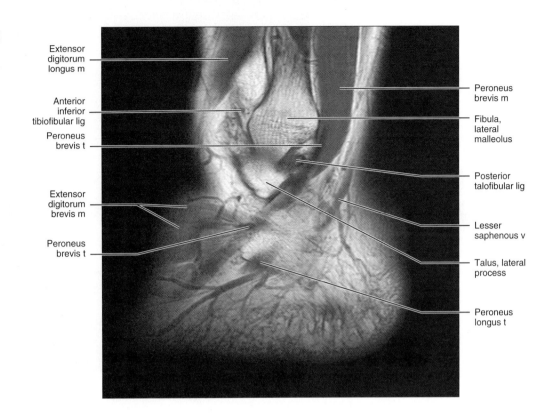

Extensor digitorum longus m

Anterior inferior tibiofibular lig

Peroneus brevis t

Extensor digitorum brevis m

Peroneus brevis t

Peroneus brevis m

Fibula, lateral malleolus

Posterior talofibular lig

Lesser saphenous v

Talus, lateral process

Peroneus longus t

Figure 14.3.4

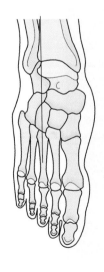

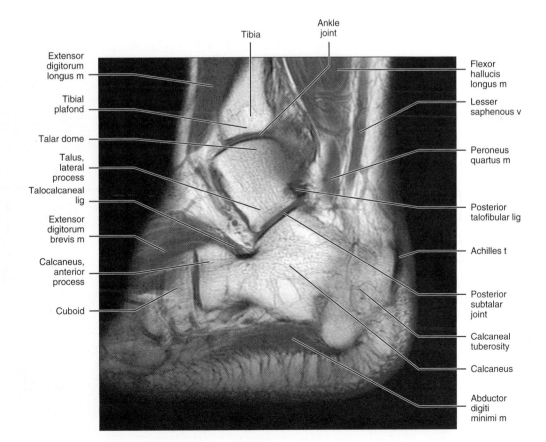

Tibia

Ankle joint

Extensor digitorum longus m

Tibial plafond

Talar dome

Talus, lateral process

Talocalcaneal lig

Extensor digitorum brevis m

Calcaneus, anterior process

Cuboid

Flexor hallucis longus m

Lesser saphenous v

Peroneus quartus m

Posterior talofibular lig

Achilles t

Posterior subtalar joint

Calcaneal tuberosity

Calcaneus

Abductor digiti minimi m

Figure 14.3.5

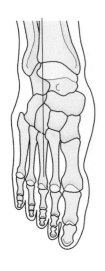

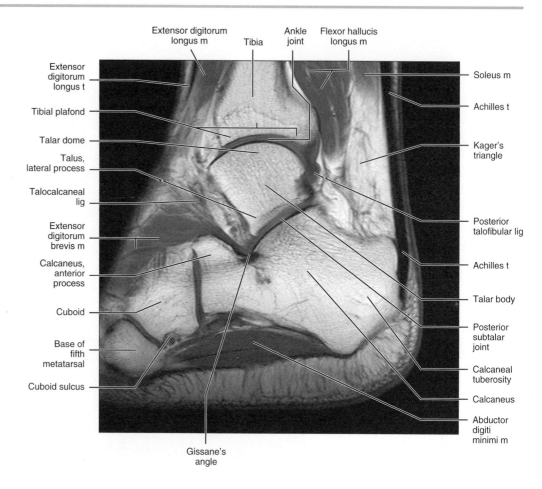

Extensor digitorum longus m

Tibia

Ankle joint

Flexor hallucis longus m

Extensor digitorum longus t

Tibial plafond

Talar dome

Talus, lateral process

Talocalcaneal lig

Extensor digitorum brevis m

Calcaneus, anterior process

Cuboid

Base of fifth metatarsal

Cuboid sulcus

Soleus m

Achilles t

Kager's triangle

Posterior talofibular lig

Achilles t

Talar body

Posterior subtalar joint

Calcaneal tuberosity

Calcaneus

Abductor digiti minimi m

Gissane's angle

Figure 14.3.6

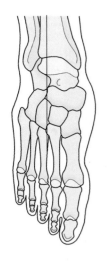

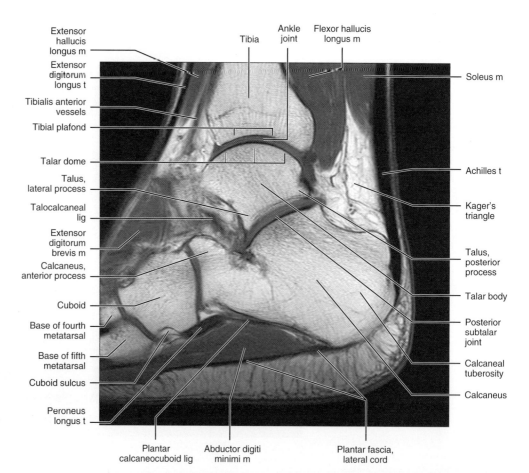

Extensor hallucis longus m

Extensor digitorum longus t

Tibialis anterior vessels

Tibial plafond

Talar dome

Talus, lateral process

Talocalcaneal lig

Extensor digitorum brevis m

Calcaneus, anterior process

Cuboid

Base of fourth metatarsal

Base of fifth metatarsal

Cuboid sulcus

Peroneus longus t

Tibia

Ankle joint

Flexor hallucis longus m

Soleus m

Achilles t

Kager's triangle

Talus, posterior process

Talar body

Posterior subtalar joint

Calcaneal tuberosity

Calcaneus

Plantar calcaneocuboid lig

Abductor digiti minimi m

Plantar fascia, lateral cord

Figure 14.3.7

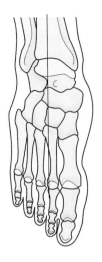

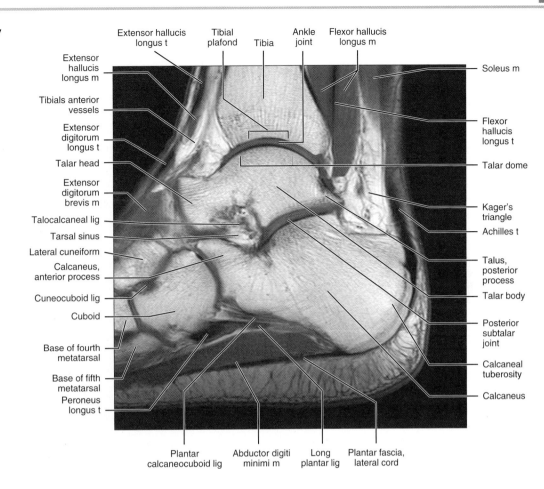

Extensor hallucis longus t   Tibial plafond   Tibia   Ankle joint   Flexor hallucis longus m

Extensor hallucis longus m

Tibials anterior vessels

Extensor digitorum longus t

Talar head

Extensor digitorum brevis m

Talocalcaneal lig

Tarsal sinus

Lateral cuneiform

Calcaneus, anterior process

Cuneocuboid lig

Cuboid

Base of fourth metatarsal

Base of fifth metatarsal

Peroneus longus t

Soleus m

Flexor hallucis longus t

Talar dome

Kager's triangle

Achilles t

Talus, posterior process

Talar body

Posterior subtalar joint

Calcaneal tuberosity

Calcaneus

Plantar calcaneocuboid lig   Abductor digiti minimi m   Long plantar lig   Plantar fascia, lateral cord

Figure 14.3.8

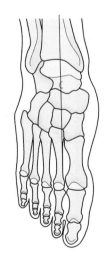

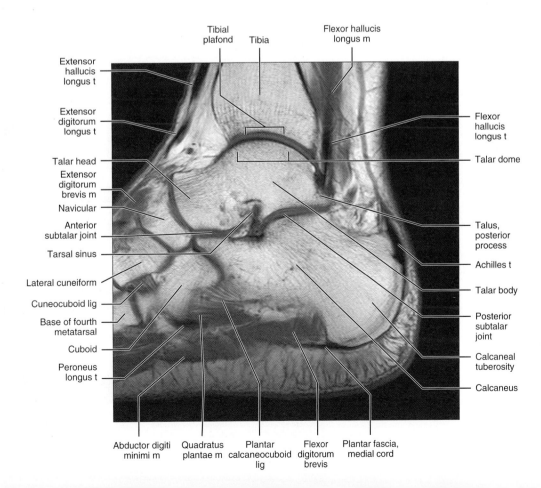

Tibial plafond   Tibia   Flexor hallucis longus m

Extensor hallucis longus t

Extensor digitorum longus t

Talar head

Extensor digitorum brevis m

Navicular

Anterior subtalar joint

Tarsal sinus

Lateral cuneiform

Cuneocuboid lig

Base of fourth metatarsal

Cuboid

Peroneus longus t

Flexor hallucis longus t

Talar dome

Talus, posterior process

Achilles t

Talar body

Posterior subtalar joint

Calcaneal tuberosity

Calcaneus

Abductor digiti minimi m   Quadratus plantae m   Plantar calcaneocuboid lig   Flexor digitorum brevis   Plantar fascia, medial cord

Figure 14.3.9

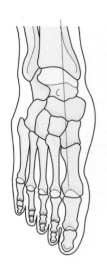

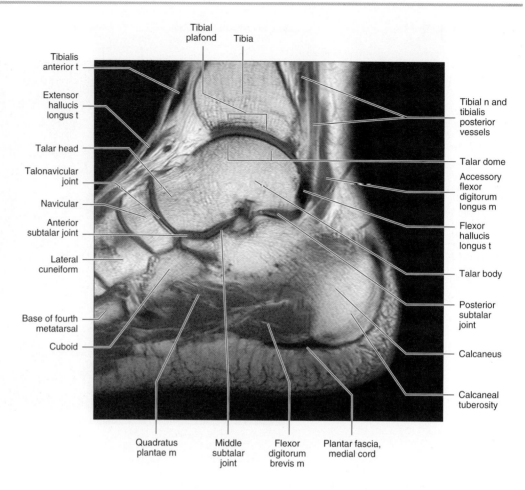

Tibial plafond

Tibia

Tibialis anterior t

Extensor hallucis longus t

Talar head

Talonavicular joint

Navicular

Anterior subtalar joint

Lateral cuneiform

Base of fourth metatarsal

Cuboid

Tibial n and tibialis posterior vessels

Talar dome

Accessory flexor digitorum longus m

Flexor hallucis longus t

Talar body

Posterior subtalar joint

Calcaneus

Calcaneal tuberosity

Quadratus plantae m

Middle subtalar joint

Flexor digitorum brevis m

Plantar fascia, medial cord

Figure 14.3.10

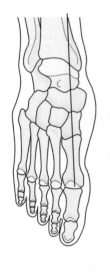

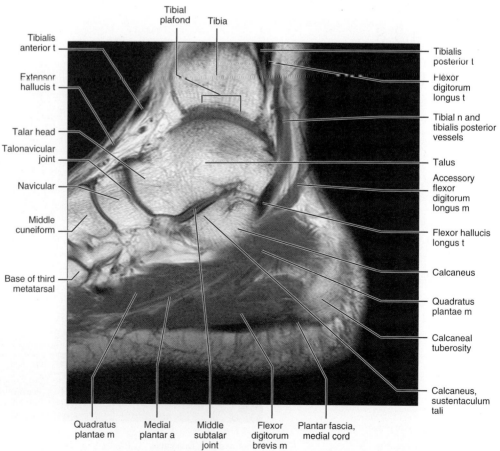

Tibial plafond

Tibia

Tibialis anterior t

Extensor hallucis t

Talar head

Talonavicular joint

Navicular

Middle cuneiform

Base of third metatarsal

Tibialis posterior t

Flexor digitorum longus t

Tibial n and tibialis posterior vessels

Talus

Accessory flexor digitorum longus m

Flexor hallucis longus t

Calcaneus

Quadratus plantae m

Calcaneal tuberosity

Calcaneus, sustentaculum tali

Quadratus plantae m

Medial plantar a

Middle subtalar joint

Flexor digitorum brevis m

Plantar fascia, medial cord

Figure 14.3.11

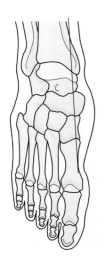

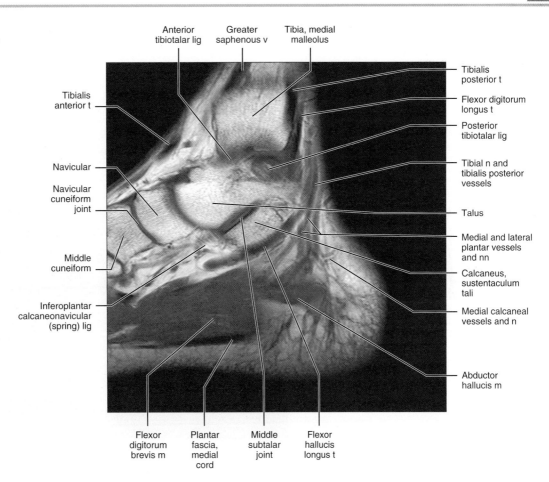

Anterior tibiotalar lig

Greater saphenous v

Tibia, medial malleolus

Tibialis anterior t

Navicular

Navicular cuneiform joint

Middle cuneiform

Inferoplantar calcaneonavicular (spring) lig

Tibialis posterior t

Flexor digitorum longus t

Posterior tibiotalar lig

Tibial n and tibialis posterior vessels

Talus

Medial and lateral plantar vessels and nn

Calcaneus, sustentaculum tali

Medial calcaneal vessels and n

Abductor hallucis m

Flexor digitorum brevis m

Plantar fascia, medial cord

Middle subtalar joint

Flexor hallucis longus t

Figure 14.3.12

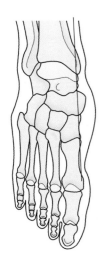

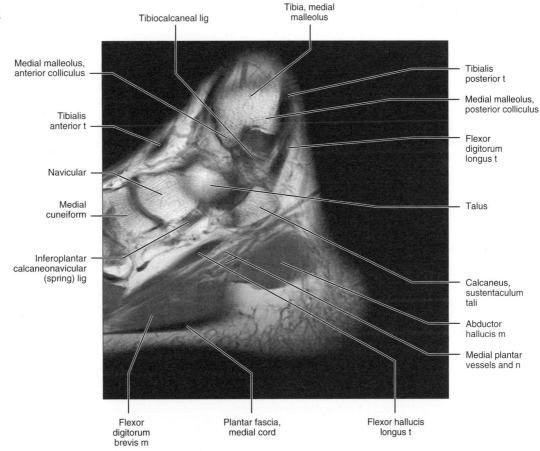

Tibiocalcaneal lig

Tibia, medial malleolus

Medial malleolus, anterior colliculus

Tibialis anterior t

Navicular

Medial cuneiform

Inferoplantar calcaneonavicular (spring) lig

Tibialis posterior t

Medial malleolus, posterior colliculus

Flexor digitorum longus t

Talus

Calcaneus, sustentaculum tali

Abductor hallucis m

Medial plantar vessels and n

Flexor digitorum brevis m

Plantar fascia, medial cord

Flexor hallucis longus t

Figure 14.3.13

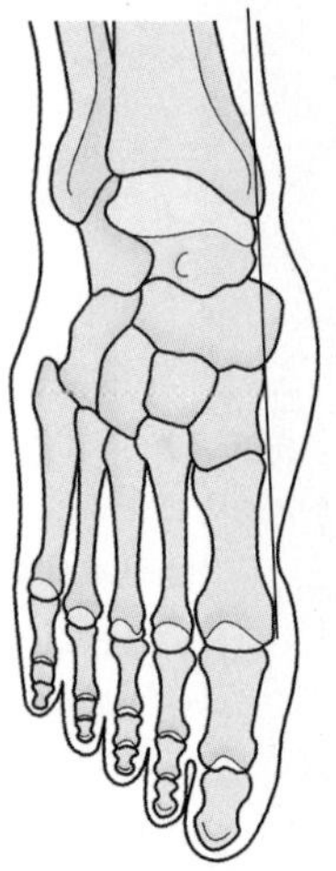

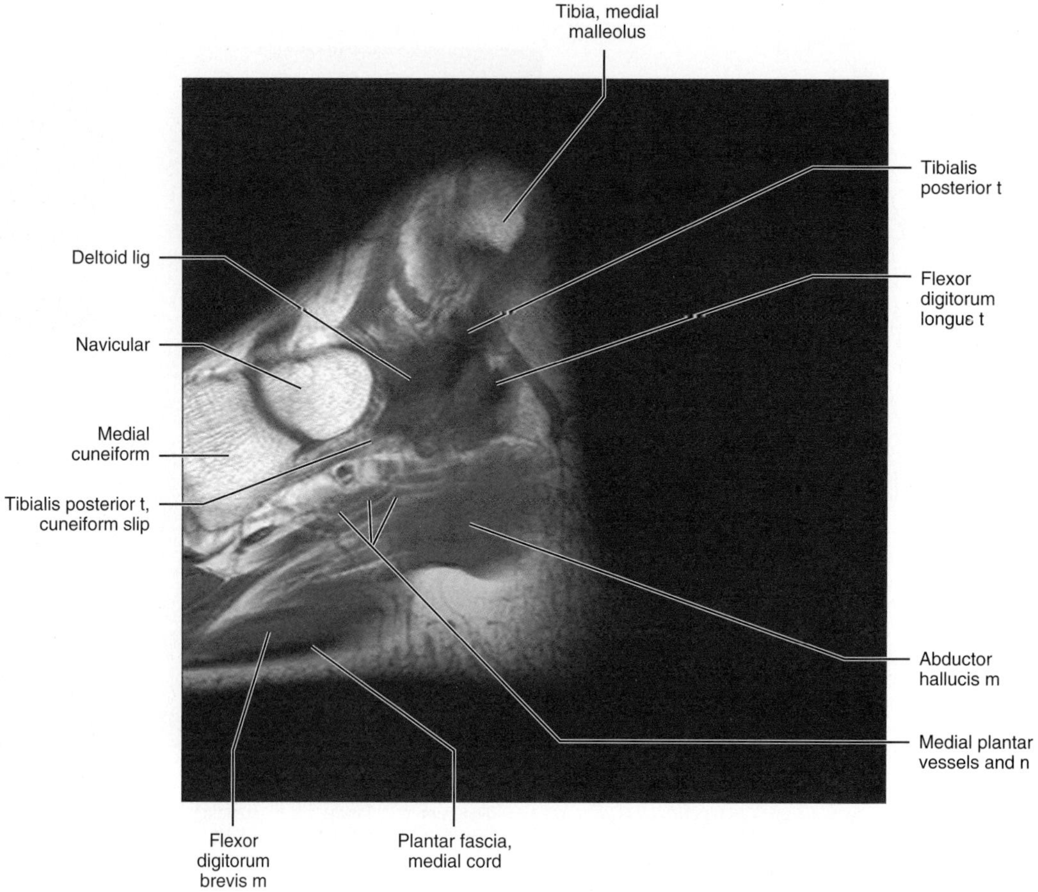

Tibia, medial malleolus

Tibialis posterior t

Deltoid lig

Flexor digitorum longus t

Navicular

Medial cuneiform

Tibialis posterior t, cuneiform slip

Abductor hallucis m

Medial plantar vessels and n

Flexor digitorum brevis m

Plantar fascia, medial cord

CORONAL
Figure 14.4.1

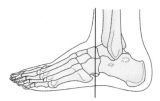

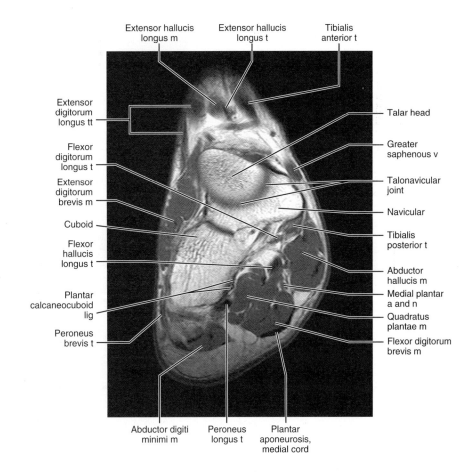

Extensor hallucis longus m
Extensor hallucis longus t
Tibialis anterior t

Extensor digitorum longus tt
Flexor digitorum longus t
Extensor digitorum brevis m
Cuboid
Flexor hallucis longus t
Plantar calcaneocuboid lig
Peroneus brevis t

Talar head
Greater saphenous v
Talonavicular joint
Navicular
Tibialis posterior t
Abductor hallucis m
Medial plantar a and n
Quadratus plantae m
Flexor digitorum brevis m

Abductor digiti minimi m
Peroneus longus t
Plantar aponeurosis, medial cord

Figure 14.4.2

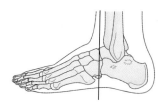

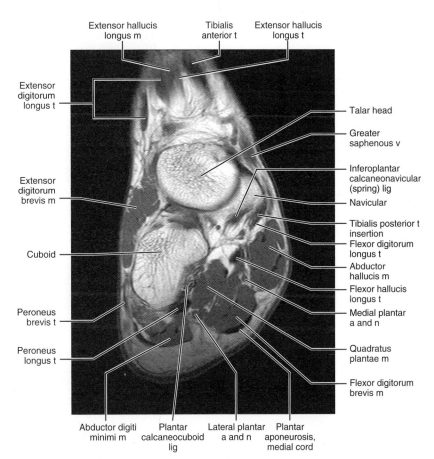

Extensor hallucis longus m
Tibialis anterior t
Extensor hallucis longus t

Extensor digitorum longus t
Extensor digitorum brevis m
Cuboid
Peroneus brevis t
Peroneus longus t

Talar head
Greater saphenous v
Inferoplantar calcaneonavicular (spring) lig
Navicular
Tibialis posterior t insertion
Flexor digitorum longus t
Abductor hallucis m
Flexor hallucis longus t
Medial plantar a and n
Quadratus plantae m
Flexor digitorum brevis m

Abductor digiti minimi m
Plantar calcaneocuboid lig
Lateral plantar a and n
Plantar aponeurosis, medial cord

Figure 14.4.3

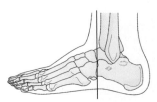

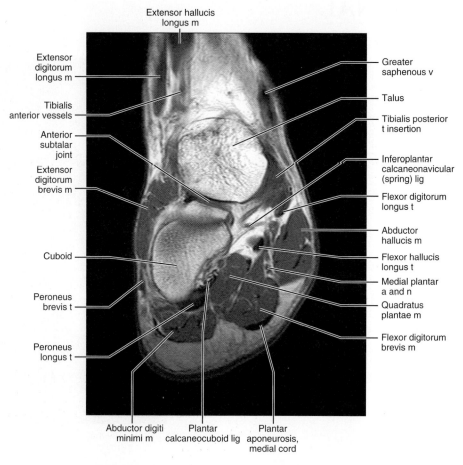

Extensor hallucis longus m

Extensor digitorum longus m

Tibialis anterior vessels

Anterior subtalar joint

Extensor digitorum brevis m

Cuboid

Peroneus brevis t

Peroneus longus t

Greater saphenous v

Talus

Tibialis posterior t insertion

Inferoplantar calcaneonavicular (spring) lig

Flexor digitorum longus t

Abductor hallucis m

Flexor hallucis longus t

Medial plantar a and n

Quadratus plantae m

Flexor digitorum brevis m

Abductor digiti minimi m

Plantar calcaneocuboid lig

Plantar aponeurosis, medial cord

Figure 14.4.4

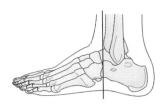

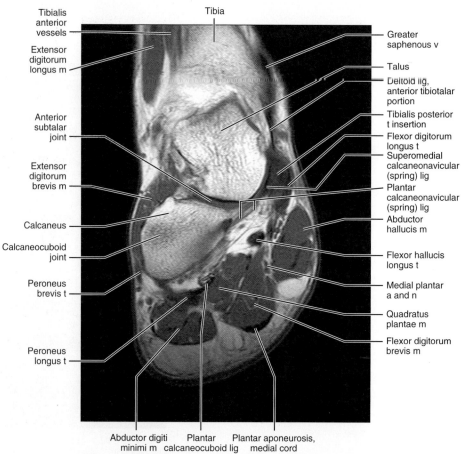

Tibia

Tibialis anterior vessels

Extensor digitorum longus m

Anterior subtalar joint

Extensor digitorum brevis m

Calcaneus

Calcaneocuboid joint

Peroneus brevis t

Peroneus longus t

Greater saphenous v

Talus

Deltoid lig, anterior tibiotalar portion

Tibialis posterior t insertion

Flexor digitorum longus t

Superomedial calcaneonavicular (spring) lig

Plantar calcaneonavicular (spring) lig

Abductor hallucis m

Flexor hallucis longus t

Medial plantar a and n

Quadratus plantae m

Flexor digitorum brevis m

Abductor digiti minimi m

Plantar calcaneocuboid lig

Plantar aponeurosis, medial cord

Figure 14.4.5

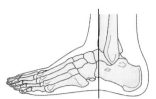

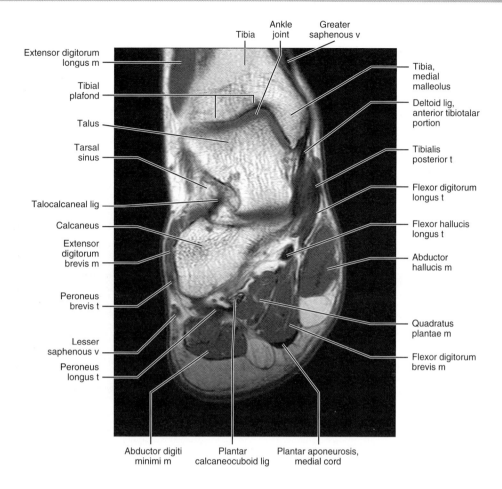

Extensor digitorum longus m

Tibial plafond

Talus

Tarsal sinus

Talocalcaneal lig

Calcaneus

Extensor digitorum brevis m

Peroneus brevis t

Lesser saphenous v

Peroneus longus t

Tibia

Ankle joint

Greater saphenous v

Tibia, medial malleolus

Deltoid lig, anterior tibiotalar portion

Tibialis posterior t

Flexor digitorum longus t

Flexor hallucis longus t

Abductor hallucis m

Quadratus plantae m

Flexor digitorum brevis m

Abductor digiti minimi m

Plantar calcaneocuboid lig

Plantar aponeurosis, medial cord

Figure 14.4.6

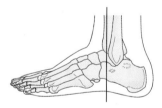

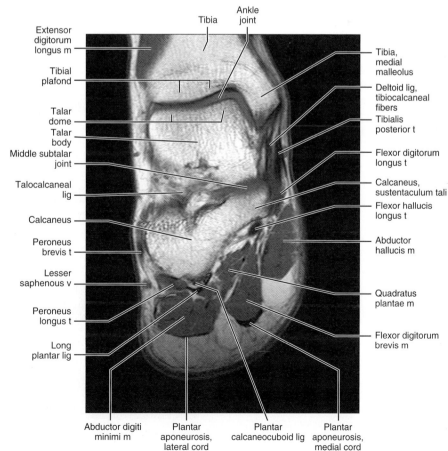

Extensor digitorum longus m

Tibial plafond

Talar dome

Talar body

Middle subtalar joint

Talocalcaneal lig

Calcaneus

Peroneus brevis t

Lesser saphenous v

Peroneus longus t

Long plantar lig

Tibia

Ankle joint

Tibia, medial malleolus

Deltoid lig, tibiocalcaneal fibers

Tibialis posterior t

Flexor digitorum longus t

Calcaneus, sustentaculum tali

Flexor hallucis longus t

Abductor hallucis m

Quadratus plantae m

Flexor digitorum brevis m

Abductor digiti minimi m

Plantar aponeurosis, lateral cord

Plantar calcaneocuboid lig

Plantar aponeurosis, medial cord

Figure 14.4.7

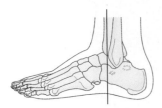

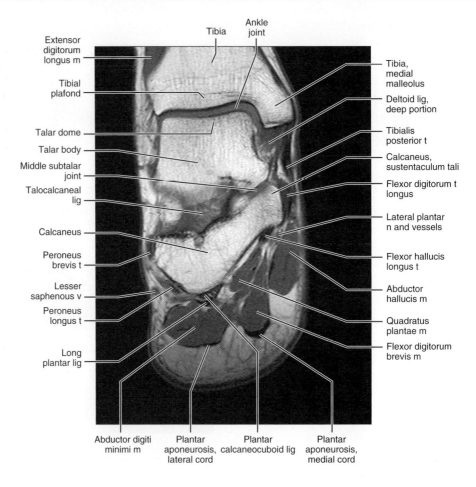

Extensor digitorum longus m

Tibial plafond

Talar dome

Talar body

Middle subtalar joint

Talocalcaneal lig

Calcaneus

Peroneus brevis t

Lesser saphenous v

Peroneus longus t

Long plantar lig

Tibia

Ankle joint

Tibia, medial malleolus

Deltoid lig, deep portion

Tibialis posterior t

Calcaneus, sustentaculum tali

Flexor digitorum t longus

Lateral plantar n and vessels

Flexor hallucis longus t

Abductor hallucis m

Quadratus plantae m

Flexor digitorum brevis m

Abductor digiti minimi m

Plantar aponeurosis, lateral cord

Plantar calcaneocuboid lig

Plantar aponeurosis, medial cord

Figure 14.4.8

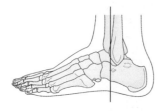

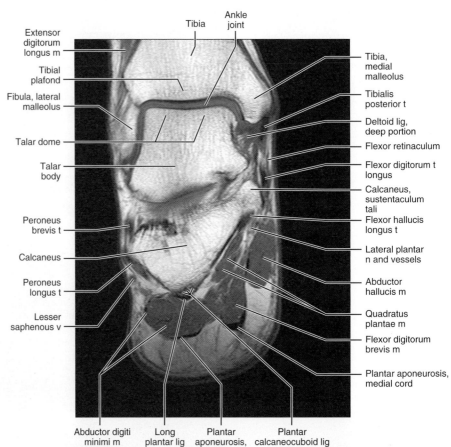

Extensor digitorum longus m

Tibial plafond

Fibula, lateral malleolus

Talar dome

Talar body

Peroneus brevis t

Calcaneus

Peroneus longus t

Lesser saphenous v

Tibia

Ankle joint

Tibia, medial malleolus

Tibialis posterior t

Deltoid lig, deep portion

Flexor retinaculum

Flexor digitorum t longus

Calcaneus, sustentaculum tali

Flexor hallucis longus t

Lateral plantar n and vessels

Abductor hallucis m

Quadratus plantae m

Flexor digitorum brevis m

Plantar aponeurosis, medial cord

Abductor digiti minimi m

Long plantar lig

Plantar aponeurosis, lateral cord

Plantar calcaneocuboid lig

Figure 14.4.9

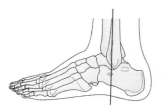

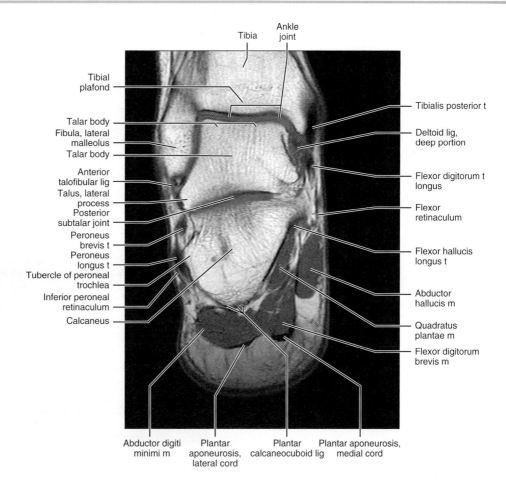

Tibia
Ankle joint
Tibial plafond
Tibialis posterior t
Talar body
Fibula, lateral malleolus
Deltoid lig, deep portion
Talar body
Flexor digitorum t longus
Anterior talofibular lig
Flexor retinaculum
Talus, lateral process
Posterior subtalar joint
Flexor hallucis longus t
Peroneus brevis t
Peroneus longus t
Tubercle of peroneal trochlea
Abductor hallucis m
Inferior peroneal retinaculum
Quadratus plantae m
Calcaneus
Flexor digitorum brevis m

Abductor digiti minimi m
Plantar aponeurosis, lateral cord
Plantar calcaneocuboid lig
Plantar aponeurosis, medial cord

Figure 14.4.10

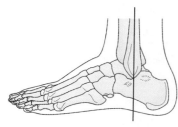

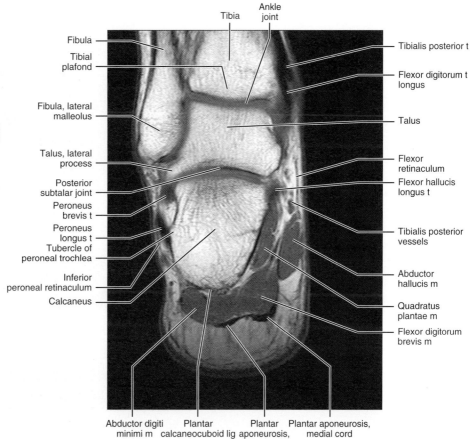

Tibia
Ankle joint
Fibula
Tibialis posterior t
Tibial plafond
Flexor digitorum t longus
Fibula, lateral malleolus
Talus
Talus, lateral process
Flexor retinaculum
Posterior subtalar joint
Flexor hallucis longus t
Peroneus brevis t
Peroneus longus t
Tibialis posterior vessels
Tubercle of peroneal trochlea
Inferior peroneal retinaculum
Abductor hallucis m
Calcaneus
Quadratus plantae m
Flexor digitorum brevis m

Abductor digiti minimi m
Plantar calcaneocuboid lig
Plantar aponeurosis, lateral cord
Plantar aponeurosis, medial cord

Figure 14.4.11

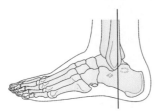

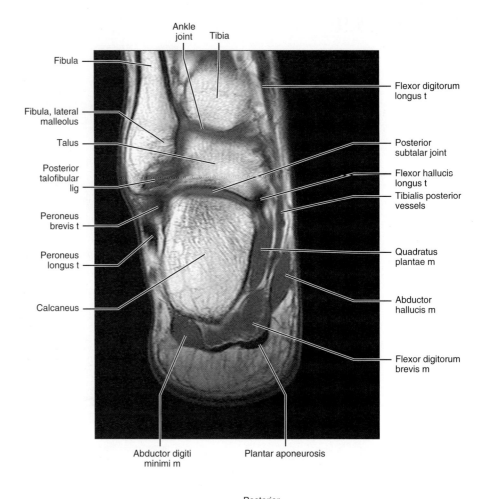

Fibula

Ankle joint

Tibia

Flexor digitorum longus t

Fibula, lateral malleolus

Talus

Posterior talofibular lig

Peroneus brevis t

Peroneus longus t

Calcaneus

Posterior subtalar joint

Flexor hallucis longus t

Tibialis posterior vessels

Quadratus plantae m

Abductor hallucis m

Flexor digitorum brevis m

Abductor digiti minimi m

Plantar aponeurosis

Figure 14.4.12

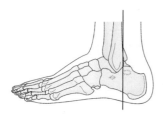

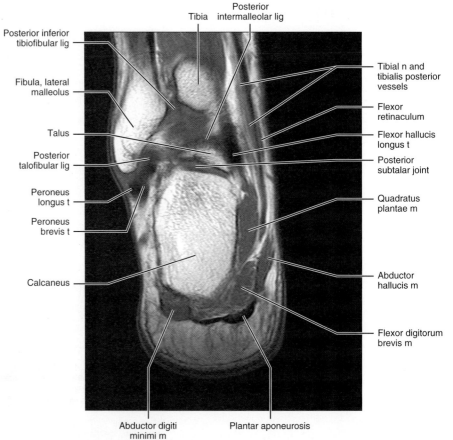

Posterior inferior tibiofibular lig

Tibia

Posterior intermalleolar lig

Fibula, lateral malleolus

Talus

Posterior talofibular lig

Peroneus longus t

Peroneus brevis t

Calcaneus

Tibial n and tibialis posterior vessels

Flexor retinaculum

Flexor hallucis longus t

Posterior subtalar joint

Quadratus plantae m

Abductor hallucis m

Flexor digitorum brevis m

Abductor digiti minimi m

Plantar aponeurosis

Figure 14.4.13

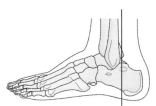

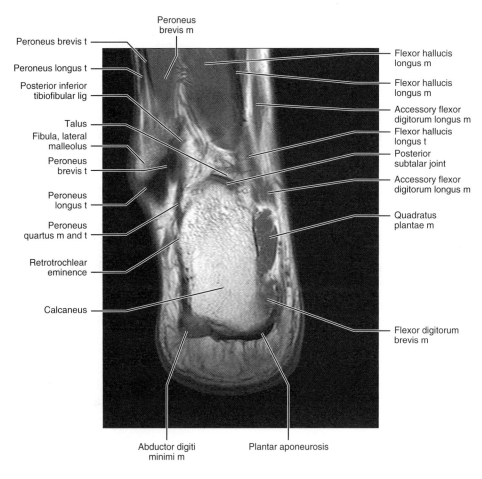

Peroneus brevis m

Peroneus brevis t

Peroneus longus t

Posterior inferior tibiofibular lig

Talus

Fibula, lateral malleolus

Peroneus brevis t

Peroneus longus t

Peroneus quartus m and t

Retrotrochlear eminence

Calcaneus

Flexor hallucis longus m

Flexor hallucis longus m

Accessory flexor digitorum longus m

Flexor hallucis longus t

Posterior subtalar joint

Accessory flexor digitorum longus m

Quadratus plantae m

Flexor digitorum brevis m

Abductor digiti minimi m

Plantar aponeurosis

Figure 14.4.14

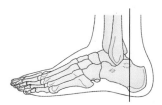

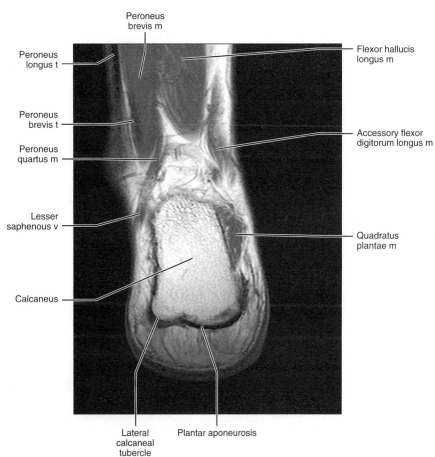

Peroneus brevis m

Peroneus longus t

Peroneus brevis t

Peroneus quartus m

Lesser saphenous v

Calcaneus

Flexor hallucis longus m

Accessory flexor digitorum longus m

Quadratus plantae m

Lateral calcaneal tubercle

Plantar aponeurosis

Figure 14.4.15

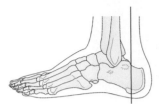

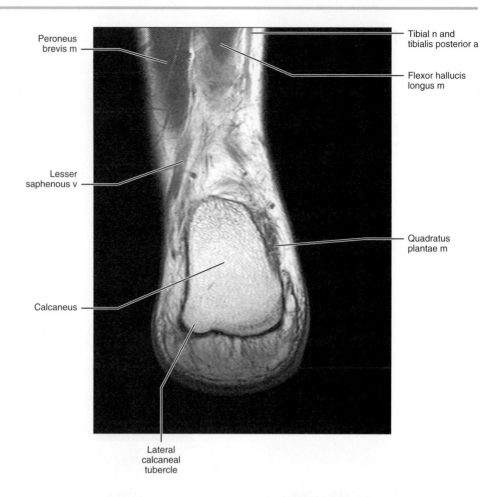

Peroneus brevis m

Tibial n and tibialis posterior a

Flexor hallucis longus m

Lesser saphenous v

Quadratus plantae m

Calcaneus

Lateral calcaneal tubercle

Figure 14.4.16

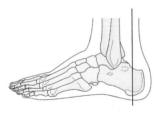

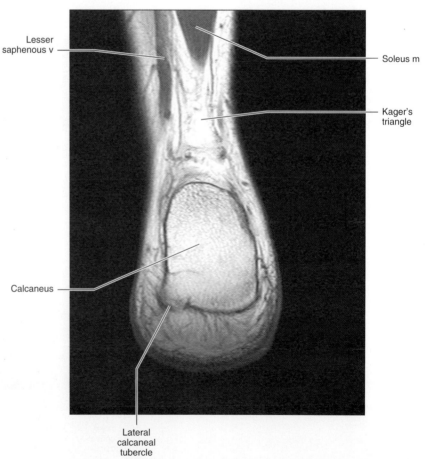

Lesser saphenous v

Soleus m

Kager's triangle

Calcaneus

Lateral calcaneal tubercle

Figure 14.4.17

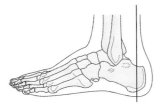

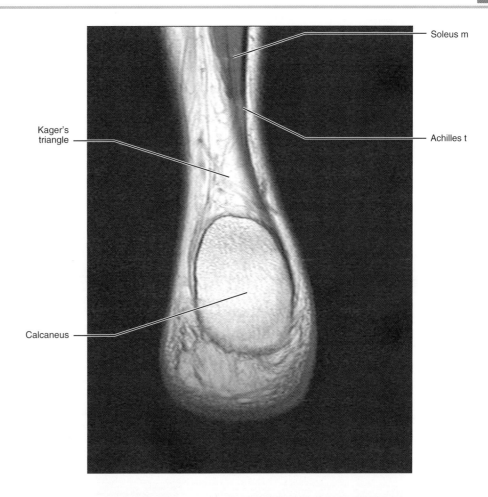

Soleus m

Kager's triangle

Achilles t

Calcaneus

Figure 14.4.18

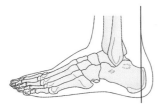

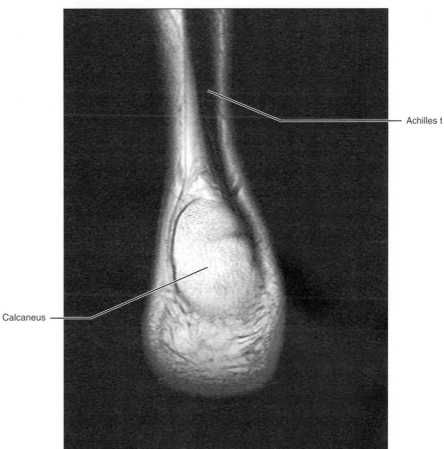

Achilles t

Calcaneus

Chapter 15

MRI of the Foot

Table 8: Muscles of the Foot

MUSCLE	ORIGIN	INSERTION	NERVE SUPPLY
Extensor digitorum brevis	Distal part of the lateral and superior surfaces of the calcaneus and the apex of the inferior extensor retinaculum	As the fiber bundles extend distally, they become grouped into four bellies. Those fibers of the most medial and largest belly are known as extensor hallucis brevis. The tendon of this muscle inserts onto the base of the first metatarsal. The remaining fiber bundles are not so distinctly isolated as described for the great toe, and their insertions are variable. The second toe inserts mainly onto the middle of the back of the base of the proximal phalanx and is often united with the tendon of the long extensor. The remaining three tendons are usually fused with the lateral margins of the corresponding tendons of the long extensor near the bases of the three middle phalanges and usually to the bases of proximal phalanges the of the corresponding toe	Deep peroneal
Flexor digitorum	Medial process of the tuber calcanei, posterior third of the plantar aponeurosis, and medial and lateral intermuscular septa	Tendons of the short (brevis) flexors pass superficial to those of the long flexor into the osteofibrous canals on the flexor surface of the digits. On the proximal phalanx of each toe, the tendon of the short flexor divides and forms an opening through which the tendon of the long flexor passes. The tendons of the short flexor insert onto the base of the middle phalanx	Surface near the medial edge of the muscle
Quadratus plantae (flexor accessorius)	Two heads: a small lateral and a large medial one. (1) Lateral head arises from an elongated tendon from the lateral process of the tuberosity of the calcaneus, and from the lateral margin of the long plantar ligament. (2) Medial head originates from the medial surface of the calcaneus in front of the tuberosity and from adjacent ligaments	The two heads are separated at their origin by a short triangular space. The heads fuse to form a single belly, but the fiber bundles of each head are separately inserted. From the lateral head, the fibers insert into the lateral margin of the flexor tendon. The medial head inserts as an aponeurosis into the deep surface of the flexor tendon	Lateral plantar nerve branch that passes obliquely across the superficial surface of the muscle, parallel with the tendon of the flexor digitorum longus

Table 8: Muscles of the Foot—Cont'd

MUSCLE	ORIGIN	INSERTION	NERVE SUPPLY
Lumbricals	Three lateral lumbricals arise from the adjacent sides of the digital tendons of the flexor digitorum longus. The first lumbrical arises on the medial margin of the second toe	Fiber bundles of each muscle converge on both sides of a tendon that becomes free near the metatarsophalangeal joint and is inserted onto the medial side of the proximal phalanx of the appropriate toe. A tendinous expansion is inserted into the aponeurosis of the extensor muscle	Three lateral lumbricals are usually supplied by branches of the deep ramus of the lateral plantar nerve. Medial lumbrical is supplied by the first common plantar digital branch of the medial plantar nerve. This nerve may supply the two more medial muscles, or the medial muscles may receive a double nerve supply
Abductor hallucis	Medial border of the medial process of the tuber calcanei, flexor retinaculum, and plantar aponeurosis	Along with the tendon of the medial belly of flexor brevis onto the base of the proximal phalanx of the great toe	Branch of the medial plantar
Flexor hallucis brevis	From the plantar surface of the lateral cuneiform and cuboid bones	The medial and lateral sides of the base of the proximal phalanx of the great toe	Branch from the medial plantar or first plantar digital. Rarely, the lateral body may receive a branch from the lateral plantar
Adductor hallucis, oblique head	Tuberosity of the cuboid and sheath of the tendon of the peroneus longus, the plantar calcaneocuboid ligament, the third cuneiform, bases of the second and third metatarsals	By a flat tendon that inserts in common with that of the flexor brevis onto the lateral part of the plantar surface of the base of the proximal phalanx, and by a slip into the aponeurosis of the long extensor muscle on the back of the great toe	Branch of the deep ramus of the lateral plantar
Adductor hallucis, transverse head	Joint capsules of the third, fourth, and fifth metatarsophalangeal joints and the deep transverse metatarsal ligaments	By a common tendon that splits and passes on each side of the tendon of the oblique head and is inserted into the sheath on the tendon of the long flexor of the great toe	Branch from the deep ramus of the lateral plantar
Abductor digiti minimi	Lateral and medial processes of the tuber calcanei and lateral and plantar surfaces of the body of the bone in front of these, lateral intermuscular septum, deep surface of the lateral plantar fascia, and fibrous band extending from the calcaneus to the lateral side of the base of the fifth metatarsal	Onto the lateral surface of the proximal phalanx of the little toe and the metatarsophalangeal capsule	Lateral plantar

Continued

Table 8: Muscles of the Foot—Cont'd

MUSCLE	ORIGIN	INSERTION	NERVE SUPPLY
Flexor digiti minimi brevis	Sheath of the peroneus longus, tuberosity of the cuboid, and base of the fifth metatarsal	By short tendinous bands onto the base of the proximal phalanx of the little toe, the capsule of the corresponding joint, and the aponeurosis on the dorsal surface of the toe	Branch from the superficial ramus of the lateral plantar
Opponens digiti minimi	An inconstant muscle, it may arise from the sheath of the peroneus longus and the tuberosity of the cuboid by a thin tendon that passes over the tuberosity of the fifth metatarsal	Onto the lateral surface of the fifth metatarsal	Branch from the nerve to the flexor brevis and the superficial ramus of the lateral plantar
Interosseous, dorsal	Each of the three lateral dorsal interosseous muscles arises from the sides of the shaft and the plantar surface of the bases of the metatarsals, bounding the space in which each lies, from the fascia covering it dorsally, and from the fibrous prolongations from the long plantar ligament. The first (medial) has a similar origin, except that its medial origin is by a tendinous slip from the peroneus longus tendon and, occasionally, by fiber bundles from the medial side of the proximal end of the first metatarsal	The first and second interosseous muscles onto each side of the base of the proximal phalanx of the second toe; the third and fourth onto the lateral side of the bases of the proximal phalanges of the third and fourth toes. Each tendon adheres to the capsule of the adjacent joint	Deep branch of the lateral plantar. The interosseous muscles of the fourth interspace are usually supplied by a branch from the superficial ramus of the lateral plantar
Interosseous, plantar	The plantar interosseous muscle arises from the proximal third of the medial plantar surface of the shaft, from the base of the metatarsal on which it lies, and from the fascial expansions of the long plantar ligament	Onto a tubercle on the medial side of the base of the proximal phalanx of the digit to which it goes	Lateral plantar

AXIAL

Figure 15.1.1

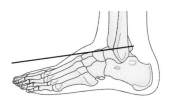

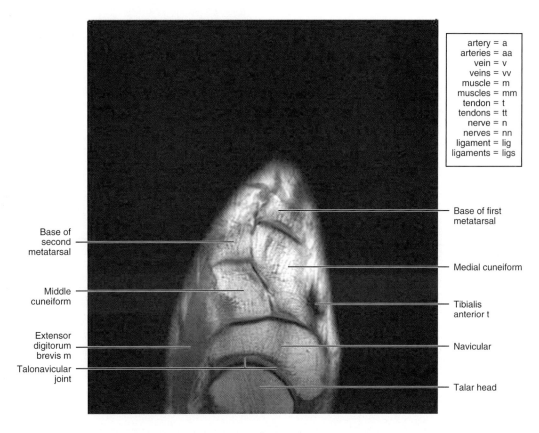

artery	= a
arteries	= aa
vein	= v
veins	= vv
muscle	= m
muscles	= mm
tendon	= t
tendons	= tt
nerve	= n
nerves	= nn
ligament	= lig
ligaments	= ligs

Base of second metatarsal

Middle cuneiform

Extensor digitorum brevis m

Talonavicular joint

Base of first metatarsal

Medial cuneiform

Tibialis anterior t

Navicular

Talar head

Figure 15.1.2

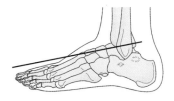

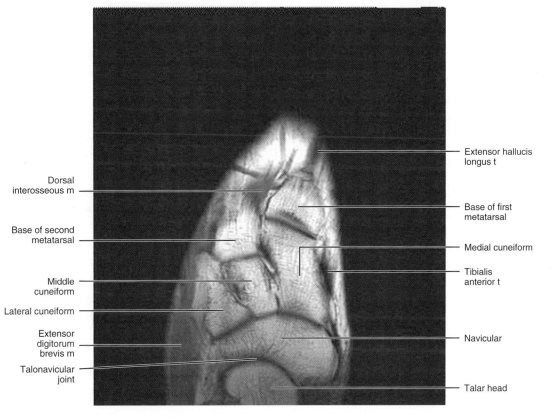

Dorsal interosseous m

Base of second metatarsal

Middle cuneiform

Lateral cuneiform

Extensor digitorum brevis m

Talonavicular joint

Extensor hallucis longus t

Base of first metatarsal

Medial cuneiform

Tibialis anterior t

Navicular

Talar head

Figure 15.1.3

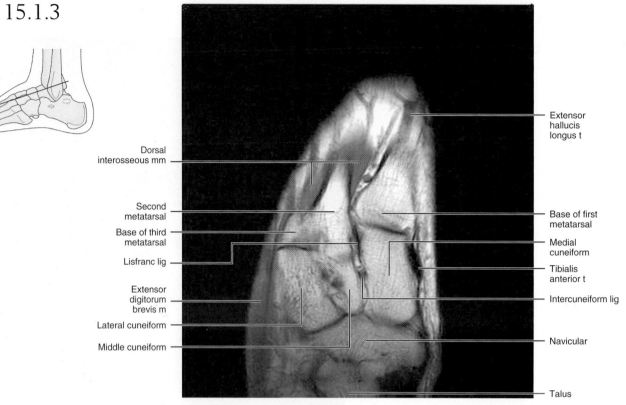

Extensor hallucis longus t

Dorsal interosseous mm

Second metatarsal

Base of first metatarsal

Base of third metatarsal

Medial cuneiform

Lisfranc lig

Tibialis anterior t

Extensor digitorum brevis m

Intercuneiform lig

Lateral cuneiform

Middle cuneiform

Navicular

Talus

Figure 15.1.4

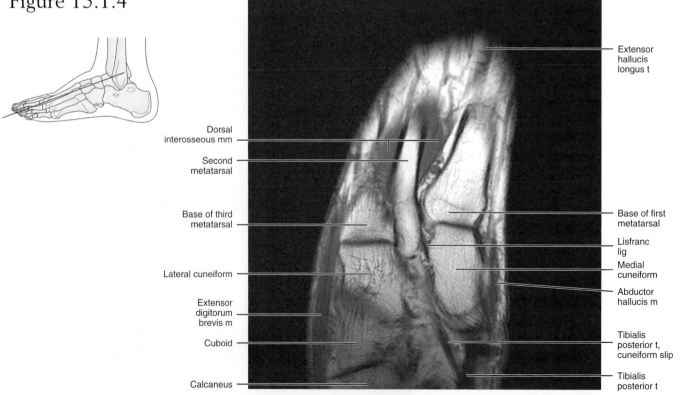

Extensor hallucis longus t

Dorsal interosseous mm

Second metatarsal

Base of third metatarsal

Base of first metatarsal

Lisfranc lig

Medial cuneiform

Lateral cuneiform

Abductor hallucis m

Extensor digitorum brevis m

Cuboid

Tibialis posterior t, cuneiform slip

Calcaneus

Tibialis posterior t

Figure 15.1.5

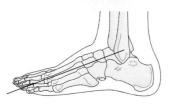

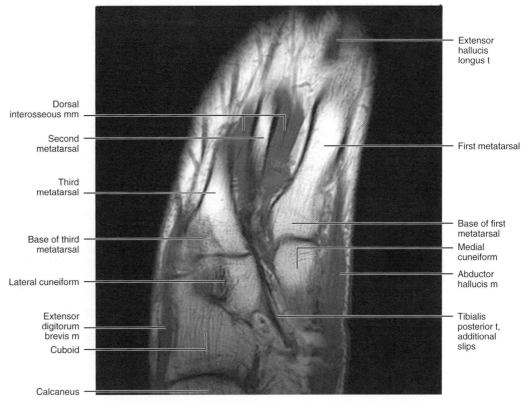

Dorsal interosseous mm

Second metatarsal

Third metatarsal

Base of third metatarsal

Lateral cuneiform

Extensor digitorum brevis m

Cuboid

Calcaneus

Extensor hallucis longus t

First metatarsal

Base of first metatarsal

Medial cuneiform

Abductor hallucis m

Tibialis posterior t, additional slips

Figure 15.1.6

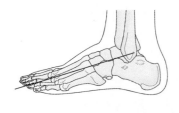

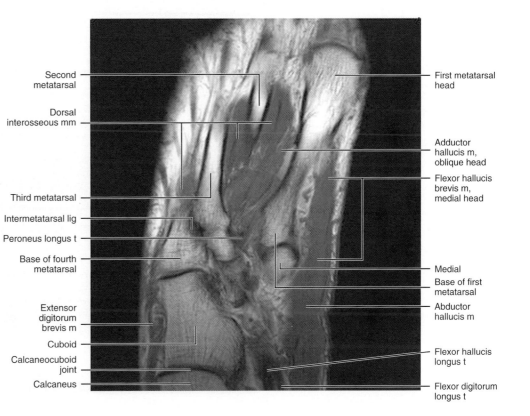

Second metatarsal

Dorsal interosseous mm

Third metatarsal

Intermetatarsal lig

Peroneus longus t

Base of fourth metatarsal

Extensor digitorum brevis m

Cuboid

Calcaneocuboid joint

Calcaneus

First metatarsal head

Adductor hallucis m, oblique head

Flexor hallucis brevis m, medial head

Medial

Base of first metatarsal

Abductor hallucis m

Flexor hallucis longus t

Flexor digitorum longus t

Figure 15.1.7

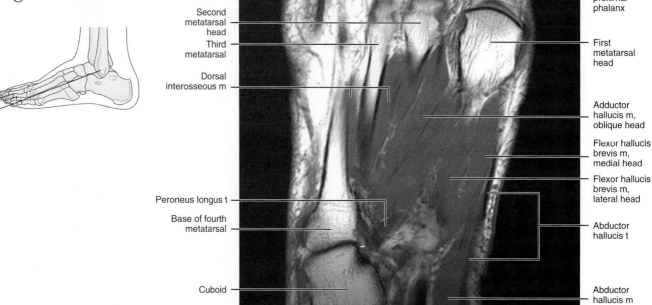

Second metatarsal head
Third metatarsal
Dorsal interosseous m
Peroneus longus t
Base of fourth metatarsal
Cuboid
Calcaneocuboid joint
Calcaneus

Great toe, proximal phalanx
First metatarsal head
Adductor hallucis m, oblique head
Flexor hallucis brevis m, medial head
Flexor hallucis brevis m, lateral head
Abductor hallucis t
Abductor hallucis m
Flexor hallucis longus t

Figure 15.1.8

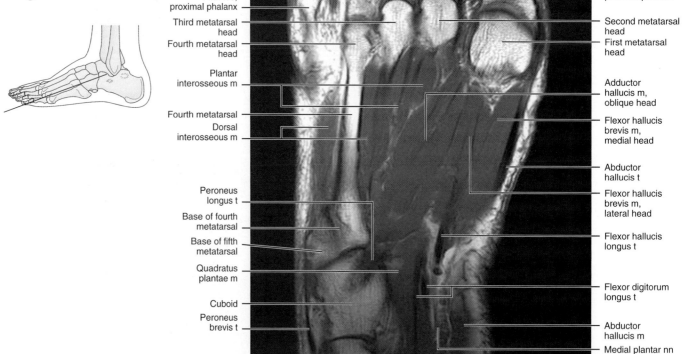

Fifth toe, proximal phalanx
Third metatarsal head
Fourth metatarsal head
Plantar interosseous m
Fourth metatarsal
Dorsal interosseous m
Peroneus longus t
Base of fourth metatarsal
Base of fifth metatarsal
Quadratus plantae m
Cuboid
Peroneus brevis t
Calcaneus

Great toe, proximal phalanx
Second metatarsal head
First metatarsal head
Adductor hallucis m, oblique head
Flexor hallucis brevis m, medial head
Abductor hallucis t
Flexor hallucis brevis m, lateral head
Flexor hallucis longus t
Flexor digitorum longus t
Abductor hallucis m
Medial plantar nn and vessels

Figure 15.1.9

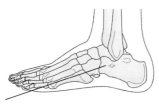

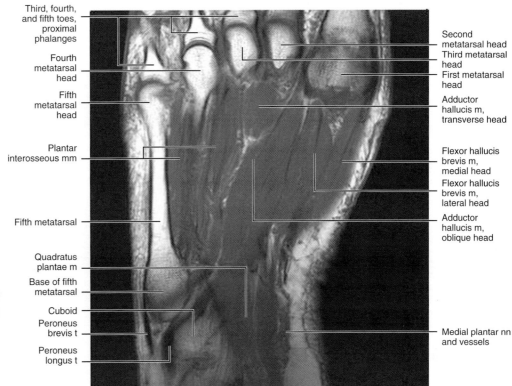

Third, fourth, and fifth toes, proximal phalanges

Fourth metatarsal head

Fifth metatarsal head

Plantar interosseous mm

Fifth metatarsal

Quadratus plantae m

Base of fifth metatarsal

Cuboid

Peroneus brevis t

Peroneus longus t

Second metatarsal head

Third metatarsal head

First metatarsal head

Adductor hallucis m, transverse head

Flexor hallucis brevis m, medial head

Flexor hallucis brevis m, lateral head

Adductor hallucis m, oblique head

Medial plantar nn and vessels

Figure 15.1.10

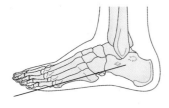

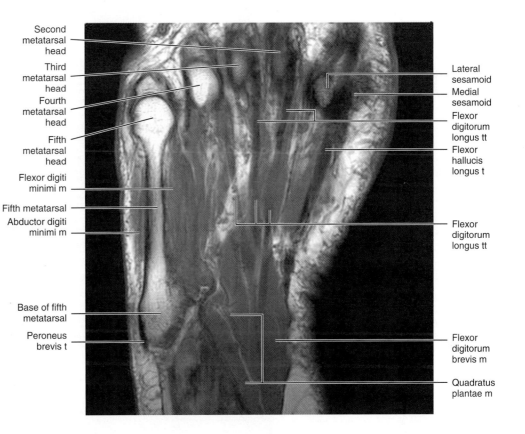

Second metatarsal head

Third metatarsal head

Fourth metatarsal head

Fifth metatarsal head

Flexor digiti minimi m

Fifth metatarsal

Abductor digiti minimi m

Base of fifth metatarsal

Peroneus brevis t

Lateral sesamoid

Medial sesamoid

Flexor digitorum longus tt

Flexor hallucis longus t

Flexor digitorum longus tt

Flexor digitorum brevis m

Quadratus plantae m

Figure 15.1.11

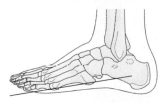

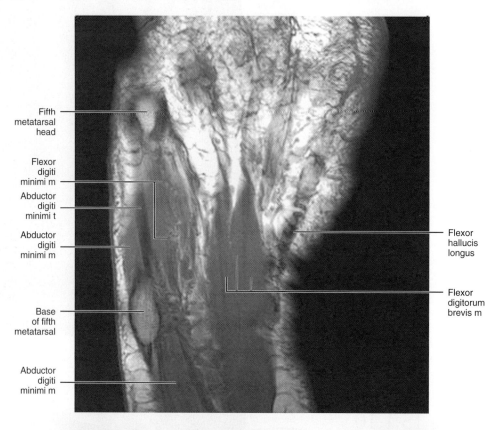

Fifth metatarsal head

Flexor digiti minimi m

Abductor digiti minimi t

Abductor digiti minimi m

Base of fifth metatarsal

Abductor digiti minimi m

Flexor hallucis longus

Flexor digitorum brevis m

Figure 15.1.12

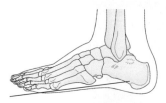

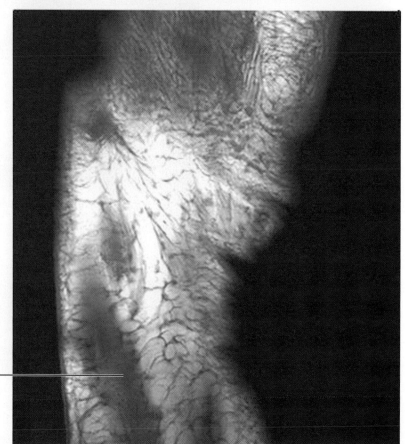

Abductor digiti minimi m

SAGITTAL
Figure 15.2.1

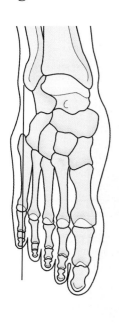

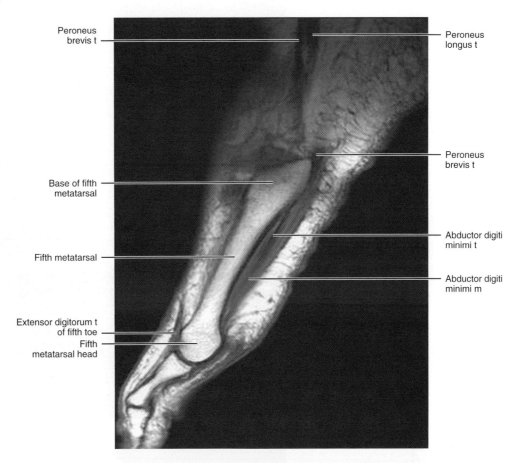

Peroneus brevis t

Peroneus longus t

Base of fifth metatarsal

Peroneus brevis t

Fifth metatarsal

Abductor digiti minimi t

Abductor digiti minimi m

Extensor digitorum t of fifth toe

Fifth metatarsal head

Figure 15.2.2

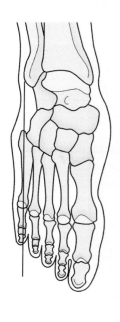

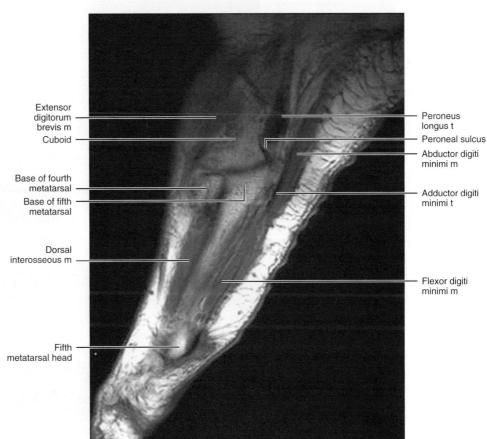

Extensor digitorum brevis m

Cuboid

Base of fourth metatarsal

Base of fifth metatarsal

Dorsal interosseous m

Fifth metatarsal head

Peroneus longus t

Peroneal sulcus

Abductor digiti minimi m

Adductor digiti minimi t

Flexor digiti minimi m

Figure 15.2.3

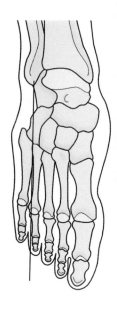

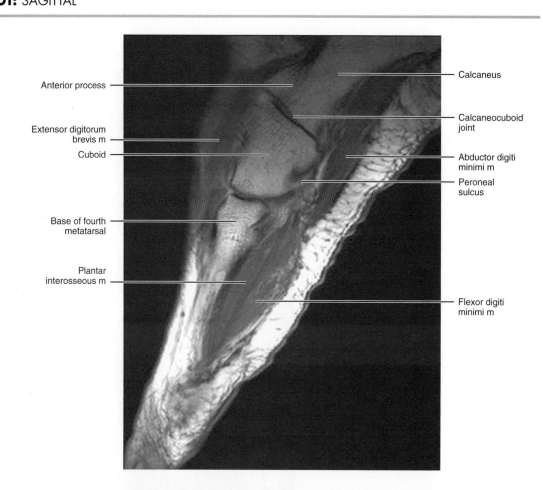

Anterior process

Extensor digitorum brevis m

Cuboid

Base of fourth metatarsal

Plantar interosseous m

Calcaneus

Calcaneocuboid joint

Abductor digiti minimi m

Peroneal sulcus

Flexor digiti minimi m

Figure 15.2.4

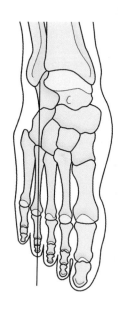

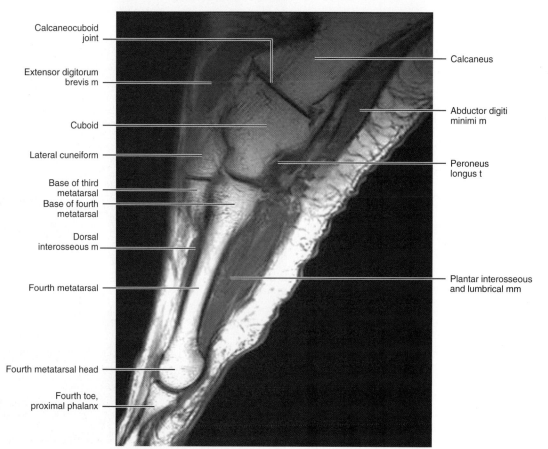

Calcaneocuboid joint

Extensor digitorum brevis m

Cuboid

Lateral cuneiform

Base of third metatarsal

Base of fourth metatarsal

Dorsal interosseous m

Fourth metatarsal

Fourth metatarsal head

Fourth toe, proximal phalanx

Calcaneus

Abductor digiti minimi m

Peroneus longus t

Plantar interosseous and lumbrical mm

Figure 15.2.5

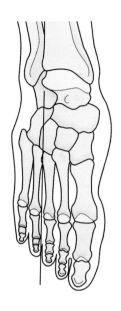

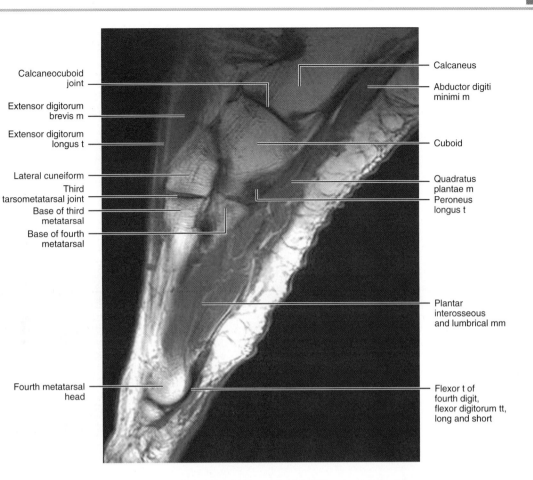

Calcaneocuboid joint

Extensor digitorum brevis m

Extensor digitorum longus t

Lateral cuneiform

Third tarsometatarsal joint

Base of third metatarsal

Base of fourth metatarsal

Fourth metatarsal head

Calcaneus

Abductor digiti minimi m

Cuboid

Quadratus plantae m

Peroneus longus t

Plantar interosseous and lumbrical mm

Flexor t of fourth digit, flexor digitorum tt, long and short

Figure 15.2.6

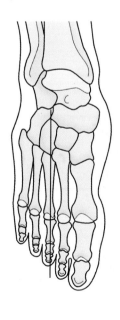

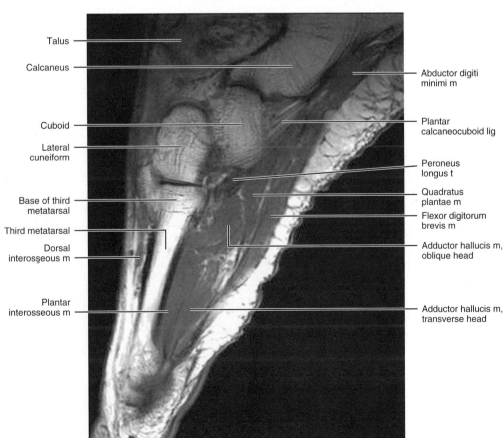

Talus

Calcaneus

Cuboid

Lateral cuneiform

Base of third metatarsal

Third metatarsal

Dorsal interosseous m

Plantar interosseous m

Abductor digiti minimi m

Plantar calcaneocuboid lig

Peroneus longus t

Quadratus plantae m

Flexor digitorum brevis m

Adductor hallucis m, oblique head

Adductor hallucis m, transverse head

Figure 15.2.7

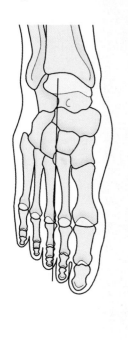

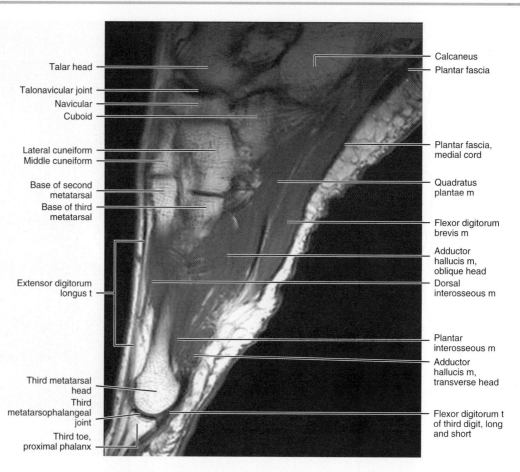

Talar head

Talonavicular joint

Navicular

Cuboid

Lateral cuneiform

Middle cuneiform

Base of second metatarsal

Base of third metatarsal

Extensor digitorum longus t

Third metatarsal head

Third metatarsophalangeal joint

Third toe, proximal phalanx

Calcaneus

Plantar fascia

Plantar fascia, medial cord

Quadratus plantae m

Flexor digitorum brevis m

Adductor hallucis m, oblique head

Dorsal interosseous m

Plantar interosseous m

Adductor hallucis m, transverse head

Flexor digitorum t of third digit, long and short

Figure 15.2.8

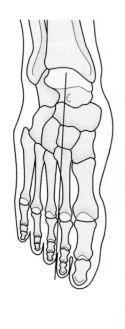

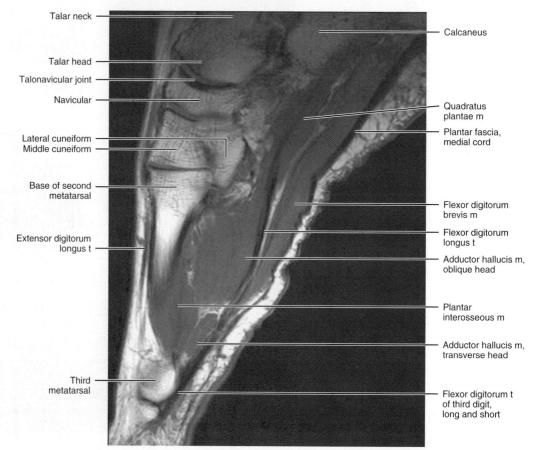

Talar neck

Talar head

Talonavicular joint

Navicular

Lateral cuneiform

Middle cuneiform

Base of second metatarsal

Extensor digitorum longus t

Third metatarsal

Calcaneus

Quadratus plantae m

Plantar fascia, medial cord

Flexor digitorum brevis m

Flexor digitorum longus t

Adductor hallucis m, oblique head

Plantar interosseous m

Adductor hallucis m, transverse head

Flexor digitorum t of third digit, long and short

Figure 15.2.9

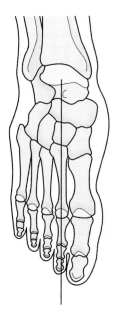

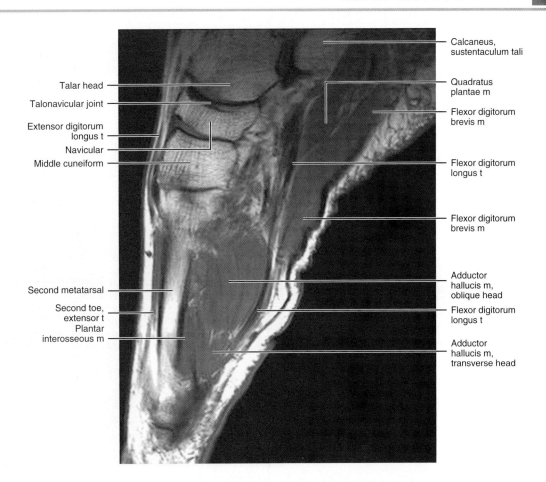

Talar head
Talonavicular joint
Extensor digitorum longus t
Navicular
Middle cuneiform

Second metatarsal
Second toe, extensor t
Plantar interosseous m

Calcaneus, sustentaculum tali
Quadratus plantae m
Flexor digitorum brevis m
Flexor digitorum longus t
Flexor digitorum brevis m
Adductor hallucis m, oblique head
Flexor digitorum longus t
Adductor hallucis m, transverse head

Figure 15.2.10

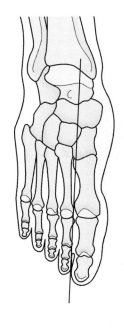

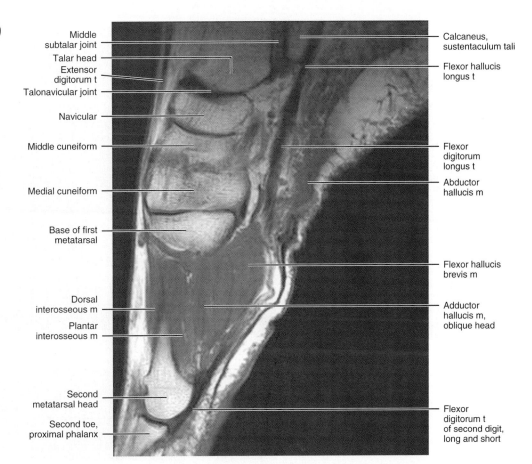

Middle subtalar joint
Talar head
Extensor digitorum t
Talonavicular joint
Navicular
Middle cuneiform
Medial cuneiform
Base of first metatarsal
Dorsal interosseous m
Plantar interosseous m
Second metatarsal head
Second toe, proximal phalanx

Calcaneus, sustentaculum tali
Flexor hallucis longus t
Flexor digitorum longus t
Abductor hallucis m
Flexor hallucis brevis m
Adductor hallucis m, oblique head
Flexor digitorum t of second digit, long and short

Figure 15.2.11

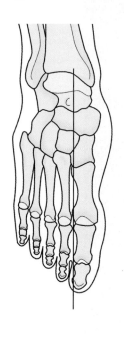

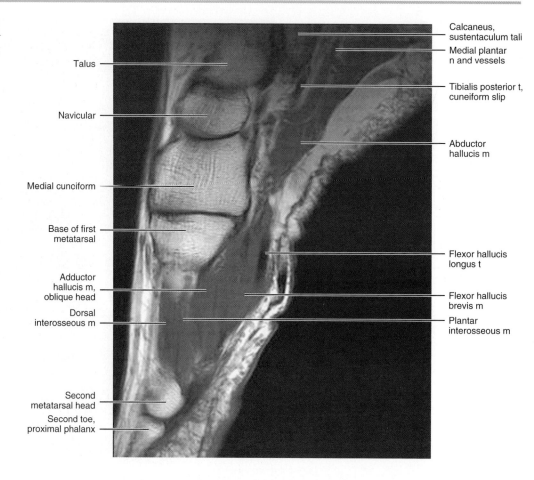

Talus

Navicular

Medial cuneiform

Base of first
metatarsal

Adductor
hallucis m,
oblique head

Dorsal
interosseous m

Second
metatarsal head

Second toe,
proximal phalanx

Calcaneus,
sustentaculum tali

Medial plantar
n and vessels

Tibialis posterior t,
cuneiform slip

Abductor
hallucis m

Flexor hallucis
longus t

Flexor hallucis
brevis m

Plantar
interosseous m

Figure 15.2.12

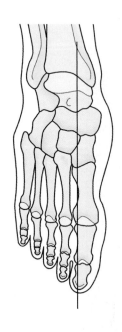

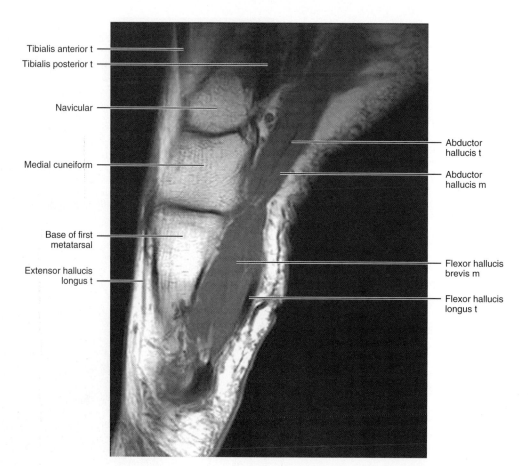

Tibialis anterior t

Tibialis posterior t

Navicular

Medial cuneiform

Base of first
metatarsal

Extensor hallucis
longus t

Abductor
hallucis t

Abductor
hallucis m

Flexor hallucis
brevis m

Flexor hallucis
longus t

Figure 15.2.13

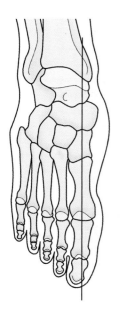

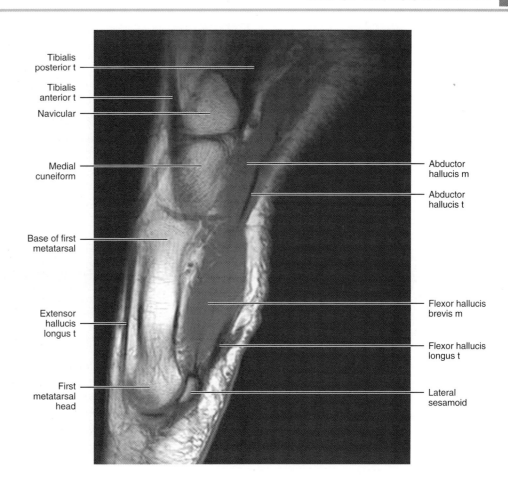

Tibialis posterior t

Tibialis anterior t

Navicular

Medial cuneiform

Base of first metatarsal

Extensor hallucis longus t

First metatarsal head

Abductor hallucis m

Abductor hallucis t

Flexor hallucis brevis m

Flexor hallucis longus t

Lateral sesamoid

Figure 15.2.14

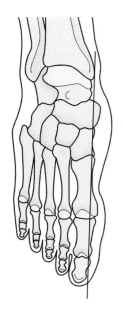

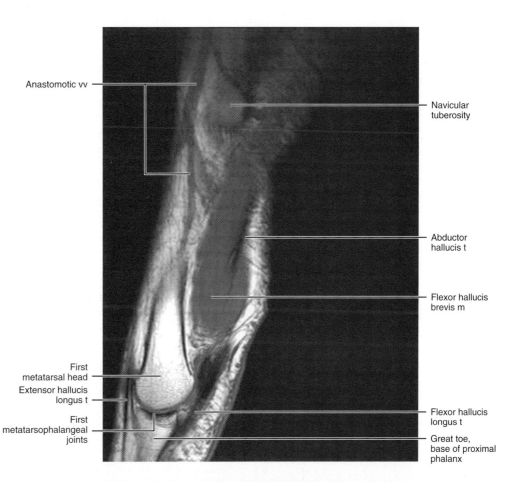

Anastomotic vv

First metatarsal head

Extensor hallucis longus t

First metatarsophalangeal joints

Navicular tuberosity

Abductor hallucis t

Flexor hallucis brevis m

Flexor hallucis longus t

Great toe, base of proximal phalanx

Figure 15.2.15

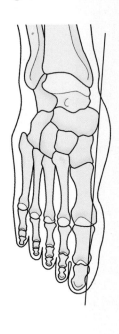

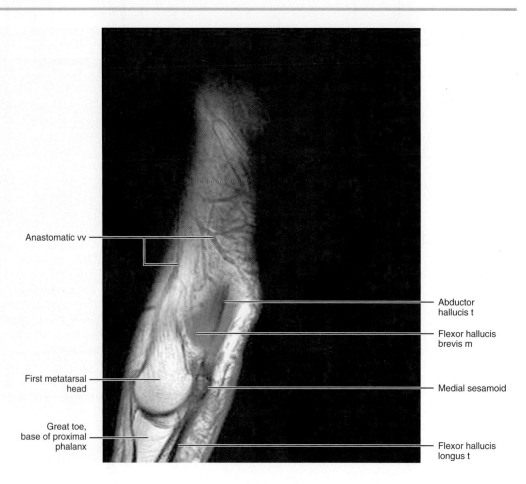

Anastomatic vv

First metatarsal head

Great toe, base of proximal phalanx

Abductor hallucis t

Flexor hallucis brevis m

Medial sesamoid

Flexor hallucis longus t

CORONAL
Figure 15.3.1

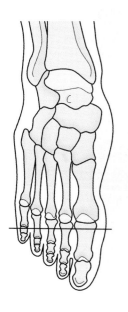

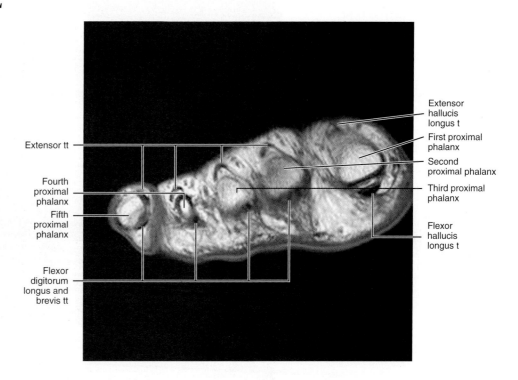

Extensor tt

Fourth
proximal
phalanx

Fifth
proximal
phalanx

Flexor
digitorum
longus and
brevis tt

Extensor
hallucis
longus t

First proximal
phalanx

Second
proximal phalanx

Third proximal
phalanx

Flexor
hallucis
longus t

Figure 15.3.2

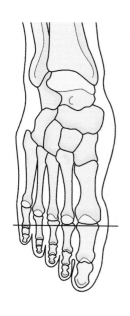

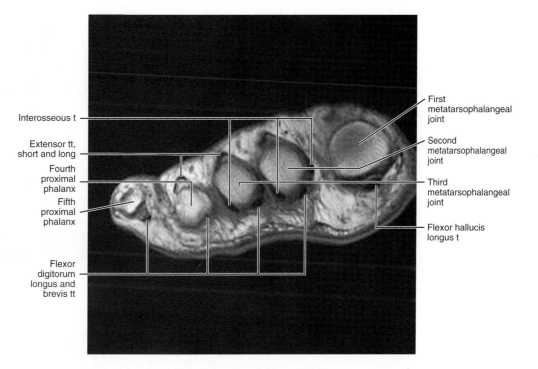

Interosseous t

Extensor tt,
short and long

Fourth
proximal
phalanx

Fifth
proximal
phalanx

Flexor
digitorum
longus and
brevis tt

First
metatarsophalangeal
joint

Second
metatarsophalangeal
joint

Third
metatarsophalangeal
joint

Flexor hallucis
longus t

Figure 15.3.3

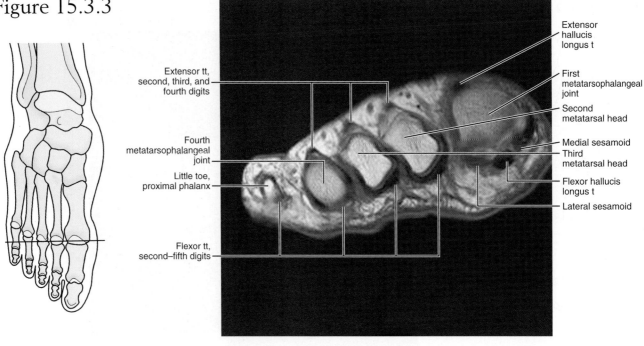

Extensor tt, second, third, and fourth digits

Extensor hallucis longus t

First metatarsophalangeal joint

Second metatarsal head

Fourth metatarsophalangeal joint

Medial sesamoid

Third metatarsal head

Little toe, proximal phalanx

Flexor hallucis longus t

Lateral sesamoid

Flexor tt, second–fifth digits

Figure 15.3.4

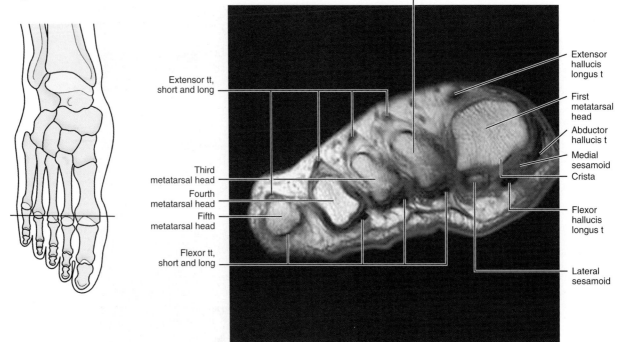

Second metatarsal head

Extensor tt, short and long

Extensor hallucis longus t

First metatarsal head

Abductor hallucis t

Medial sesamoid

Crista

Third metatarsal head

Fourth metatarsal head

Fifth metatarsal head

Flexor hallucis longus t

Flexor tt, short and long

Lateral sesamoid

Figure 15.3.5

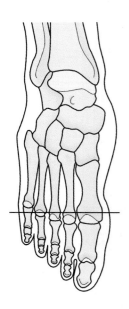

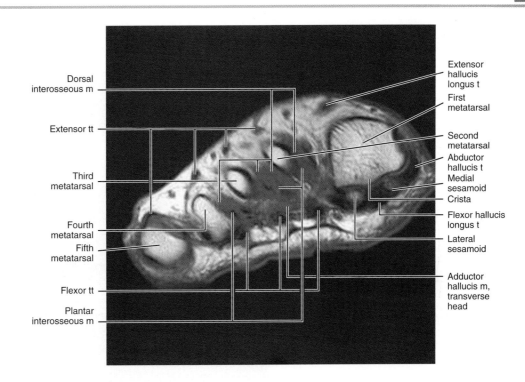

Dorsal interosseous m

Extensor tt

Third metatarsal

Fourth metatarsal

Fifth metatarsal

Flexor tt

Plantar interosseous m

Extensor hallucis longus t

First metatarsal

Second metatarsal

Abductor hallucis t

Medial sesamoid

Crista

Flexor hallucis longus t

Lateral sesamoid

Adductor hallucis m, transverse head

Figure 15.3.6

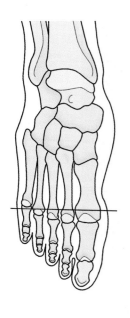

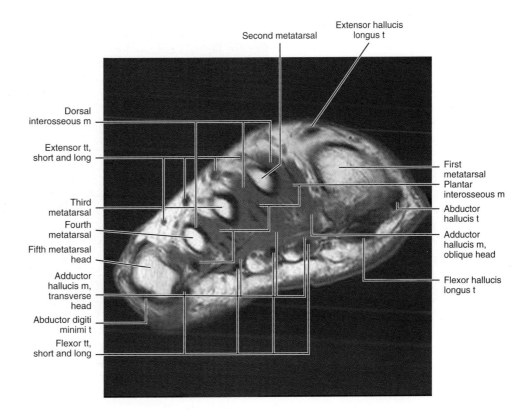

Second metatarsal

Extensor hallucis longus t

Dorsal interosseous m

Extensor tt, short and long

Third metatarsal

Fourth metatarsal

Fifth metatarsal head

Adductor hallucis m, transverse head

Abductor digiti minimi t

Flexor tt, short and long

First metatarsal

Plantar interosseous m

Abductor hallucis t

Adductor hallucis m, oblique head

Flexor hallucis longus t

Figure 15.3.7

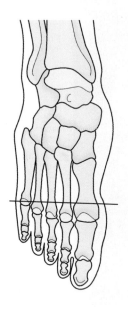

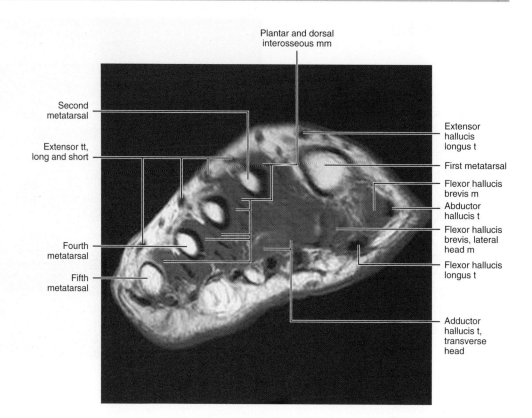

Plantar and dorsal
interosseous mm

Second
metatarsal

Extensor tt,
long and short

Fourth
metatarsal

Fifth
metatarsal

Extensor
hallucis
longus t

First metatarsal

Flexor hallucis
brevis m

Abductor
hallucis t

Flexor hallucis
brevis, lateral
head m

Flexor hallucis
longus t

Adductor
hallucis t,
transverse
head

Figure 15.3.8

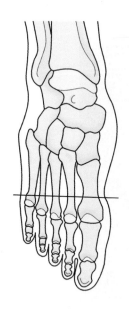

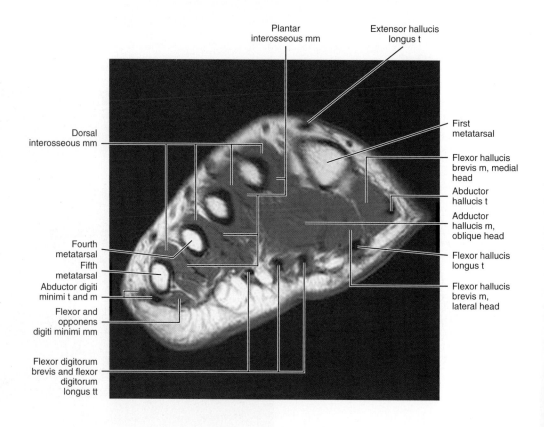

Plantar
interosseous mm

Extensor hallucis
longus t

Dorsal
interosseous mm

Fourth
metatarsal

Fifth
metatarsal

Abductor digiti
minimi t and m

Flexor and
opponens
digiti minimi mm

Flexor digitorum
brevis and flexor
digitorum
longus tt

First
metatarsal

Flexor hallucis
brevis m, medial
head

Abductor
hallucis t

Adductor
hallucis m,
oblique head

Flexor hallucis
longus t

Flexor hallucis
brevis m,
lateral head

Figure 15.3.9

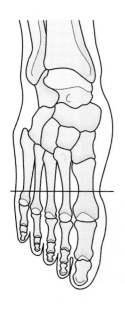

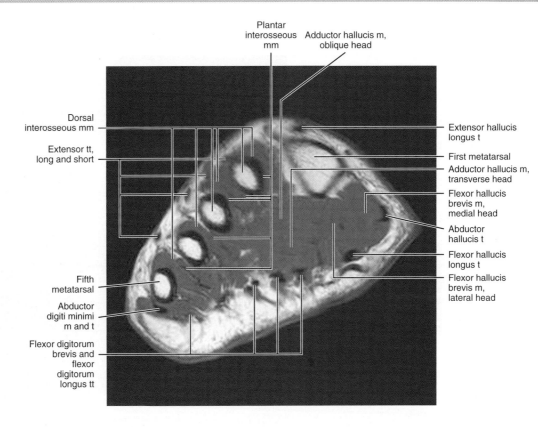

Plantar
interosseous
mm

Adductor hallucis m,
oblique head

Dorsal
interosseous mm

Extensor tt,
long and short

Fifth
metatarsal

Abductor
digiti minimi
m and t

Flexor digitorum
brevis and
flexor
digitorum
longus tt

Extensor hallucis
longus t

First metatarsal

Adductor hallucis m,
transverse head

Flexor hallucis
brevis m,
medial head

Abductor
hallucis t

Flexor hallucis
longus t

Flexor hallucis
brevis m,
lateral head

Figure 15.3.10

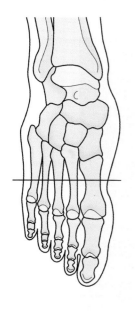

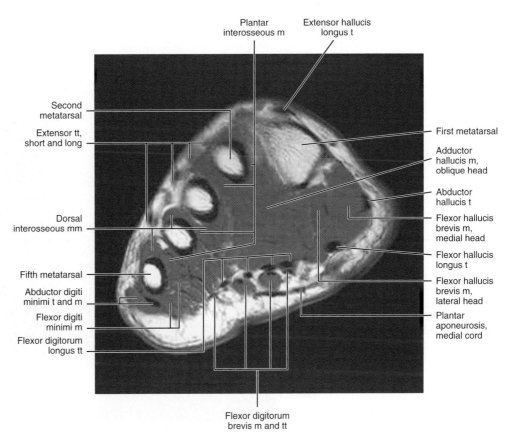

Plantar
interosseous m

Extensor hallucis
longus t

Second
metatarsal

Extensor tt,
short and long

Dorsal
interosseous mm

Fifth metatarsal

Abductor digiti
minimi t and m

Flexor digiti
minimi m

Flexor digitorum
longus tt

First metatarsal

Adductor
hallucis m,
oblique head

Abductor
hallucis t

Flexor hallucis
brevis m,
medial head

Flexor hallucis
longus t

Flexor hallucis
brevis m,
lateral head

Plantar
aponeurosis,
medial cord

Flexor digitorum
brevis m and tt

Figure 15.3.11

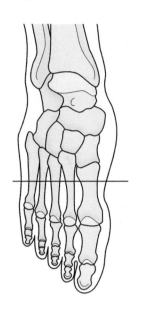

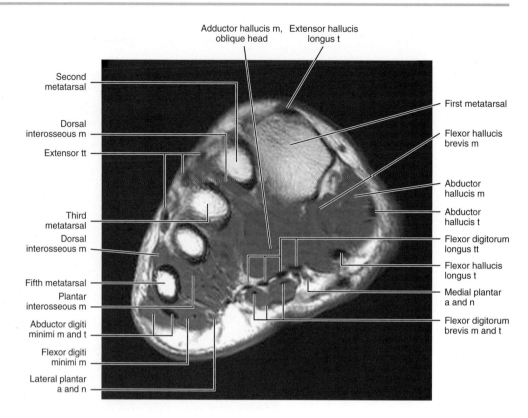

Adductor hallucis m, oblique head

Extensor hallucis longus t

Second metatarsal

Dorsal interosseous m

Extensor tt

Third metatarsal

Dorsal interosseous m

Fifth metatarsal

Plantar interosseous m

Abductor digiti minimi m and t

Flexor digiti minimi m

Lateral plantar a and n

First metatarsal

Flexor hallucis brevis m

Abductor hallucis m

Abductor hallucis t

Flexor digitorum longus tt

Flexor hallucis longus t

Medial plantar a and n

Flexor digitorum brevis m and t

Figure 15.3.12

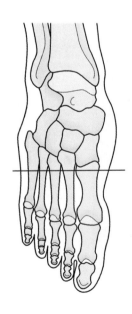

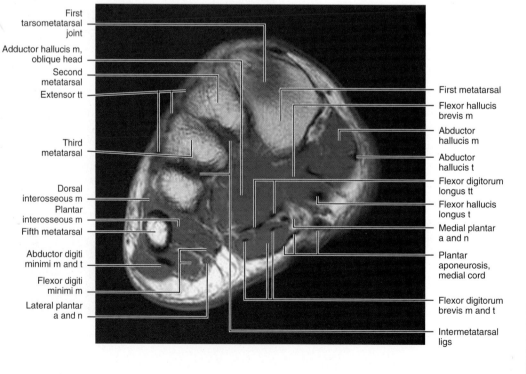

First tarsometatarsal joint

Adductor hallucis m, oblique head

Second metatarsal

Extensor tt

Third metatarsal

Dorsal interosseous m

Plantar interosseous m

Fifth metatarsal

Abductor digiti minimi m and t

Flexor digiti minimi m

Lateral plantar a and n

First metatarsal

Flexor hallucis brevis m

Abductor hallucis m

Abductor hallucis t

Flexor digitorum longus tt

Flexor hallucis longus t

Medial plantar a and n

Plantar aponeurosis, medial cord

Flexor digitorum brevis m and t

Intermetatarsal ligs

Figure 15.3.13

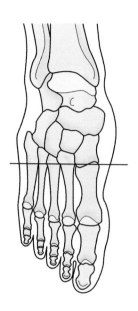

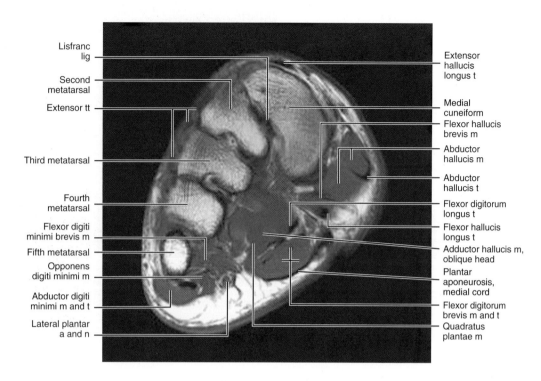

Lisfranc lig
Second metatarsal
Extensor tt
Third metatarsal
Fourth metatarsal
Flexor digiti minimi brevis m
Fifth metatarsal
Opponens digiti minimi m
Abductor digiti minimi m and t
Lateral plantar a and n

Extensor hallucis longus t
Medial cuneiform
Flexor hallucis brevis m
Abductor hallucis m
Abductor hallucis t
Flexor digitorum longus t
Flexor hallucis longus t
Adductor hallucis m, oblique head
Plantar aponeurosis, medial cord
Flexor digitorum brevis m and t
Quadratus plantae m

Figure 15.3.14

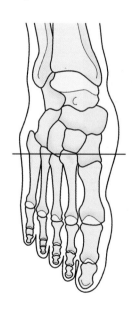

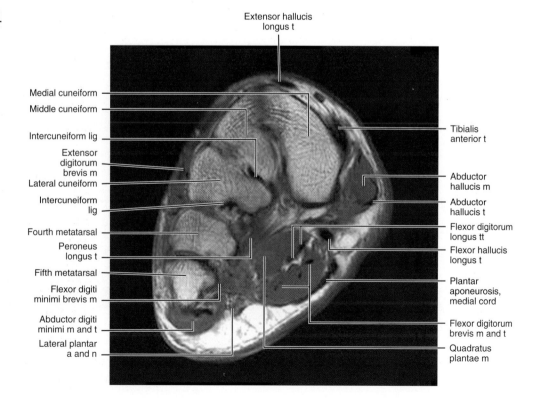

Extensor hallucis longus t

Medial cuneiform
Middle cuneiform
Intercuneiform lig
Extensor digitorum brevis m
Lateral cuneiform
Intercuneiform lig
Fourth metatarsal
Peroneus longus t
Fifth metatarsal
Flexor digiti minimi brevis m
Abductor digiti minimi m and t
Lateral plantar a and n

Tibialis anterior t
Abductor hallucis m
Abductor hallucis t
Flexor digitorum longus tt
Flexor hallucis longus t
Plantar aponeurosis, medial cord
Flexor digitorum brevis m and t
Quadratus plantae m

Figure 15.3.15

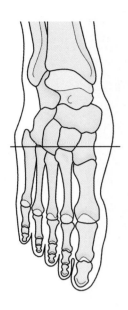

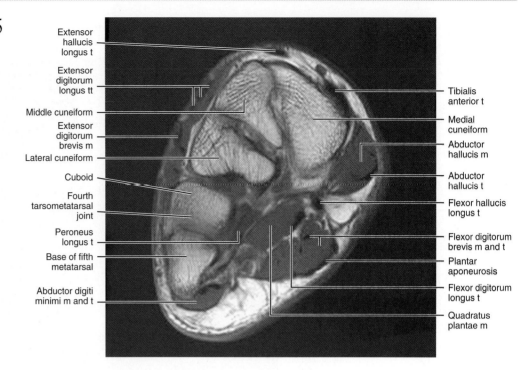

Extensor hallucis longus t
Extensor digitorum longus tt
Middle cuneiform
Extensor digitorum brevis m
Lateral cuneiform
Cuboid
Fourth tarsometatarsal joint
Peroneus longus t
Base of fifth metatarsal
Abductor digiti minimi m and t

Tibialis anterior t
Medial cuneiform
Abductor hallucis m
Abductor hallucis t
Flexor hallucis longus t
Flexor digitorum brevis m and t
Plantar aponeurosis
Flexor digitorum longus t
Quadratus plantae m

Figure 15.3.16

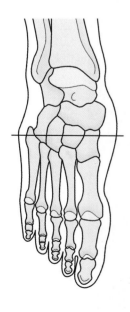

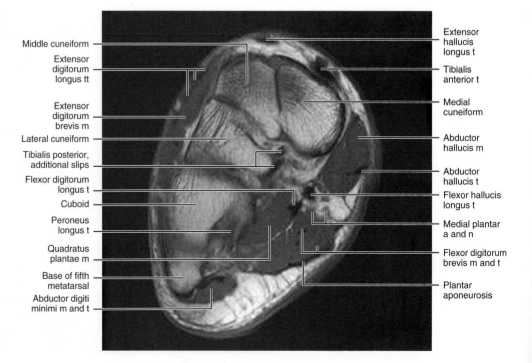

Middle cuneiform
Extensor digitorum longus tt
Extensor digitorum brevis m
Lateral cuneiform
Tibialis posterior, additional slips
Flexor digitorum longus t
Cuboid
Peroneus longus t
Quadratus plantae m
Base of fifth metatarsal
Abductor digiti minimi m and t

Extensor hallucis longus t
Tibialis anterior t
Medial cuneiform
Abductor hallucis m
Abductor hallucis t
Flexor hallucis longus t
Medial plantar a and n
Flexor digitorum brevis m and t
Plantar aponeurosis

Figure 15.3.17

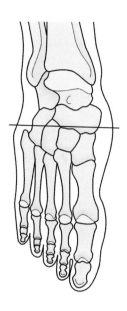

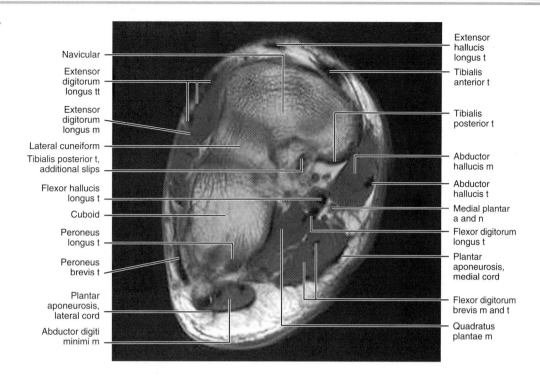

Navicular

Extensor digitorum longus tt

Extensor digitorum longus m

Lateral cuneiform

Tibialis posterior t, additional slips

Flexor hallucis longus t

Cuboid

Peroneus longus t

Peroneus brevis t

Plantar aponeurosis, lateral cord

Abductor digiti minimi m

Extensor hallucis longus t

Tibialis anterior t

Tibialis posterior t

Abductor hallucis m

Abductor hallucis t

Medial plantar a and n

Flexor digitorum longus t

Plantar aponeurosis, medial cord

Flexor digitorum brevis m and t

Quadratus plantae m

Figure 15.3.18

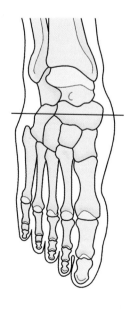

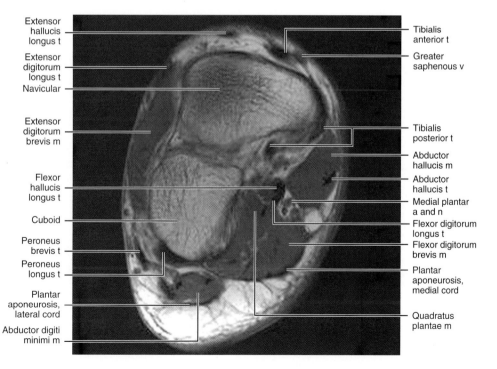

Extensor hallucis longus t

Extensor digitorum longus t

Navicular

Extensor digitorum brevis m

Flexor hallucis longus t

Cuboid

Peroneus brevis t

Peroneus longus t

Plantar aponeurosis, lateral cord

Abductor digiti minimi m

Tibialis anterior t

Greater saphenous v

Tibialis posterior t

Abductor hallucis m

Abductor hallucis t

Medial plantar a and n

Flexor digitorum longus t

Flexor digitorum brevis m

Plantar aponeurosis, medial cord

Quadratus plantae m

Spine and Back

Table 9: Muscles of the Back

MUSCLE	ORIGIN	INSERTION	NERVE SUPPLY
Trapezius	Medial third of the superior nuchal line, external occipital protuberance, ligamentum nuchae, spinous processes of the seventh cervical and thoracic vertebrae, and corresponding supraspinous ligaments	Lateral third of the posterior surface of the clavicle, medial side of the acromion, and upper border of the spine of the scapula	Accessory and cervical plexus
Rhomboideus major	Spinous processes and corresponding supraspinous ligaments of the first four thoracic vertebrae	Medial border of the scapula below the scapular spine	Dorsal scapular
Rhomboideus minor	Spinous processes of the sixth and seventh cervical vertebrae	Medial margin of the scapula above the scapular spine	Dorsal scapular
Levator scapulae	Posterior tubercles of the transverse processes of the four upper cervical vertebrae	Superior angle of the scapula	Dorsal scapular
Serratus posterior superior	From spinous processes of the two lower cervical and two upper thoracic vertebrae	Onto the lateral side of the angles of the second to fifth ribs	First to fourth intercostal
Serratus posterior inferior	With latissimus dorsi, from the spinous processes of the two lower thoracic and two upper lumbar vertebrae	Onto the lower borders of the last four ribs	Ninth to twelfth intercostal
Serratus anterior	From the center of the lateral aspect of the first eight or nine ribs	Superior and inferior angles and intervening medial margin of the scapula	Long thoracic from brachial plexus
Deltoid	Lateral third of the clavicle, lateral border of the acromion process, lower border of the scapular spine	Lateral side of the shaft of the humerus above its middle	Axillary from fifth and sixth cervical nerves through brachial plexus
Latissimus dorsi	Spinous processes of the lower five or six thoracic and lumbar vertebrae, median ridge of the sacrum, and outer lip of the iliac crest	With teres major, onto the posterior lip of the bicipital groove of the humerus	Thoracodorsal
Infraspinatus	Infraspinous fossa of the scapula	Middle facet of the great tubercle of the humerus	Suprascapular from fifth to sixth cervical
Supraspinatus	Supraspinous fossa of the scapula	Great tubercle of the humerus	Suprascapular from fifth to sixth cervical

Table 9: Muscles of the Back—Cont'd

MUSCLE	ORIGIN	INSERTION	NERVE SUPPLY
Teres major	Inferior angle and lower third of the border of the scapula	Medial border of the intertubercular groove of the humerus	Lower subscapular from fifth and sixth cervical
Teres minor	Upper two thirds of the lateral border of the scapula	Lower facet of the great tuberosity of the humerus	Axillary from fifth and sixth cervical
Spinalis capitis	Rarely a separate muscle; it arises with the semispinalis capitis from the upper thoracic spinous process	Inserts with the semispinalis capitis on the occiput	Branches of the dorsal primary divisions of the spinal nerves
Spinalis cervicis	Spinous processes of the sixth and seventh cervical vertebrae	Spinous processes of the axis and the third cervical vertebra	Dorsal branches of cervical
Spinalis thoracis	Spinous processes of the upper lumbar and two lower thoracic vertebrae	Spinous processes of the middle and upper thoracic vertebrae	Dorsal branches of thoracic and upper lumbar
Iliocostalis cervicis	Angles of the upper six ribs	Transverse processes of the middle cervical vertebrae	Dorsal branches of upper thoracic
Iliocostalis thoracis	Medial side of the angles of the lower six ribs	Angles of the upper six ribs	Dorsal branches of thoracic
Iliocostalis lumborum	With erector spinae, from the sacrum, ilium, and spines of the lumbar vertebrae	Angles of the lower six ribs	Dorsal branches of thoracic and lumbar nerves
Longissimus capitis	From the transverse processes of the upper thoracic and transverse and articular processes of the lower and middle cervical vertebrae	Onto the mastoid process	Dorsal branches of cervical
Longissimus cervicis	Transverse processes of the upper thoracic vertebrae	Transverse processes of the middle and upper cervical vertebrae	Dorsal branches of lower cervical and upper thoracic
Longissimus thoracis	With the iliocostalis and from the transverse processes of the lower thoracic vertebrae	By lateral slips onto most or all of the ribs between the angles and the tubercles and onto the tips of the transverse processes of the upper lumbar vertebrae, and by medial slips into the accessory processes of the upper lumbar and transverse processes of the thoracic vertebrae	Dorsal branches of thoracic and lumbar

Continued

Table 9: Muscles of the Back—Cont'd

MUSCLE	ORIGIN	INSERTION	NERVE SUPPLY
Splenius capitis	From the ligamentum nuchae of the last four cervical vertebrae and the supraspinous ligament of first and second thoracic vertebrae	Lateral half of the superior nuchal line and mastoid process	Dorsal branches of second to sixth cervical
Splenius cervicis	From the supraspinous ligament and the spinous processes of the third to fifth thoracic vertebrae	Posterior tubercles of the transverse processes of the first and second (sometimes third) cervical vertebrae	Dorsal branches of fourth to eighth cervical
Semispinalis capitis	Transverse processes of the five or six upper thoracic and articular processes of the four lower cervical vertebrae	Occipital bone between the superior and inferior nuchal lines	Dorsal branches of cervical
Semispinalis cervicis	Transverse processes of the second to fifth thoracic vertebrae	Spinous processes of the axis and the third to fifth cervical vertebrae	Dorsal branches of cervical and thoracic
Semispinalis thoracis	Transverse processes of the fifth to eleventh thoracic vertebrae	Spinous processes of the first four thoracic and fifth and seventh cervical vertebrae	Dorsal branches of cervical and thoracic
Multifidus	From the sacrum, the sacroiliac ligament, mammillary processes of the lumbar vertebrae, transverse processes of the thoracic vertebrae, and articular processes of the last four cervical vertebrae	Onto the spinous processes of all the vertebrae, up to and including the axis	Dorsal branches of spinal
Rotatores	Primarily developed in the thoracic region from the transverse processes of the vertebrae	Into the root of the spinous processes of the next two or three vertebrae above	Dorsal branches of spinal
Interspinales cervicis	Tubercle of the spinous process of the cervical vertebrae	Tubercle of the spinous process of the next superior vertebra	Dorsal branches of cervical
Interspinales thoracis	Often poorly developed or absent between the spinous processes of the thoracic vertebrae	Spinous processes of thoracic vertebrae	Dorsal branches of thoracic
Interspinales lumborum	Superior margin of the lumbar spinous processes	Inferior margin of the next superior spinous process	Dorsal branches of lumbar
Intertransversarii anteriores cervicis	Anterior tubercle of the cervical transverse process	Anterior tubercle of the next superior transverse process	Ventral branch of cervical

Table 9: Muscles of the Back—Cont'd

MUSCLE	ORIGIN	INSERTION	NERVE SUPPLY
Intertransversarii laterales lumbar	Transverse processes of the lumbar vertebrae	Next superior transverse process	Ventral branches of lumbar
Intertransversarii thoracis	Transverse processes of the thoracic vertebrae	Next superior transverse process	Dorsal branches of thoracic

Chapter 16

MRI of the Thoracic Spine

AXIAL

Figure 16.1.1

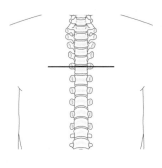

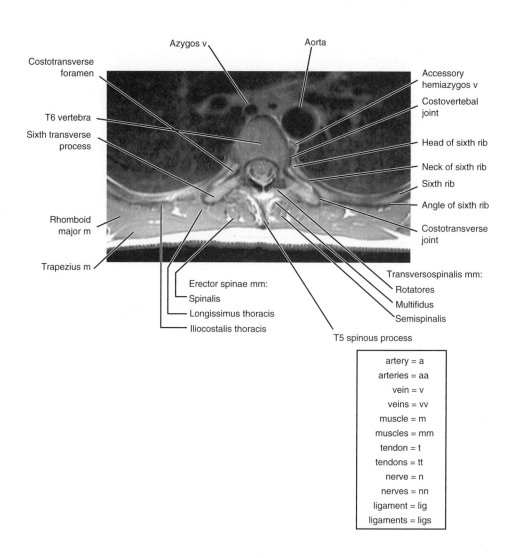

Azygos v

Aorta

Costotransverse foramen

T6 vertebra

Sixth transverse process

Accessory hemiazygos v

Costovertebal joint

Head of sixth rib

Neck of sixth rib

Sixth rib

Angle of sixth rib

Costotransverse joint

Rhomboid major m

Trapezius m

Erector spinae mm:

Spinalis

Longissimus thoracis

Iliocostalis thoracis

T5 spinous process

Transversospinalis mm:

Rotatores

Multifidus

Semispinalis

artery = a
arteries = aa
vein = v
veins = vv
muscle = m
muscles = mm
tendon = t
tendons = tt
nerve = n
nerves = nn
ligament = lig
ligaments = ligs

Figure 16.1.2

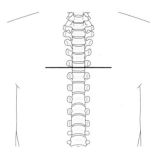

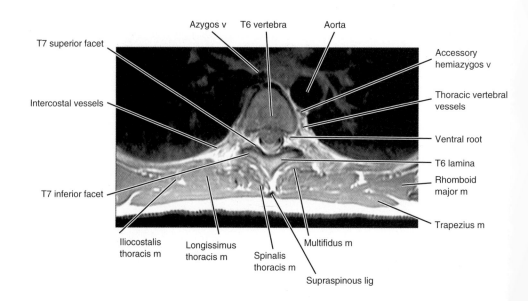

Azygos v   T6 vertebra   Aorta

T7 superior facet

Intercostal vessels

T7 inferior facet

Accessory hemiazygos v

Thoracic vertebral vessels

Ventral root

T6 lamina

Rhomboid major m

Trapezius m

Iliocostalis thoracis m

Longissimus thoracis m

Spinalis thoracis m

Multifidus m

Supraspinous lig

Figure 16.1.3

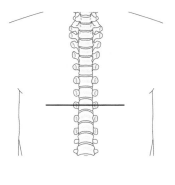

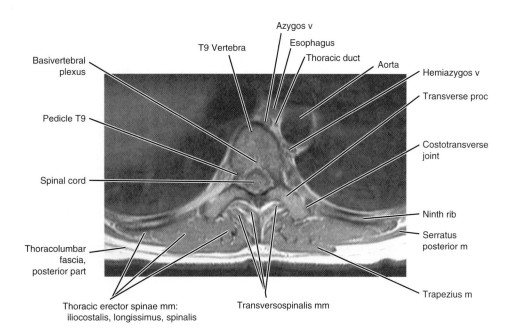

Azygos v
T9 Vertebra
Esophagus
Thoracic duct
Aorta
Basivertebral plexus
Hemiazygos v
Transverse proc
Pedicle T9
Costotransverse joint
Spinal cord
Ninth rib
Serratus posterior m
Thoracolumbar fascia, posterior part
Trapezius m
Thoracic erector spinae mm: iliocostalis, longissimus, spinalis
Transversospinalis mm

Figure 16.1.4

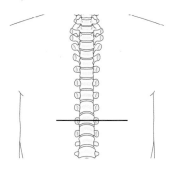

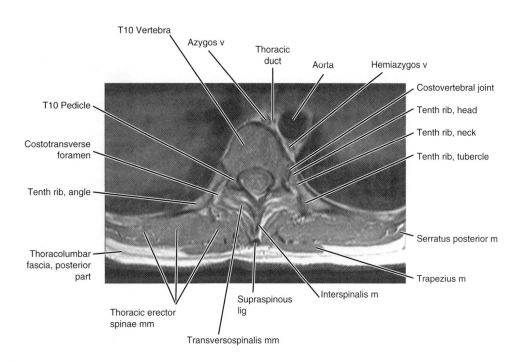

T10 Vertebra
Azygos v
Thoracic duct
Aorta
Hemiazygos v
T10 Pedicle
Costovertebral joint
Tenth rib, head
Costotransverse foramen
Tenth rib, neck
Tenth rib, tubercle
Tenth rib, angle
Thoracolumbar fascia, posterior part
Serratus posterior m
Trapezius m
Thoracic erector spinae mm
Supraspinous lig
Interspinalis m
Transversospinalis mm

SAGITTAL

Figure 16.2.1

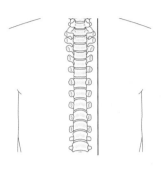

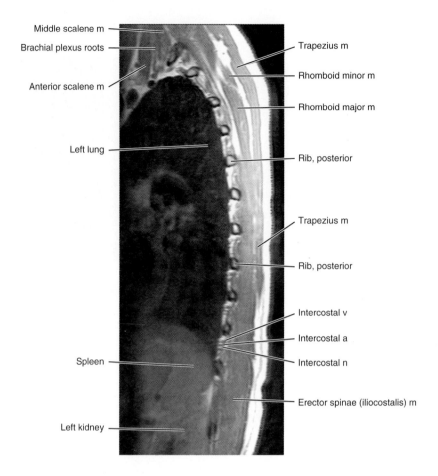

Middle scalene m

Brachial plexus roots

Anterior scalene m

Left lung

Spleen

Left kidney

Trapezius m

Rhomboid minor m

Rhomboid major m

Rib, posterior

Trapezius m

Rib, posterior

Intercostal v

Intercostal a

Intercostal n

Erector spinae (iliocostalis) m

Figure 16.2.2

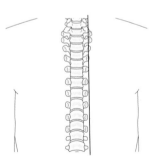

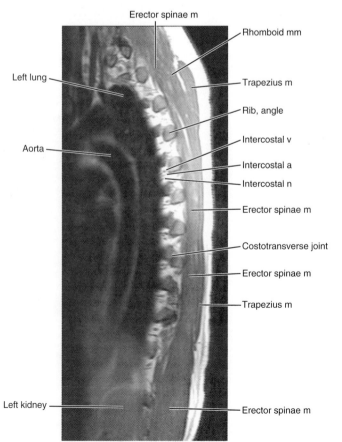

Erector spinae m

Left lung

Aorta

Left kidney

Rhomboid mm

Trapezius m

Rib, angle

Intercostal v

Intercostal a

Intercostal n

Erector spinae m

Costotransverse joint

Erector spinae m

Trapezius m

Erector spinae m

Figure 16.2.3

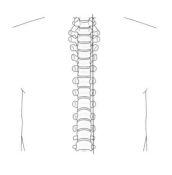

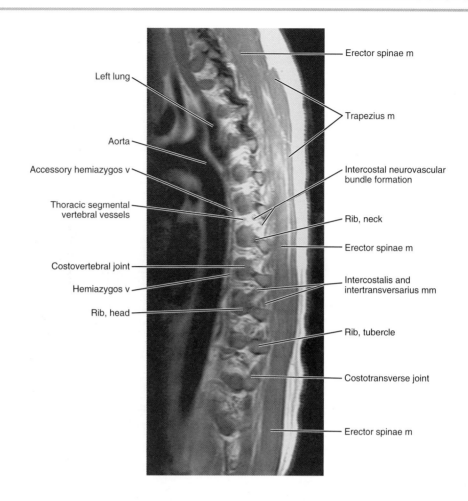

Left lung

Aorta

Accessory hemiazygos v

Thoracic segmental vertebral vessels

Costovertebral joint

Hemiazygos v

Rib, head

Erector spinae m

Trapezius m

Intercostal neurovascular bundle formation

Rib, neck

Erector spinae m

Intercostalis and intertransversarius mm

Rib, tubercle

Costotransverse joint

Erector spinae m

Figure 16.2.4

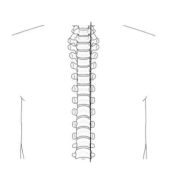

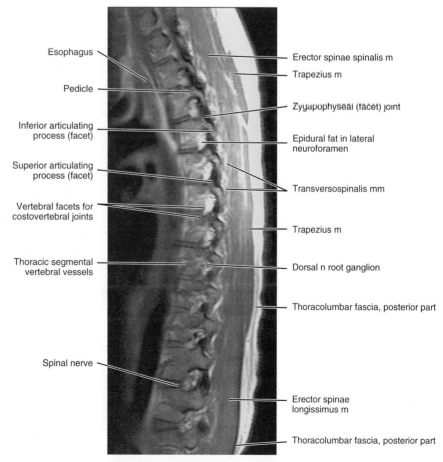

Esophagus

Pedicle

Inferior articulating process (facet)

Superior articulating process (facet)

Vertebral facets for costovertebral joints

Thoracic segmental vertebral vessels

Spinal nerve

Erector spinae spinalis m

Trapezius m

Zygapophyseal (facet) joint

Epidural fat in lateral neuroforamen

Transversospinalis mm

Trapezius m

Dorsal n root ganglion

Thoracolumbar fascia, posterior part

Erector spinae longissimus m

Thoracolumbar fascia, posterior part

Figure 16.2.5

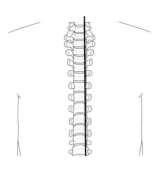

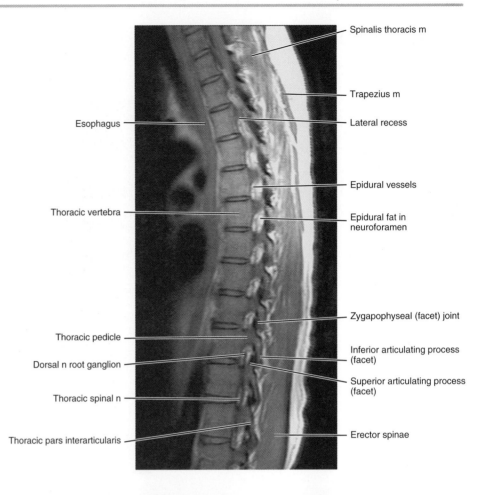

Spinalis thoracis m

Trapezius m

Lateral recess

Esophagus

Epidural vessels

Thoracic vertebra

Epidural fat in neuroforamen

Zygapophyseal (facet) joint

Thoracic pedicle

Inferior articulating process (facet)

Dorsal n root ganglion

Superior articulating process (facet)

Thoracic spinal n

Erector spinae

Thoracic pars interarticularis

Figure 16.2.6

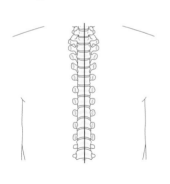

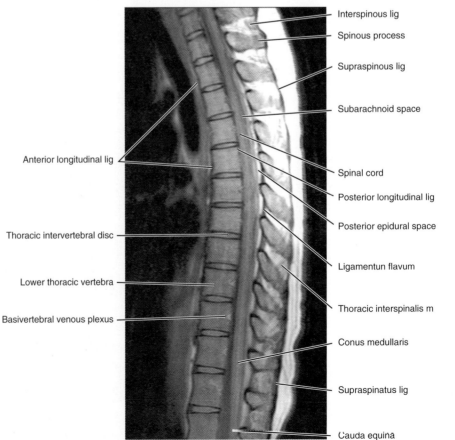

Interspinous lig

Spinous process

Supraspinous lig

Subarachnoid space

Anterior longitudinal lig

Spinal cord

Posterior longitudinal lig

Posterior epidural space

Thoracic intervertebral disc

Ligamentun flavum

Lower thoracic vertebra

Thoracic interspinalis m

Basivertebral venous plexus

Conus medullaris

Supraspinatus lig

Cauda equina

CORONAL
Figure 16.3.1

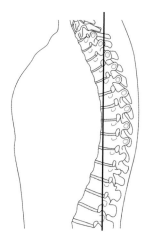

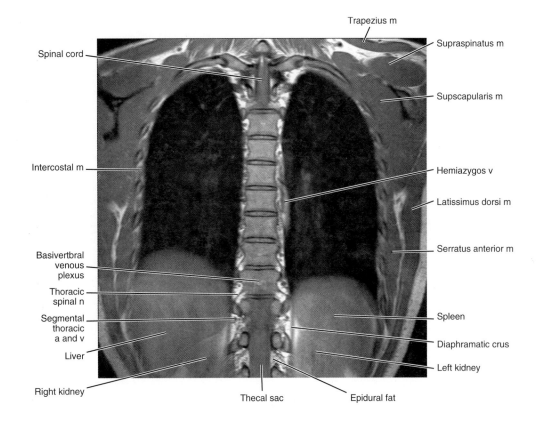

Spinal cord

Trapezius m

Supraspinatus m

Supscapularis m

Intercostal m

Hemiazygos v

Latissimus dorsi m

Serratus anterior m

Basivertbral venous plexus

Thoracic spinal n

Segmental thoracic a and v

Spleen

Diaphramatic crus

Liver

Left kidney

Right kidney

Thecal sac

Epidural fat

Figure 16.3.2

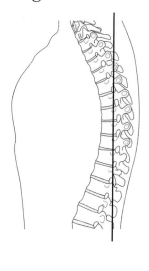

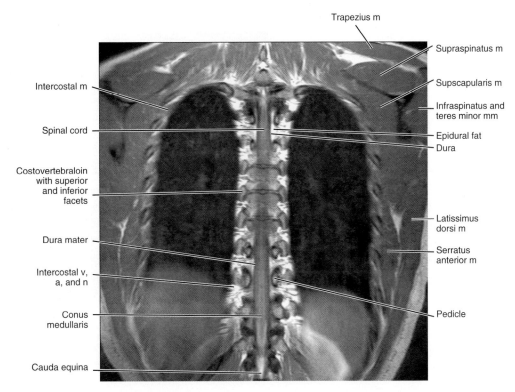

Trapezius m

Supraspinatus m

Supscapularis m

Intercostal m

Infraspinatus and teres minor mm

Spinal cord

Epidural fat

Dura

Costovertebraloin with superior and inferior facets

Dura mater

Latissimus dorsi m

Serratus anterior m

Intercostal v, a, and n

Conus medullaris

Pedicle

Cauda equina

Figure 16.3.3

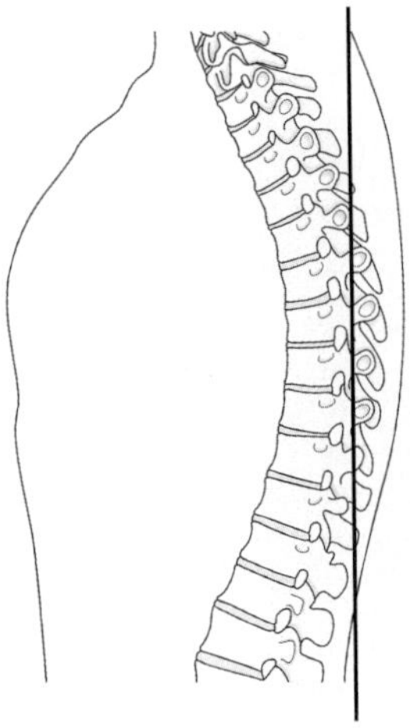

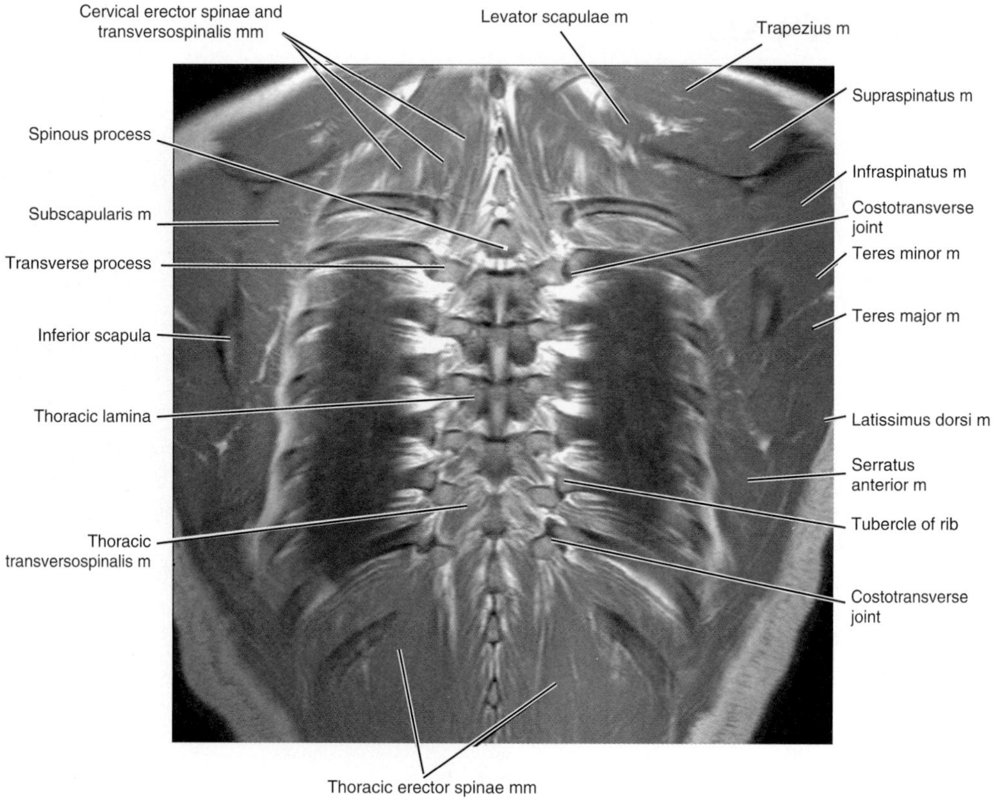

Cervical erector spinae and transversospinalis mm

Levator scapulae m

Trapezius m

Spinous process

Suprapinatus m

Subscapularis m

Infraspinatus m

Transverse process

Costotransverse joint

Inferior scapula

Teres minor m

Thoracic lamina

Teres major m

Thoracic transversospinalis m

Latissimus dorsi m

Serratus anterior m

Tubercle of rib

Costotransverse joint

Thoracic erector spinae mm

Figure 16.3.4

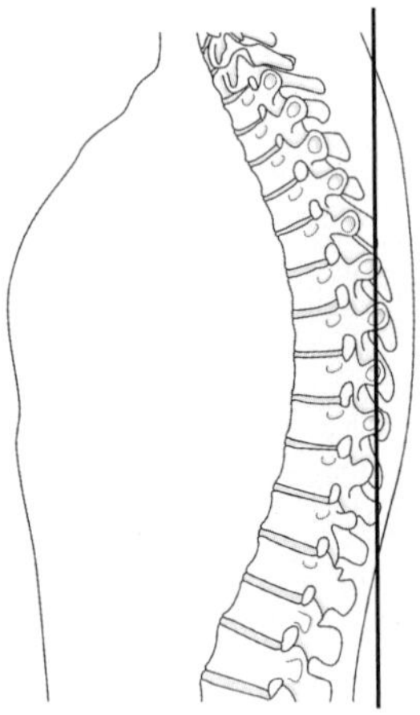

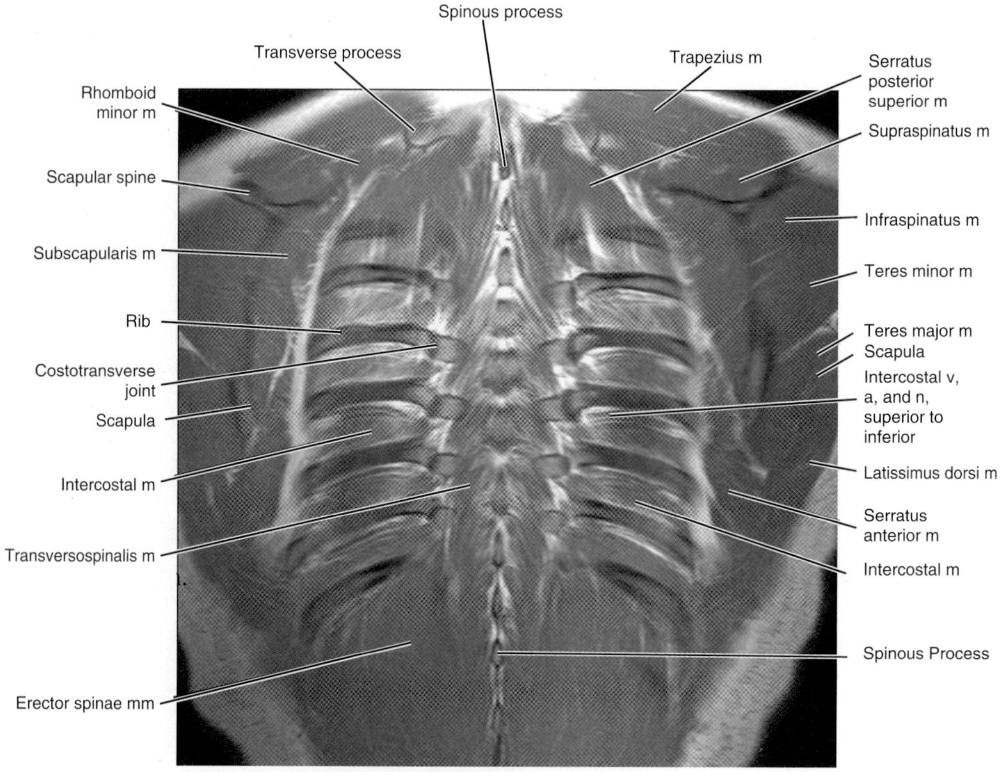

Spinous process

Transverse process

Trapezius m

Serratus posterior superior m

Rhomboid minor m

Supraspinatus m

Scapular spine

Infraspinatus m

Subscapularis m

Teres minor m

Rib

Teres major m
Scapula

Costotransverse joint

Intercostal v, a, and n, superior to inferior

Scapula

Latissimus dorsi m

Intercostal m

Serratus anterior m

Transversospinalis m

Intercostal m

Erector spinae mm

Spinous Process

Figure 16.3.5

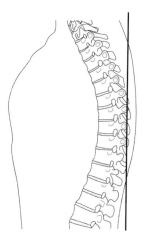

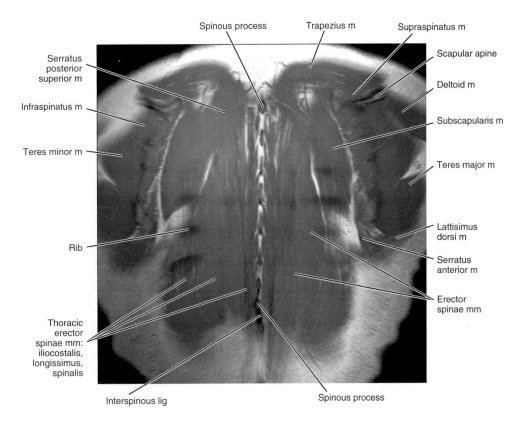

Spinous process
Trapezius m
Supraspinatus m
Serratus posterior superior m
Scapular apine
Infraspinatus m
Deltoid m
Subscapularis m
Teres minor m
Teres major m
Rib
Lattisimus dorsi m
Serratus anterior m
Erector spinae mm
Thoracic erector spinae mm: iliocostalis, longissimus, spinalis
Interspinous lig
Spinous process

Figure 16.3.6

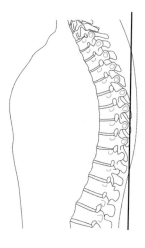

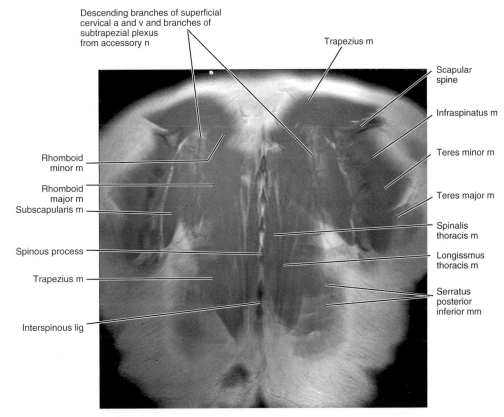

Descending branches of superficial cervical a and v and branches of subtrapezial plexus from accessory n
Trapezius m
Scapular spine
Infraspinatus m
Rhomboid minor m
Teres minor m
Rhomboid major m
Subscapularis m
Teres major m
Spinalis thoracis m
Spinous process
Longissmus thoracis m
Trapezius m
Serratus posterior inferior mm
Interspinous lig

Figure 16.3.7

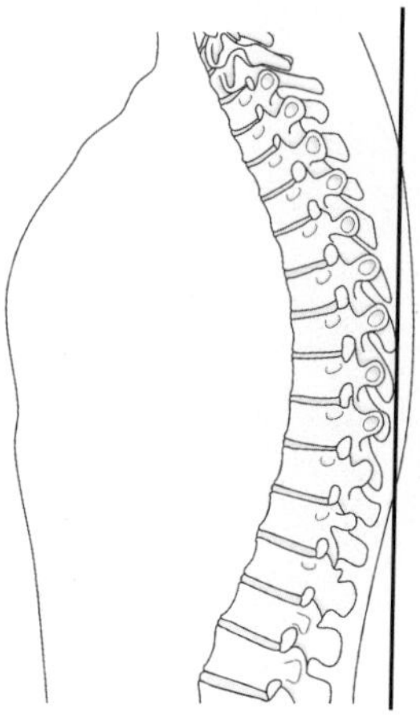

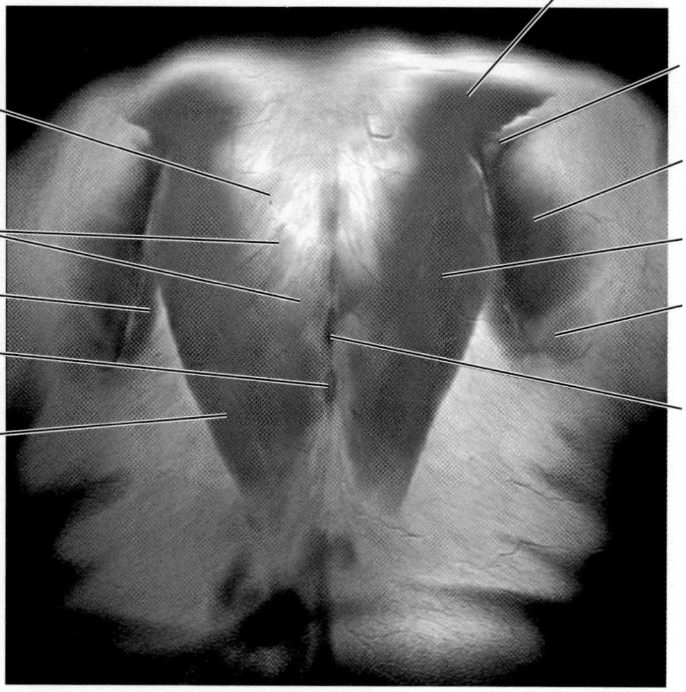

Trapezius m

Scapular spine

Rhomboid
major m

Infraspinatus
and teres
minor mm

Serratus
posterior
superior mm

Trapezius m

Subscapularis m

Teres major m

Spinous process

Supraspinous lig

Trapezius m

Chapter 17

MRI of the Lumbar Spine

AXIAL

Figure 17.1.1

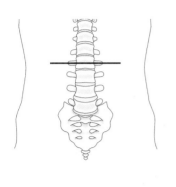

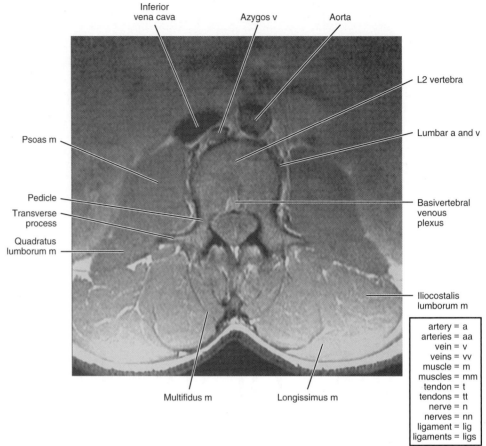

Inferior vena cava
Azygos v
Aorta
L2 vertebra
Lumbar a and v
Psoas m
Pedicle
Transverse process
Quadratus lumborum m
Basivertebral venous plexus
Iliocostalis lumborum m
Multifidus m
Longissimus m

artery = a
arteries = aa
vein = v
veins = vv
muscle = m
muscles = mm
tendon = t
tendons = tt
nerve = n
nerves = nn
ligament = lig
ligaments = ligs

Figure 17.1.2

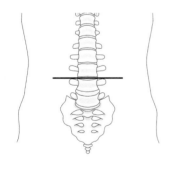

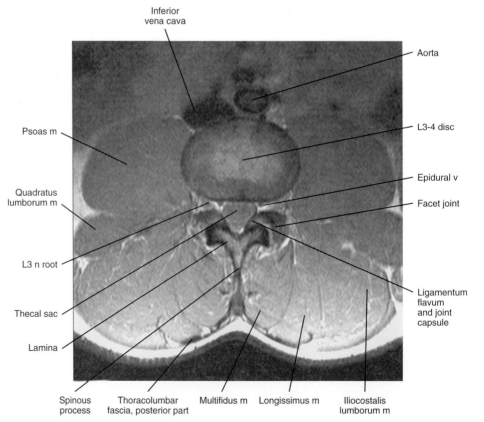

Inferior vena cava
Aorta
L3-4 disc
Psoas m
Epidural v
Facet joint
Quadratus lumborum m
L3 n root
Thecal sac
Lamina
Ligamentum flavum and joint capsule
Spinous process
Thoracolumbar fascia, posterior part
Multifidus m
Longissimus m
Iliocostalis lumborum m

Figure 17.1.3

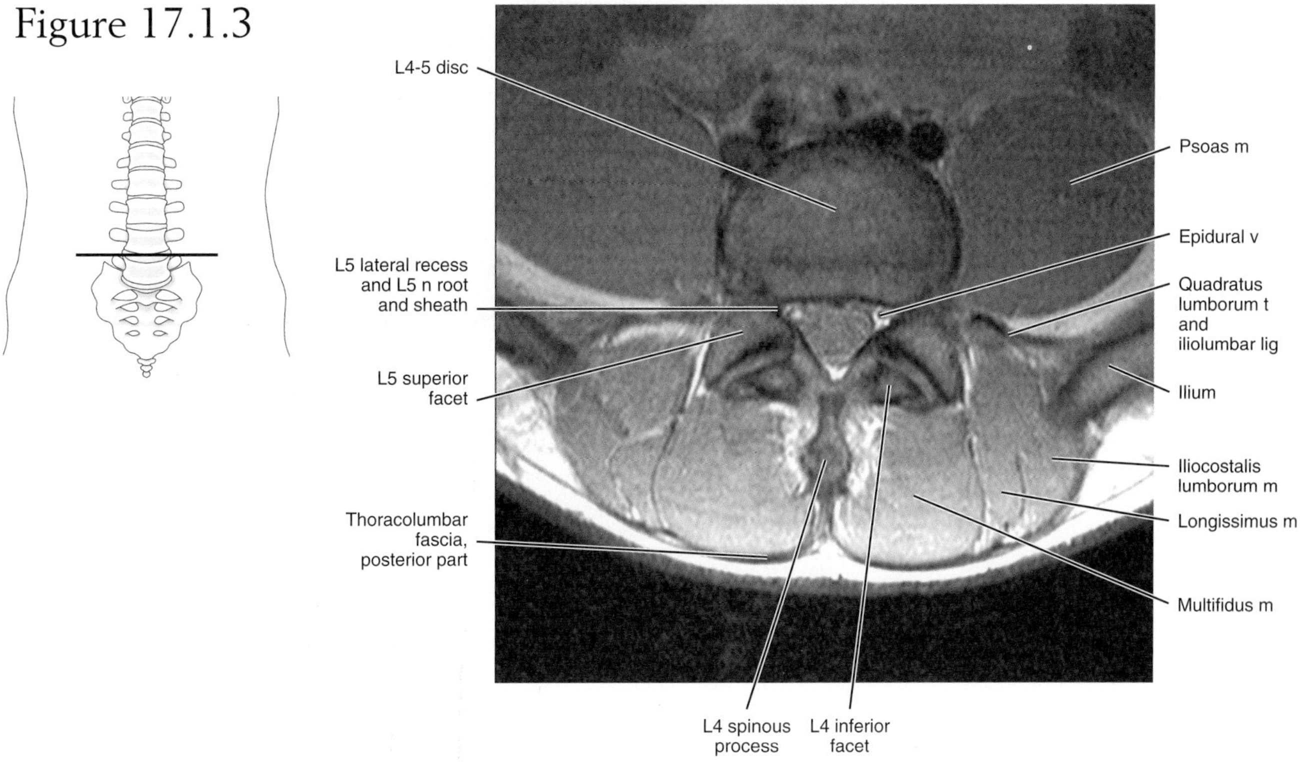

L4-5 disc

Psoas m

L5 lateral recess
and L5 n root
and sheath

Epidural v

Quadratus
lumborum t
and
iliolumbar lig

L5 superior
facet

Ilium

Iliocostalis
lumborum m

Longissimus m

Thoracolumbar
fascia,
posterior part

Multifidus m

L4 spinous
process

L4 inferior
facet

Figure 17.1.4

Left common
iliac v

Left common
iliac a

Psoas m

L5 vertebra

Iliacus m

Left L5
pedicle

Iliac crest

Left L5
transverse
process

Lumbosacral
trunk nn

Iliocostalis
lumborum m

Gluteus
medius m

Longissimus m

Thecal sac

Multifidus m

Spinous
process

Thoracolumbar fascia,
posterior part

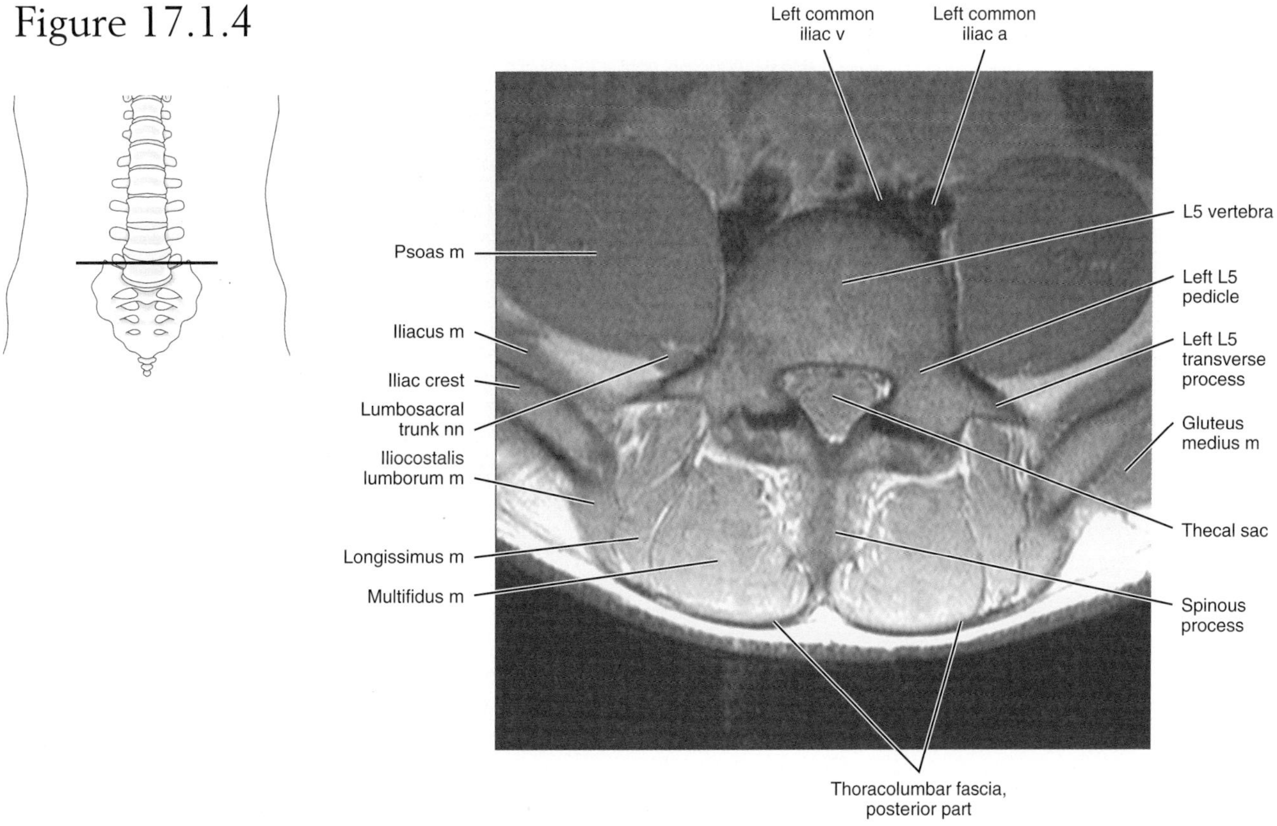

Figure 17.1.5

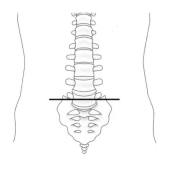
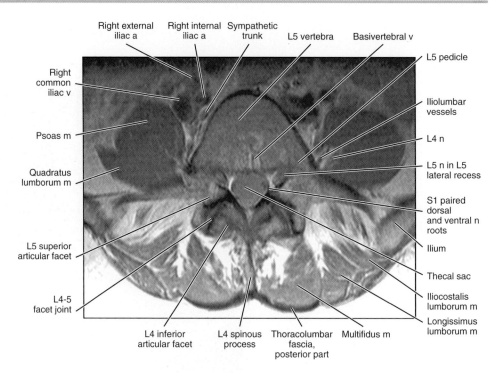

Right external iliac a — Right internal iliac a — Sympathetic trunk — L5 vertebra — Basivertebral v

Right common iliac v

Psoas m

Quadratus lumborum m

L5 superior articular facet

L4-5 facet joint

L5 pedicle

Iliolumbar vessels

L4 n

L5 n in L5 lateral recess

S1 paired dorsal and ventral n roots

Ilium

Thecal sac

Iliocostalis lumborum m

Longissimus lumborum m

L4 inferior articular facet — L4 spinous process — Thoracolumbar fascia, posterior part — Multifidus m

Figure 17.1.6

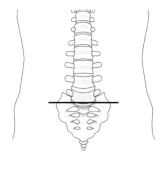
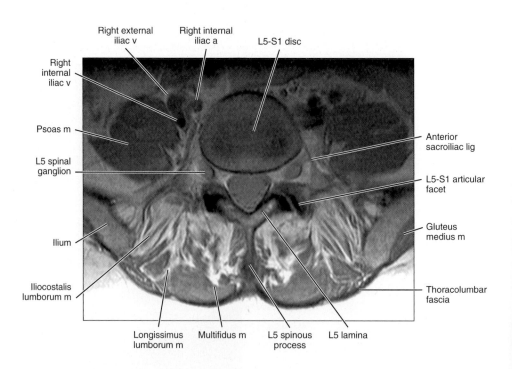

Right external iliac v — Right internal iliac a — L5-S1 disc

Right internal iliac v

Psoas m

L5 spinal ganglion

Ilium

Iliocostalis lumborum m

Anterior sacroiliac lig

L5-S1 articular facet

Gluteus medius m

Thoracolumbar fascia

Longissimus lumborum m — Multifidus m — L5 spinous process — L5 lamina

Figure 17.1.7

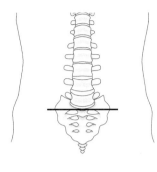

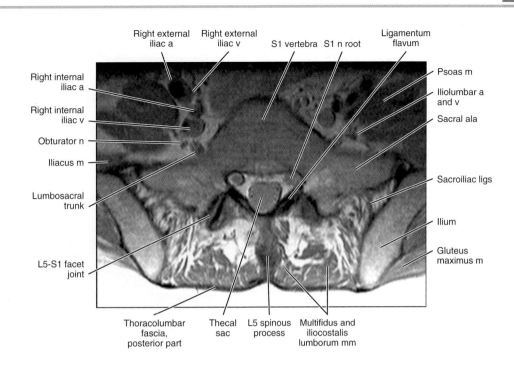

Right external iliac a

Right external iliac v

S1 vertebra

S1 n root

Ligamentum flavum

Right internal iliac a

Right internal iliac v

Obturator n

Iliacus m

Lumbosacral trunk

L5-S1 facet joint

Psoas m

Iliolumbar a and v

Sacral ala

Sacroiliac ligs

Ilium

Gluteus maximus m

Thoracolumbar fascia, posterior part

Thecal sac

L5 spinous process

Multifidus and iliocostalis lumborum mm

Figure 17.1.8

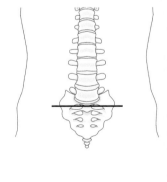

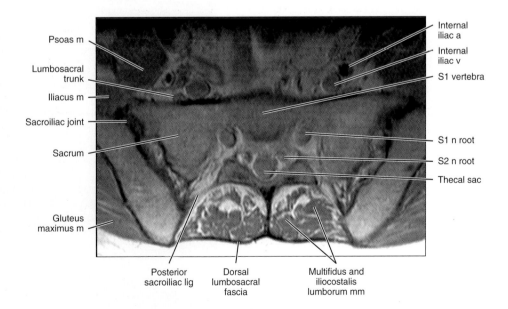

Psoas m

Lumbosacral trunk

Iliacus m

Sacroiliac joint

Sacrum

Gluteus maximus m

Internal iliac a

Internal iliac v

S1 vertebra

S1 n root

S2 n root

Thecal sac

Posterior sacroiliac lig

Dorsal lumbosacral fascia

Multifidus and iliocostalis lumborum mm

SAGITTAL
Figure 17.2.1

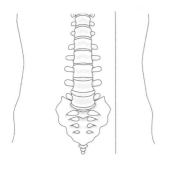

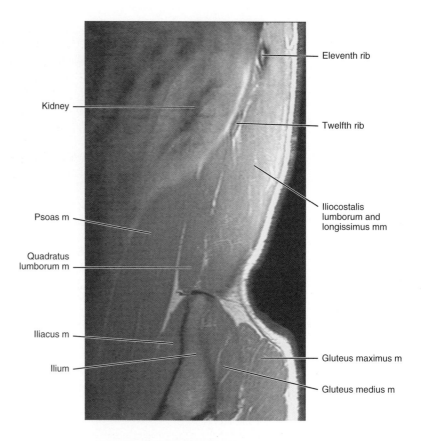

Eleventh rib

Twelfth rib

Iliocostalis lumborum and longissimus mm

Kidney

Psoas m

Quadratus lumborum m

Iliacus m

Ilium

Gluteus maximus m

Gluteus medius m

Figure 17.2.2

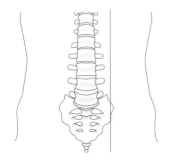

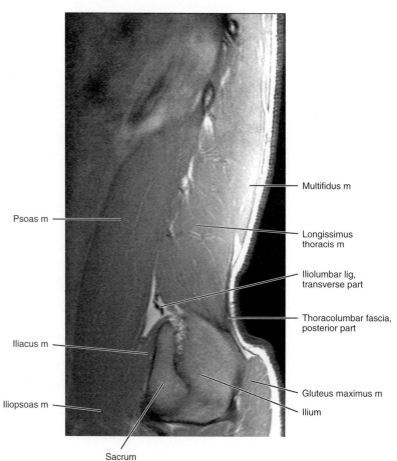

Multifidus m

Psoas m

Longissimus thoracis m

Iliolumbar lig, transverse part

Thoracolumbar fascia, posterior part

Iliacus m

Iliopsoas m

Gluteus maximus m

Ilium

Sacrum

Figure 17.2.3

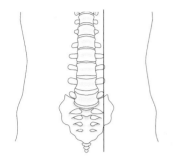

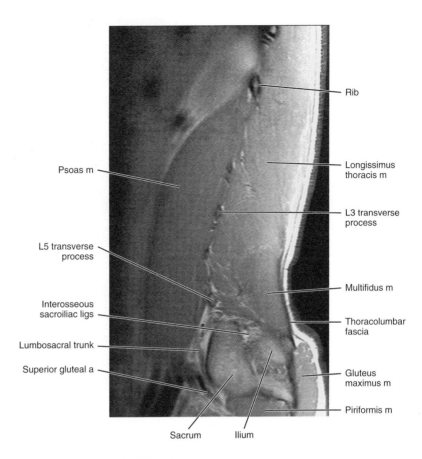

Rib

Longissimus
thoracis m

L3 transverse
process

Multifidus m

Thoracolumbar
fascia

Gluteus
maximus m

Piriformis m

Psoas m

L5 transverse
process

Interosseous
sacroiliac ligs

Lumbosacral trunk

Superior gluteal a

Sacrum   Ilium

Figure 17.2.4

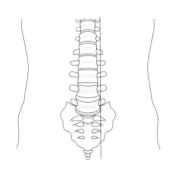

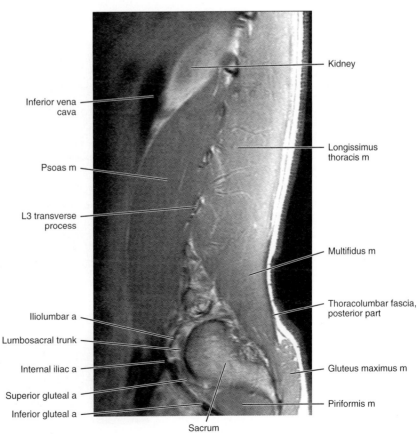

Kidney

Longissimus
thoracis m

Multifidus m

Thoracolumbar fascia,
posterior part

Gluteus maximus m

Piriformis m

Inferior vena
cava

Psoas m

L3 transverse
process

Iliolumbar a

Lumbosacral trunk

Internal iliac a

Superior gluteal a

Inferior gluteal a

Sacrum

Figure 17.2.5

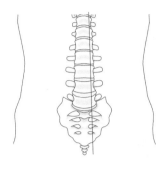

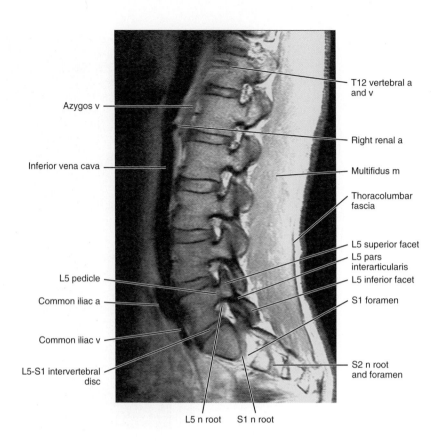

Azygos v

Inferior vena cava

L5 pedicle

Common iliac a

Common iliac v

L5-S1 intervertebral disc

L5 n root   S1 n root

T12 vertebral a and v

Right renal a

Multifidus m

Thoracolumbar fascia

L5 superior facet

L5 pars interarticularis

L5 inferior facet

S1 foramen

S2 n root and foramen

Figure 17.2.6

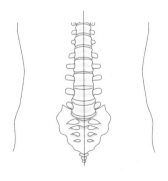

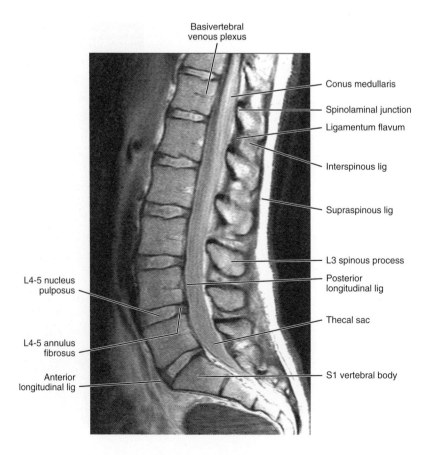

Basivertebral venous plexus

Conus medullaris

Spinolaminal junction

Ligamentum flavum

Interspinous lig

Supraspinous lig

L3 spinous process

Posterior longitudinal lig

Thecal sac

S1 vertebral body

L4-5 nucleus pulposus

L4-5 annulus fibrosus

Anterior longitudinal lig

CORONAL
Figure 17.3.1

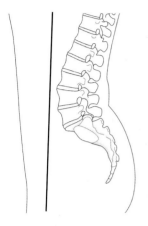

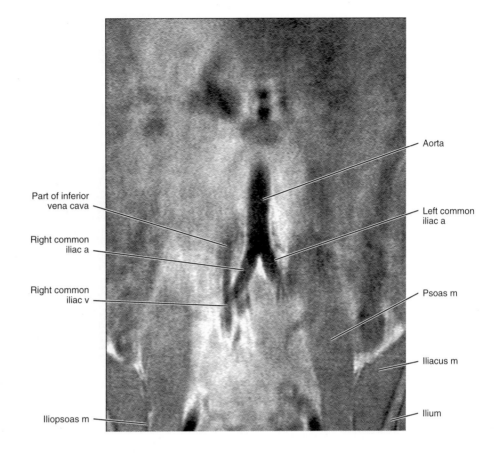

Aorta

Part of inferior vena cava

Left common iliac a

Right common iliac a

Right common iliac v

Psoas m

Iliacus m

Iliopsoas m

Ilium

Figure 17.3.2

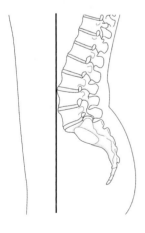

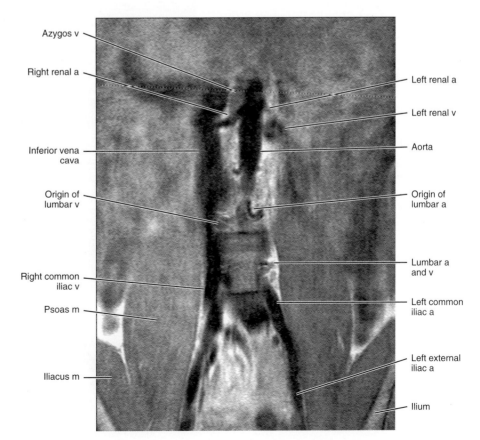

Azygos v

Right renal a

Left renal a

Left renal v

Inferior vena cava

Aorta

Origin of lumbar v

Origin of lumbar a

Lumbar a and v

Right common iliac v

Left common iliac a

Psoas m

Left external iliac a

Iliacus m

Ilium

Figure 17.3.3

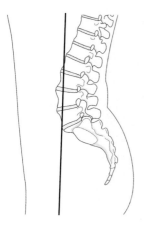

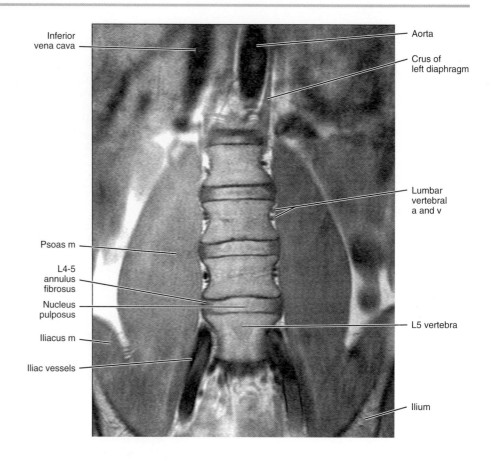

Inferior vena cava

Aorta

Crus of left diaphragm

Lumbar vertebral a and v

Psoas m

L4-5 annulus fibrosus

Nucleus pulposus

Iliacus m

Iliac vessels

L5 vertebra

Ilium

Figure 17.3.4

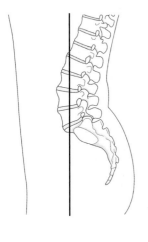

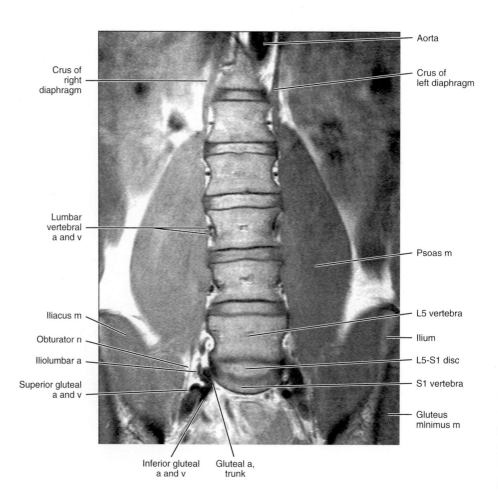

Crus of right diaphragm

Aorta

Crus of left diaphragm

Lumbar vertebral a and v

Psoas m

Iliacus m

L5 vertebra

Obturator n

Ilium

Iliolumbar a

L5-S1 disc

Superior gluteal a and v

S1 vertebra

Gluteus mlnimus m

Inferior gluteal a and v

Gluteal a, trunk

Figure 17.3.5

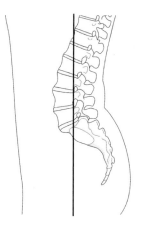

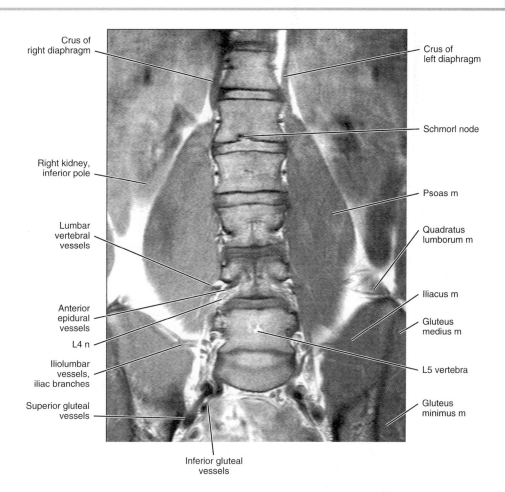

Crus of
right diaphragm

Crus of
left diaphragm

Schmorl node

Right kidney,
inferior pole

Psoas m

Lumbar
vertebral
vessels

Quadratus
lumborum m

Iliacus m

Anterior
epidural
vessels

Gluteus
medius m

L4 n

Iliolumbar
vessels,
iliac branches

L5 vertebra

Superior gluteal
vessels

Gluteus
minimus m

Inferior gluteal
vessels

Figure 17.3.6

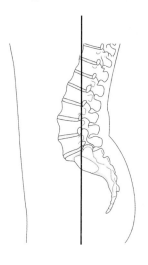

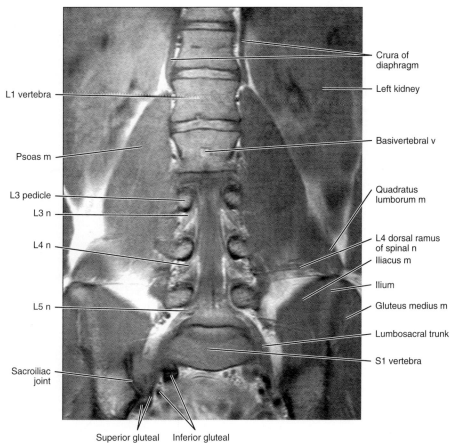

Crura of
diaphragm

L1 vertebra

Left kidney

Psoas m

Basivertebral v

L3 pedicle

Quadratus
lumborum m

L3 n

L4 dorsal ramus
of spinal n

L4 n

Iliacus m

Ilium

Gluteus medius m

L5 n

Lumbosacral trunk

S1 vertebra

Sacroiliac
joint

Superior gluteal   Inferior gluteal
vessels   vessels

Figure 17.3.7

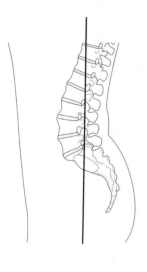

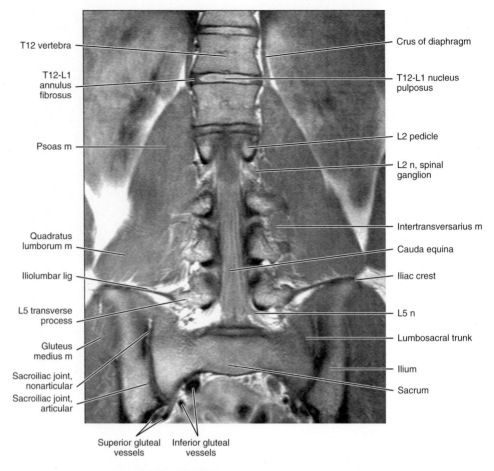

T12 vertebra

T12-L1 annulus fibrosus

Psoas m

Quadratus lumborum m

Iliolumbar lig

L5 transverse process

Gluteus medius m

Sacroiliac joint, nonarticular

Sacroiliac joint, articular

Crus of diaphragm

T12-L1 nucleus pulposus

L2 pedicle

L2 n, spinal ganglion

Intertransversarius m

Cauda equina

Iliac crest

L5 n

Lumbosacral trunk

Ilium

Sacrum

Superior gluteal vessels

Inferior gluteal vessels

Figure 17.3.8

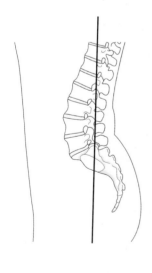

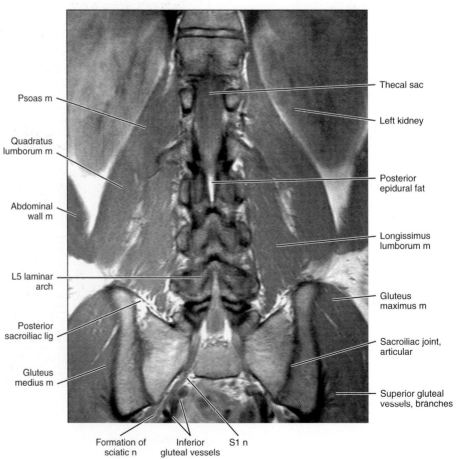

Psoas m

Quadratus lumborum m

Abdominal wall m

L5 laminar arch

Posterior sacroiliac lig

Gluteus medius m

Thecal sac

Left kidney

Posterior epidural fat

Longissimus lumborum m

Gluteus maximus m

Sacroiliac joint, articular

Superior gluteal vessels, branches

Formation of sciatic n

Inferior gluteal vessels

S1 n

Figure 17.3.9

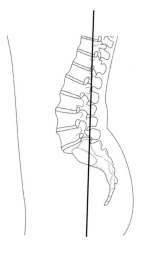

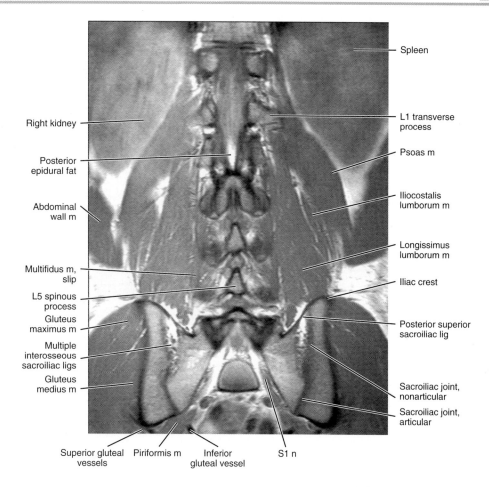

Right kidney

Posterior epidural fat

Abdominal wall m

Multifidus m, slip

L5 spinous process

Gluteus maximus m

Multiple interosseous sacroiliac ligs

Gluteus medius m

Spleen

L1 transverse process

Psoas m

Iliocostalis lumborum m

Longissimus lumborum m

Iliac crest

Posterior superior sacroiliac lig

Sacroiliac joint, nonarticular

Sacroiliac joint, articular

Superior gluteal vessels

Piriformis m

Inferior gluteal vessel

S1 n

Figure 17.3.10

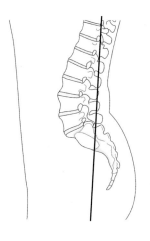

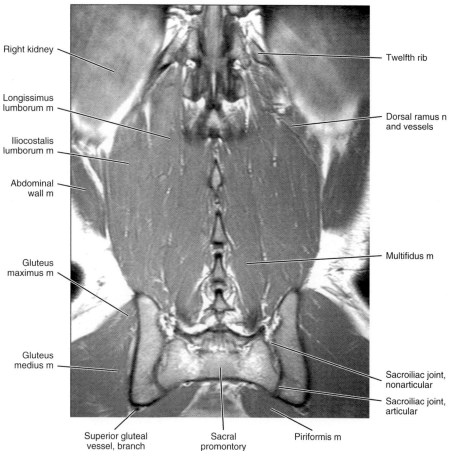

Right kidney

Longissimus lumborum m

Iliocostalis lumborum m

Abdominal wall m

Gluteus maximus m

Gluteus medius m

Twelfth rib

Dorsal ramus n and vessels

Multifidus m

Sacroiliac joint, nonarticular

Sacroiliac joint, articular

Superior gluteal vessel, branch

Sacral promontory

Piriformis m

Figure 17.3.11

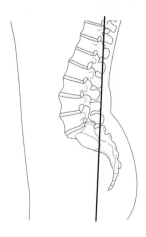

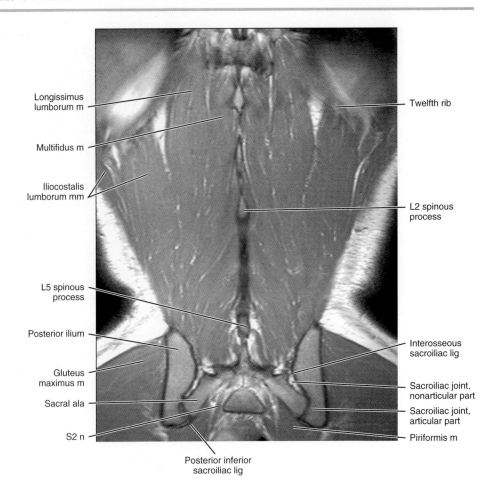

Longissimus lumborum m

Multifidus m

Iliocostalis lumborum mm

L5 spinous process

Posterior ilium

Gluteus maximus m

Sacral ala

S2 n

Posterior inferior sacroiliac lig

Twelfth rib

L2 spinous process

Interosseous sacroiliac lig

Sacroiliac joint, nonarticular part

Sacroiliac joint, articular part

Piriformis m

Thorax

Chapter 18

CT of the Thorax

AXIAL

Figure 18.1.1

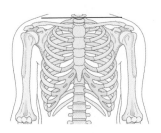

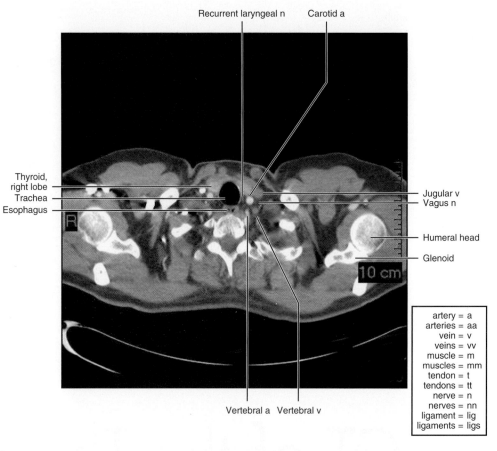

Recurrent laryngeal n   Carotid a

Thyroid, right lobe
Trachea
Esophagus

Jugular v
Vagus n

Humeral head
Glenoid

10 cm

Vertebral a   Vertebral v

artery =	a
arteries =	aa
vein =	v
veins =	vv
muscle =	m
muscles =	mm
tendon =	t
tendons =	tt
nerve =	n
nerves =	nn
ligament =	lig
ligaments =	ligs

Figure 18.1.2

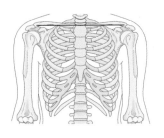

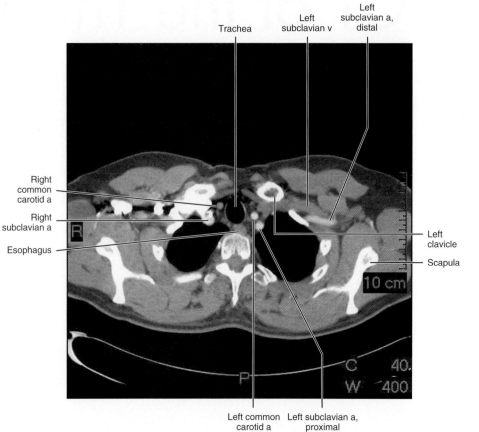

Trachea   Left subclavian v   Left subclavian a, distal

Right common carotid a
Right subclavian a
Esophagus

Left clavicle
Scapula

10 cm

C 40.
W 400

Left common carotid a   Left subclavian a, proximal

Figure 18.1.3

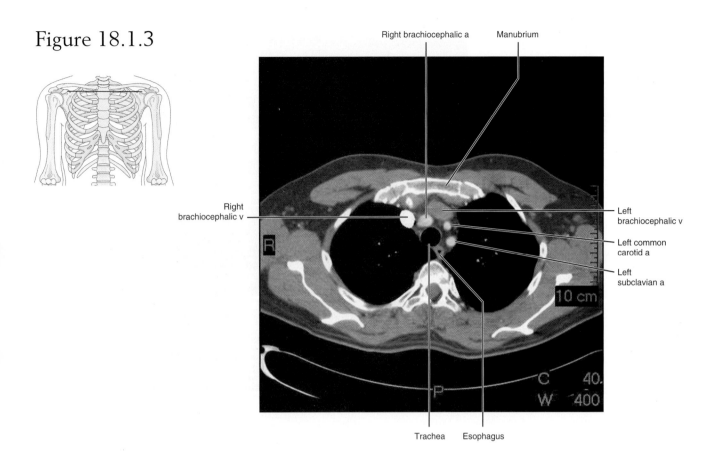

Right brachiocephalic a   Manubrium

Right
brachiocephalic v

Left
brachiocephalic v

Left common
carotid a

Left
subclavian a

10 cm

R

C 40.
W 400

Trachea   Esophagus

Figure 18.1.4

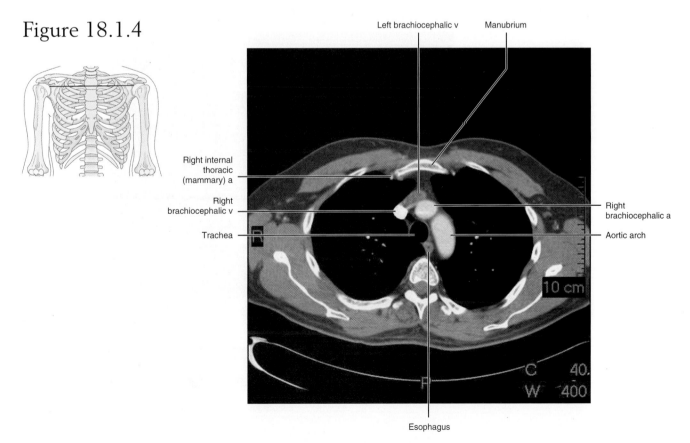

Left brachiocephalic v   Manubrium

Right internal
thoracic
(mammary) a

Right
brachiocephalic v

Right
brachiocephalic a

Trachea

Aortic arch

10 cm

C 40.
W 400

Esophagus

Figure 18.1.5

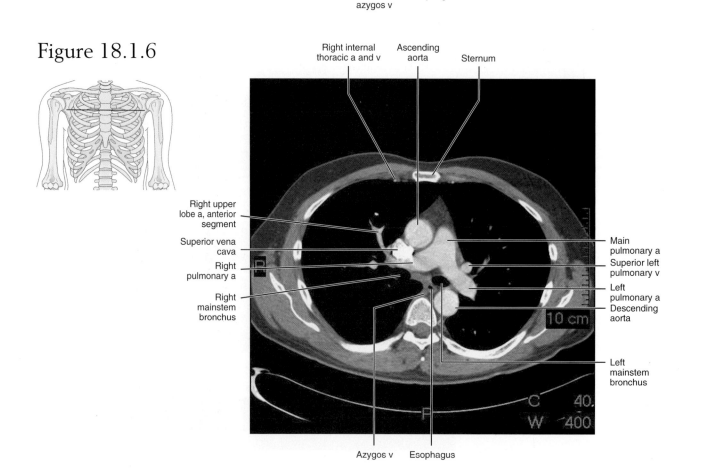

Left internal thoracic (mammary) v

Left internal thoracic (mammary) a

Superior vena cava

Right scapula

Ascending aortic arch

Tracheal carina

Descending aortic arch

10 cm

C 40.
W 400

Arch of azygos v

Esophagus

Figure 18.1.6

Right internal thoracic a and v

Ascending aorta

Sternum

Right upper lobe a, anterior segment

Superior vena cava

Right pulmonary a

Right mainstem bronchus

Main pulmonary a

Superior left pulmonary v

Left pulmonary a

Descending aorta

10 cm

Left mainstem bronchus

C 40.
W 400

Azygos v

Esophagus

Figure 18.1.7

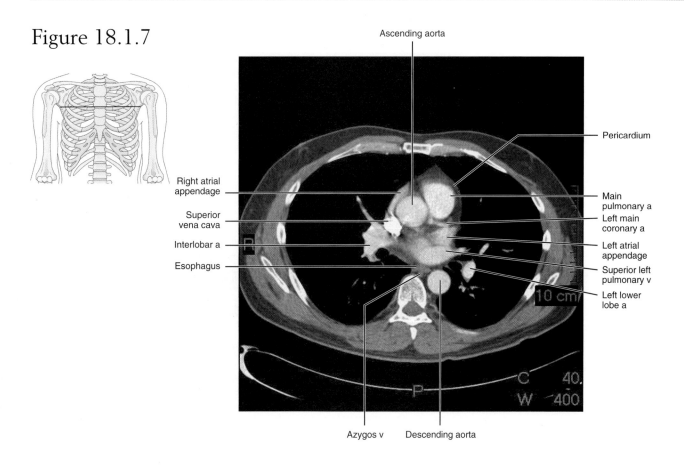

Ascending aorta

Pericardium

Right atrial appendage

Main pulmonary a

Superior vena cava

Left main coronary a

Interlobar a

Left atrial appendage

Esophagus

Superior left pulmonary v

Left lower lobe a

Azygos v   Descending aorta

Figure 18.1.8

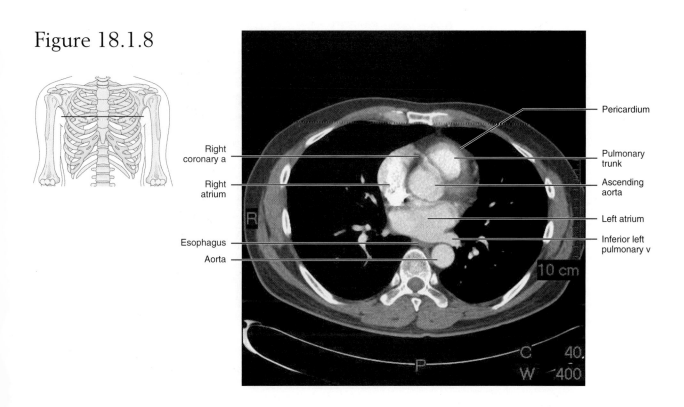

Pericardium

Right coronary a

Pulmonary trunk

Right atrium

Ascending aorta

Left atrium

Esophagus

Inferior left pulmonary v

Aorta

Figure 18.1.9

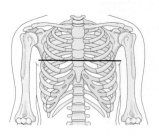

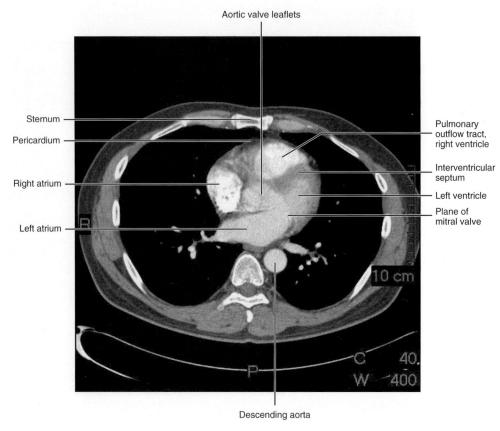

Aortic valve leaflets

Sternum

Pericardium

Right atrium

Left atrium

Pulmonary outflow tract, right ventricle

Interventricular septum

Left ventricle

Plane of mitral valve

10 cm

C 40.
W 400

Descending aorta

Figure 18.1.10

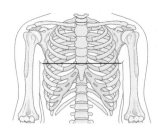

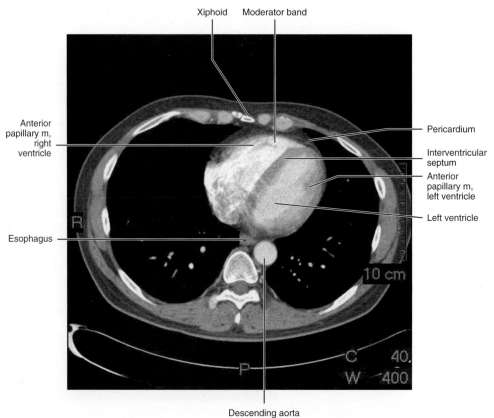

Xiphoid   Moderator band

Anterior papillary m, right ventricle

Esophagus

Pericardium

Interventricular septum

Anterior papillary m, left ventricle

Left ventricle

10 cm

C 40.
W 400

Descending aorta

Figure 18.1.11

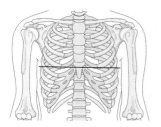

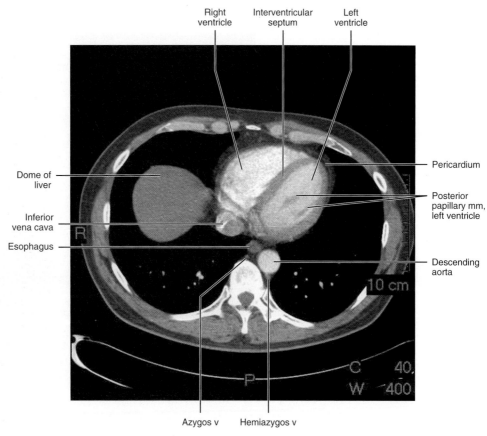

Right ventricle · Interventricular septum · Left ventricle

Dome of liver

Inferior vena cava

Esophagus

Pericardium

Posterior papillary mm, left ventricle

Descending aorta

Azygos v · Hemiazygos v

Figure 18.1.12

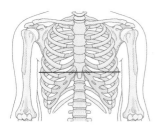

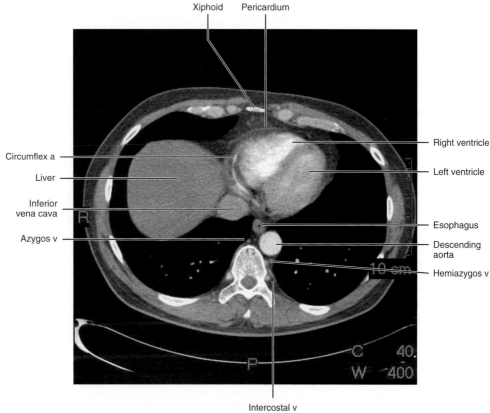

Xiphoid · Pericardium

Circumflex a

Liver

Inferior vena cava

Azygos v

Right ventricle

Left ventricle

Esophagus

Descending aorta

Hemiazygos v

Intercostal v

Figure 18.1.13

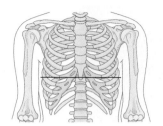

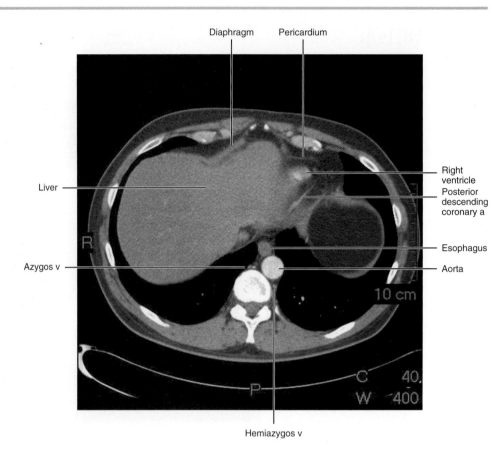

SAGITTAL
Figure 18.2.1A

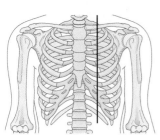

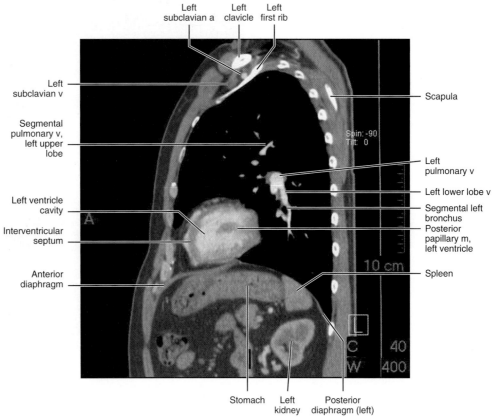

Left subclavian a

Left clavicle

Left first rib

Left subclavian v

Scapula

Segmental pulmonary v, left upper lobe

Spin: -90
Tilt: 0

Left pulmonary v

Left lower lobe v

Left ventricle cavity

Segmental left bronchus

Interventricular septum

Posterior papillary m, left ventricle

10 cm

Anterior diaphragm

Spleen

A

L
C 40
W 400

Stomach

Left kidney

Posterior diaphragm (left)

Figure 18.2.1B

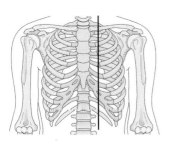

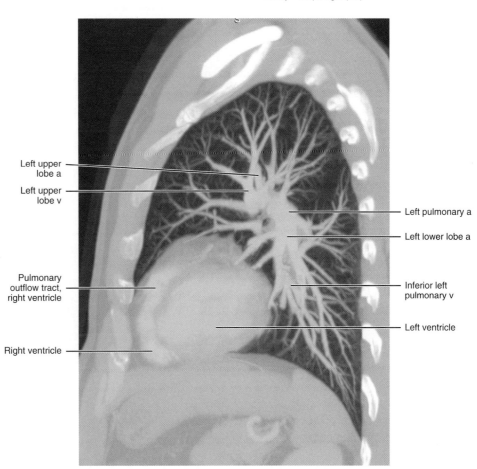

Left upper lobe a

Left upper lobe v

Left pulmonary a

Left lower lobe a

Pulmonary outflow tract, right ventricle

Inferior left pulmonary v

Left ventricle

Right ventricle

Figure 18.2.2

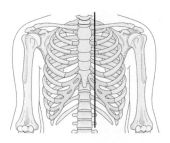

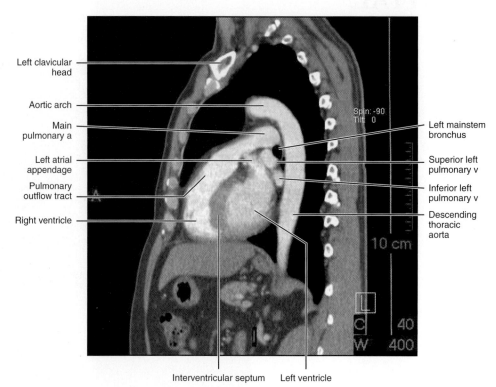

Left clavicular head

Aortic arch

Main pulmonary a

Left atrial appendage

Pulmonary outflow tract

Right ventricle

Left mainstem bronchus

Superior left pulmonary v

Inferior left pulmonary v

Descending thoracic aorta

10 cm

40

400

Interventricular septum   Left ventricle

Figure 18.2.3

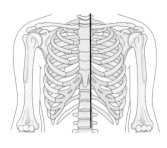

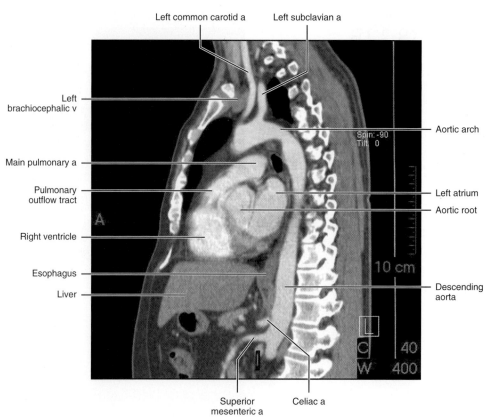

Left common carotid a   Left subclavian a

Left brachiocephalic v

Main pulmonary a

Pulmonary outflow tract

Right ventricle

Esophagus

Liver

Aortic arch

Left atrium

Aortic root

Descending aorta

10 cm

40

400

Superior mesenteric a   Celiac a

Figure 18.2.4

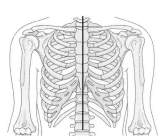

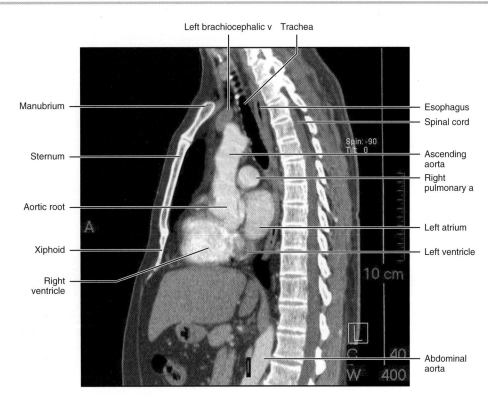

Left brachiocephalic v   Trachea

Manubrium

Sternum

Aortic root

Xiphoid

Right ventricle

Esophagus

Spinal cord

Ascending aorta

Right pulmonary a

Left atrium

Left ventricle

10 cm

Abdominal aorta

Figure 18.2.5

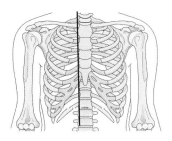

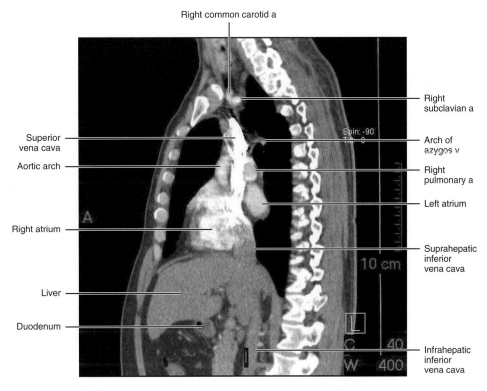

Right common carotid a

Superior vena cava

Aortic arch

Right atrium

Liver

Duodenum

Right subclavian a

Arch of azygos v

Right pulmonary a

Left atrium

Suprahepatic inferior vena cava

10 cm

Infrahepatic inferior vena cava

Figure 18.2.6

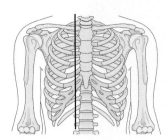

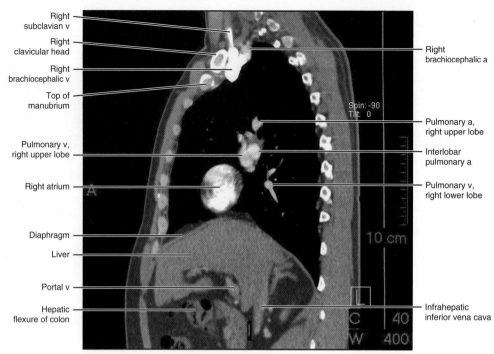

Right subclavian v

Right clavicular head

Right brachiocephalic v

Top of manubrium

Pulmonary v, right upper lobe

Right atrium

Diaphragm

Liver

Portal v

Hepatic flexure of colon

Right brachiocephalic a

Pulmonary a, right upper lobe

Interlobar pulmonary a

Pulmonary v, right lower lobe

Infrahepatic inferior vena cava

Spin: -90
Tilt: 0

10 cm

C 40
W 400

CORONAL
Figure 18.3.1

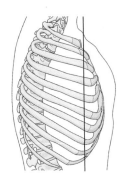

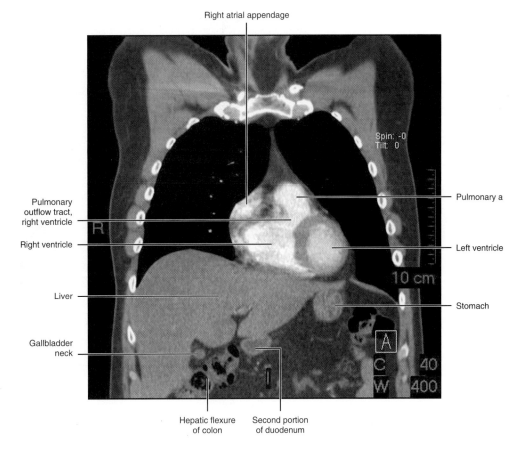

Right atrial appendage

Pulmonary outflow tract, right ventricle

Right ventricle

Liver

Gallbladder neck

Pulmonary a

Left ventricle

Stomach

Hepatic flexure of colon

Second portion of duodenum

Figure 18.3.2

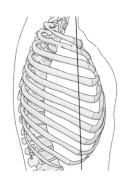

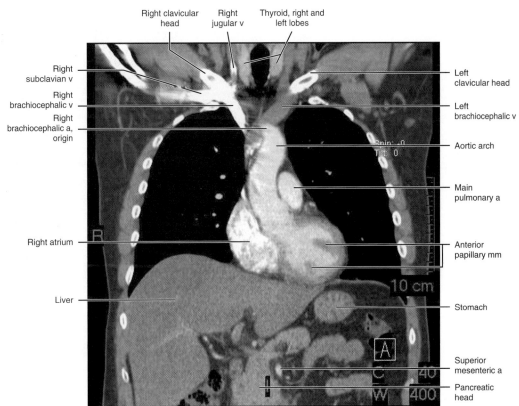

Right clavicular head

Right jugular v

Thyroid, right and left lobes

Right subclavian v

Right brachiocephalic v

Right brachiocephalic a, origin

Right atrium

Liver

Left clavicular head

Left brachiocephalic v

Aortic arch

Main pulmonary a

Anterior papillary mm

Stomach

Superior mesenteric a

Pancreatic head

Figure 18.3.3A

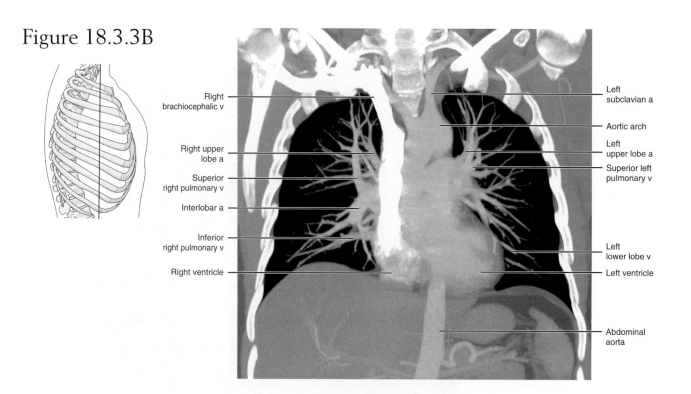

Right common carotid a
Trachea
Left common carotid a

Right subclavian v

Left jugular v

Left subclavian v

Right brachiocephalic v

Left brachiocephalic v

Right brachiocephalic a

Left common carotid a, origin

Aortic arch

Superior vena cava

Main pulmonary a

Left circumflex a

Right atrium

Left ventricular papillary m

10 cm

Splenic a

Portal v

Splenic v

Superior mesenteric a

Plane of aortic valve

Figure 18.3.3B

Right brachiocephalic v

Left subclavian a

Aortic arch

Right upper lobe a

Left upper lobe a

Superior right pulmonary v

Superior left pulmonary v

Interlobar a

Inferior right pulmonary v

Left lower lobe v

Right ventricle

Left ventricle

Abdominal aorta

Figure 18.3.4

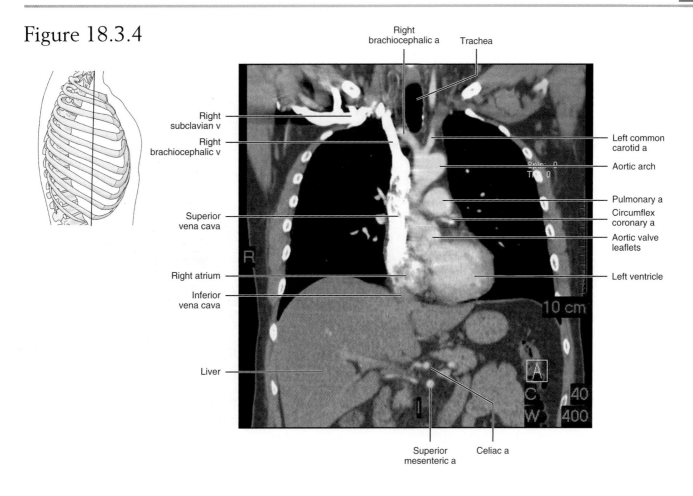

Right brachiocephalic a

Trachea

Right subclavian v

Right brachiocephalic v

Left common carotid a

Aortic arch

Pulmonary a

Circumflex coronary a

Aortic valve leaflets

Superior vena cava

Right atrium

Inferior vena cava

Left ventricle

Liver

Superior mesenteric a

Celiac a

Figure 18.3.5

Esophagus

Trachea

Right upper lobe a

Right pulmonary a

Left subclavian a

Aortic arch

Pulmonary v, left upper lobe

Left atrium

Plane of mitral valve

Suprahepatic inferior vena cava

Intrahepatic inferior vena cava

Infrahepatic inferior vena cava

Celiac a

Superior mesenteric a

Abdominal aorta

Right renal v

Figure 18.3.6A

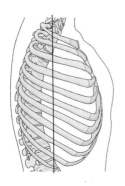

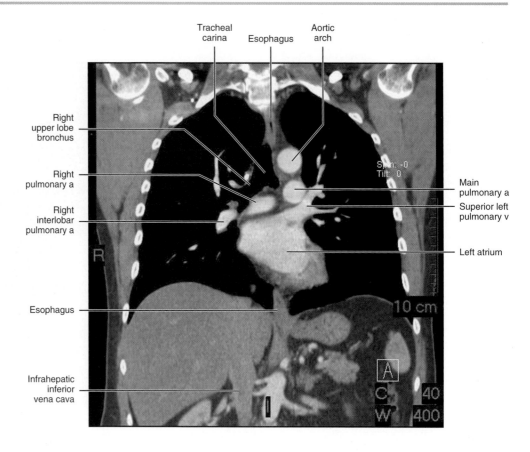

Tracheal carina
Esophagus
Aortic arch
Right upper lobe bronchus
Right pulmonary a
Right interlobar pulmonary a
Main pulmonary a
Superior left pulmonary v
Left atrium
Esophagus
Infrahepatic inferior vena cava
Spin: -0
Tilt: 0
10 cm
A
C 40
W 400
R

Figure 18.3.6B

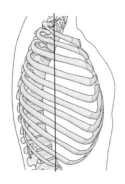

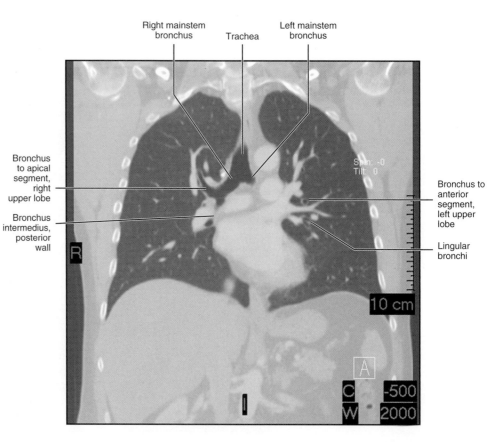

Right mainstem bronchus
Trachea
Left mainstem bronchus
Bronchus to apical segment, right upper lobe
Bronchus to anterior segment, left upper lobe
Bronchus intermedius, posterior wall
Lingular bronchi
Spin: -0
Tilt: 0
10 cm
A
C -500
W 2000
R

Figure 18.3.7A

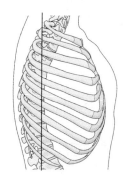

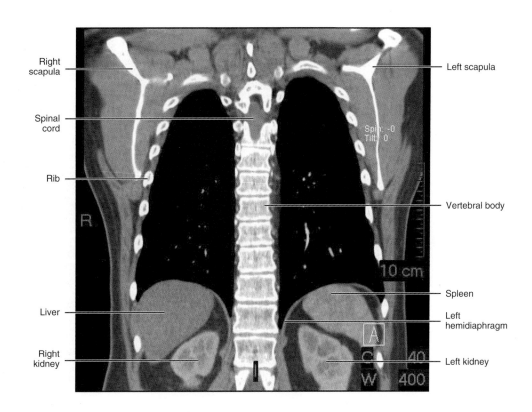

Right scapula — Left scapula

Spinal cord

Rib — Vertebral body

R

10 cm

Liver — Spleen

Right kidney — Left hemidiaphragm

Left kidney

Figure 18.3.7B

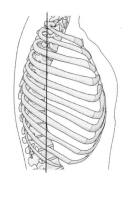

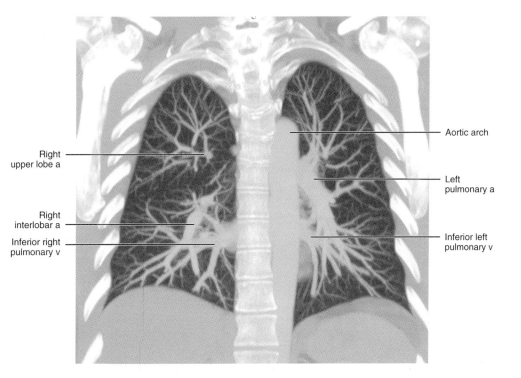

Right upper lobe a — Aortic arch

Left pulmonary a

Right interlobar a

Inferior right pulmonary v — Inferior left pulmonary v

Figure 18.3.8

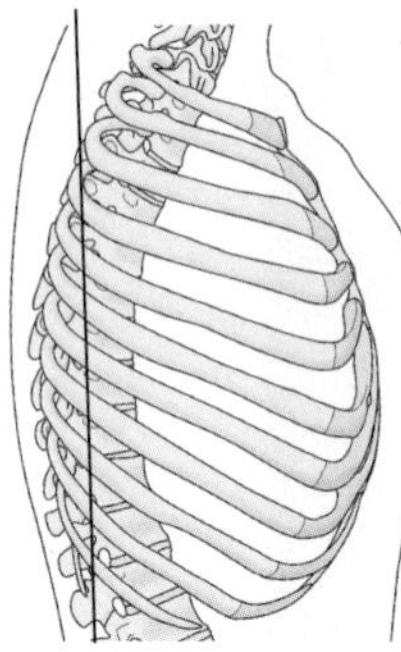

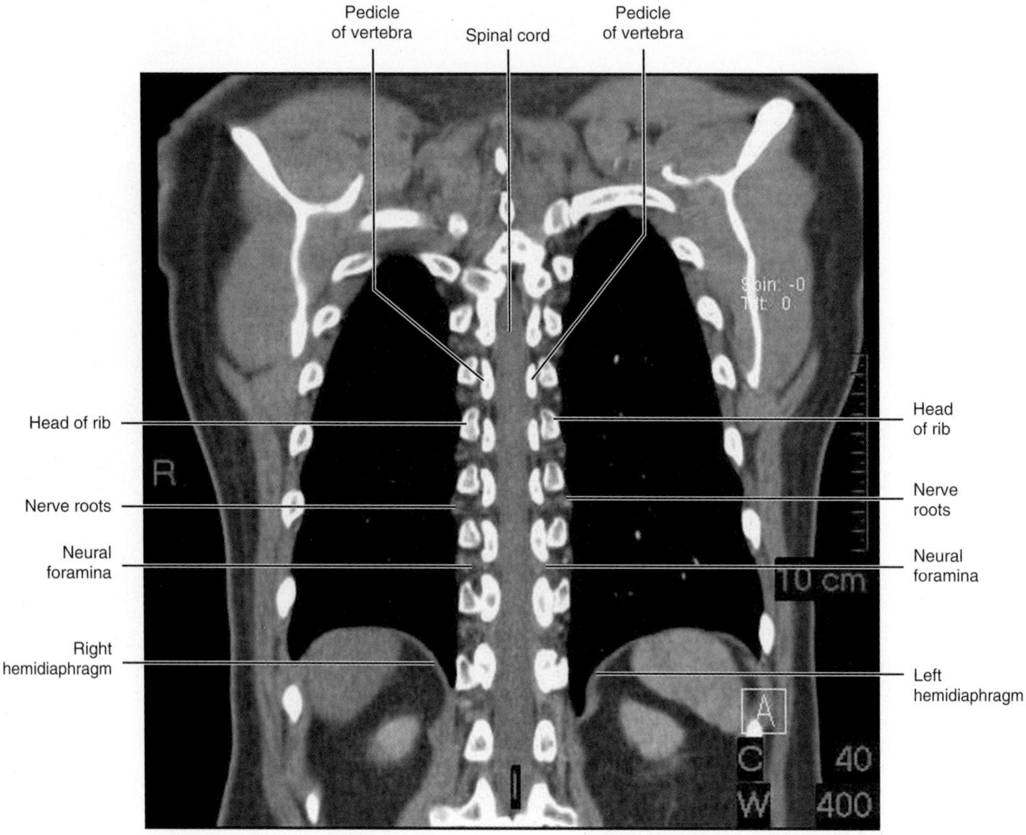

Pedicle of vertebra

Spinal cord

Pedicle of vertebra

Head of rib

Head of rib

Nerve roots

Nerve roots

Neural foramina

Neural foramina

Right hemidiaphragm

Left hemidiaphragm

R

10 cm

Spin: -0
Tilt: 0

A
C   40
W   400

Chapter 19

MRI of the Heart

AXIAL

Figure 19.1.1

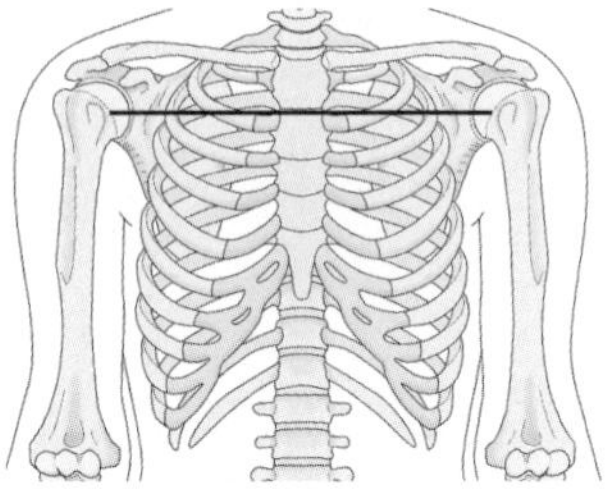

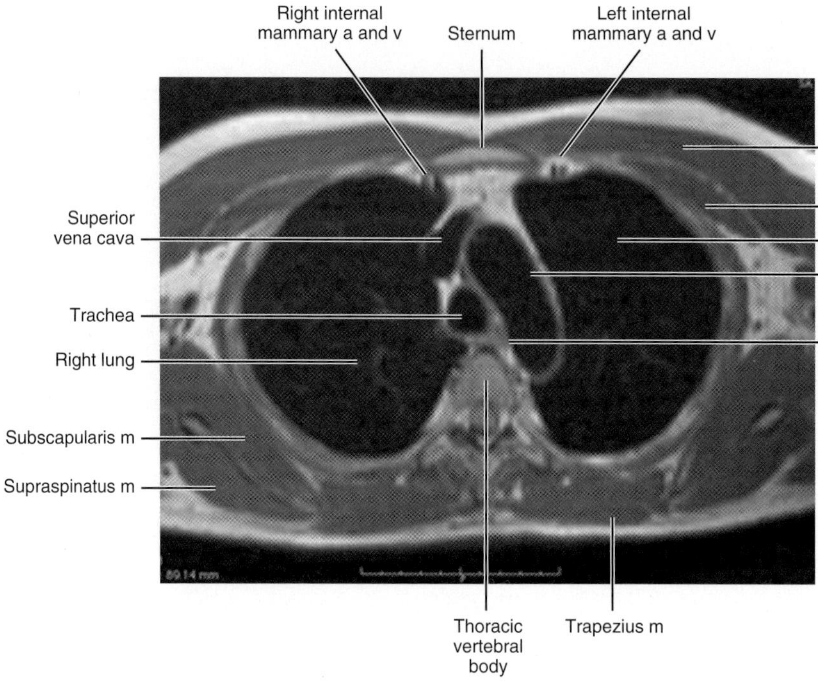

Right internal mammary a and v
Sternum
Left internal mammary a and v

Superior vena cava

Trachea

Right lung

Subscapularis m

Supraspinatus m

Pectoralis major m

Pectoralis minor m

Left lung

Aortic arch

Esophagus

artery = a
arteries = aa
vein = v
veins = vv
muscle = m
muscles = mm
tendon = t
tendons = tt
nerve = n
nerves = nn
ligament = lig
ligaments = ligs

Thoracic vertebral body

Trapezius m

Figure 19.1.2

Superior vena cava

Carina

Right lung

Ascending aorta

Left lung

Descending aorta

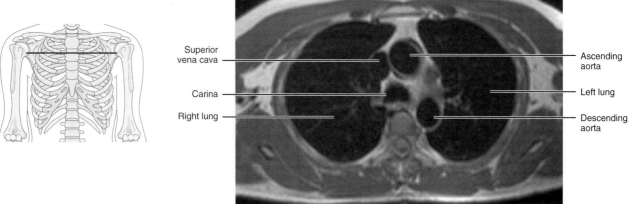

Figure 19.1.3

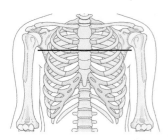

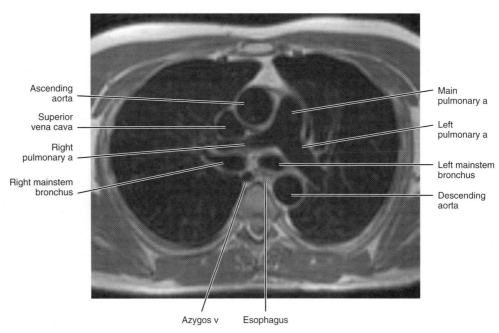

Ascending aorta
Superior vena cava
Right pulmonary a
Right mainstem bronchus

Main pulmonary a
Left pulmonary a
Left mainstem bronchus
Descending aorta

Azygos v   Esophagus

Figure 19.1.4

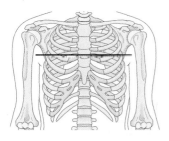

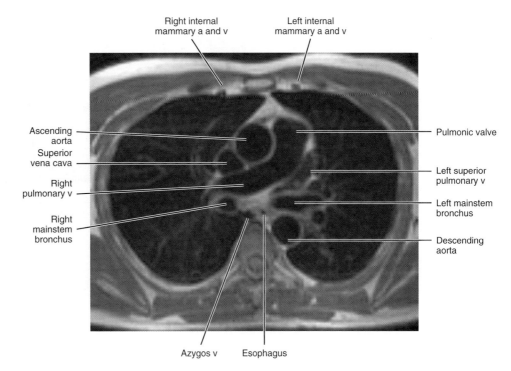

Right internal mammary a and v
Left internal mammary a and v

Ascending aorta
Superior vena cava
Right pulmonary v
Right mainstem bronchus

Pulmonic valve
Left superior pulmonary v
Left mainstem bronchus
Descending aorta

Azygos v   Esophagus

Figure 19.1.5

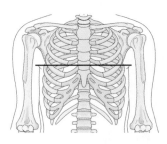

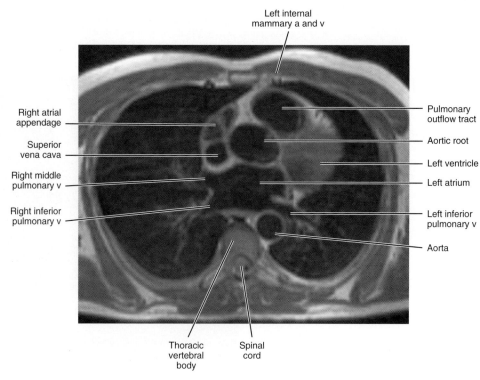

Left internal mammary a and v

Right atrial appendage

Superior vena cava

Right middle pulmonary v

Right inferior pulmonary v

Pulmonary outflow tract

Aortic root

Left ventricle

Left atrium

Left inferior pulmonary v

Aorta

Thoracic vertebral body

Spinal cord

Figure 19.1.6

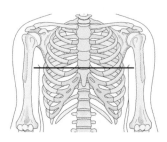

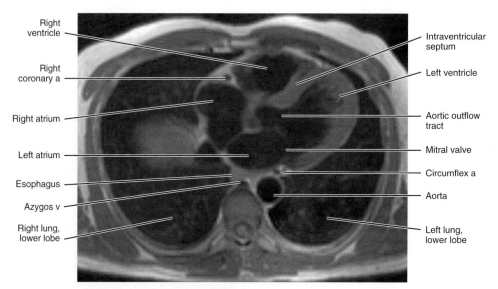

Right ventricle

Right coronary a

Right atrium

Left atrium

Esophagus

Azygos v

Right lung, lower lobe

Intraventricular septum

Left ventricle

Aortic outflow tract

Mitral valve

Circumflex a

Aorta

Left lung, lower lobe

Figure 19.1.7

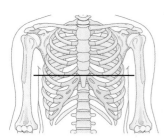

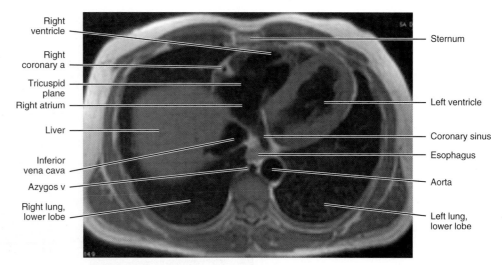

Right ventricle

Right coronary a

Tricuspid plane

Right atrium

Liver

Inferior vena cava

Azygos v

Right lung, lower lobe

Sternum

Left ventricle

Coronary sinus

Esophagus

Aorta

Left lung, lower lobe

SAGITTAL

Figure 19.2.1

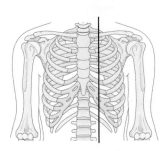

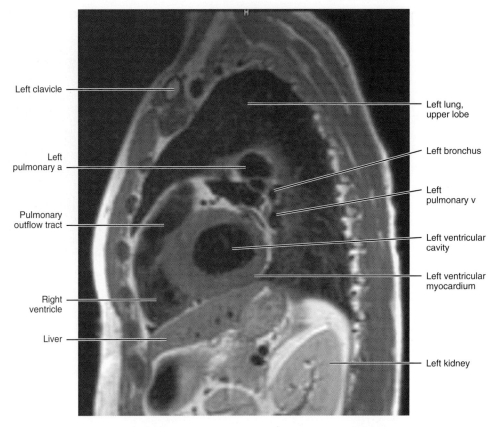

Left clavicle

Left pulmonary a

Pulmonary outflow tract

Right ventricle

Liver

Left lung, upper lobe

Left bronchus

Left pulmonary v

Left ventricular cavity

Left ventricular myocardium

Left kidney

Figure 19.2.2

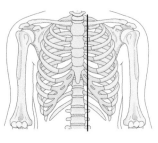

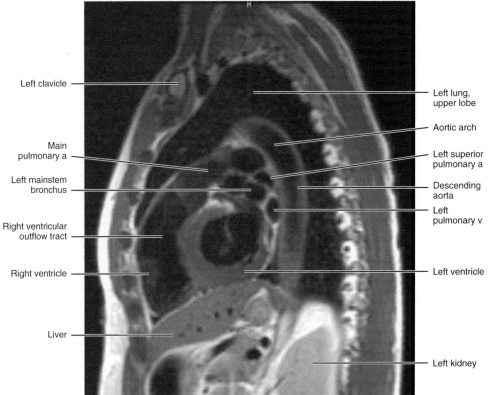

Left clavicle

Main pulmonary a

Left mainstem bronchus

Right ventricular outflow tract

Right ventricle

Liver

Left lung, upper lobe

Aortic arch

Left superior pulmonary a

Descending aorta

Left pulmonary v

Left ventricle

Left kidney

Figure 19.2.3

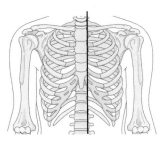

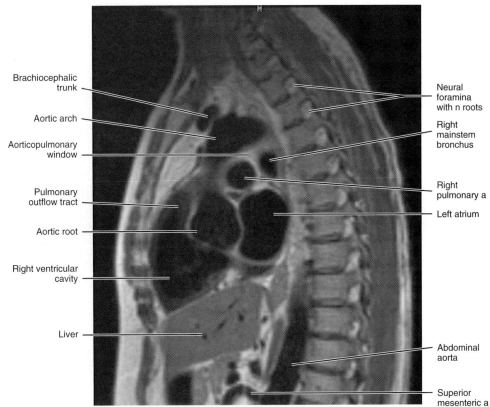

Brachiocephalic trunk

Aortic arch

Aorticopulmonary window

Pulmonary outflow tract

Aortic root

Right ventricular cavity

Liver

Neural foramina with n roots

Right mainstem bronchus

Right pulmonary a

Left atrium

Abdominal aorta

Superior mesenteric a

Figure 19.2.4

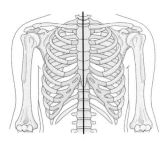

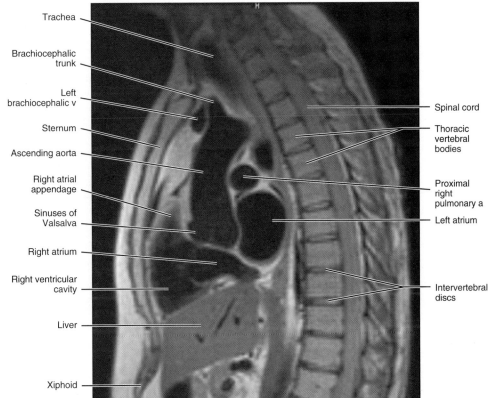

Trachea

Brachiocephalic trunk

Left brachiocephalic v

Sternum

Ascending aorta

Right atrial appendage

Sinuses of Valsalva

Right atrium

Right ventricular cavity

Liver

Xiphoid

Spinal cord

Thoracic vertebral bodies

Proximal right pulmonary a

Left atrium

Intervertebral discs

Figure 19.2.5

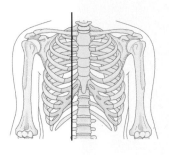

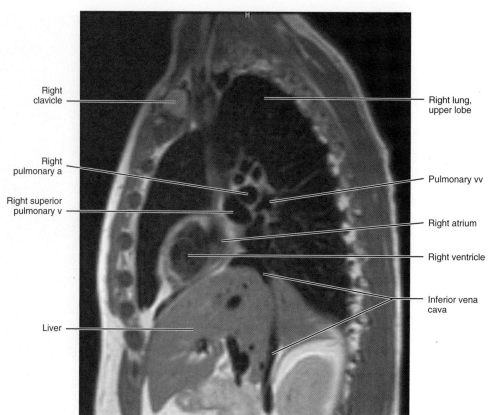

Right clavicle

Right pulmonary a

Right superior pulmonary v

Liver

Right lung, upper lobe

Pulmonary vv

Right atrium

Right ventricle

Inferior vena cava

CORONAL
Figure 19.3.1

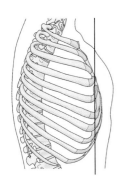

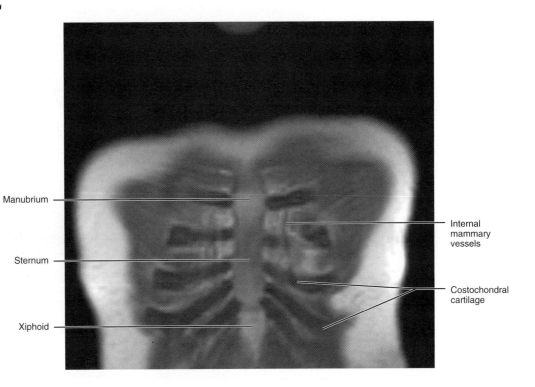

Manubrium

Sternum

Xiphoid

Internal mammary vessels

Costochondral cartilage

Figure 19.3.2

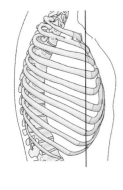

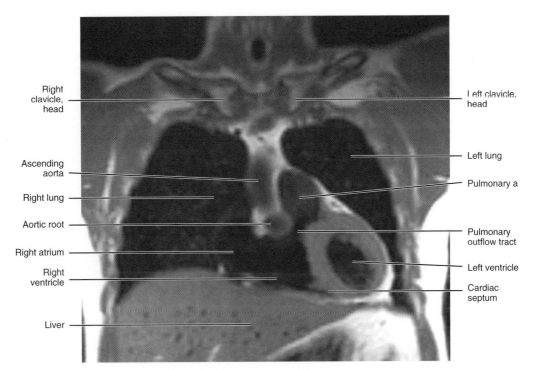

Right clavicle, head

Ascending aorta

Right lung

Aortic root

Right atrium

Right ventricle

Liver

Left clavicle, head

Left lung

Pulmonary a

Pulmonary outflow tract

Left ventricle

Cardiac septum

Figure 19.3.3

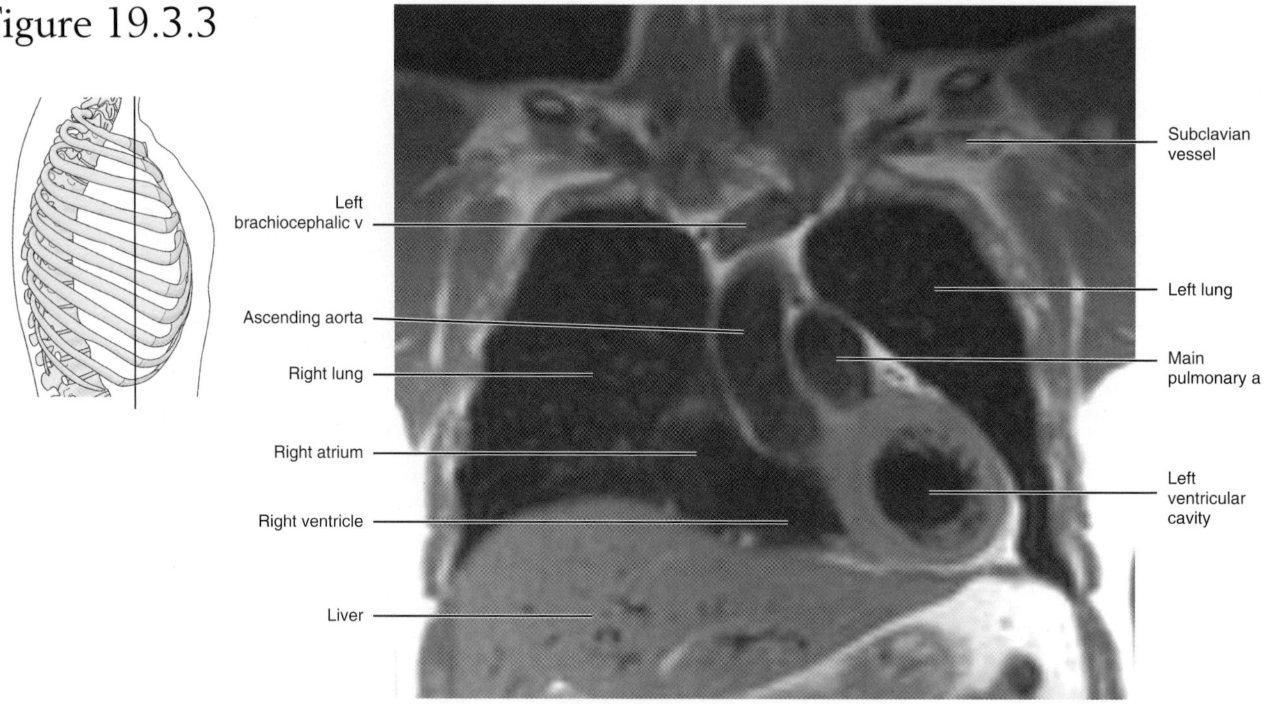

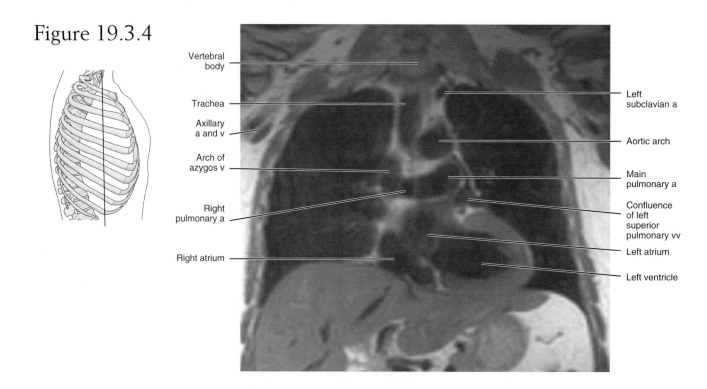

Left brachiocephalic v

Ascending aorta

Right lung

Right atrium

Right ventricle

Liver

Subclavian vessel

Left lung

Main pulmonary a

Left ventricular cavity

Figure 19.3.4

Vertebral body

Trachea

Axillary a and v

Arch of azygos v

Right pulmonary a

Right atrium

Left subclavian a

Aortic arch

Main pulmonary a

Confluence of left superior pulmonary vv

Left atrium

Left ventricle

Figure 19.3.5

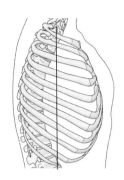

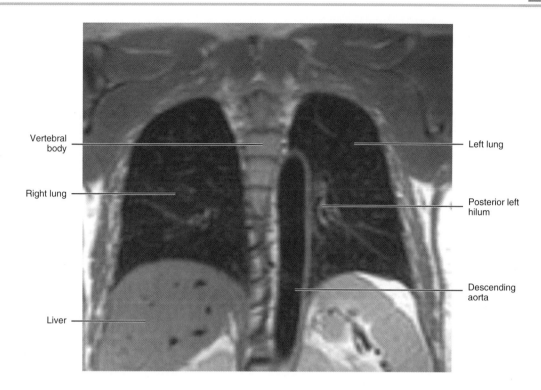

Vertebral body

Right lung

Liver

Left lung

Posterior left hilum

Descending aorta

Abdomen

Table 10: Muscles of the Abdominal Wall

MUSCLE	ORIGIN	INSERTION	NERVE SUPPLY
Rectus abdominis	Crest and symphysis of the pubis	Xiphoid process and fifth to seventh costal cartilages	Branches of the lower thoracic
External oblique (obliquus externus abdominis)	Fifth to twelfth ribs	Anterior half of the iliac crest, inguinal ligament, and anterior layer of the sheath of the rectus abdominis	Ventral branches of the lower thoracic
Internal oblique (obliquus internus abdominis)	Iliac fascia deep to the lateral part of the inguinal ligament, the anterior half of the iliac crest, and the lumbar fascia	Tenth to twelfth ribs and sheath of the rectus abdominis; some fibers from the inguinal ligament terminate in the falx inguinalis	Lower thoracic
Transversus abdominis	Seventh to twelfth costal cartilages, lumbar fascia, iliac crest, and inguinal ligament	Xiphoid cartilage and linea alba and through the falx inguinalis, pubic tubercle, and pecten	Lower thoracic

Chapter 20

CT of the Abdomen

AXIAL
Figure 20.1.1

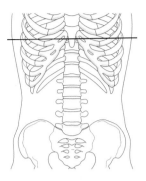

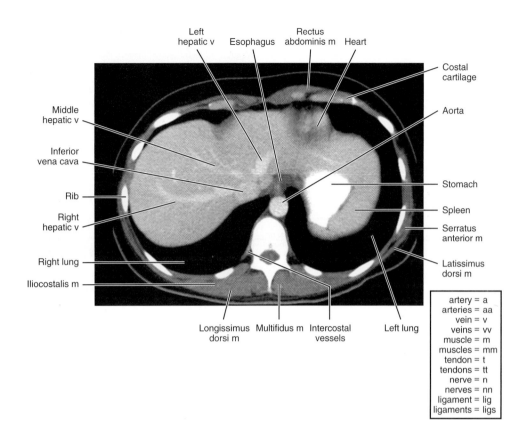

Left hepatic v
Esophagus
Rectus abdominis m
Heart
Costal cartilage
Aorta
Middle hepatic v
Inferior vena cava
Rib
Right hepatic v
Right lung
Iliocostalis m
Stomach
Spleen
Serratus anterior m
Latissimus dorsi m
Longissimus dorsi m
Multifidus m
Intercostal vessels
Left lung

artery = a
arteries = aa
vein = v
veins = vv
muscle = m
muscles = mm
tendon = t
tendons = tt
nerve = n
nerves = nn
ligament = lig
ligaments = ligs

Figure 20.1.2

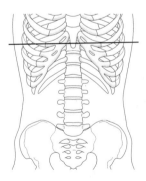

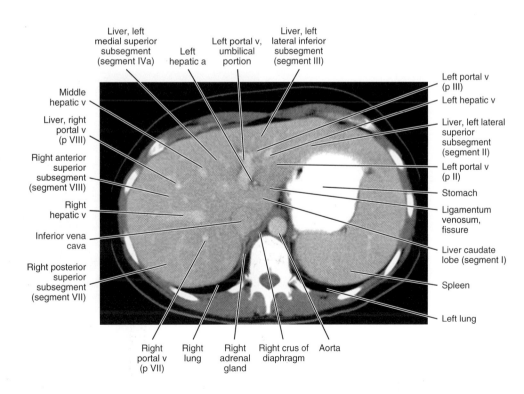

Liver, left medial superior subsegment (segment IVa)
Left hepatic a
Left portal v, umbilical portion
Liver, left lateral inferior subsegment (segment III)
Left portal v (p III)
Left hepatic v
Middle hepatic v
Liver, right portal v (p VIII)
Right anterior superior subsegment (segment VIII)
Right hepatic v
Inferior vena cava
Right posterior superior subsegment (segment VII)
Liver, left lateral superior subsegment (segment II)
Left portal v (p II)
Stomach
Ligamentum venosum, fissure
Liver caudate lobe (segment I)
Spleen
Left lung
Right portal v (p VII)
Right lung
Right adrenal gland
Right crus of diaphragm
Aorta

Figure 20.1.3

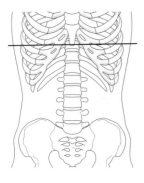

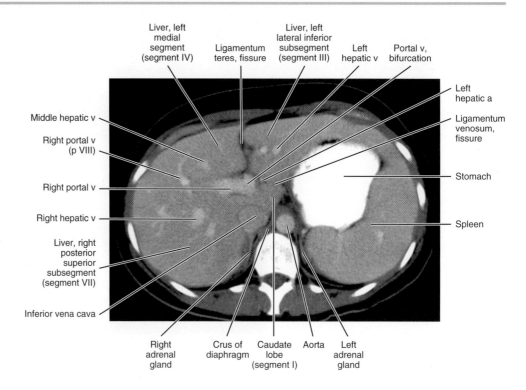

Liver, left medial segment (segment IV)
Ligamentum teres, fissure
Liver, left lateral inferior subsegment (segment III)
Left hepatic v
Portal v, bifurcation
Left hepatic a
Ligamentum venosum, fissure
Stomach
Spleen

Middle hepatic v
Right portal v (p VIII)
Right portal v
Right hepatic v
Liver, right posterior superior subsegment (segment VII)
Inferior vena cava

Right adrenal gland
Crus of diaphragm
Caudate lobe (segment I)
Aorta
Left adrenal gland

Figure 20.1.4

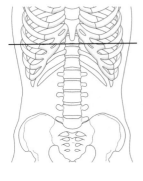

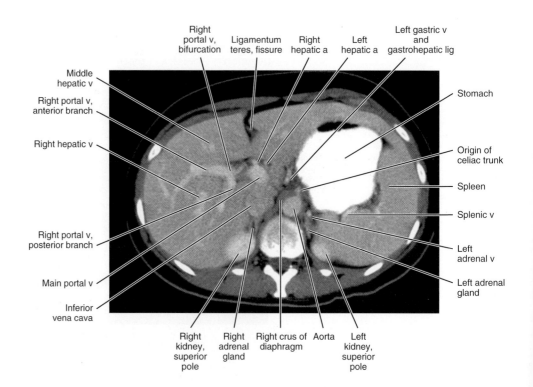

Right portal v, bifurcation
Ligamentum teres, fissure
Right hepatic a
Left hepatic a
Left gastric v and gastrohepatic lig
Stomach
Origin of celiac trunk
Spleen
Splenic v
Left adrenal v
Left adrenal gland

Middle hepatic v
Right portal v, anterior branch
Right hepatic v
Right portal v, posterior branch
Main portal v
Inferior vena cava

Right kidney, superior pole
Right adrenal gland
Right crus of diaphragm
Aorta
Left kidney, superior pole

Figure 20.1.5

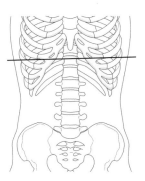

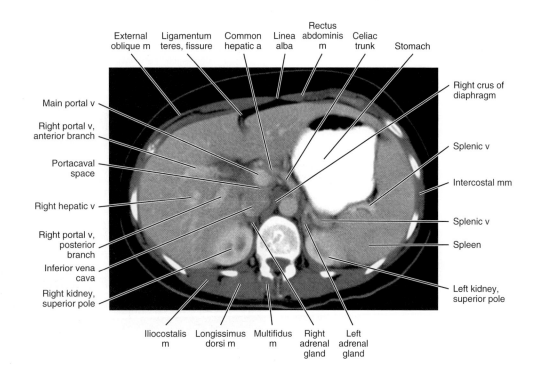

External oblique m
Ligamentum teres, fissure
Common hepatic a
Linea alba
Rectus abdominis m
Celiac trunk
Stomach
Right crus of diaphragm
Splenic v
Intercostal mm
Splenic v
Spleen
Left kidney, superior pole
Main portal v
Right portal v, anterior branch
Portacaval space
Right hepatic v
Right portal v, posterior branch
Inferior vena cava
Right kidney, superior pole
Iliocostalis m
Longissimus dorsi m
Multifidus m
Right adrenal gland
Left adrenal gland

Figure 20.1.6

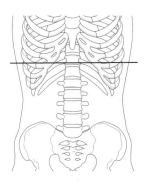

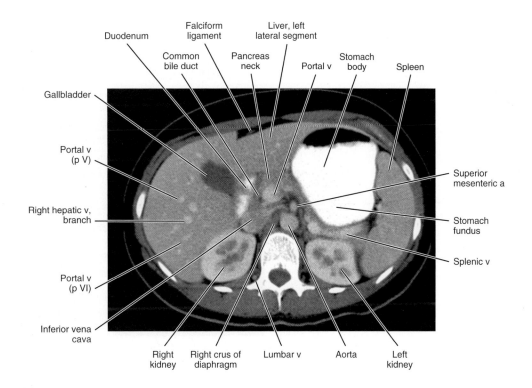

Duodenum
Falciform ligament
Liver, left lateral segment
Common bile duct
Pancreas neck
Portal v
Stomach body
Spleen
Gallbladder
Portal v (p V)
Right hepatic v, branch
Portal v (p VI)
Inferior vena cava
Superior mesenteric a
Stomach fundus
Splenic v
Right kidney
Right crus of diaphragm
Lumbar v
Aorta
Left kidney

Figure 20.1.7

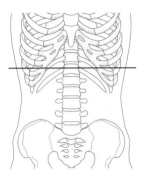

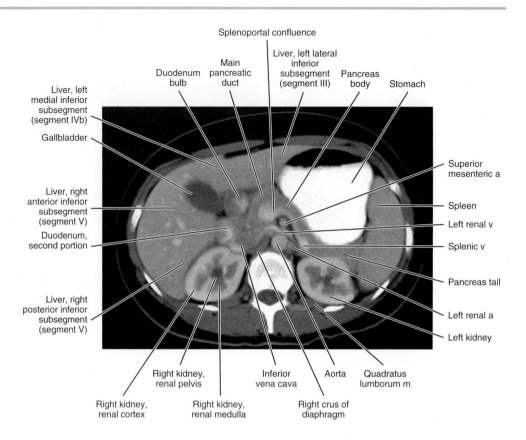

Splenoportal confluence

Duodenum bulb

Main pancreatic duct

Liver, left lateral inferior subsegment (segment III)

Pancreas body

Stomach

Liver, left medial inferior subsegment (segment IVb)

Gallbladder

Superior mesenteric a

Spleen

Left renal v

Liver, right anterior inferior subsegment (segment V)

Duodenum, second portion

Splenic v

Pancreas tail

Liver, right posterior inferior subsegment (segment V)

Left renal a

Left kidney

Right kidney, renal pelvis

Inferior vena cava

Aorta

Quadratus lumborum m

Right kidney, renal cortex

Right kidney, renal medulla

Right crus of diaphragm

Figure 20.1.8

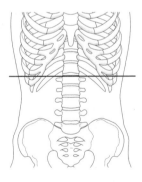

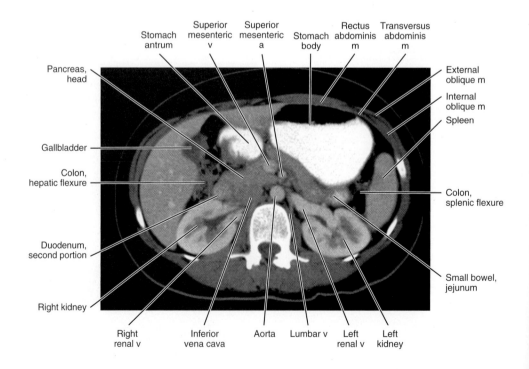

Stomach antrum

Superior mesenteric v

Superior mesenteric a

Stomach body

Rectus abdominis m

Transversus abdominis m

Pancreas, head

External oblique m

Internal oblique m

Spleen

Gallbladder

Colon, hepatic flexure

Colon, splenic flexure

Duodenum, second portion

Small bowel, jejunum

Right kidney

Right renal v

Inferior vena cava

Aorta

Lumbar v

Left renal v

Left kidney

Figure 20.1.9

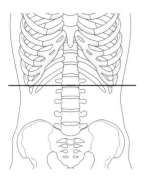

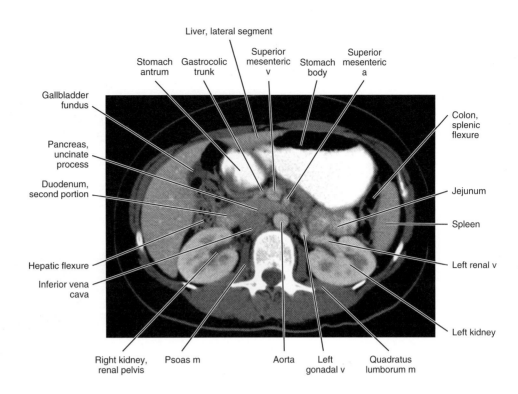

Liver, lateral segment
Stomach antrum
Gastrocolic trunk
Superior mesenteric v
Stomach body
Superior mesenteric a
Gallbladder fundus
Pancreas, uncinate process
Duodenum, second portion
Hepatic flexure
Inferior vena cava
Colon, splenic flexure
Jejunum
Spleen
Left renal v
Left kidney
Right kidney, renal pelvis
Psoas m
Aorta
Left gonadal v
Quadratus lumborum m

Figure 20.1.10

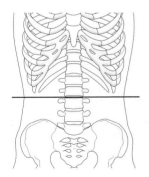

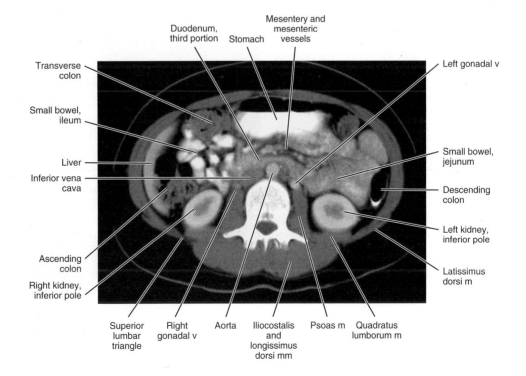

Duodenum, third portion
Stomach
Mesentery and mesenteric vessels
Left gonadal v
Transverse colon
Small bowel, ileum
Liver
Inferior vena cava
Small bowel, jejunum
Descending colon
Left kidney, inferior pole
Latissimus dorsi m
Ascending colon
Right kidney, inferior pole
Superior lumbar triangle
Right gonadal v
Aorta
Iliocostalis and longissimus dorsi mm
Psoas m
Quadratus lumborum m

Figure 20.1.11

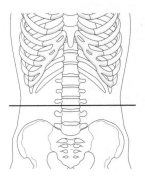

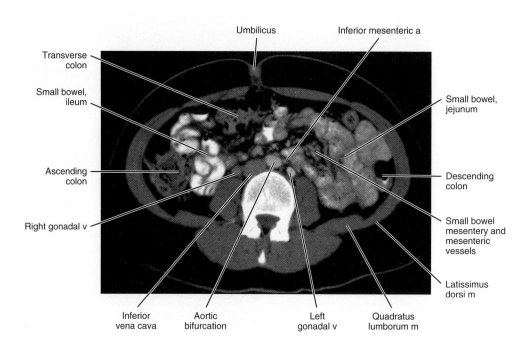

Umbilicus — Inferior mesenteric a

Transverse colon

Small bowel, ileum

Ascending colon

Right gonadal v

Small bowel, jejunum

Descending colon

Small bowel mesentery and mesenteric vessels

Latissimus dorsi m

Inferior vena cava — Aortic bifurcation — Left gonadal v — Quadratus lumborum m

Figure 20.1.12

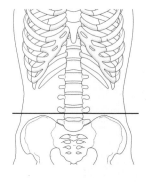

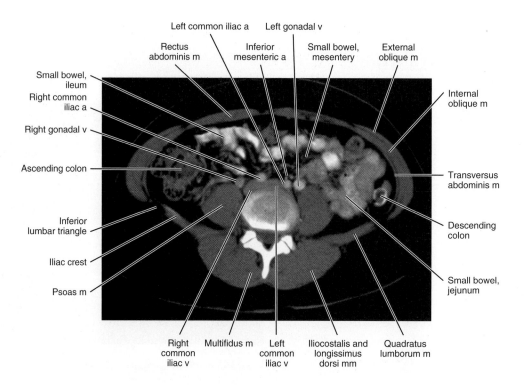

Left common iliac a — Left gonadal v

Rectus abdominis m — Inferior mesenteric a — Small bowel, mesentery — External oblique m

Small bowel, ileum

Right common iliac a

Right gonadal v

Ascending colon

Inferior lumbar triangle

Iliac crest

Psoas m

Internal oblique m

Transversus abdominis m

Descending colon

Small bowel, jejunum

Right common iliac v — Multifidus m — Left common iliac v — Iliocostalis and longissimus dorsi mm — Quadratus lumborum m

SAGITTAL

Figure 20.2.1

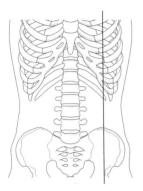

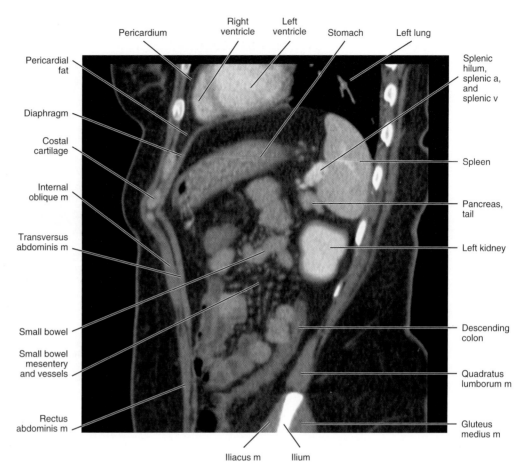

Pericardium · Right ventricle · Left ventricle · Stomach · Left lung

Pericardial fat · Splenic hilum, splenic a, and splenic v

Diaphragm · Spleen

Costal cartilage · Pancreas, tail

Internal oblique m · Left kidney

Transversus abdominis m

Small bowel · Descending colon

Small bowel mesentery and vessels · Quadratus lumborum m

Rectus abdominis m · Gluteus medius m

Iliacus m · Ilium

Figure 20.2.2

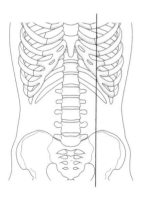

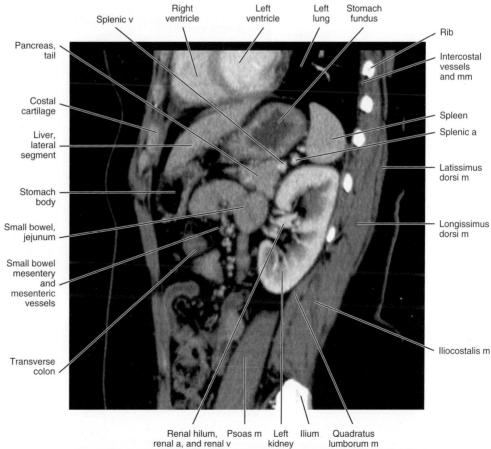

Splenic v · Right ventricle · Left ventricle · Left lung · Stomach fundus · Rib

Pancreas, tail · Intercostal vessels and mm

Costal cartilage · Spleen

Liver, lateral segment · Splenic a

Latissimus dorsi m

Stomach body · Longissimus dorsi m

Small bowel, jejunum

Small bowel mesentery and mesenteric vessels

Iliocostalis m

Transverse colon

Renal hilum, renal a, and renal v · Psoas m · Left kidney · Ilium · Quadratus lumborum m

Figure 20.2.3

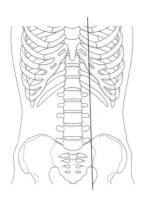

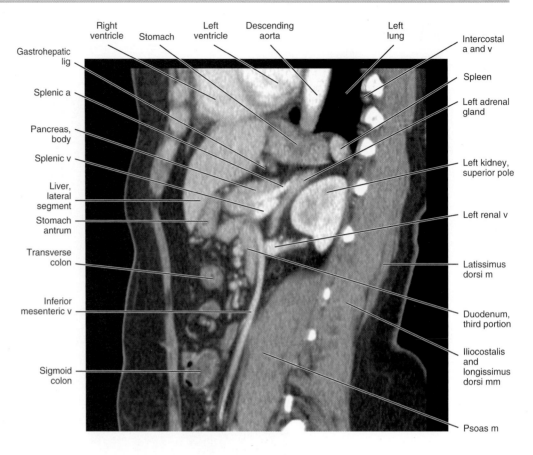

Right ventricle

Stomach

Left ventricle

Descending aorta

Left lung

Gastrohepatic lig

Intercostal a and v

Splenic a

Spleen

Pancreas, body

Left adrenal gland

Splenic v

Left kidney, superior pole

Liver, lateral segment

Left renal v

Stomach antrum

Transverse colon

Latissimus dorsi m

Inferior mesenteric v

Duodenum, third portion

Iliocostalis and longissimus dorsi mm

Sigmoid colon

Psoas m

Figure 20.2.4

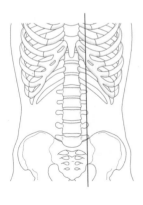

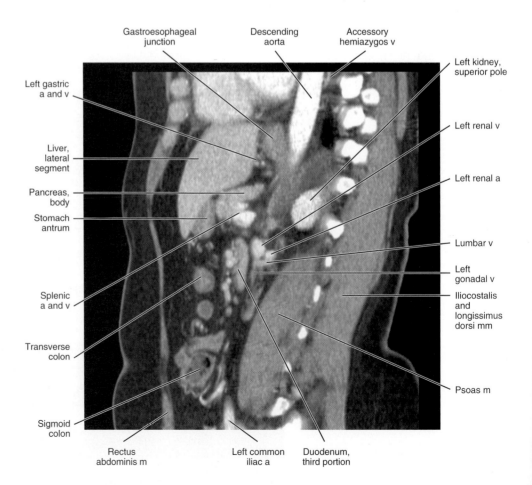

Gastroesophageal junction

Descending aorta

Accessory hemiazygos v

Left kidney, superior pole

Left gastric a and v

Left renal v

Liver, lateral segment

Left renal a

Pancreas, body

Stomach antrum

Lumbar v

Left gonadal v

Splenic a and v

Iliocostalis and longissimus dorsi mm

Transverse colon

Psoas m

Sigmoid colon

Rectus abdominis m

Left common iliac a

Duodenum, third portion

Figure 20.2.5

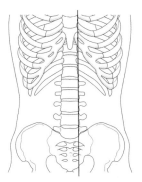

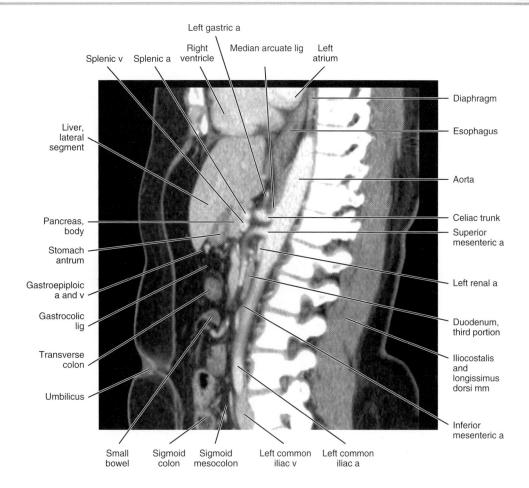

Left gastric a

Splenic v · Splenic a · Right ventricle · Median arcuate lig · Left atrium

Diaphragm

Esophagus

Liver, lateral segment

Aorta

Celiac trunk

Pancreas, body

Superior mesenteric a

Stomach antrum

Left renal a

Gastroepiploic a and v

Gastrocolic lig

Duodenum, third portion

Transverse colon

Iliocostalis and longissimus dorsi mm

Umbilicus

Inferior mesenteric a

Small bowel · Sigmoid colon · Sigmoid mesocolon · Left common iliac v · Left common iliac a

Figure 20.2.6

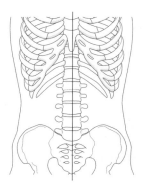

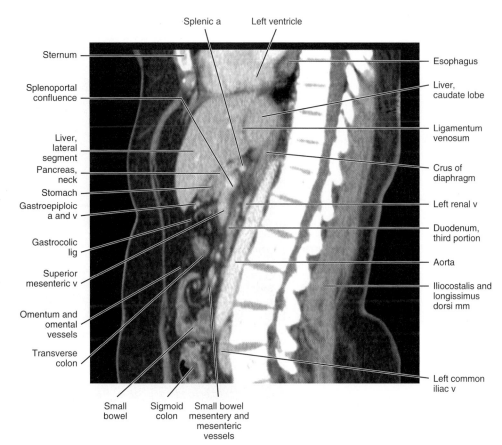

Splenic a · Left ventricle

Sternum

Esophagus

Splenoportal confluence

Liver, caudate lobe

Ligamentum venosum

Liver, lateral segment

Pancreas, neck

Crus of diaphragm

Stomach

Left renal v

Gastroepiploic a and v

Gastrocolic lig

Duodenum, third portion

Aorta

Superior mesenteric v

Iliocostalis and longissimus dorsi mm

Omentum and omental vessels

Transverse colon

Left common iliac v

Small bowel · Sigmoid colon · Small bowel mesentery and mesenteric vessels

Figure 20.2.7

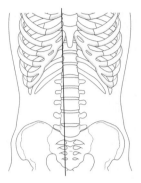

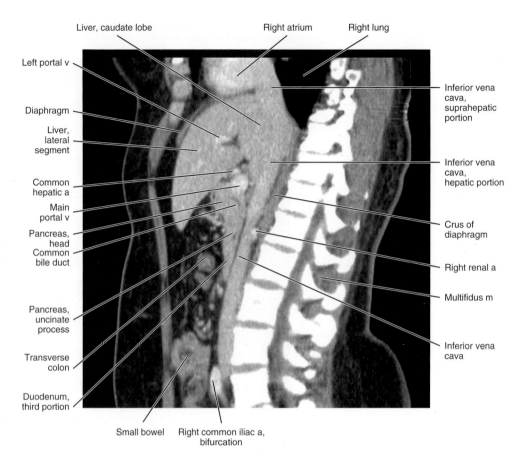

Liver, caudate lobe
Right atrium
Right lung
Left portal v
Diaphragm
Liver, lateral segment
Common hepatic a
Main portal v
Pancreas, head
Common bile duct
Pancreas, uncinate process
Transverse colon
Duodenum, third portion
Inferior vena cava, suprahepatic portion
Inferior vena cava, hepatic portion
Crus of diaphragm
Right renal a
Multifidus m
Inferior vena cava
Small bowel
Right common iliac a, bifurcation

Figure 20.2.8

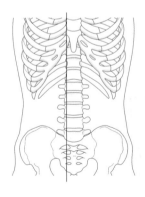

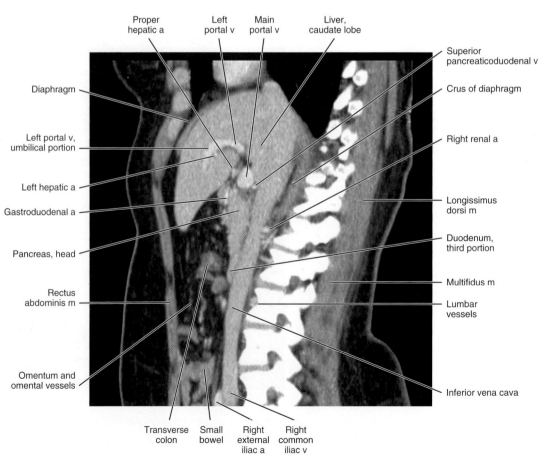

Proper hepatic a
Left portal v
Main portal v
Liver, caudate lobe
Diaphragm
Left portal v, umbilical portion
Left hepatic a
Gastroduodenal a
Pancreas, head
Rectus abdominis m
Omentum and omental vessels
Superior pancreaticoduodenal v
Crus of diaphragm
Right renal a
Longissimus dorsi m
Duodenum, third portion
Multifidus m
Lumbar vessels
Inferior vena cava
Transverse colon
Small bowel
Right external iliac a
Right common iliac v

Figure 20.2.9

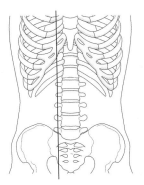

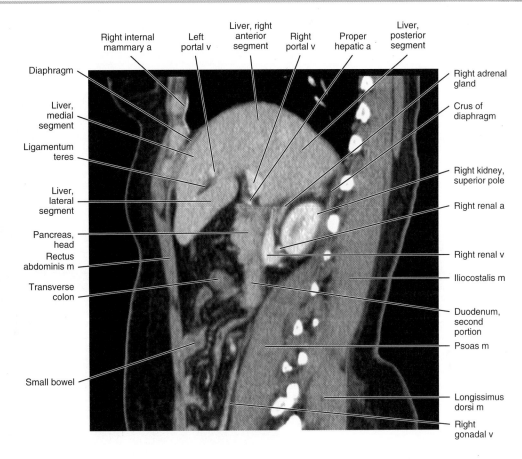

Right internal mammary a

Left portal v

Liver, right anterior segment

Right portal v

Proper hepatic a

Liver, posterior segment

Diaphragm

Liver, medial segment

Ligamentum teres

Liver, lateral segment

Pancreas, head

Rectus abdominis m

Transverse colon

Small bowel

Right adrenal gland

Crus of diaphragm

Right kidney, superior pole

Right renal a

Right renal v

Iliocostalis m

Duodenum, second portion

Psoas m

Longissimus dorsi m

Right gonadal v

Figure 20.2.10

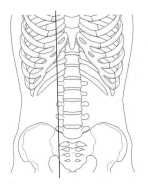

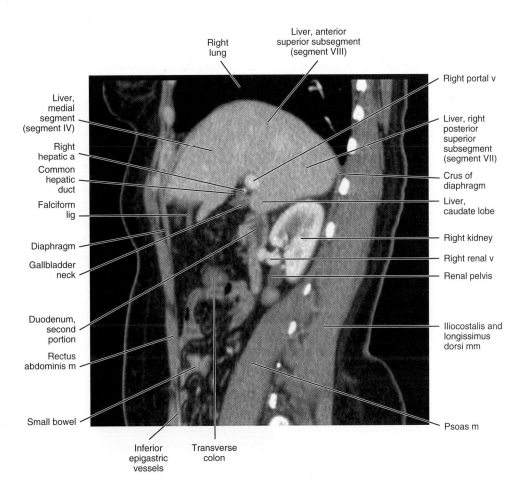

Right lung

Liver, anterior superior subsegment (segment VIII)

Right portal v

Liver, medial segment (segment IV)

Right hepatic a

Common hepatic duct

Falciform lig

Diaphragm

Gallbladder neck

Duodenum, second portion

Rectus abdominis m

Small bowel

Inferior epigastric vessels

Transverse colon

Liver, right posterior superior subsegment (segment VII)

Crus of diaphragm

Liver, caudate lobe

Right kidney

Right renal v

Renal pelvis

Iliocostalis and longissimus dorsi mm

Psoas m

Figure 20.2.11

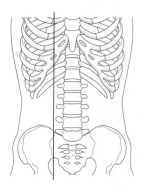

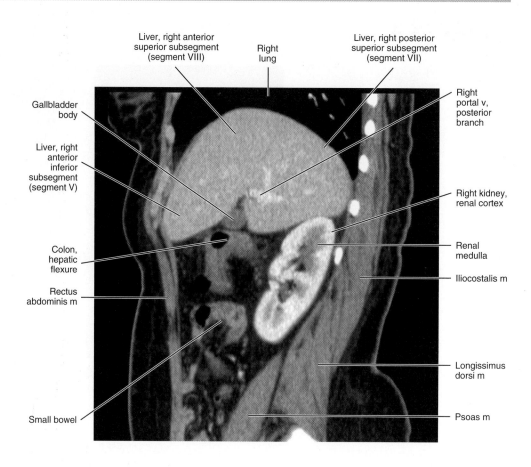

Liver, right anterior superior subsegment (segment VIII)

Right lung

Liver, right posterior superior subsegment (segment VII)

Gallbladder body

Right portal v, posterior branch

Liver, right anterior inferior subsegment (segment V)

Right kidney, renal cortex

Colon, hepatic flexure

Renal medulla

Rectus abdominis m

Iliocostalis m

Longissimus dorsi m

Small bowel

Psoas m

Figure 20.2.12

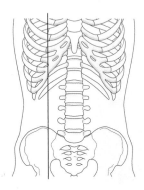

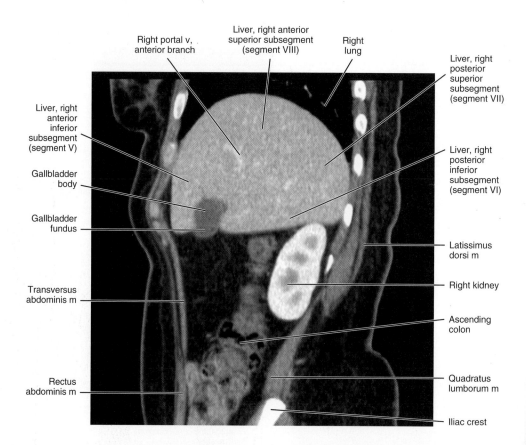

Right portal v, anterior branch

Liver, right anterior superior subsegment (segment VIII)

Right lung

Liver, right posterior superior subsegment (segment VII)

Liver, right anterior inferior subsegment (segment V)

Liver, right posterior inferior subsegment (segment VI)

Gallbladder body

Gallbladder fundus

Latissimus dorsi m

Right kidney

Transversus abdominis m

Ascending colon

Quadratus lumborum m

Rectus abdominis m

Iliac crest

CORONAL
Figure 20.3.1

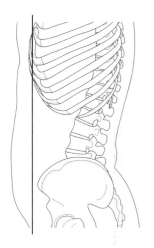

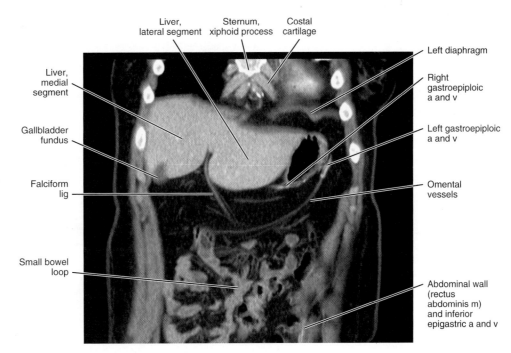

Liver, lateral segment
Sternum, xiphoid process
Costal cartilage
Left diaphragm
Right gastroepiploic a and v
Left gastroepiploic a and v
Liver, medial segment
Omental vessels
Gallbladder fundus
Falciform lig
Small bowel loop
Abdominal wall (rectus abdominis m) and inferior epigastric a and v

Figure 20.3.2

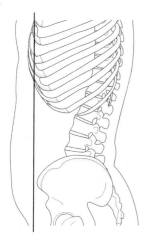

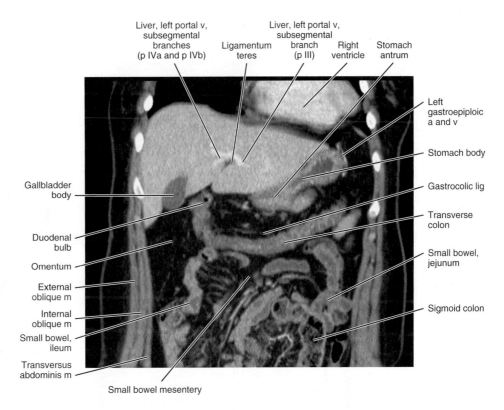

Liver, left portal v, subsegmental branches (p IVa and p IVb)
Ligamentum teres
Liver, left portal v, subsegmental branch (p III)
Right ventricle
Stomach antrum
Left gastroepiploic a and v
Stomach body
Gallbladder body
Gastrocolic lig
Transverse colon
Duodenal bulb
Small bowel, jejunum
Omentum
External oblique m
Internal oblique m
Sigmoid colon
Small bowel, ileum
Transversus abdominis m
Small bowel mesentery

Figure 20.3.3

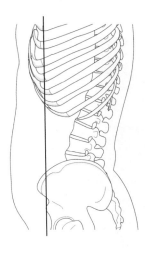

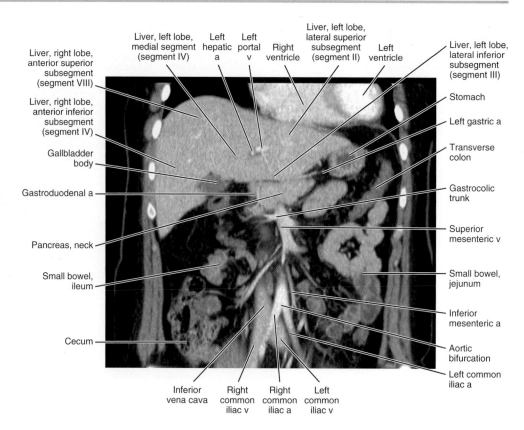

Liver, right lobe, anterior superior subsegment (segment VIII)

Liver, right lobe, anterior inferior subsegment (segment IV)

Gallbladder body

Gastroduodenal a

Pancreas, neck

Small bowel, ileum

Cecum

Liver, left lobe, medial segment (segment IV)

Left hepatic a

Left portal v

Right ventricle

Liver, left lobe, lateral superior subsegment (segment II)

Left ventricle

Liver, left lobe, lateral inferior subsegment (segment III)

Stomach

Left gastric a

Transverse colon

Gastrocolic trunk

Superior mesenteric v

Small bowel, jejunum

Inferior mesenteric a

Aortic bifurcation

Left common iliac a

Inferior vena cava

Right common iliac v

Right common iliac a

Left common iliac v

Figure 20.3.4

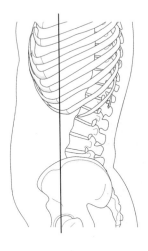

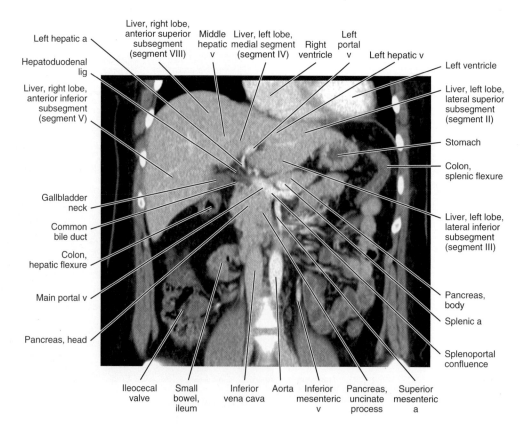

Left hepatic a

Hepatoduodenal lig

Liver, right lobe, anterior inferior subsegment (segment V)

Gallbladder neck

Common bile duct

Colon, hepatic flexure

Main portal v

Pancreas, head

Liver, right lobe, anterior superior subsegment (segment VIII)

Middle hepatic v

Liver, left lobe, medial segment (segment IV)

Right ventricle

Left portal v

Left hepatic v

Left ventricle

Liver, left lobe, lateral superior subsegment (segment II)

Stomach

Colon, splenic flexure

Liver, left lobe, lateral inferior subsegment (segment III)

Pancreas, body

Splenic a

Splenoportal confluence

Ileocecal valve

Small bowel, ileum

Inferior vena cava

Aorta

Inferior mesenteric v

Pancreas, uncinate process

Superior mesenteric a

Figure 20.3.5

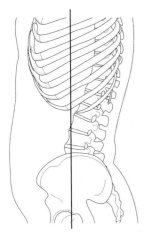

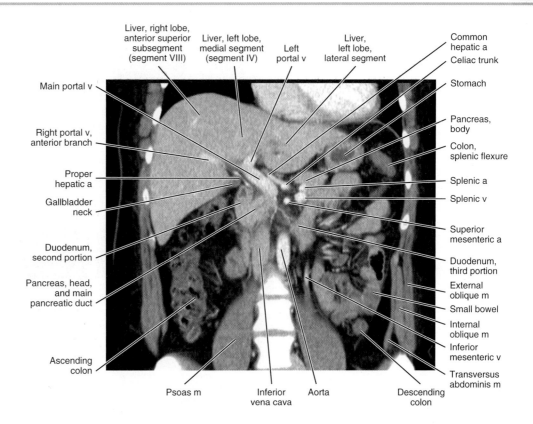

Liver, right lobe, anterior superior subsegment (segment VIII)

Liver, left lobe, medial segment (segment IV)

Left portal v

Liver, left lobe, lateral segment

Common hepatic a

Celiac trunk

Stomach

Pancreas, body

Colon, splenic flexure

Splenic a

Splenic v

Superior mesenteric a

Duodenum, third portion

External oblique m

Small bowel

Internal oblique m

Inferior mesenteric v

Transversus abdominis m

Descending colon

Main portal v

Right portal v, anterior branch

Proper hepatic a

Gallbladder neck

Duodenum, second portion

Pancreas, head, and main pancreatic duct

Ascending colon

Psoas m

Inferior vena cava

Aorta

Figure 20.3.6

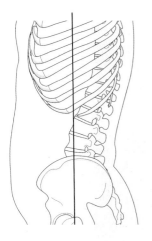

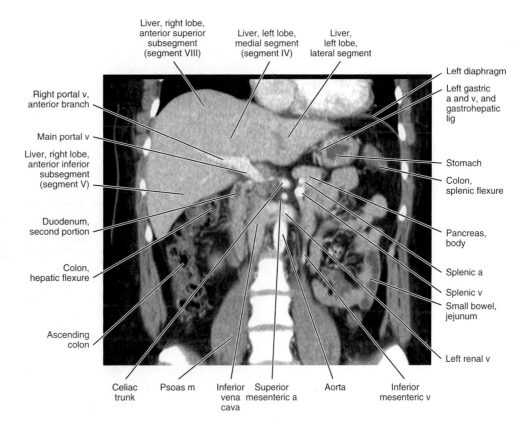

Liver, right lobe, anterior superior subsegment (segment VIII)

Liver, left lobe, medial segment (segment IV)

Liver, left lobe, lateral segment

Left diaphragm

Left gastric a and v, and gastrohepatic lig

Stomach

Colon, splenic flexure

Pancreas, body

Splenic a

Splenic v

Small bowel, jejunum

Left renal v

Right portal v, anterior branch

Main portal v

Liver, right lobe, anterior inferior subsegment (segment V)

Duodenum, second portion

Colon, hepatic flexure

Ascending colon

Celiac trunk

Psoas m

Inferior vena cava

Superior mesenteric a

Aorta

Inferior mesenteric v

Figure 20.3.7

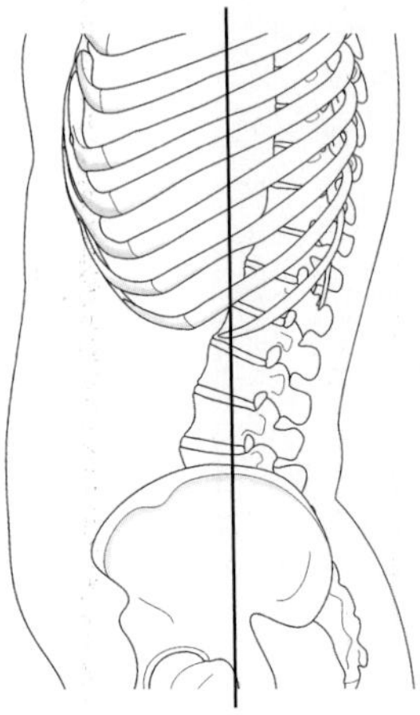

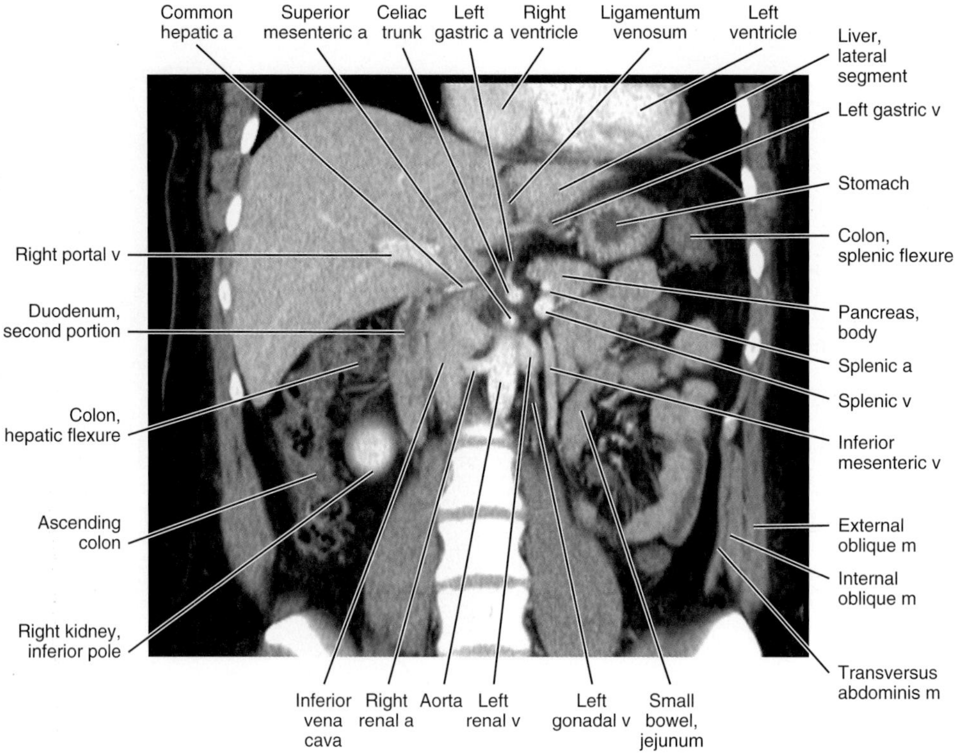

Common hepatic a
Superior mesenteric a
Celiac trunk
Left gastric a
Right ventricle
Ligamentum venosum
Left ventricle
Liver, lateral segment
Left gastric v
Stomach
Colon, splenic flexure
Pancreas, body
Splenic a
Splenic v
Inferior mesenteric v
External oblique m
Internal oblique m
Transversus abdominis m

Right portal v
Duodenum, second portion
Colon, hepatic flexure
Ascending colon
Right kidney, inferior pole

Inferior vena cava
Right renal a
Aorta
Left renal v
Left gonadal v
Small bowel, jejunum

Figure 20.3.8

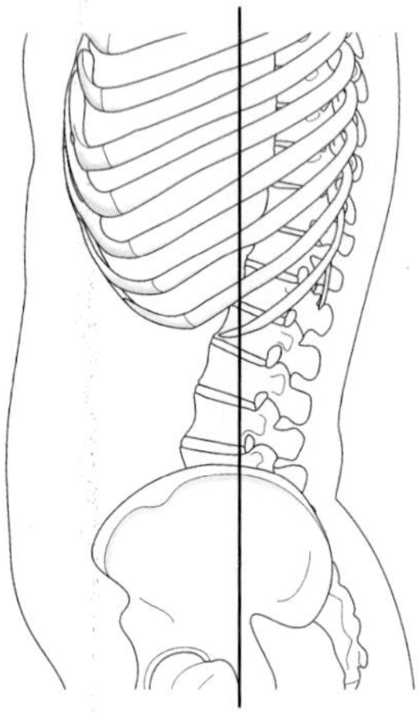

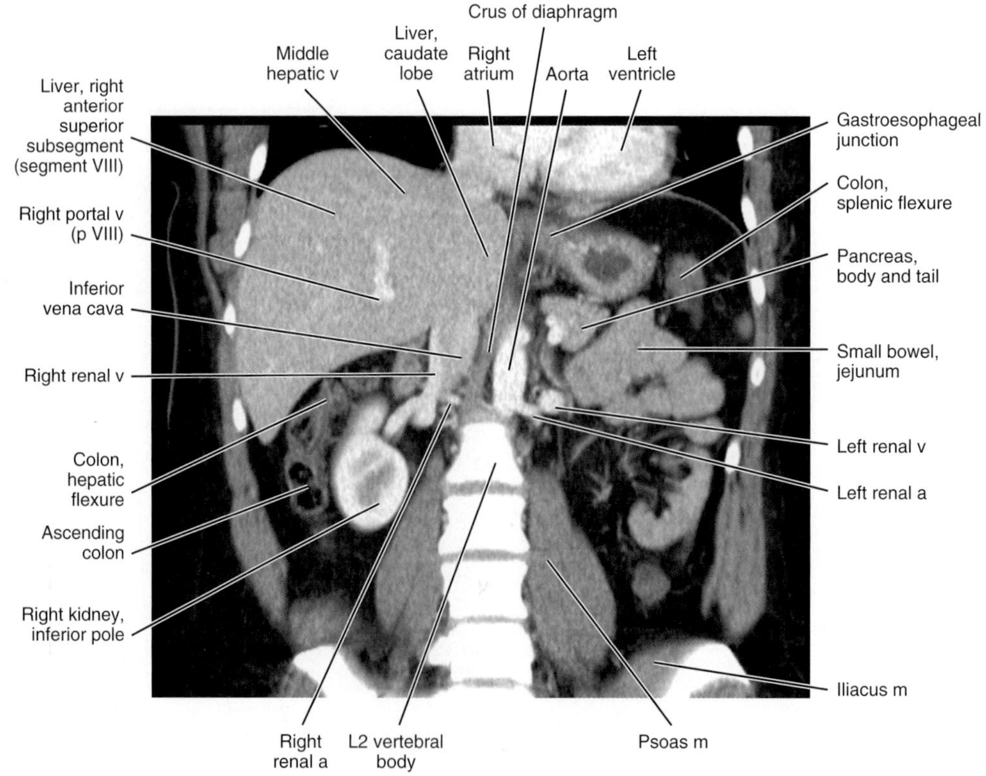

Crus of diaphragm
Liver, caudate lobe
Right atrium
Aorta
Left ventricle
Middle hepatic v

Liver, right anterior superior subsegment (segment VIII)
Right portal v (p VIII)
Inferior vena cava
Right renal v
Colon, hepatic flexure
Ascending colon
Right kidney, inferior pole

Gastroesophageal junction
Colon, splenic flexure
Pancreas, body and tail
Small bowel, jejunum
Left renal v
Left renal a
Iliacus m

Right renal a
L2 vertebral body
Psoas m

Figure 20.3.9

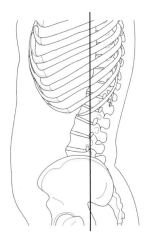

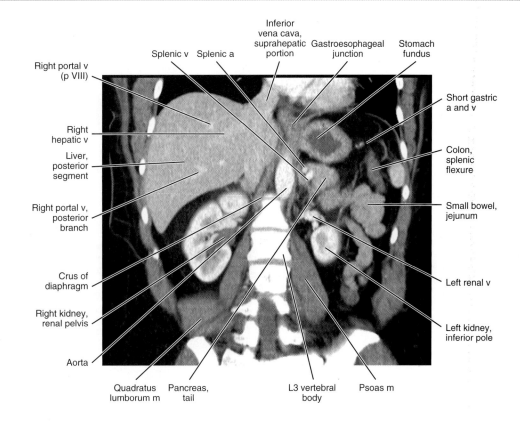

Right portal v (p VIII)

Splenic v   Splenic a

Inferior vena cava, suprahepatic portion

Gastroesophageal junction

Stomach fundus

Right hepatic v

Short gastric a and v

Liver, posterior segment

Colon, splenic flexure

Right portal v, posterior branch

Small bowel, jejunum

Crus of diaphragm

Left renal v

Right kidney, renal pelvis

Left kidney, inferior pole

Aorta

Quadratus lumborum m   Pancreas, tail   L3 vertebral body   Psoas m

Figure 20.3.10

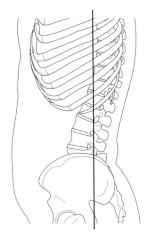

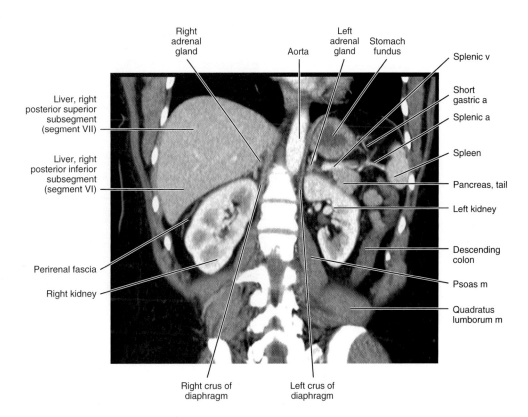

Right adrenal gland

Aorta

Left adrenal gland

Stomach fundus

Splenic v

Liver, right posterior superior subsegment (segment VII)

Short gastric a

Splenic a

Liver, right posterior inferior subsegment (segment VI)

Spleen

Pancreas, tail

Left kidney

Descending colon

Perirenal fascia

Psoas m

Right kidney

Quadratus lumborum m

Right crus of diaphragm   Left crus of diaphragm

Figure 20.3.11

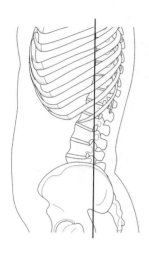

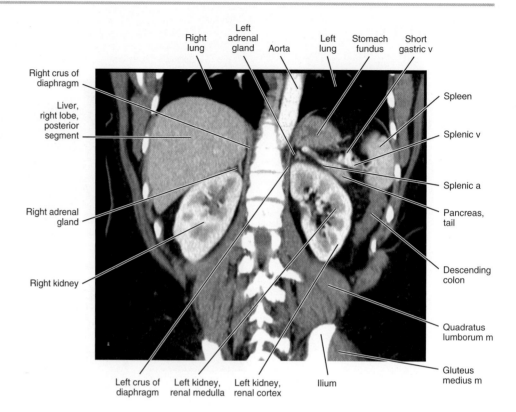

Right lung

Left adrenal gland

Aorta

Left lung

Stomach fundus

Short gastric v

Right crus of diaphragm

Liver, right lobe, posterior segment

Right adrenal gland

Right kidney

Spleen

Splenic v

Splenic a

Pancreas, tail

Descending colon

Quadratus lumborum m

Gluteus medius m

Left crus of diaphragm

Left kidney, renal medulla

Left kidney, renal cortex

Ilium

Figure 20.3.12

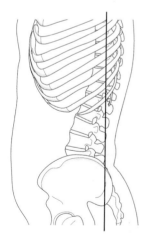

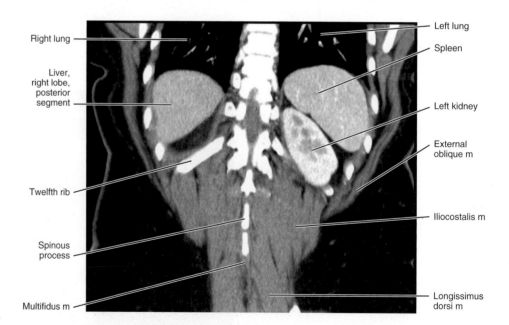

Right lung

Liver, right lobe, posterior segment

Twelfth rib

Spinous process

Multifidus m

Left lung

Spleen

Left kidney

External oblique m

Iliocostalis m

Longissimus dorsi m

Chapter 21

MRI of the Abdomen

AXIAL
Figure 21.1.1

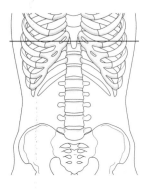

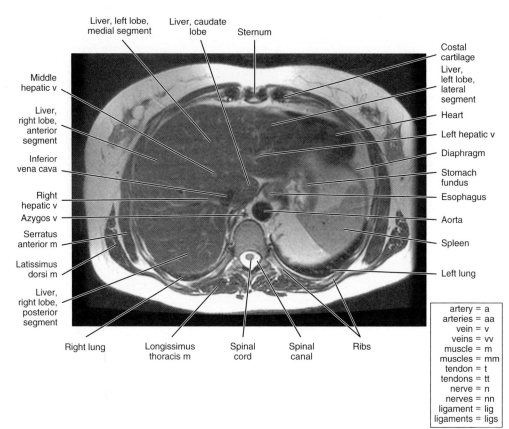

Liver, left lobe, medial segment
Liver, caudate lobe
Sternum
Costal cartilage
Liver, left lobe, lateral segment
Heart
Left hepatic v
Diaphragm
Stomach fundus
Esophagus
Aorta
Spleen
Left lung

Middle hepatic v
Liver, right lobe, anterior segment
Inferior vena cava
Right hepatic v
Azygos v
Serratus anterior m
Latissimus dorsi m
Liver, right lobe, posterior segment

Right lung
Longissimus thoracis m
Spinal cord
Spinal canal
Ribs

artery = a
arteries = aa
vein = v
veins = vv
muscle = m
muscles = mm
tendon = t
tendons = tt
nerve = n
nerves = nn
ligament = lig
ligaments = ligs

Figure 21.1.2

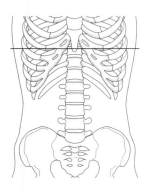

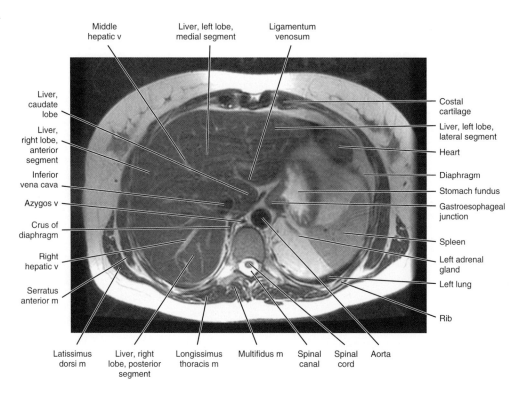

Middle hepatic v
Liver, left lobe, medial segment
Ligamentum venosum
Costal cartilage
Liver, left lobe, lateral segment
Heart
Diaphragm
Stomach fundus
Gastroesophageal junction
Spleen
Left adrenal gland
Left lung
Rib

Liver, caudate lobe
Liver, right lobe, anterior segment
Inferior vena cava
Azygos v
Crus of diaphragm
Right hepatic v
Serratus anterior m

Latissimus dorsi m
Liver, right lobe, posterior segment
Longissimus thoracis m
Multifidus m
Spinal canal
Spinal cord
Aorta

Figure 21.1.3

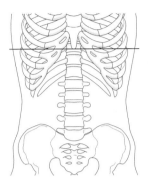

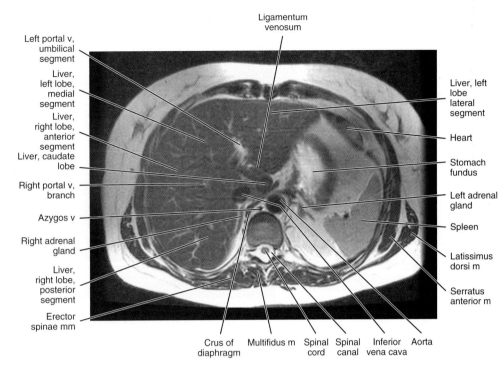

Ligamentum venosum

Left portal v, umbilical segment

Liver, left lobe, medial segment

Liver, right lobe, anterior segment

Liver, caudate lobe

Right portal v, branch

Azygos v

Right adrenal gland

Liver, right lobe, posterior segment

Erector spinae mm

Liver, left lobe lateral segment

Heart

Stomach fundus

Left adrenal gland

Spleen

Latissimus dorsi m

Serratus anterior m

Crus of diaphragm

Multifidus m

Spinal cord

Spinal canal

Inferior vena cava

Aorta

Figure 21.1.4

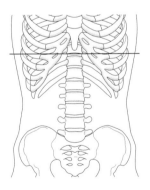

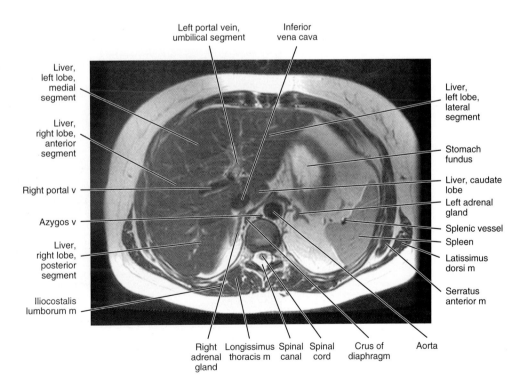

Left portal vein, umbilical segment

Inferior vena cava

Liver, left lobe, medial segment

Liver, right lobe, anterior segment

Right portal v

Azygos v

Liver, right lobe, posterior segment

Iliocostalis lumborum m

Liver, left lobe, lateral segment

Stomach fundus

Liver, caudate lobe

Left adrenal gland

Splenic vessel

Spleen

Latissimus dorsi m

Serratus anterior m

Right adrenal gland

Longissimus thoracis m

Spinal canal

Spinal cord

Crus of diaphragm

Aorta

Figure 21.1.5

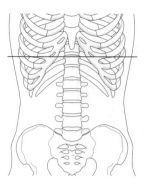

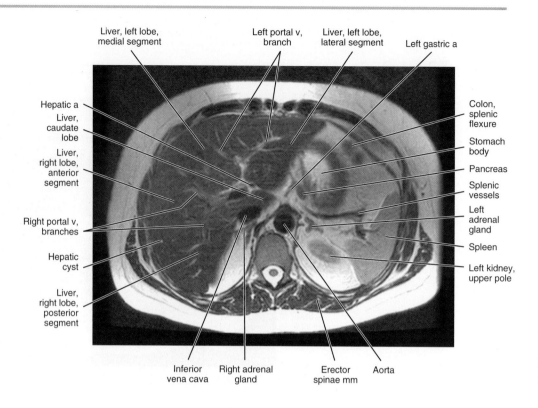

Liver, left lobe, medial segment

Left portal v, branch

Liver, left lobe, lateral segment

Left gastric a

Hepatic a

Liver, caudate lobe

Liver, right lobe, anterior segment

Right portal v, branches

Hepatic cyst

Liver, right lobe, posterior segment

Colon, splenic flexure

Stomach body

Pancreas

Splenic vessels

Left adrenal gland

Spleen

Left kidney, upper pole

Inferior vena cava

Right adrenal gland

Erector spinae mm

Aorta

Figure 21.1.6

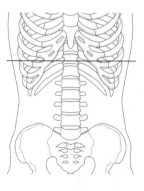

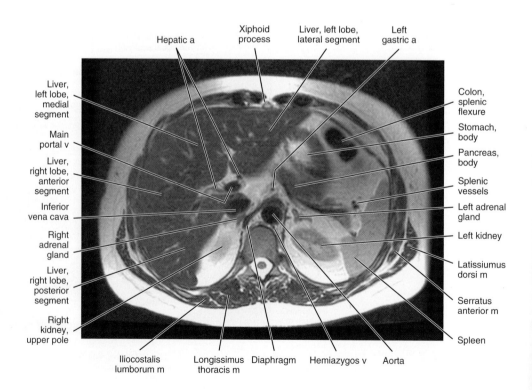

Hepatic a

Xiphoid process

Liver, left lobe, lateral segment

Left gastric a

Liver, left lobe, medial segment

Main portal v

Liver, right lobe, anterior segment

Inferior vena cava

Right adrenal gland

Liver, right lobe, posterior segment

Right kidney, upper pole

Colon, splenic flexure

Stomach, body

Pancreas, body

Splenic vessels

Left adrenal gland

Left kidney

Latissiumus dorsi m

Serratus anterior m

Spleen

Iliocostalis lumborum m

Longissimus thoracis m

Diaphragm

Hemiazygos v

Aorta

Figure 21.1.7

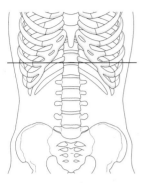

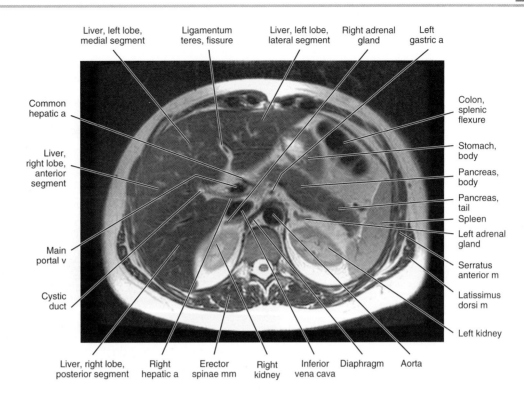

Liver, left lobe, medial segment — Ligamentum teres, fissure — Liver, left lobe, lateral segment — Right adrenal gland — Left gastric a

Common hepatic a

Liver, right lobe, anterior segment

Main portal v

Cystic duct

Colon, splenic flexure

Stomach, body

Pancreas, body

Pancreas, tail

Spleen

Left adrenal gland

Serratus anterior m

Latissimus dorsi m

Left kidney

Liver, right lobe, posterior segment — Right hepatic a — Erector spinae mm — Right kidney — Inferior vena cava — Diaphragm — Aorta

Figure 21.1.8

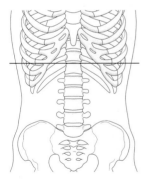

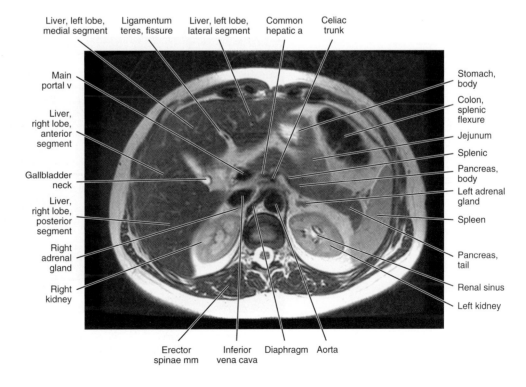

Liver, left lobe, medial segment — Ligamentum teres, fissure — Liver, left lobe, lateral segment — Common hepatic a — Celiac trunk

Main portal v

Liver, right lobe, anterior segment

Gallbladder neck

Liver, right lobe, posterior segment

Right adrenal gland

Right kidney

Stomach, body

Colon, splenic flexure

Jejunum

Splenic

Pancreas, body

Left adrenal gland

Spleen

Pancreas, tail

Renal sinus

Left kidney

Erector spinae mm — Inferior vena cava — Diaphragm — Aorta

Figure 21.1.9

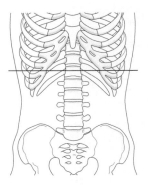

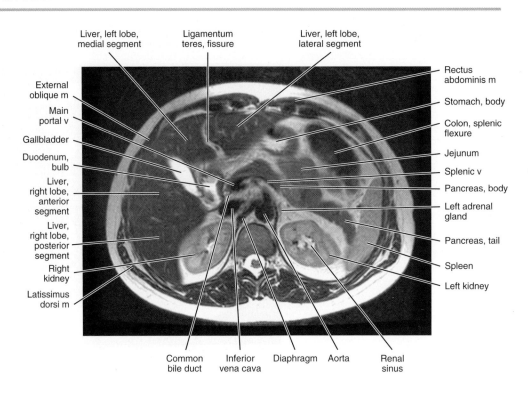

Liver, left lobe, medial segment
Ligamentum teres, fissure
Liver, left lobe, lateral segment
External oblique m
Main portal v
Gallbladder
Duodenum, bulb
Liver, right lobe, anterior segment
Liver, right lobe, posterior segment
Right kidney
Latissimus dorsi m
Rectus abdominis m
Stomach, body
Colon, splenic flexure
Jejunum
Splenic v
Pancreas, body
Left adrenal gland
Pancreas, tail
Spleen
Left kidney
Common bile duct
Inferior vena cava
Diaphragm
Aorta
Renal sinus

Figure 21.1.10

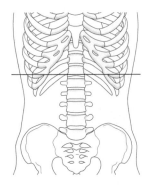

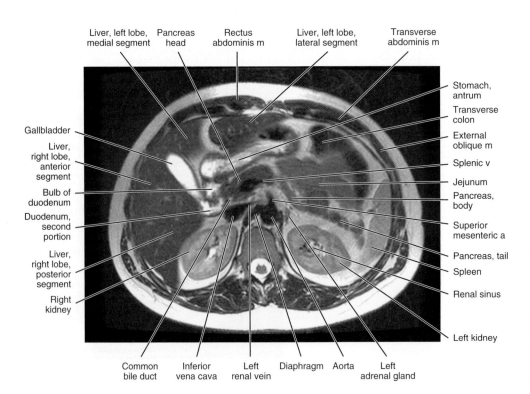

Liver, left lobe, medial segment
Pancreas head
Rectus abdominis m
Liver, left lobe, lateral segment
Transverse abdominis m
Gallbladder
Liver, right lobe, anterior segment
Bulb of duodenum
Duodenum, second portion
Liver, right lobe, posterior segment
Right kidney
Stomach, antrum
Transverse colon
External oblique m
Splenic v
Jejunum
Pancreas, body
Superior mesenteric a
Pancreas, tail
Spleen
Renal sinus
Left kidney
Common bile duct
Inferior vena cava
Left renal vein
Diaphragm
Aorta
Left adrenal gland

Figure 21.1.11

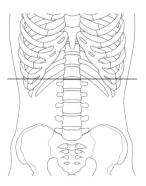

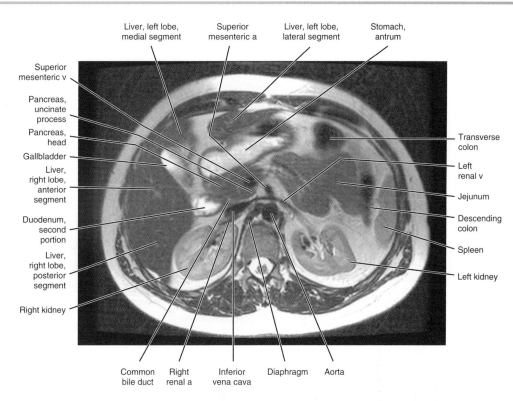

Liver, left lobe, medial segment
Superior mesenteric a
Liver, left lobe, lateral segment
Stomach, antrum
Superior mesenteric v
Pancreas, uncinate process
Pancreas, head
Gallbladder
Liver, right lobe, anterior segment
Duodenum, second portion
Liver, right lobe, posterior segment
Right kidney
Transverse colon
Left renal v
Jejunum
Descending colon
Spleen
Left kidney
Common bile duct
Right renal a
Inferior vena cava
Diaphragm
Aorta

Figure 21.1.12

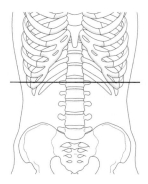

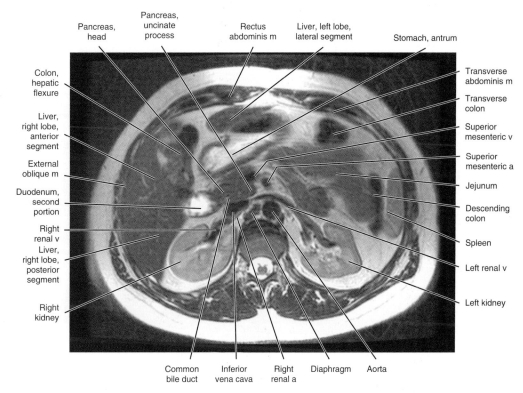

Pancreas, head
Pancreas, uncinate process
Rectus abdominis m
Liver, left lobe, lateral segment
Stomach, antrum
Colon, hepatic flexure
Liver, right lobe, anterior segment
External oblique m
Duodenum, second portion
Right renal v
Liver, right lobe, posterior segment
Right kidney
Transverse abdominis m
Transverse colon
Superior mesenteric v
Superior mesenteric a
Jejunum
Descending colon
Spleen
Left renal v
Left kidney
Common bile duct
Inferior vena cava
Right renal a
Diaphragm
Aorta

Figure 21.1.13

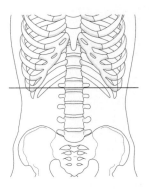

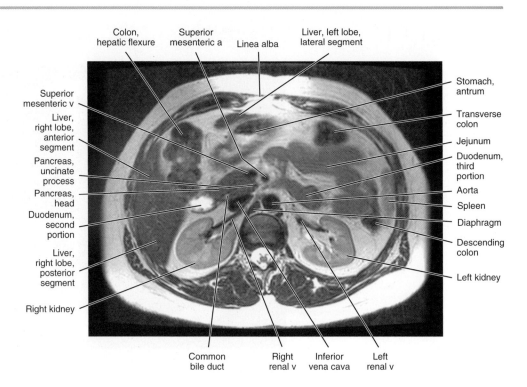

Colon, hepatic flexure

Superior mesenteric a

Linea alba

Liver, left lobe, lateral segment

Superior mesenteric v

Liver, right lobe, anterior segment

Pancreas, uncinate process

Pancreas, head

Duodenum, second portion

Liver, right lobe, posterior segment

Right kidney

Stomach, antrum

Transverse colon

Jejunum

Duodenum, third portion

Aorta

Spleen

Diaphragm

Descending colon

Left kidney

Common bile duct

Right renal v

Inferior vena cava

Left renal v

Figure 21.1.14

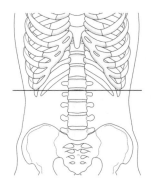

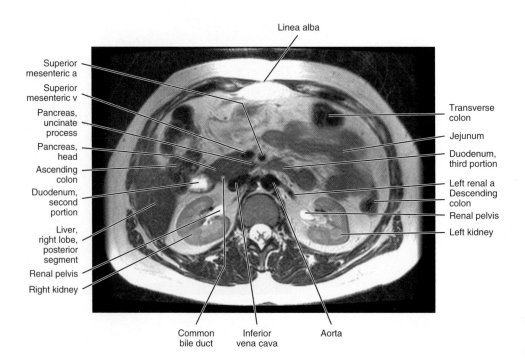

Linea alba

Superior mesenteric a

Superior mesenteric v

Pancreas, uncinate process

Pancreas, head

Ascending colon

Duodenum, second portion

Liver, right lobe, posterior segment

Renal pelvis

Right kidney

Transverse colon

Jejunum

Duodenum, third portion

Left renal a

Descending colon

Renal pelvis

Left kidney

Common bile duct

Inferior vena cava

Aorta

Figure 21.1.15

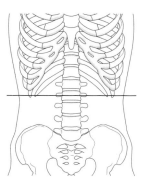

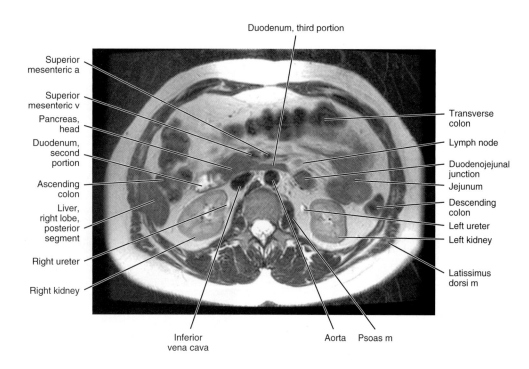

Duodenum, third portion

Superior mesenteric a

Superior mesenteric v

Pancreas, head

Duodenum, second portion

Ascending colon

Liver, right lobe, posterior segment

Right ureter

Right kidney

Transverse colon

Lymph node

Duodenojejunal junction

Jejunum

Descending colon

Left ureter

Left kidney

Latissimus dorsi m

Inferior vena cava

Aorta   Psoas m

Figure 21.1.16

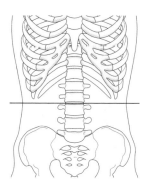

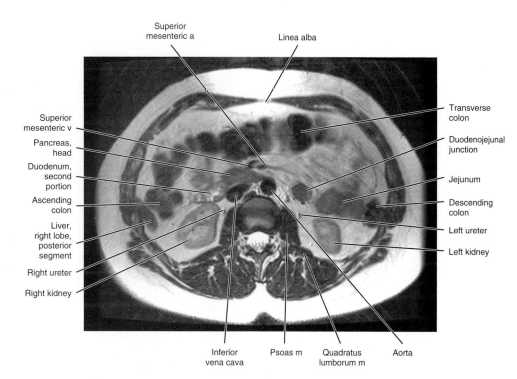

Superior mesenteric a

Linea alba

Superior mesenteric v

Pancreas, head

Duodenum, second portion

Ascending colon

Liver, right lobe, posterior segment

Right ureter

Right kidney

Transverse colon

Duodenojejunal junction

Jejunum

Descending colon

Left ureter

Left kidney

Inferior vena cava

Psoas m

Quadratus lumborum m

Aorta

SAGITTAL

Figure 21.2.1

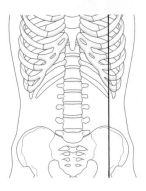

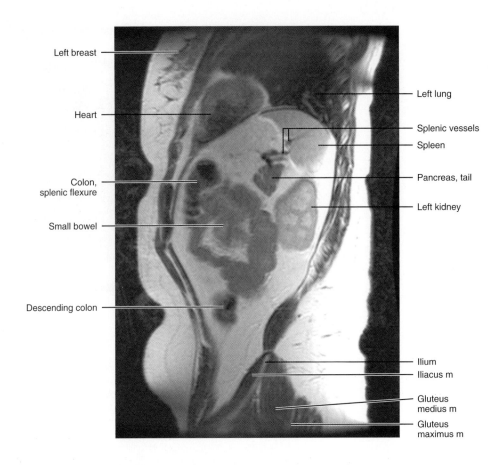

Left breast

Heart

Colon,
splenic flexure

Small bowel

Descending colon

Left lung

Splenic vessels

Spleen

Pancreas, tail

Left kidney

Ilium

Iliacus m

Gluteus
medius m

Gluteus
maximus m

Figure 21.2.2

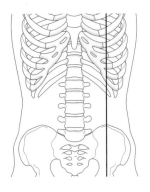

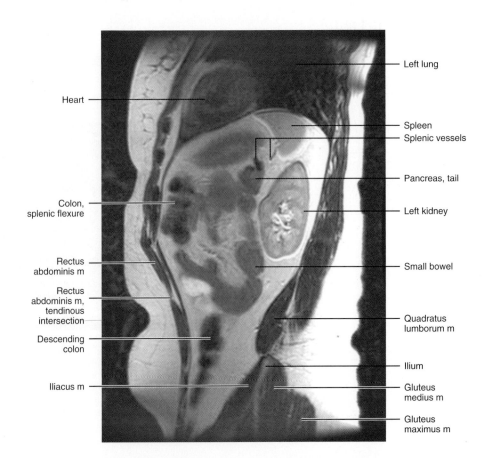

Heart

Colon,
splenic flexure

Rectus
abdominis m

Rectus
abdominis m,
tendinous
intersection

Descending
colon

Iliacus m

Left lung

Spleen
Splenic vessels

Pancreas, tail

Left kidney

Small bowel

Quadratus
lumborum m

Ilium

Gluteus
medius m

Gluteus
maximus m

Figure 21.2.3

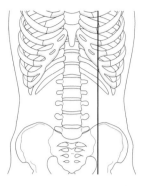

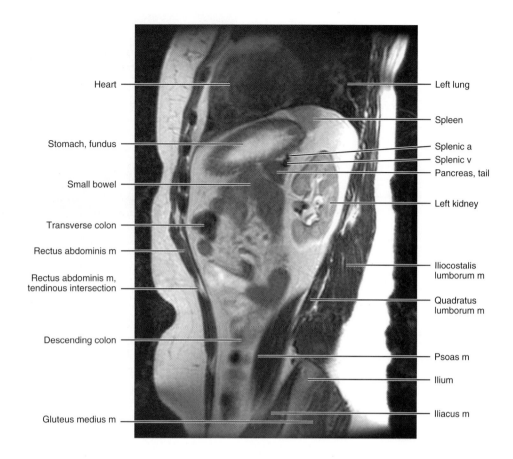

Heart

Stomach, fundus

Small bowel

Transverse colon

Rectus abdominis m

Rectus abdominis m, tendinous intersection

Descending colon

Gluteus medius m

Left lung

Spleen

Splenic a

Splenic v

Pancreas, tail

Left kidney

Iliocostalis lumborum m

Quadratus lumborum m

Psoas m

Ilium

Iliacus m

Figure 21.2.4

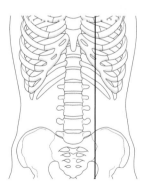

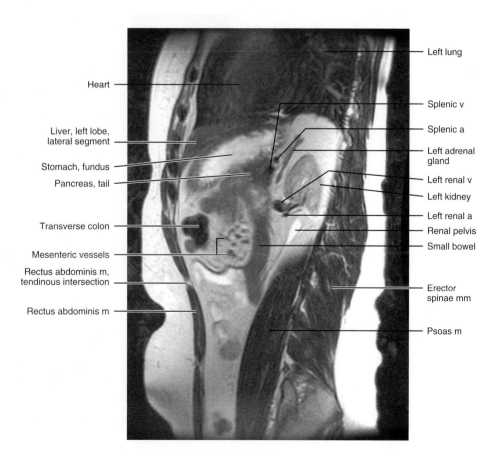

Heart

Liver, left lobe, lateral segment

Stomach, fundus

Pancreas, tail

Transverse colon

Mesenteric vessels

Rectus abdominis m, tendinous intersection

Rectus abdominis m

Left lung

Splenic v

Splenic a

Left adrenal gland

Left renal v

Left kidney

Left renal a

Renal pelvis

Small bowel

Erector spinae mm

Psoas m

Figure 21.2.5

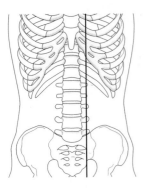

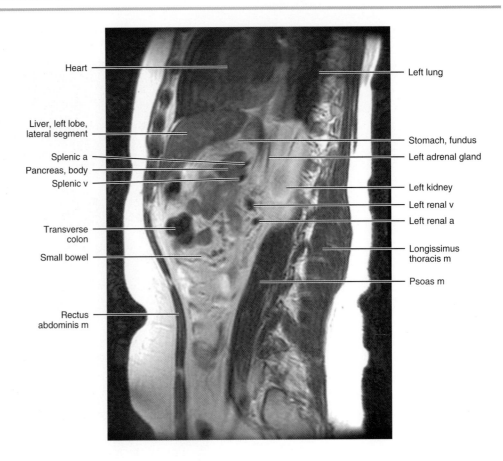

Heart

Left lung

Liver, left lobe, lateral segment

Stomach, fundus

Splenic a

Left adrenal gland

Pancreas, body

Splenic v

Left kidney

Left renal v

Left renal a

Transverse colon

Small bowel

Longissimus thoracis m

Psoas m

Rectus abdominis m

Figure 21.2.6

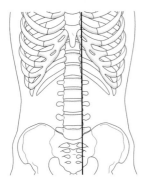

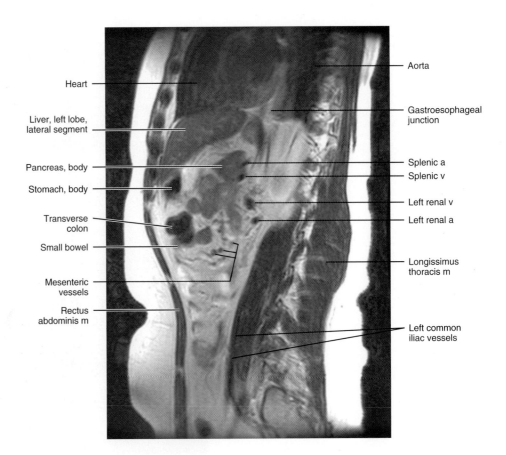

Aorta

Heart

Gastroesophageal junction

Liver, left lobe, lateral segment

Pancreas, body

Splenic a

Splenic v

Stomach, body

Left renal v

Transverse colon

Left renal a

Small bowel

Mesenteric vessels

Longissimus thoracis m

Rectus abdominis m

Left common iliac vessels

Figure 21.2.7

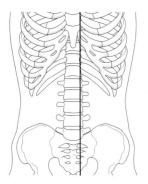

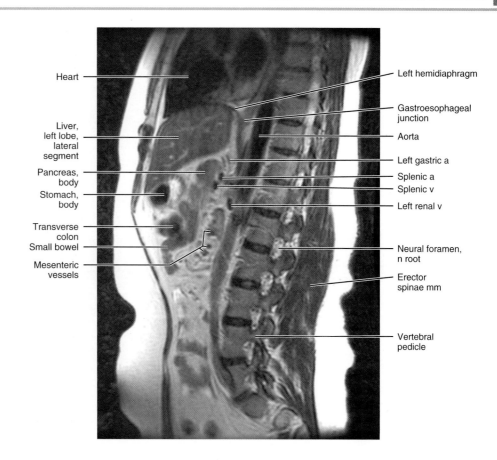

Heart

Liver,
left lobe,
lateral
segment

Pancreas,
body

Stomach,
body

Transverse
colon

Small bowel

Mesenteric
vessels

Left hemidiaphragm

Gastroesophageal
junction

Aorta

Left gastric a

Splenic a

Splenic v

Left renal v

Neural foramen,
n root

Erector
spinae mm

Vertebral
pedicle

Figure 21.2.8

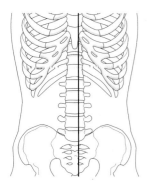

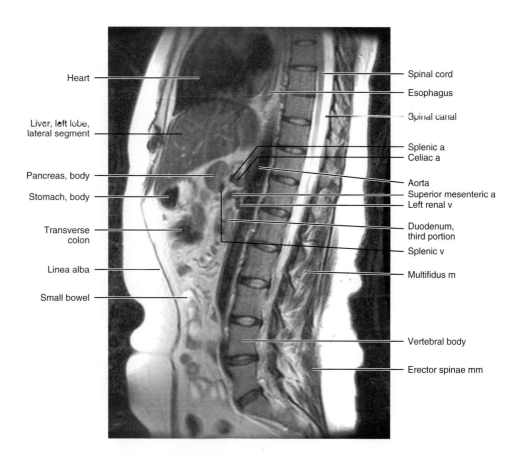

Heart

Liver, left lobe,
lateral segment

Pancreas, body

Stomach, body

Transverse
colon

Linea alba

Small bowel

Spinal cord

Esophagus

Spinal canal

Splenic a

Celiac a

Aorta

Superior mesenteric a

Left renal v

Duodenum,
third portion

Splenic v

Multifidus m

Vertebral body

Erector spinae mm

Figure 21.2.9

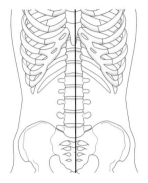

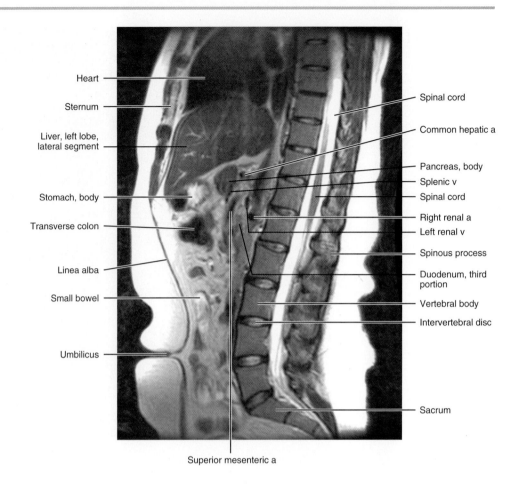

Heart

Sternum

Liver, left lobe, lateral segment

Stomach, body

Transverse colon

Linea alba

Small bowel

Umbilicus

Spinal cord

Common hepatic a

Pancreas, body

Splenic v

Spinal cord

Right renal a

Left renal v

Spinous process

Duodenum, third portion

Vertebral body

Intervertebral disc

Sacrum

Superior mesenteric a

Figure 21.2.10

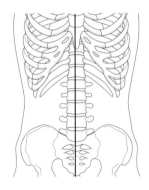

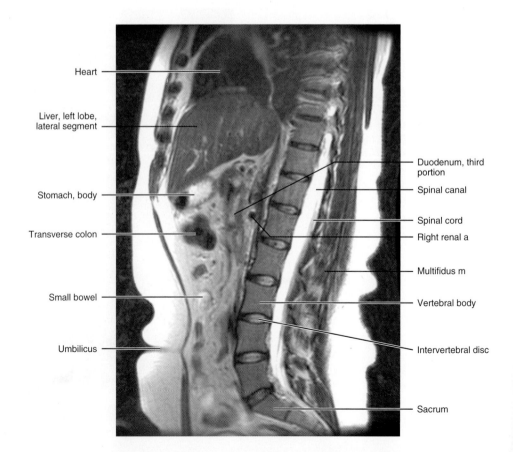

Heart

Liver, left lobe, lateral segment

Stomach, body

Transverse colon

Small bowel

Umbilicus

Duodenum, third portion

Spinal canal

Spinal cord

Right renal a

Multifidus m

Vertebral body

Intervertebral disc

Sacrum

Figure 21.2.11

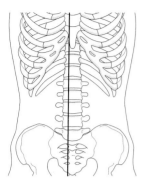

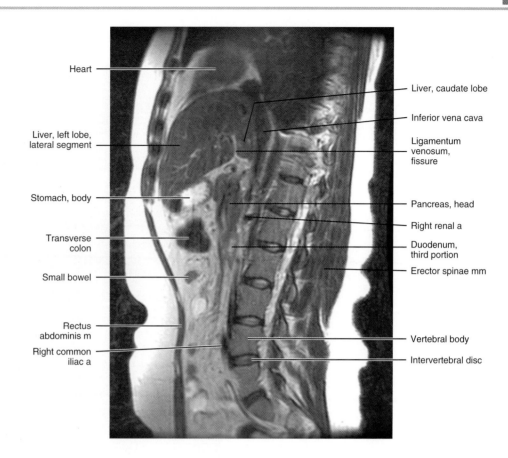

Heart

Liver, caudate lobe

Inferior vena cava

Liver, left lobe,
lateral segment

Ligamentum
venosum,
fissure

Stomach, body

Pancreas, head

Right renal a

Transverse
colon

Duodenum,
third portion

Small bowel

Erector spinae mm

Rectus
abdominis m

Vertebral body

Right common
iliac a

Intervertebral disc

Figure 21.2.12

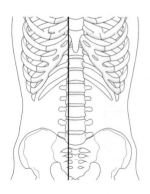

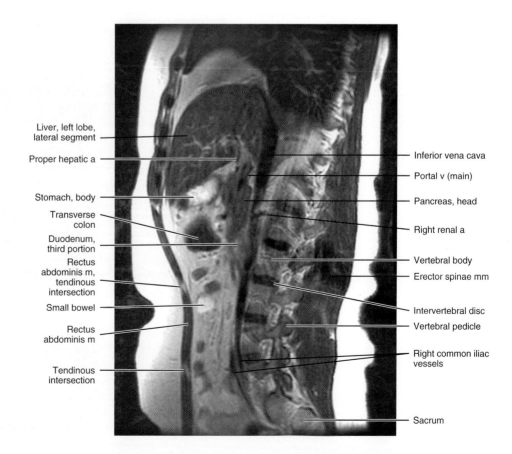

Liver, left lobe,
lateral segment

Inferior vena cava

Proper hepatic a

Portal v (main)

Stomach, body

Pancreas, head

Transverse
colon

Right renal a

Duodenum,
third portion

Rectus
abdominis m,
tendinous
intersection

Vertebral body

Erector spinae mm

Small bowel

Intervertebral disc

Rectus
abdominis m

Vertebral pedicle

Right common
iliac vessels

Tendinous
intersection

Sacrum

Figure 21.2.13

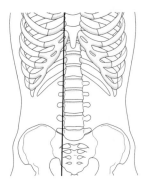

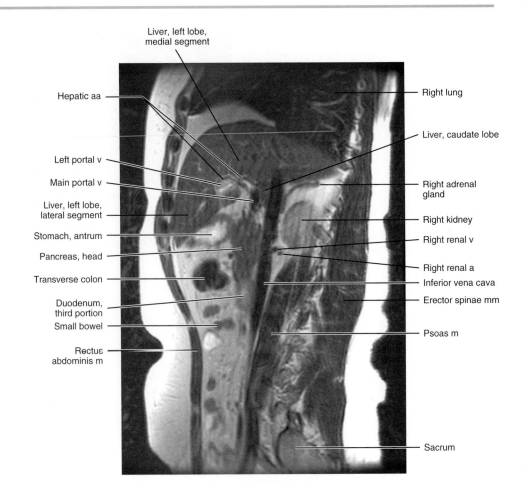

Liver, left lobe, medial segment

Hepatic aa

Left portal v

Main portal v

Liver, left lobe, lateral segment

Stomach, antrum

Pancreas, head

Transverse colon

Duodenum, third portion

Small bowel

Rectus abdominis m

Right lung

Liver, caudate lobe

Right adrenal gland

Right kidney

Right renal v

Right renal a

Inferior vena cava

Erector spinae mm

Psoas m

Sacrum

Figure 21.2.14

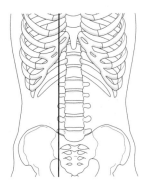

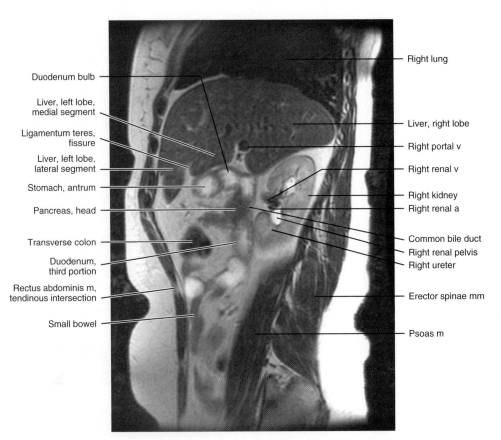

Duodenum bulb

Liver, left lobe, medial segment

Ligamentum teres, fissure

Liver, left lobe, lateral segment

Stomach, antrum

Pancreas, head

Transverse colon

Duodenum, third portion

Rectus abdominis m, tendinous intersection

Small bowel

Right lung

Liver, right lobe

Right portal v

Right renal v

Right kidney

Right renal a

Common bile duct

Right renal pelvis

Right ureter

Erector spinae mm

Psoas m

Figure 21.2.15

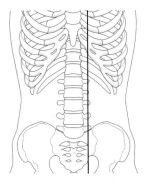

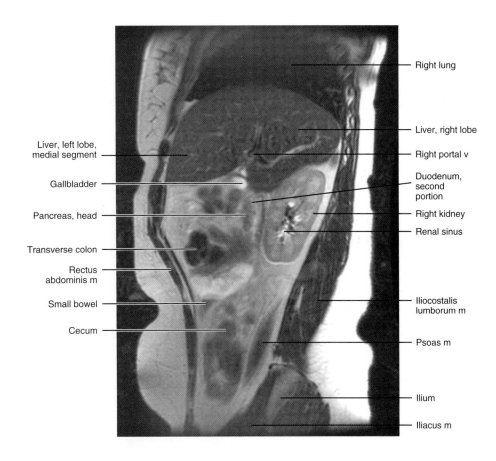

Right lung

Liver, right lobe

Right portal v

Duodenum, second portion

Right kidney

Renal sinus

Liver, left lobe, medial segment

Gallbladder

Pancreas, head

Transverse colon

Rectus abdominis m

Small bowel

Cecum

Iliocostalis lumborum m

Psoas m

Ilium

Iliacus m

Figure 21.2.16

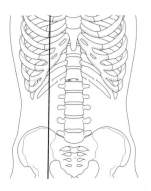

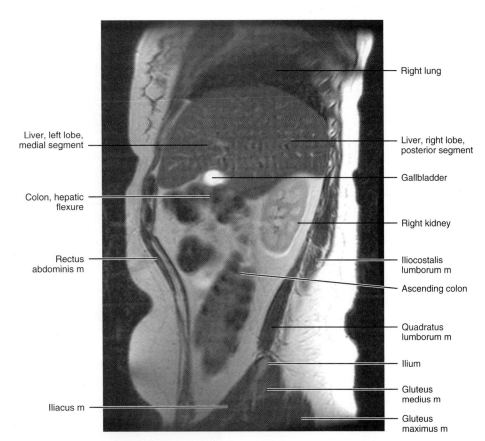

Right lung

Liver, right lobe, posterior segment

Gallbladder

Right kidney

Iliocostalis lumborum m

Ascending colon

Quadratus lumborum m

Ilium

Gluteus medius m

Gluteus maximus m

Liver, left lobe, medial segment

Colon, hepatic flexure

Rectus abdominis m

Iliacus m

CORONAL
Figure 21.3.1

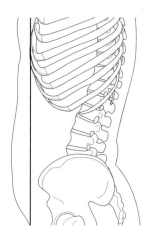

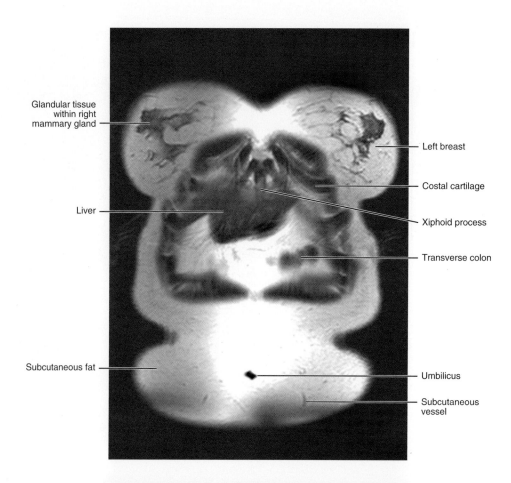

Glandular tissue within right mammary gland

Left breast

Costal cartilage

Liver

Xiphoid process

Transverse colon

Subcutaneous fat

Umbilicus

Subcutaneous vessel

Figure 21.3.2

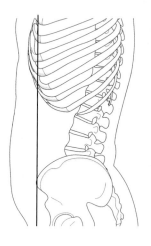

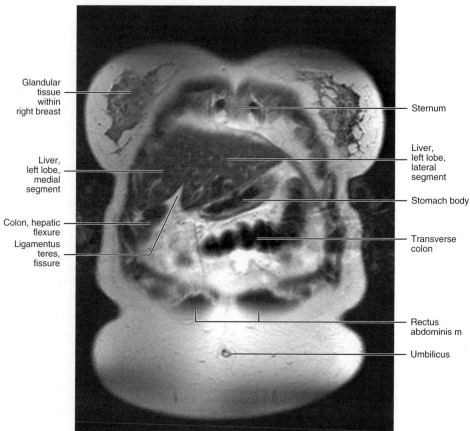

Glandular tissue within right breast

Sternum

Liver, left lobe, medial segment

Liver, left lobe, lateral segment

Colon, hepatic flexure

Stomach body

Ligamentus teres, fissure

Transverse colon

Rectus abdominis m

Umbilicus

Figure 21.3.3

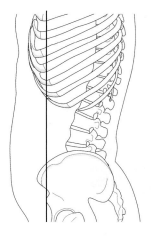

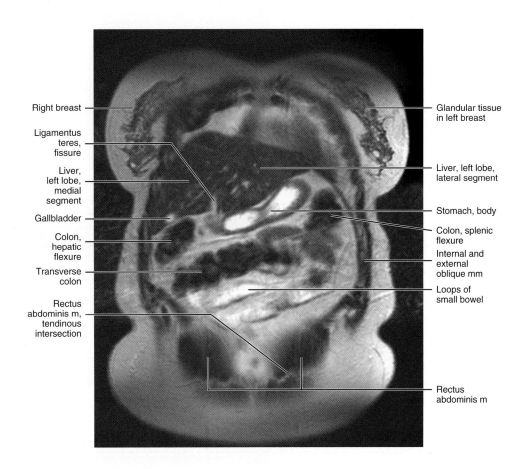

Right breast

Ligamentus teres, fissure

Liver, left lobe, medial segment

Gallbladder

Colon, hepatic flexure

Transverse colon

Rectus abdominis m, tendinous intersection

Glandular tissue in left breast

Liver, left lobe, lateral segment

Stomach, body

Colon, splenic flexure

Internal and external oblique mm

Loops of small bowel

Rectus abdominis m

Figure 21.3.4

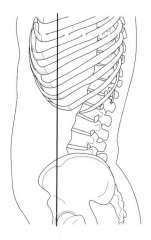

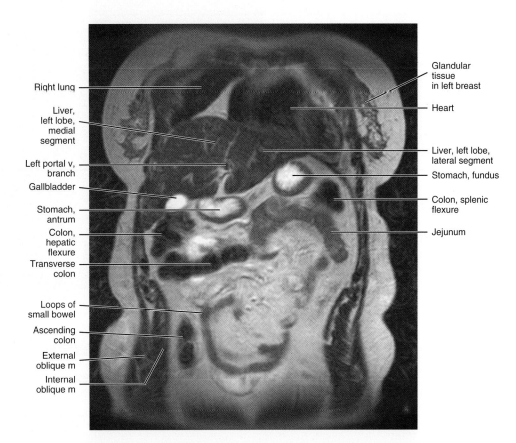

Right lung

Liver, left lobe, medial segment

Left portal v, branch

Gallbladder

Stomach, antrum

Colon, hepatic flexure

Transverse colon

Loops of small bowel

Ascending colon

External oblique m

Internal oblique m

Glandular tissue in left breast

Heart

Liver, left lobe, lateral segment

Stomach, fundus

Colon, splenic flexure

Jejunum

Figure 21.3.5

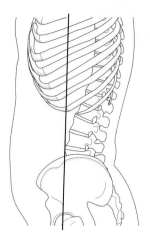

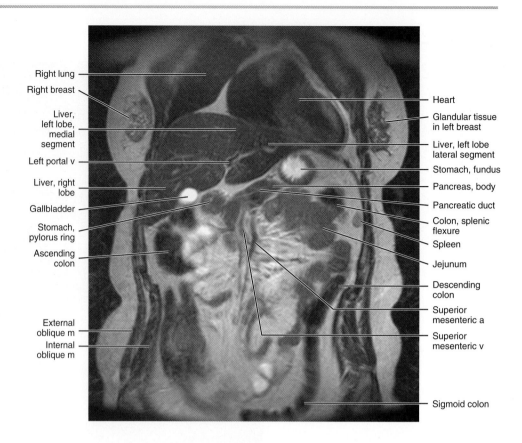

Right lung

Right breast

Liver, left lobe, medial segment

Left portal v

Liver, right lobe

Gallbladder

Stomach, pylorus ring

Ascending colon

External oblique m

Internal oblique m

Heart

Glandular tissue in left breast

Liver, left lobe lateral segment

Stomach, fundus

Pancreas, body

Pancreatic duct

Colon, splenic flexure

Spleen

Jejunum

Descending colon

Superior mesenteric a

Superior mesenteric v

Sigmoid colon

Figure 21.3.6

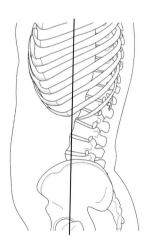

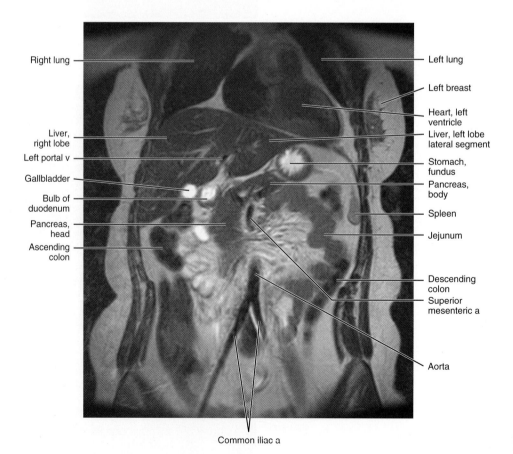

Right lung

Liver, right lobe

Left portal v

Gallbladder

Bulb of duodenum

Pancreas, head

Ascending colon

Left lung

Left breast

Heart, left ventricle

Liver, left lobe lateral segment

Stomach, fundus

Pancreas, body

Spleen

Jejunum

Descending colon

Superior mesenteric a

Aorta

Common iliac a

Figure 21.3.7

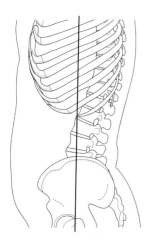

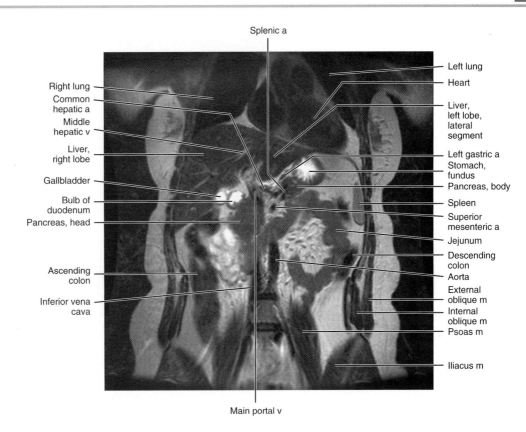

Splenic a

Right lung
Common hepatic a
Middle hepatic v
Liver, right lobe
Gallbladder
Bulb of duodenum
Pancreas, head
Ascending colon
Inferior vena cava

Left lung
Heart
Liver, left lobe, lateral segment
Left gastric a
Stomach, fundus
Pancreas, body
Spleen
Superior mesenteric a
Jejunum
Descending colon
Aorta
External oblique m
Internal oblique m
Psoas m
Iliacus m

Main portal v

Figure 21.3.8

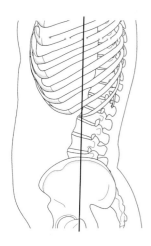

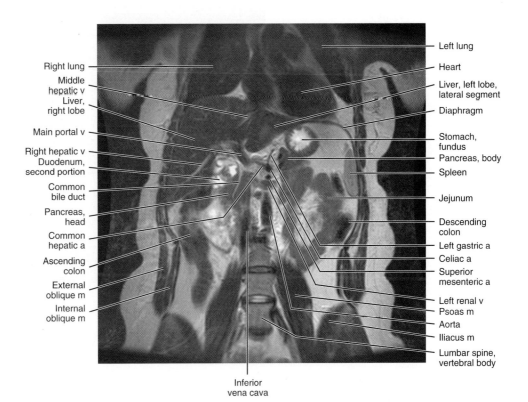

Right lung
Middle hepatic v
Liver, right lobe
Main portal v
Right hepatic v
Duodenum, second portion
Common bile duct
Pancreas, head
Common hepatic a
Ascending colon
External oblique m
Internal oblique m

Left lung
Heart
Liver, left lobe, lateral segment
Diaphragm
Stomach, fundus
Pancreas, body
Spleen
Jejunum
Descending colon
Left gastric a
Celiac a
Superior mesenteric a
Left renal v
Psoas m
Aorta
Iliacus m
Lumbar spine, vertebral body

Inferior vena cava

Figure 21.3.9

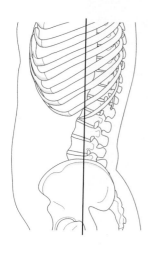

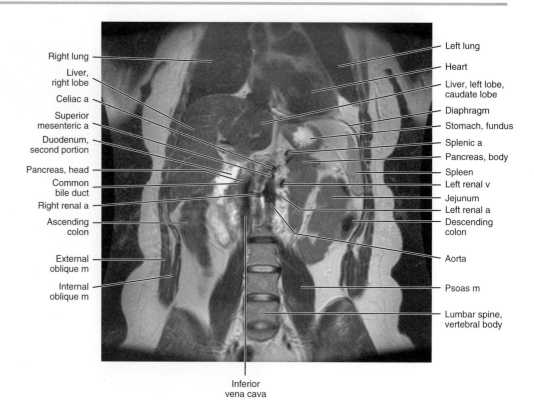

Right lung
Liver, right lobe
Celiac a
Superior mesenteric a
Duodenum, second portion
Pancreas, head
Common bile duct
Right renal a
Ascending colon
External oblique m
Internal oblique m

Left lung
Heart
Liver, left lobe, caudate lobe
Diaphragm
Stomach, fundus
Splenic a
Pancreas, body
Spleen
Left renal v
Jejunum
Left renal a
Descending colon
Aorta
Psoas m
Lumbar spine, vertebral body

Inferior vena cava

Figure 21.3.10

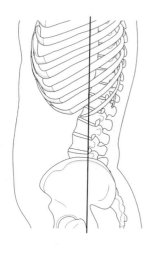

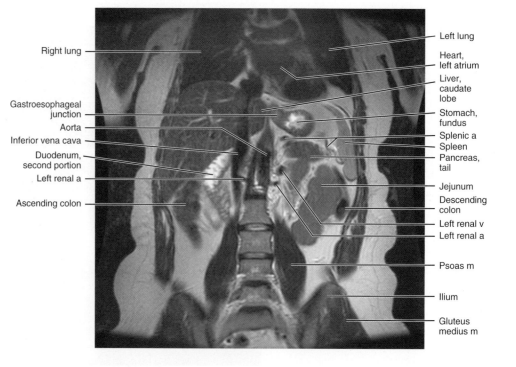

Right lung
Gastroesophageal junction
Aorta
Inferior vena cava
Duodenum, second portion
Left renal a
Ascending colon

Left lung
Heart, left atrium
Liver, caudate lobe
Stomach, fundus
Splenic a
Spleen
Pancreas, tail
Jejunum
Descending colon
Left renal v
Left renal a
Psoas m
Ilium
Gluteus medius m

Figure 21.3.11

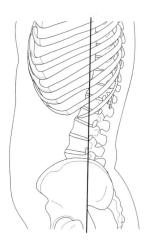

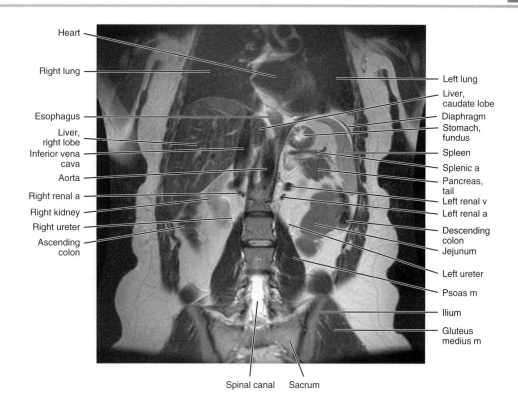

Heart
Right lung
Esophagus
Liver, right lobe
Inferior vena cava
Aorta
Right renal a
Right kidney
Right ureter
Ascending colon

Left lung
Liver, caudate lobe
Diaphragm
Stomach, fundus
Spleen
Splenic a
Pancreas, tail
Left renal v
Left renal a
Descending colon
Jejunum
Left ureter
Psoas m
Ilium
Gluteus medius m

Spinal canal   Sacrum

Figure 21.3.12

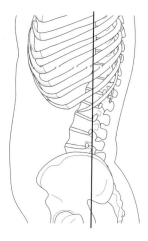

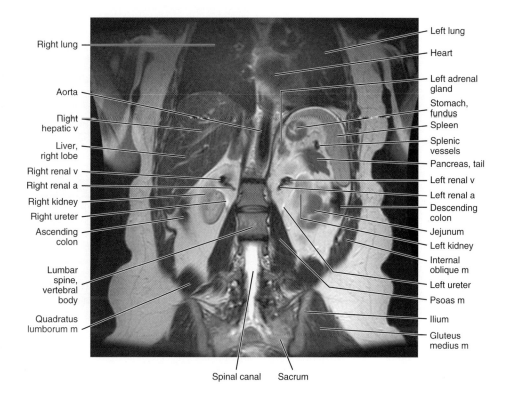

Right lung
Aorta
Right hepatic v
Liver, right lobe
Right renal v
Right renal a
Right kidney
Right ureter
Ascending colon
Lumbar spine, vertebral body
Quadratus lumborum m

Left lung
Heart
Left adrenal gland
Stomach, fundus
Spleen
Splenic vessels
Pancreas, tail
Left renal v
Left renal a
Descending colon
Jejunum
Left kidney
Internal oblique m
Left ureter
Psoas m
Ilium
Gluteus medius m

Spinal canal   Sacrum

Figure 21.3.13

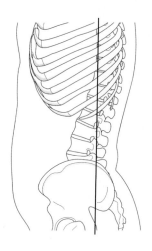

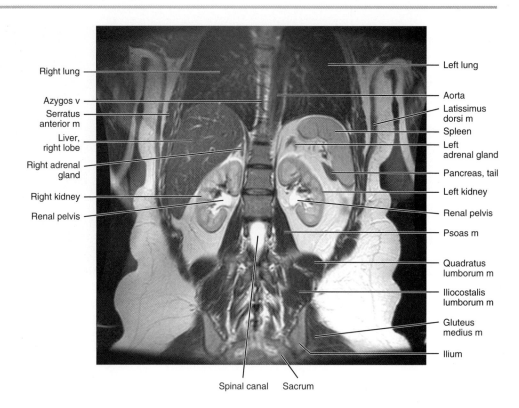

Right lung

Azygos v

Serratus
anterior m

Liver,
right lobe

Right adrenal
gland

Right kidney

Renal pelvis

Left lung

Aorta

Latissimus
dorsi m

Spleen

Left
adrenal gland

Pancreas, tail

Left kidney

Renal pelvis

Psoas m

Quadratus
lumborum m

Iliocostalis
lumborum m

Gluteus
medius m

Ilium

Spinal canal   Sacrum

Figure 21.3.14

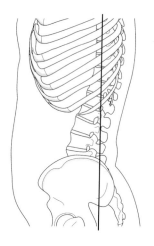

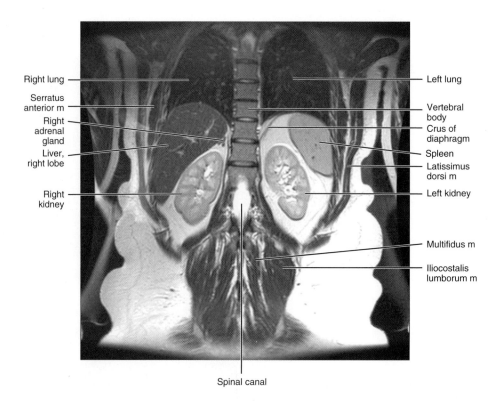

Right lung

Serratus
anterior m

Right
adrenal
gland

Liver,
right lobe

Right
kidney

Left lung

Vertebral
body

Crus of
diaphragm

Spleen

Latissimus
dorsi m

Left kidney

Multifidus m

Iliocostalis
lumborum m

Spinal canal

Figure 21.3.15

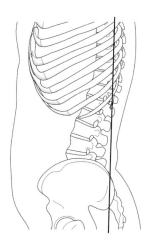

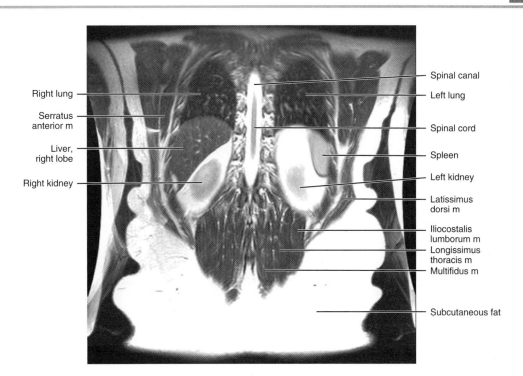

Right lung

Serratus anterior m

Liver, right lobe

Right kidney

Spinal canal

Left lung

Spinal cord

Spleen

Left kidney

Latissimus dorsi m

Iliocostalis lumborum m

Longissimus thoracis m

Multifidus m

Subcutaneous fat

Figure 21.3.16

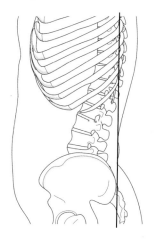

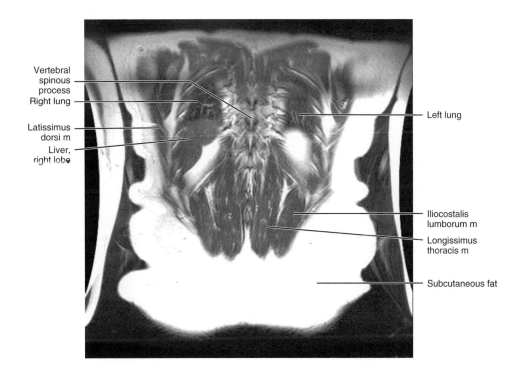

Vertebral spinous process

Right lung

Latissimus dorsi m

Liver, right lobe

Left lung

Iliocostalis lumborum m

Longissimus thoracis m

Subcutaneous fat

Pelvis

Chapter 22

CT of the Male Pelvis

AXIAL

Figure 22.1.1

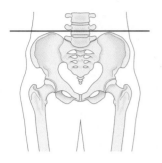

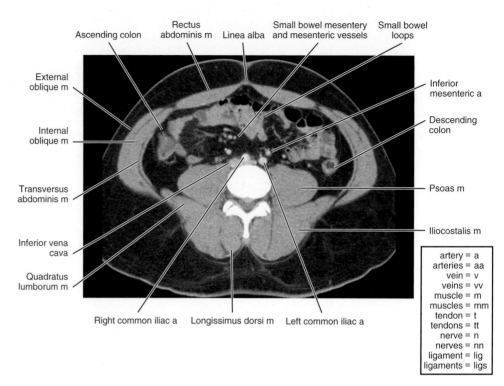

Ascending colon

Rectus abdominis m

Linea alba

Small bowel mesentery and mesenteric vessels

Small bowel loops

External oblique m

Internal oblique m

Transversus abdominis m

Inferior vena cava

Quadratus lumborum m

Inferior mesenteric a

Descending colon

Psoas m

Iliocostalis m

Right common iliac a

Longissimus dorsi m

Left common iliac a

artery	= a
arteries	= aa
vein	= v
veins	= vv
muscle	= m
muscles	= mm
tendon	= t
tendons	= tt
nerve	= n
nerves	= nn
ligament	= lig
ligaments	= ligs

Figure 22.1.2

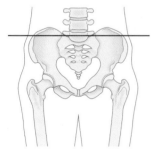

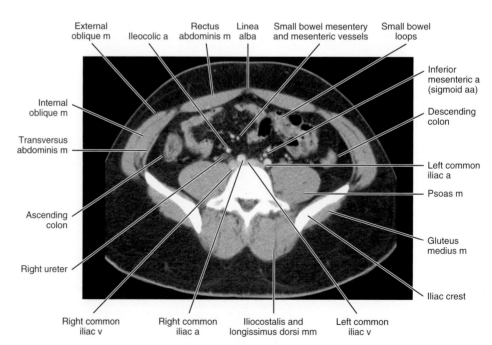

External oblique m

Ileocolic a

Rectus abdominis m

Linea alba

Small bowel mesentery and mesenteric vessels

Small bowel loops

Internal oblique m

Transversus abdominis m

Ascending colon

Right ureter

Inferior mesenteric a (sigmoid aa)

Descending colon

Left common iliac a

Psoas m

Gluteus medius m

Iliac crest

Right common iliac v

Right common iliac a

Iliocostalis and longissimus dorsi mm

Left common iliac v

Figure 22.1.3

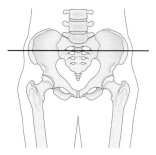

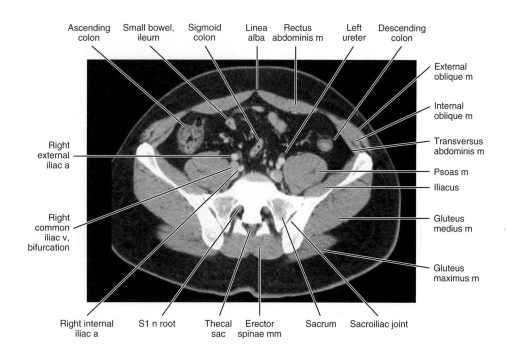

Ascending colon — Small bowel, ileum — Sigmoid colon — Linea alba — Rectus abdominis m — Left ureter — Descending colon

External oblique m

Internal oblique m

Transversus abdominis m

Psoas m

Iliacus

Gluteus medius m

Gluteus maximus m

Right external iliac a

Right common iliac v, bifurcation

Right internal iliac a — S1 n root — Thecal sac — Erector spinae mm — Sacrum — Sacroiliac joint

Figure 22.1.4

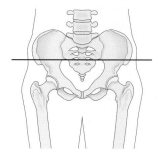

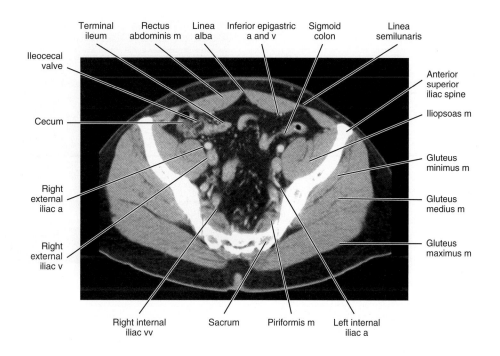

Terminal ileum — Rectus abdominis m — Linea alba — Inferior epigastric a and v — Sigmoid colon — Linea semilunaris

Ileocecal valve

Cecum

Anterior superior iliac spine

Iliopsoas m

Gluteus minimus m

Gluteus medius m

Gluteus maximus m

Right external iliac a

Right external iliac v

Right internal iliac vv — Sacrum — Piriformis m — Left internal iliac a

Figure 22.1.5

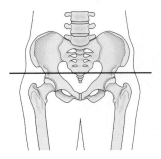

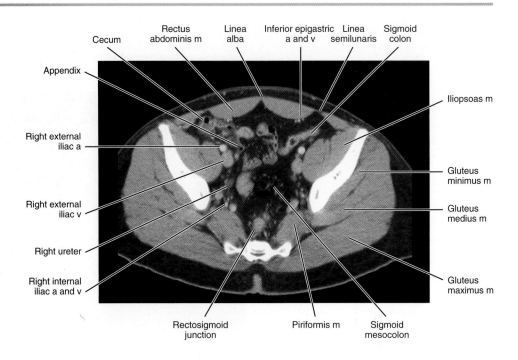

Cecum · Rectus abdominis m · Linea alba · Inferior epigastric a and v · Linea semilunaris · Sigmoid colon

Appendix

Right external iliac a

Right external iliac v

Right ureter

Right internal iliac a and v

Iliopsoas m

Gluteus minimus m

Gluteus medius m

Gluteus maximus m

Rectosigmoid junction · Piriformis m · Sigmoid mesocolon

Figure 22.1.6

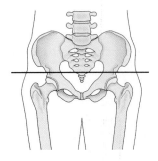

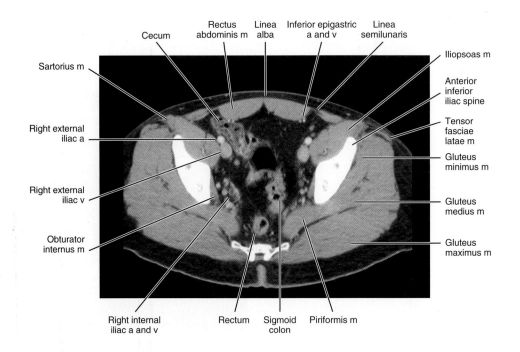

Cecum · Rectus abdominis m · Linea alba · Inferior epigastric a and v · Linea semilunaris

Sartorius m

Right external iliac a

Right external iliac v

Obturator internus m

Iliopsoas m

Anterior inferior iliac spine

Tensor fasciae latae m

Gluteus minimus m

Gluteus medius m

Gluteus maximus m

Right internal iliac a and v · Rectum · Sigmoid colon · Piriformis m

Figure 22.1.7

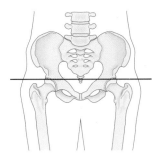

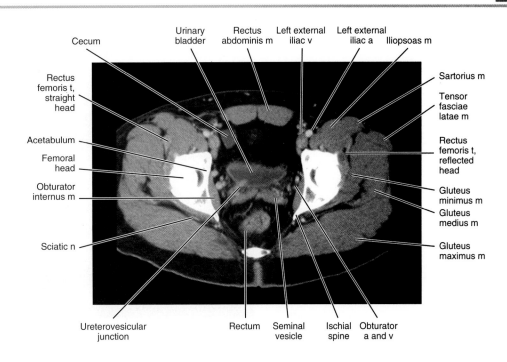

Cecum

Urinary bladder

Rectus abdominis m

Left external iliac v

Left external iliac a

Iliopsoas m

Rectus femoris t, straight head

Sartorius m

Tensor fasciae latae m

Acetabulum

Rectus femoris t, reflected head

Femoral head

Gluteus minimus m

Obturator internus m

Gluteus medius m

Sciatic n

Gluteus maximus m

Ureterovesicular junction

Rectum

Seminal vesicle

Ischial spine

Obturator a and v

Figure 22.1.8

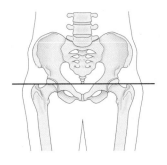

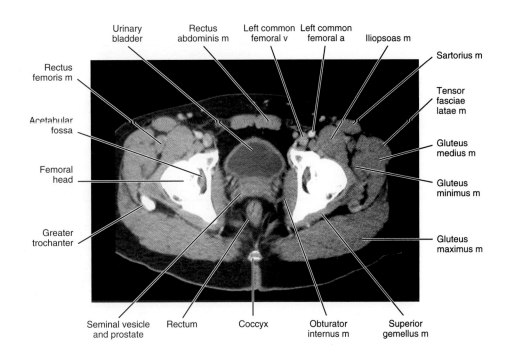

Urinary bladder

Rectus abdominis m

Left common femoral v

Left common femoral a

Iliopsoas m

Rectus femoris m

Sartorius m

Tensor fasciae latae m

Acetabular fossa

Gluteus medius m

Femoral head

Gluteus minimus m

Greater trochanter

Gluteus maximus m

Seminal vesicle and prostate

Rectum

Coccyx

Obturator internus m

Superior gemellus m

Figure 22.1.9

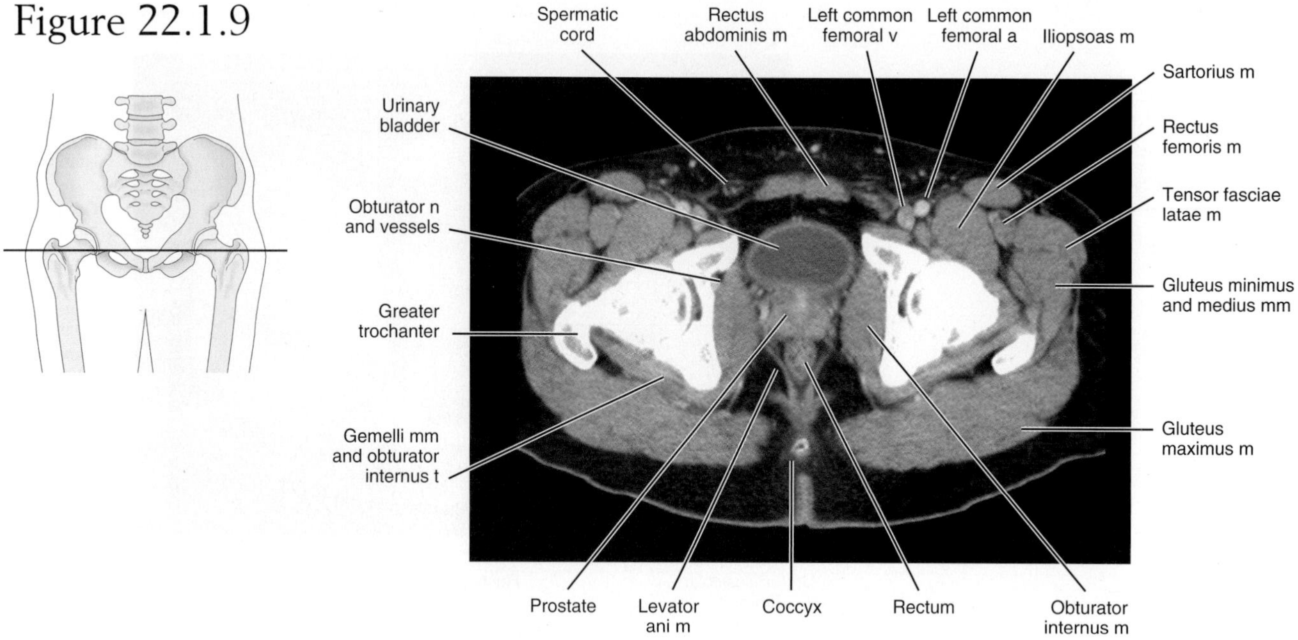

Spermatic cord
Rectus abdominis m
Left common femoral v
Left common femoral a
Iliopsoas m
Sartorius m
Rectus femoris m
Tensor fasciae latae m
Gluteus minimus and medius mm
Urinary bladder
Obturator n and vessels
Greater trochanter
Gemelli mm and obturator internus t
Gluteus maximus m
Prostate
Levator ani m
Coccyx
Rectum
Obturator internus m

Figure 22.1.10

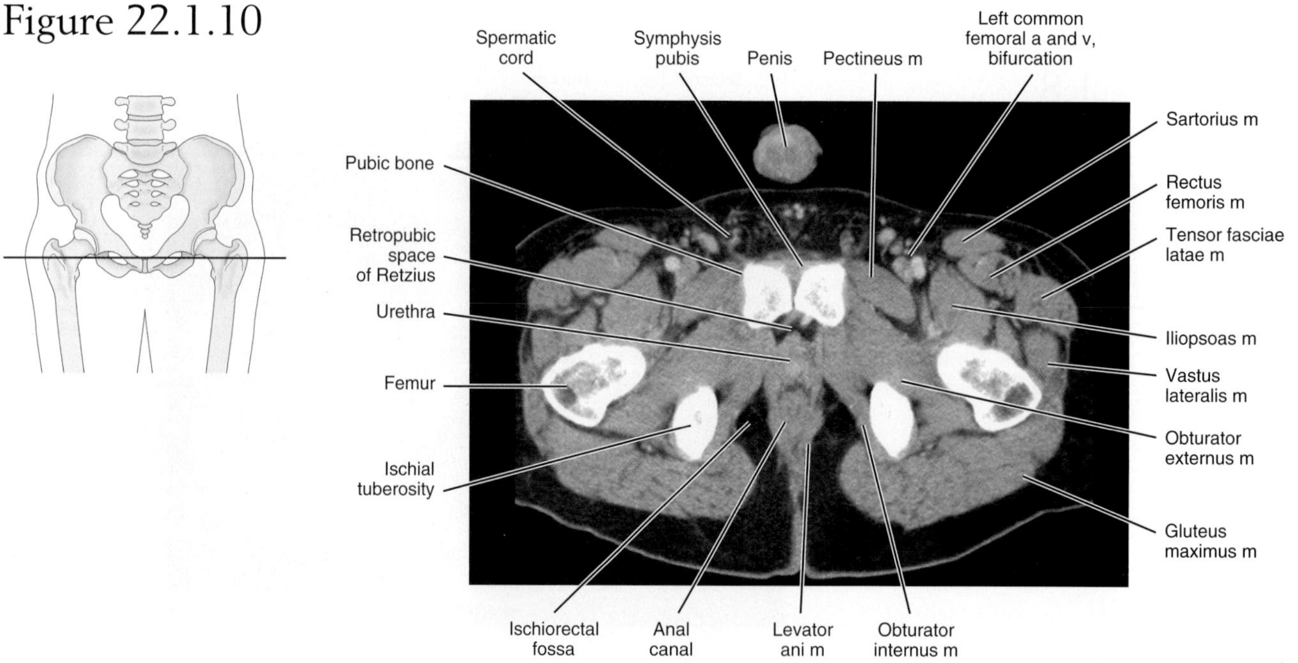

Spermatic cord
Symphysis pubis
Penis
Pectineus m
Left common femoral a and v, bifurcation
Sartorius m
Rectus femoris m
Tensor fasciae latae m
Pubic bone
Retropubic space of Retzius
Urethra
Femur
Ischial tuberosity
Iliopsoas m
Vastus lateralis m
Obturator externus m
Gluteus maximus m
Ischiorectal fossa
Anal canal
Levator ani m
Obturator internus m

Figure 22.1.11

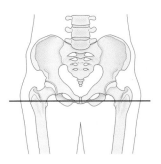

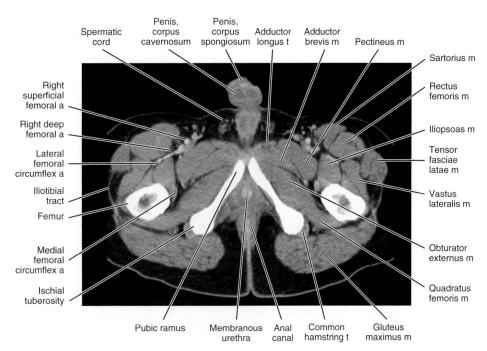

Spermatic cord
Penis, corpus cavernosum
Penis, corpus spongiosum
Adductor longus t
Adductor brevis m
Pectineus m
Sartorius m
Rectus femoris m
Iliopsoas m
Tensor fasciae latae m
Vastus lateralis m
Obturator externus m
Quadratus femoris m
Right superficial femoral a
Right deep femoral a
Lateral femoral circumflex a
Iliotibial tract
Femur
Medial femoral circumflex a
Ischial tuberosity
Pubic ramus
Membranous urethra
Anal canal
Common hamstring t
Gluteus maximus m

Figure 22.1.12

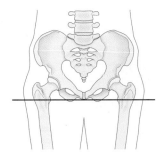

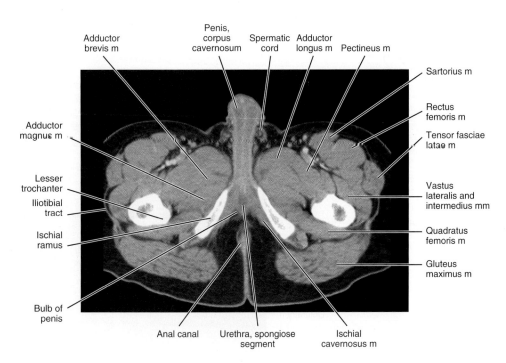

Adductor brevis m
Penis, corpus cavernosum
Spermatic cord
Adductor longus m
Pectineus m
Sartorius m
Rectus femoris m
Tensor fasciae latae m
Vastus lateralis and intermedius mm
Quadratus femoris m
Gluteus maximus m
Adductor magnus m
Lesser trochanter
Iliotibial tract
Ischial ramus
Bulb of penis
Anal canal
Urethra, spongiose segment
Ischial cavernosus m

SAGITTAL

Figure 22.2.1

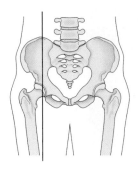

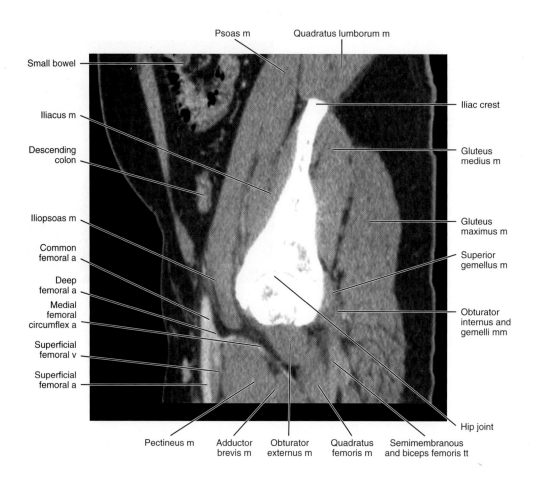

Small bowel

Iliacus m

Descending colon

Iliopsoas m

Common femoral a

Deep femoral a

Medial femoral circumflex a

Superficial femoral v

Superficial femoral a

Psoas m

Quadratus lumborum m

Iliac crest

Gluteus medius m

Gluteus maximus m

Superior gemellus m

Obturator internus and gemelli mm

Hip joint

Pectineus m

Adductor brevis m

Obturator externus m

Quadratus femoris m

Semimembranous and biceps femoris tt

Figure 22.2.2

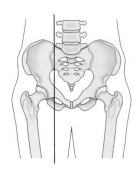

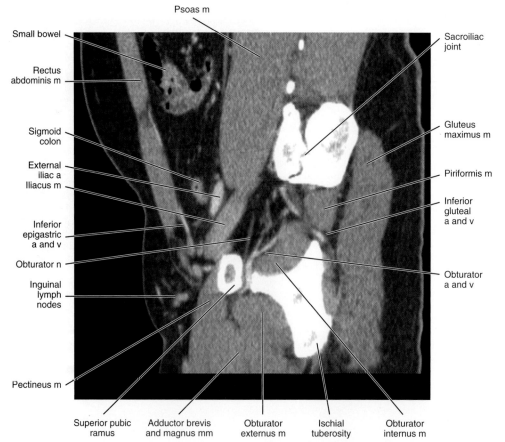

Small bowel

Rectus abdominis m

Sigmoid colon

External iliac a
Iliacus m

Inferior epigastric a and v

Obturator n

Inguinal lymph nodes

Pectineus m

Psoas m

Sacroiliac joint

Gluteus maximus m

Piriformis m

Inferior gluteal a and v

Obturator a and v

Superior pubic ramus

Adductor brevis and magnus mm

Obturator externus m

Ischial tuberosity

Obturator internus m

Figure 22.2.3

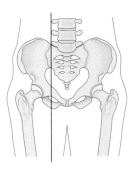

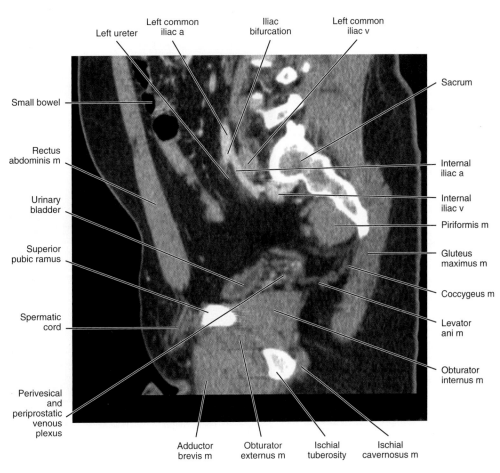

Left ureter

Left common
iliac a

Iliac
bifurcation

Left common
iliac v

Small bowel

Rectus
abdominis m

Urinary
bladder

Superior
pubic ramus

Spermatic
cord

Perivesical
and
periprostatic
venous
plexus

Sacrum

Internal
iliac a

Internal
iliac v

Piriformis m

Gluteus
maximus m

Coccygeus m

Levator
ani m

Obturator
internus m

Adductor
brevis m

Obturator
externus m

Ischial
tuberosity

Ischial
cavernosus m

Figure 22.2.4

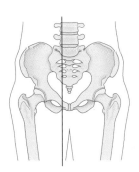

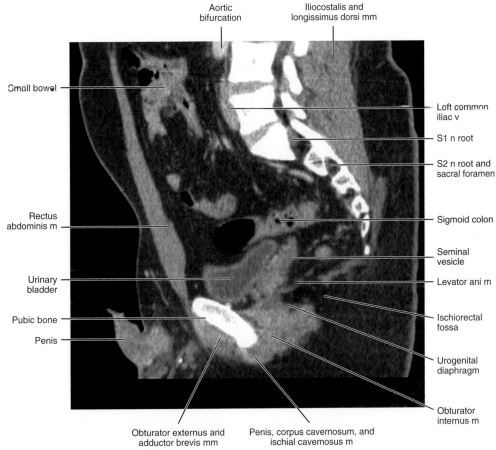

Aortic
bifurcation

Iliocostalis and
longissimus dorsi mm

Small bowel

Rectus
abdominis m

Urinary
bladder

Pubic bone

Penis

Left common
iliac v

S1 n root

S2 n root and
sacral foramen

Sigmoid colon

Seminal
vesicle

Levator ani m

Ischiorectal
fossa

Urogenital
diaphragm

Obturator
internus m

Obturator externus and
adductor brevis mm

Penis, corpus cavernosum, and
ischial cavernosus m

Figure 22.2.5

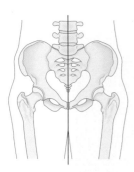

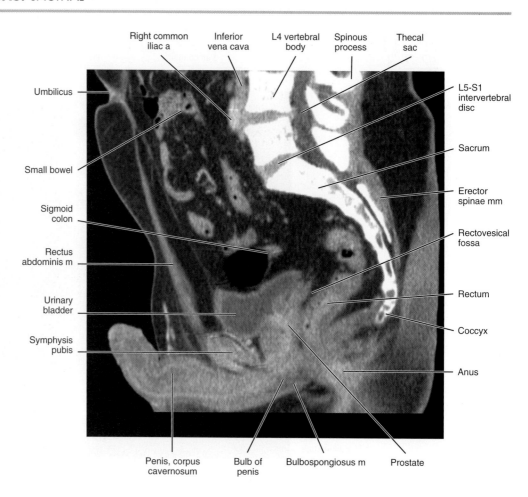

Umbilicus

Small bowel

Sigmoid colon

Rectus abdominis m

Urinary bladder

Symphysis pubis

Right common iliac a

Inferior vena cava

L4 vertebral body

Spinous process

Thecal sac

L5-S1 intervertebral disc

Sacrum

Erector spinae mm

Rectovesical fossa

Rectum

Coccyx

Anus

Penis, corpus cavernosum

Bulb of penis

Bulbospongiosus m

Prostate

CORONAL
Figure 22.3.1

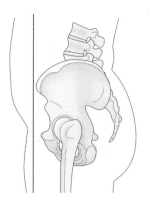

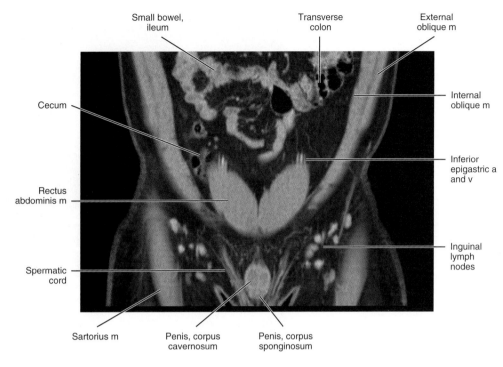

Small bowel, ileum

Transverse colon

External oblique m

Cecum

Internal oblique m

Inferior epigastric a and v

Rectus abdominis m

Inguinal lymph nodes

Spermatic cord

Sartorius m

Penis, corpus cavernosum

Penis, corpus sponginosum

Figure 22.3.2

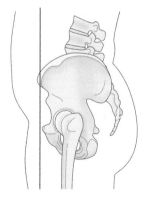

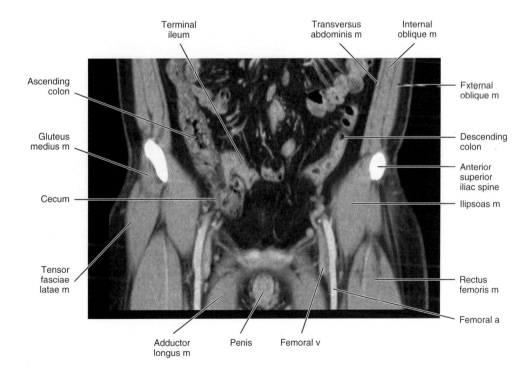

Terminal ileum

Transversus abdominis m

Internal oblique m

Ascending colon

Fxternal oblique m

Gluteus medius m

Descending colon

Anterior superior iliac spine

Cecum

Ilipsoas m

Tensor fasciae latae m

Rectus femoris m

Femoral a

Adductor longus m

Penis

Femoral v

Figure 22.3.3

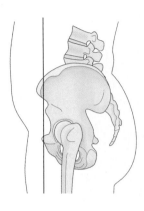

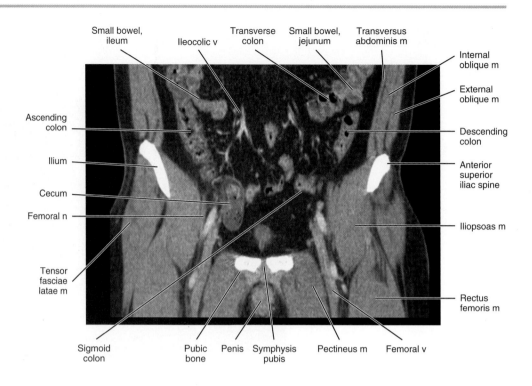

Small bowel, ileum — Ileocolic v — Transverse colon — Small bowel, jejunum — Transversus abdominis m

Internal oblique m

External oblique m

Ascending colon

Descending colon

Ilium

Anterior superior iliac spine

Cecum

Femoral n

Iliopsoas m

Tensor fasciae latae m

Rectus femoris m

Sigmoid colon — Pubic bone — Penis — Symphysis pubis — Pectineus m — Femoral v

Figure 22.3.4

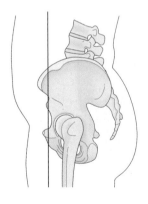

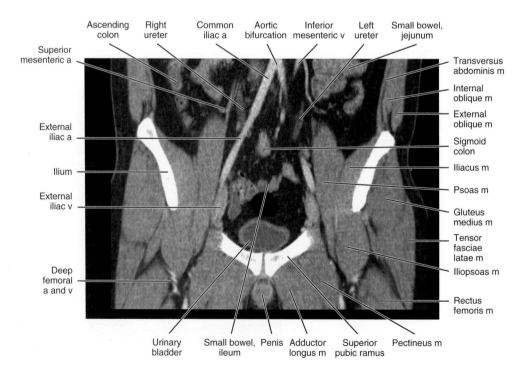

Ascending colon — Right ureter — Common iliac a — Aortic bifurcation — Inferior mesenteric v — Left ureter — Small bowel, jejunum

Superior mesenteric a

Transversus abdominis m

Internal oblique m

External iliac a

External oblique m

Sigmoid colon

Ilium

Iliacus m

External iliac v

Psoas m

Gluteus medius m

Tensor fasciae latae m

Iliopsoas m

Deep femoral a and v

Rectus femoris m

Urinary bladder — Small bowel, ileum — Penis — Adductor longus m — Superior pubic ramus — Pectineus m

Figure 22.3.5

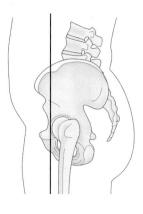

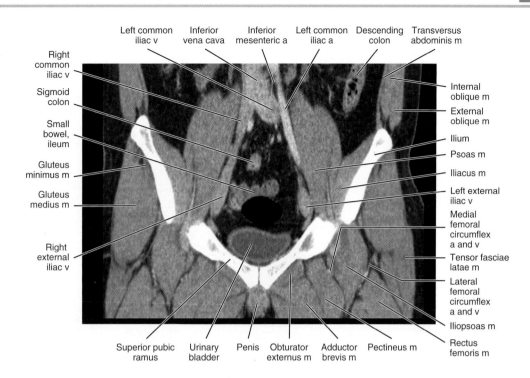

Right common iliac v
Sigmoid colon
Small bowel, ileum
Gluteus minimus m
Gluteus medius m
Right external iliac v

Left common iliac v
Inferior vena cava
Inferior mesenteric a
Left common iliac a
Descending colon
Transversus abdominis m

Internal oblique m
External oblique m
Ilium
Psoas m
Iliacus m
Left external iliac v
Medial femoral circumflex a and v
Tensor fasciae latae m
Lateral femoral circumflex a and v
Iliopsoas m
Rectus femoris m

Superior pubic ramus
Urinary bladder
Penis
Obturator externus m
Adductor brevis m
Pectineus m

Figure 22.3.6

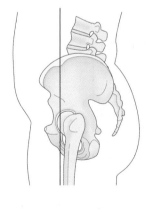

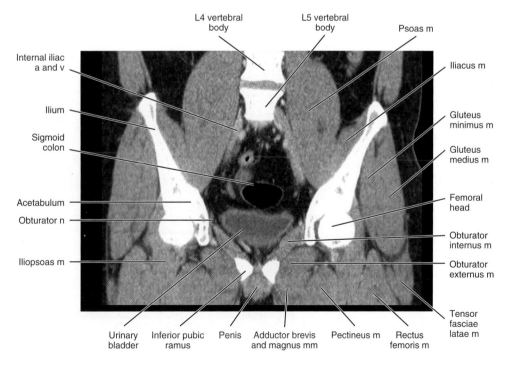

L4 vertebral body
L5 vertebral body
Psoas m

Internal iliac a and v
Ilium
Sigmoid colon
Acetabulum
Obturator n
Iliopsoas m

Iliacus m
Gluteus minimus m
Gluteus medius m
Femoral head
Obturator internus m
Obturator externus m
Tensor fasciae latae m

Urinary bladder
Inferior pubic ramus
Penis
Adductor brevis and magnus mm
Pectineus m
Rectus femoris m

Figure 22.3.7

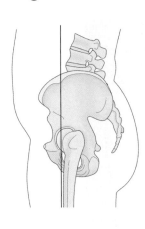

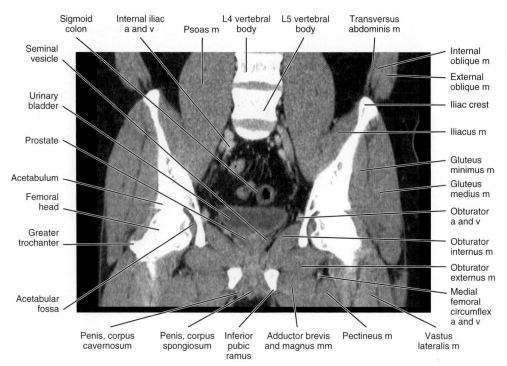

Sigmoid colon — Internal iliac a and v — Psoas m — L4 vertebral body — L5 vertebral body — Transversus abdominis m

Seminal vesicle — Urinary bladder — Prostate — Acetabulum — Femoral head — Greater trochanter — Acetabular fossa

Internal oblique m — External oblique m — Iliac crest — Iliacus m — Gluteus minimus m — Gluteus medius m — Obturator a and v — Obturator internus m — Obturator externus m — Medial femoral circumflex a and v

Penis, corpus cavernosum — Penis, corpus spongiosum — Inferior pubic ramus — Adductor brevis and magnus mm — Pectineus m — Vastus lateralis m

Figure 22.3.8

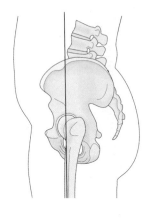

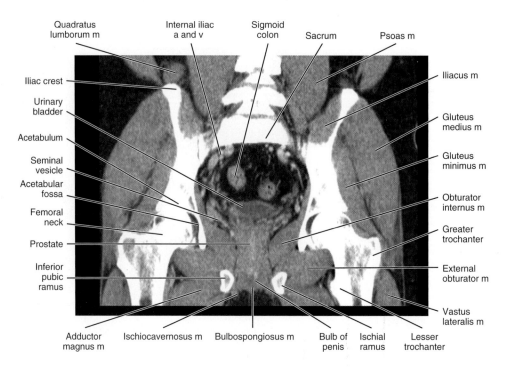

Quadratus lumborum m — Internal iliac a and v — Sigmoid colon — Sacrum — Psoas m

Iliac crest — Urinary bladder — Acetabulum — Seminal vesicle — Acetabular fossa — Femoral neck — Prostate — Inferior pubic ramus

Iliacus m — Gluteus medius m — Gluteus minimus m — Obturator internus m — Greater trochanter — External obturator m — Vastus lateralis m

Adductor magnus m — Ischiocavernosus m — Bulbospongiosus m — Bulb of penis — Ischial ramus — Lesser trochanter

Figure 22.3.9

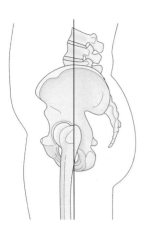

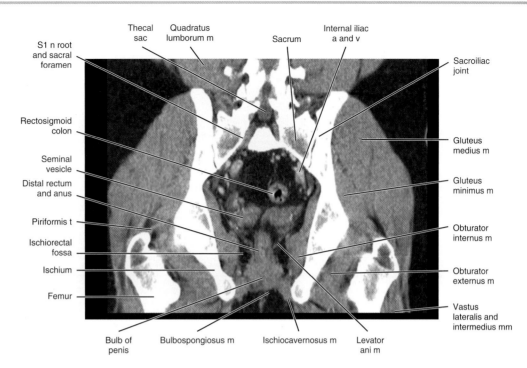

Thecal sac · Quadratus lumborum m · Sacrum · Internal iliac a and v

S1 n root and sacral foramen · Sacroiliac joint

Rectosigmoid colon · Gluteus medius m

Seminal vesicle · Gluteus minimus m

Distal rectum and anus · Obturator internus m

Piriformis t · Obturator externus m

Ischiorectal fossa · Vastus lateralis and intermedius mm

Ischium

Femur

Bulb of penis · Bulbospongiosus m · Ischiocavernosus m · Levator ani m

Figure 22.3.10

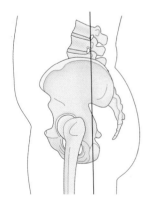

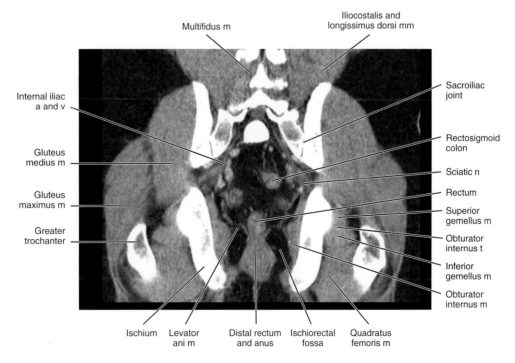

Multifidus m · Iliocostalis and longissimus dorsi mm

Internal iliac a and v · Sacroiliac joint

Gluteus medius m · Rectosigmoid colon

Gluteus maximus m · Sciatic n

Greater trochanter · Rectum

Superior gemellus m

Obturator internus t

Inferior gemellus m

Obturator internus m

Ischium · Levator ani m · Distal rectum and anus · Ischiorectal fossa · Quadratus femoris m

Figure 22.3.11

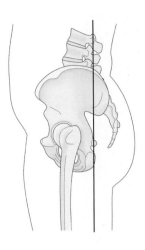

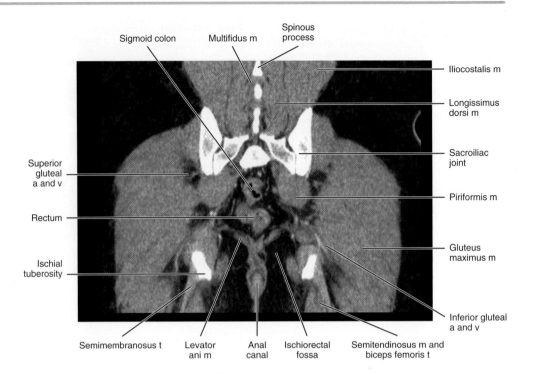

Sigmoid colon

Multifidus m

Spinous process

Iliocostalis m

Longissimus dorsi m

Sacroiliac joint

Superior gluteal a and v

Piriformis m

Rectum

Ischial tuberosity

Gluteus maximus m

Inferior gluteal a and v

Semimembranosus t

Levator ani m

Anal canal

Ischiorectal fossa

Semitendinosus m and biceps femoris t

Chapter 23

CT of the Female Pelvis

AXIAL

Figure 23.1.1

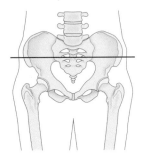

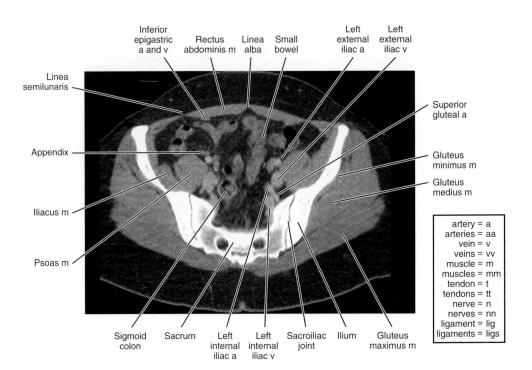

Labels (Figure 23.1.1):
Inferior epigastric a and v · Rectus abdominis m · Linea alba · Small bowel · Left external iliac a · Left external iliac v · Linea semilunaris · Superior gluteal a · Appendix · Gluteus minimus m · Gluteus medius m · Iliacus m · Psoas m · Sigmoid colon · Sacrum · Left internal iliac a · Left internal iliac v · Sacroiliac joint · Ilium · Gluteus maximus m

artery	= a
arteries	= aa
vein	= v
veins	= vv
muscle	= m
muscles	= mm
tendon	= t
tendons	= tt
nerve	= n
nerves	= nn
ligament	= lig
ligaments	= ligs

Figure 23.1.2

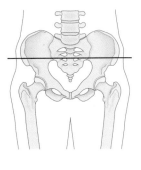

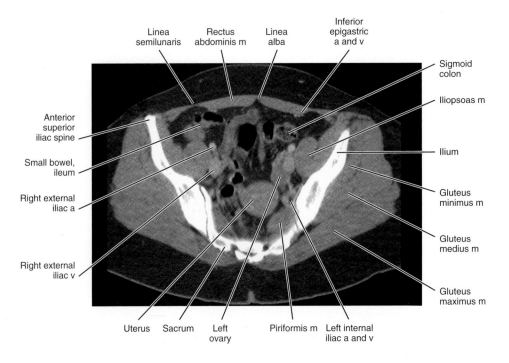

Labels (Figure 23.1.2):
Linea semilunaris · Rectus abdominis m · Linea alba · Inferior epigastric a and v · Sigmoid colon · Iliopsoas m · Anterior superior iliac spine · Ilium · Small bowel, ileum · Gluteus minimus m · Right external iliac a · Gluteus medius m · Right external iliac v · Gluteus maximus m · Uterus · Sacrum · Left ovary · Piriformis m · Left internal iliac a and v

Figure 23.1.3

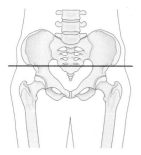

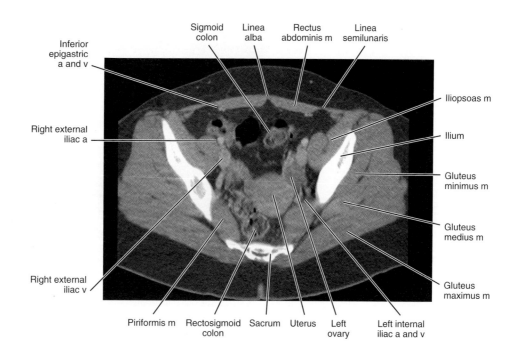

Inferior epigastric a and v

Sigmoid colon

Linea alba

Rectus abdominis m

Linea semilunaris

Iliopsoas m

Ilium

Right external iliac a

Gluteus minimus m

Gluteus medius m

Gluteus maximus m

Right external iliac v

Piriformis m   Rectosigmoid colon   Sacrum   Uterus   Left ovary   Left internal iliac a and v

Figure 23.1.4

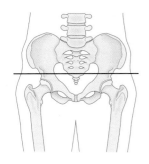

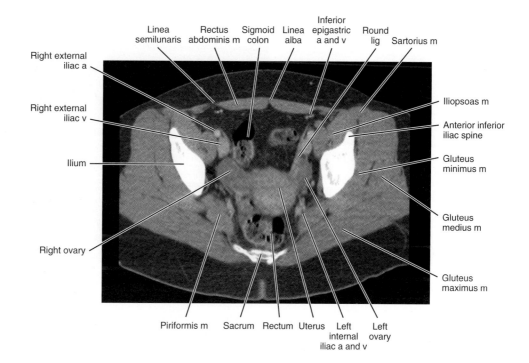

Linea semilunaris

Rectus abdominis m

Sigmoid colon

Linea alba

Inferior epigastric a and v

Round lig

Sartorius m

Right external iliac a

Iliopsoas m

Right external iliac v

Anterior inferior iliac spine

Gluteus minimus m

Ilium

Gluteus medius m

Right ovary

Gluteus maximus m

Piriformis m   Sacrum   Rectum   Uterus   Left internal iliac a and v   Left ovary

Figure 23.1.5

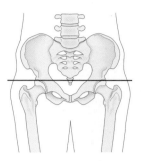

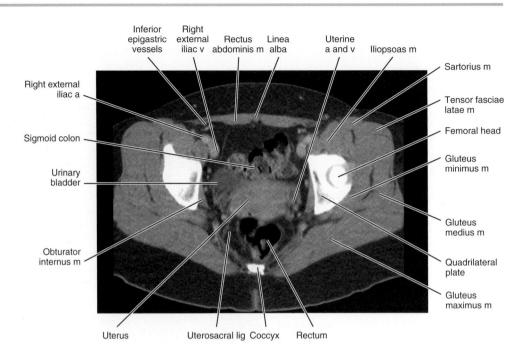

Inferior epigastric vessels · Right external iliac v · Rectus abdominis m · Linea alba · Uterine a and v · Iliopsoas m · Sartorius m · Tensor fasciae latae m · Femoral head · Gluteus minimus m · Gluteus medius m · Quadrilateral plate · Gluteus maximus m · Right external iliac a · Sigmoid colon · Urinary bladder · Obturator internus m · Uterus · Uterosacral lig · Coccyx · Rectum

Figure 23.1.6

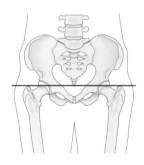

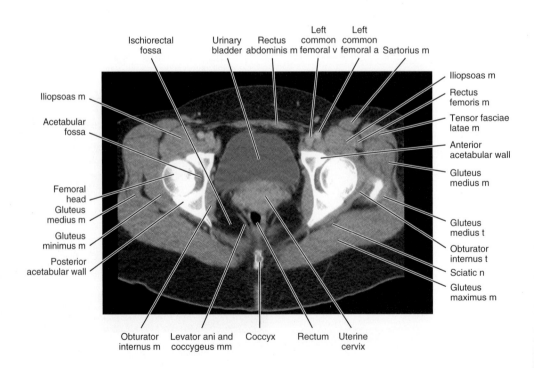

Ischiorectal fossa · Urinary bladder · Rectus abdominis m · Left common femoral v · Left common femoral a · Sartorius m · Iliopsoas m · Rectus femoris m · Tensor fasciae latae m · Anterior acetabular wall · Gluteus medius m · Gluteus medius t · Obturator internus t · Sciatic n · Gluteus maximus m · Iliopsoas m · Acetabular fossa · Femoral head · Gluteus medius m · Gluteus minimus m · Posterior acetabular wall · Obturator internus m · Levator ani and coccygeus mm · Coccyx · Rectum · Uterine cervix

Figure 23.1.7

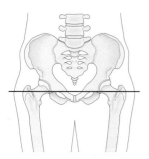

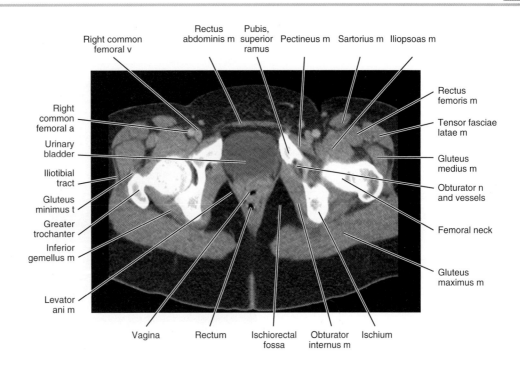

Right common femoral v

Rectus abdominis m

Pubis, superior ramus

Pectineus m

Sartorius m

Iliopsoas m

Right common femoral a

Urinary bladder

Iliotibial tract

Gluteus minimus t

Greater trochanter

Inferior gemellus m

Levator ani m

Rectus femoris m

Tensor fasciae latae m

Gluteus medius m

Obturator n and vessels

Femoral neck

Gluteus maximus m

Vagina

Rectum

Ischiorectal fossa

Obturator internus m

Ischium

Figure 23.1.8

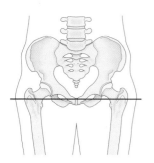

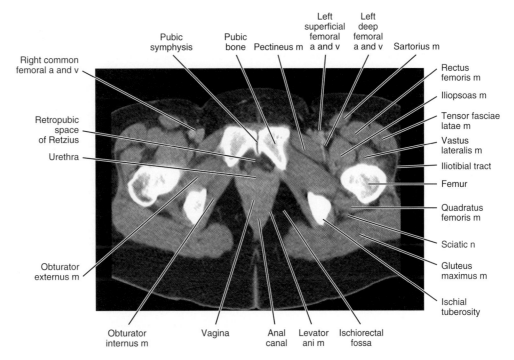

Pubic symphysis

Pubic bone

Pectineus m

Left superficial femoral a and v

Left deep femoral a and v

Sartorius m

Right common femoral a and v

Retropubic space of Retzius

Urethra

Obturator externus m

Rectus femoris m

Iliopsoas m

Tensor fasciae latae m

Vastus lateralis m

Iliotibial tract

Femur

Quadratus femoris m

Sciatic n

Gluteus maximus m

Ischial tuberosity

Obturator internus m

Vagina

Anal canal

Levator ani m

Ischiorectal fossa

Figure 23.1.9

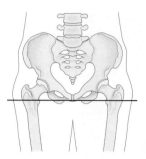

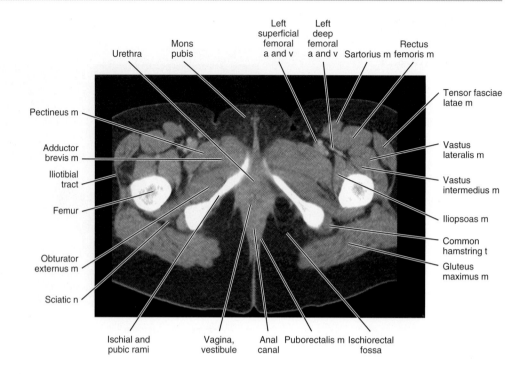

Urethra

Mons pubis

Left superficial femoral a and v

Left deep femoral a and v

Sartorius m

Rectus femoris m

Tensor fasciae latae m

Pectineus m

Vastus lateralis m

Adductor brevis m

Vastus intermedius m

Iliotibial tract

Femur

Iliopsoas m

Common hamstring t

Obturator externus m

Gluteus maximus m

Sciatic n

Ischial and pubic rami

Vagina, vestibule

Anal canal

Puborectalis m

Ischiorectal fossa

SAGITTAL
Figure 23.2.1

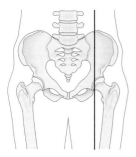

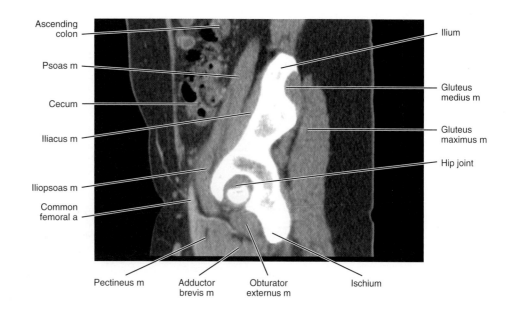

Ascending colon

Psoas m

Cecum

Iliacus m

Iliopsoas m

Common femoral a

Ilium

Gluteus medius m

Gluteus maximus m

Hip joint

Pectineus m

Adductor brevis m

Obturator externus m

Ischium

Figure 23.2.2

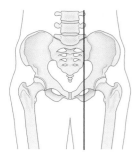

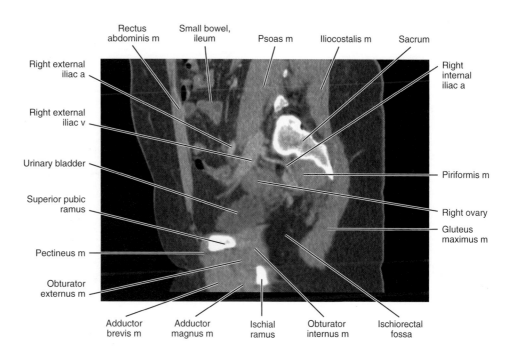

Rectus abdominis m

Small bowel, ileum

Psoas m

Iliocostalis m

Sacrum

Right external iliac a

Right external iliac v

Urinary bladder

Superior pubic ramus

Pectineus m

Obturator externus m

Right internal iliac a

Piriformis m

Right ovary

Gluteus maximus m

Adductor brevis m

Adductor magnus m

Ischial ramus

Obturator internus m

Ischiorectal fossa

Figure 23.2.3

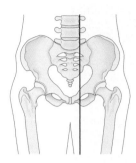

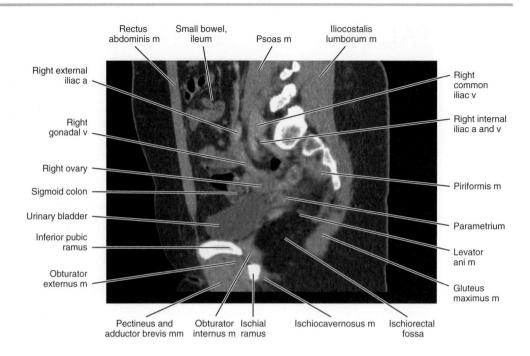

Rectus abdominis m — Small bowel, ileum — Psoas m — Iliocostalis lumborum m

Right external iliac a

Right common iliac v

Right gonadal v

Right internal iliac a and v

Right ovary

Sigmoid colon

Piriformis m

Urinary bladder

Parametrium

Inferior pubic ramus

Levator ani m

Obturator externus m

Gluteus maximus m

Pectineus and adductor brevis mm — Obturator internus m — Ischial ramus — Ischiocavernosus m — Ischiorectal fossa

Figure 23.2.4

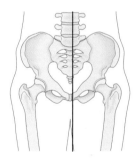

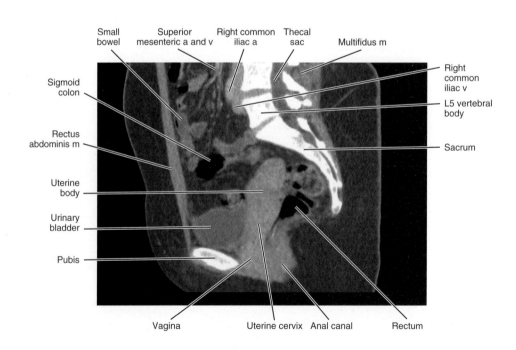

Small bowel — Superior mesenteric a and v — Right common iliac a — Thecal sac — Multifidus m

Sigmoid colon

Right common iliac v

L5 vertebral body

Rectus abdominis m

Sacrum

Uterine body

Urinary bladder

Pubis

Vagina — Uterine cervix — Anal canal — Rectum

Figure 23.2.5

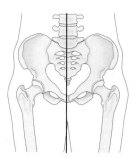

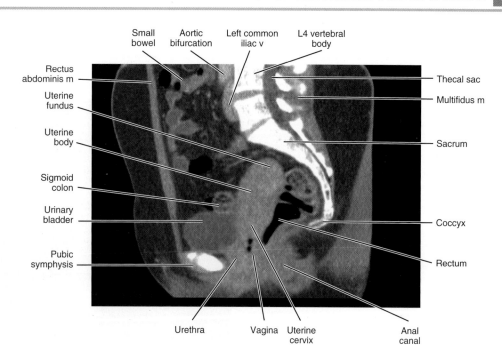

Small bowel

Aortic bifurcation

Left common iliac v

L4 vertebral body

Rectus abdominis m

Uterine fundus

Uterine body

Sigmoid colon

Urinary bladder

Pubic symphysis

Thecal sac

Multifidus m

Sacrum

Coccyx

Rectum

Urethra

Vagina

Uterine cervix

Anal canal

CORONAL

Figure 23.3.1

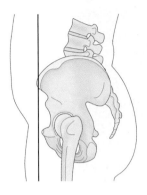

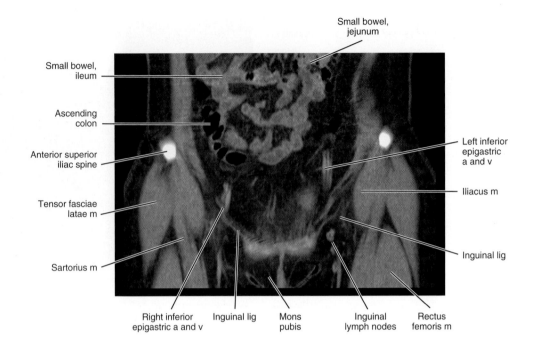

Small bowel, jejunum

Small bowel, ileum

Ascending colon

Anterior superior iliac spine

Tensor fasciae latae m

Sartorius m

Left inferior epigastric a and v

Iliacus m

Inguinal lig

Right inferior epigastric a and v

Inguinal lig

Mons pubis

Inguinal lymph nodes

Rectus femoris m

Figure 23.3.2

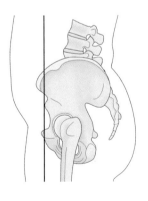

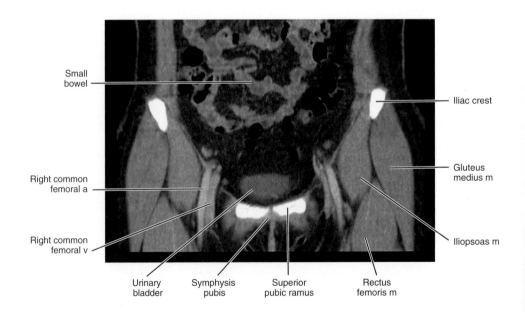

Small bowel

Iliac crest

Right common femoral a

Gluteus medius m

Right common femoral v

Iliopsoas m

Urinary bladder

Symphysis pubis

Superior pubic ramus

Rectus femoris m

Figure 23.3.3

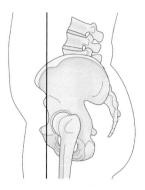

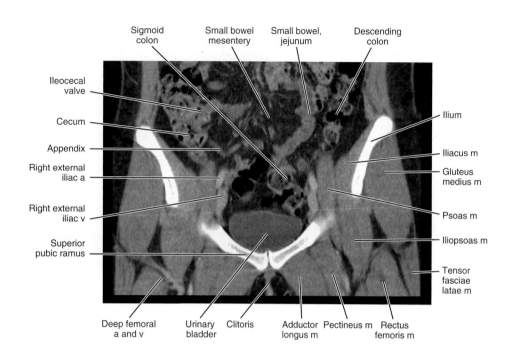

Sigmoid colon

Small bowel mesentery

Small bowel, jejunum

Descending colon

Ileocecal valve

Cecum

Appendix

Right external iliac a

Right external iliac v

Superior pubic ramus

Ilium

Iliacus m

Gluteus medius m

Psoas m

Iliopsoas m

Tensor fasciae latae m

Deep femoral a and v

Urinary bladder

Clitoris

Adductor longus m

Pectineus m

Rectus femoris m

Figure 23.3.4

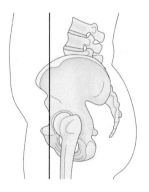

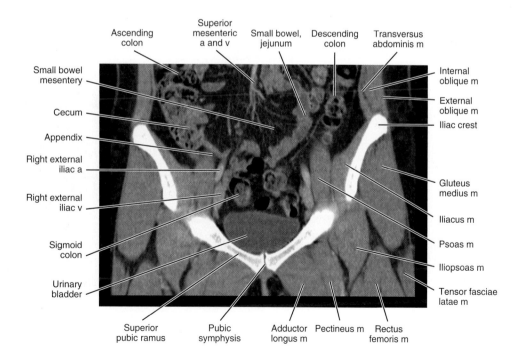

Ascending colon

Superior mesenteric a and v

Small bowel, jejunum

Descending colon

Transversus abdominis m

Small bowel mesentery

Cecum

Appendix

Right external iliac a

Right external iliac v

Sigmoid colon

Urinary bladder

Internal oblique m

External oblique m

Iliac crest

Gluteus medius m

Iliacus m

Psoas m

Iliopsoas m

Tensor fasciae latae m

Superior pubic ramus

Pubic symphysis

Adductor longus m

Pectineus m

Rectus femoris m

Figure 23.3.5

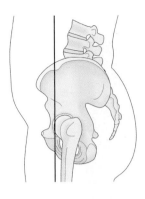

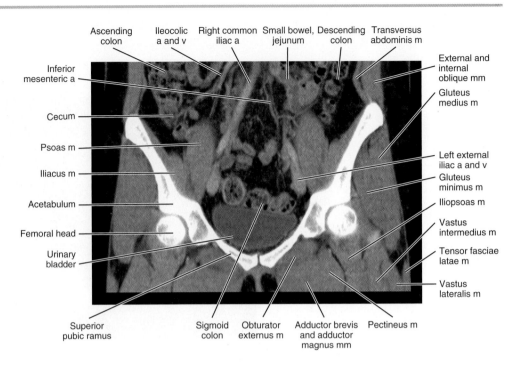

Inferior mesenteric a — Ascending colon — Ileocolic a and v — Right common iliac a — Small bowel, jejunum — Descending colon — Transversus abdominis m — External and internal oblique mm — Gluteus medius m — Cecum — Psoas m — Iliacus m — Acetabulum — Femoral head — Urinary bladder — Left external iliac a and v — Gluteus minimus m — Iliopsoas m — Vastus intermedius m — Tensor fasciae latae m — Vastus lateralis m

Superior pubic ramus — Sigmoid colon — Obturator externus m — Adductor brevis and adductor magnus mm — Pectineus m

Figure 23.3.6

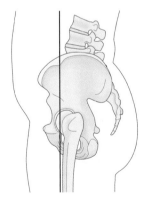

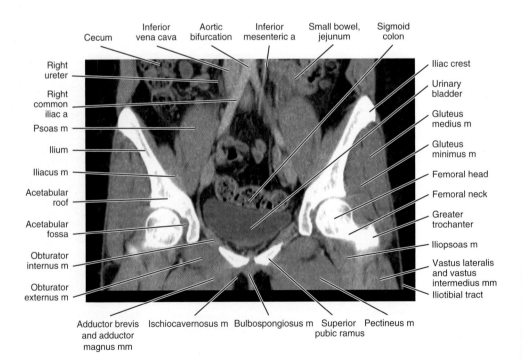

Cecum — Inferior vena cava — Aortic bifurcation — Inferior mesenteric a — Small bowel, jejunum — Sigmoid colon — Right ureter — Iliac crest — Right common iliac a — Urinary bladder — Psoas m — Gluteus medius m — Ilium — Gluteus minimus m — Iliacus m — Femoral head — Acetabular roof — Femoral neck — Acetabular fossa — Greater trochanter — Obturator internus m — Iliopsoas m — Obturator externus m — Vastus lateralis and vastus intermedius mm — Iliotibial tract

Adductor brevis and adductor magnus mm — Ischiocavernosus m — Bulbospongiosus m — Superior pubic ramus — Pectineus m

Figure 23.3.7

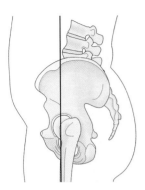

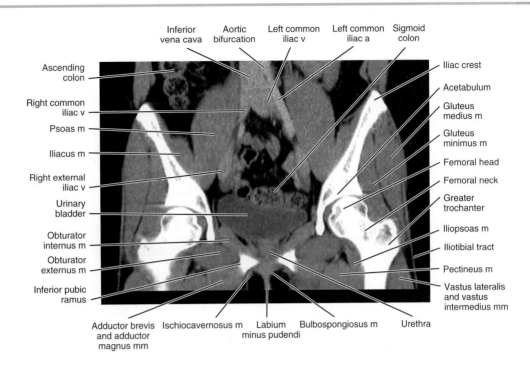

Inferior vena cava
Aortic bifurcation
Left common iliac v
Left common iliac a
Sigmoid colon

Ascending colon

Right common iliac v

Psoas m

Iliacus m

Right external iliac v

Urinary bladder

Obturator internus m

Obturator externus m

Inferior pubic ramus

Iliac crest

Acetabulum

Gluteus medius m

Gluteus minimus m

Femoral head

Femoral neck

Greater trochanter

Iliopsoas m

Iliotibial tract

Pectineus m

Vastus lateralis and vastus intermedius mm

Adductor brevis and adductor magnus mm
Ischiocavernosus m
Labium minus pudendi
Bulbospongiosus m
Urethra

Figure 23.3.8

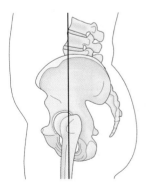

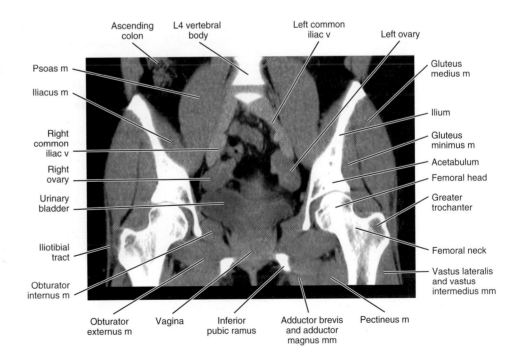

Ascending colon
L4 vertebral body
Left common iliac v
Left ovary

Psoas m

Iliacus m

Right common iliac v

Right ovary

Urinary bladder

Iliotibial tract

Obturator internus m

Gluteus medius m

Ilium

Gluteus minimus m

Acetabulum

Femoral head

Greater trochanter

Femoral neck

Vastus lateralis and vastus intermedius mm

Obturator externus m
Vagina
Inferior pubic ramus
Adductor brevis and adductor magnus mm
Pectineus m

Figure 23.3.9

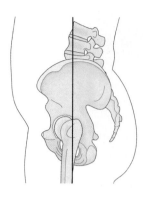

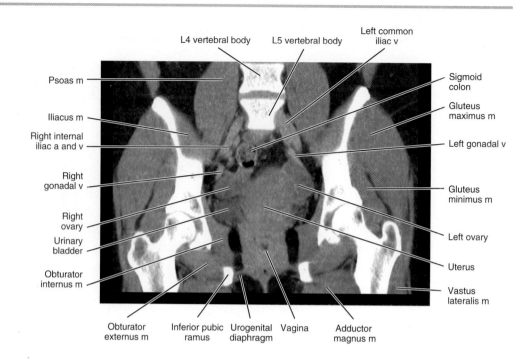

L4 vertebral body
L5 vertebral body
Left common iliac v
Psoas m
Sigmoid colon
Iliacus m
Gluteus maximus m
Right internal iliac a and v
Left gonadal v
Right gonadal v
Gluteus minimus m
Right ovary
Urinary bladder
Left ovary
Obturator internus m
Uterus
Vastus lateralis m
Obturator externus m
Inferior pubic ramus
Urogenital diaphragm
Vagina
Adductor magnus m

Figure 23.3.10

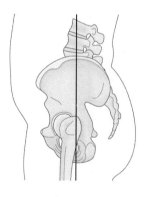

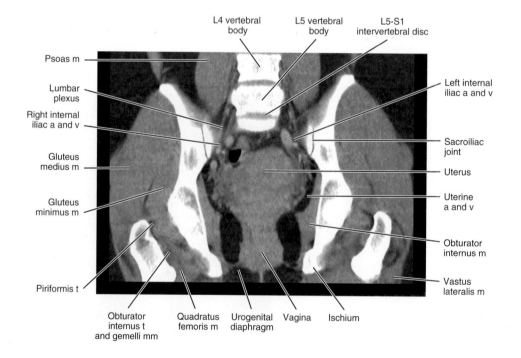

L4 vertebral body
L5 vertebral body
L5-S1 intervertebral disc
Psoas m
Lumbar plexus
Left internal iliac a and v
Right internal iliac a and v
Sacroiliac joint
Gluteus medius m
Uterus
Gluteus minimus m
Uterine a and v
Obturator internus m
Piriformis t
Vastus lateralis m
Obturator internus t and gemelli mm
Quadratus femoris m
Urogenital diaphragm
Vagina
Ischium

Figure 23.3.11

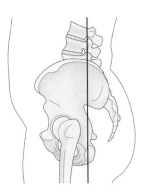

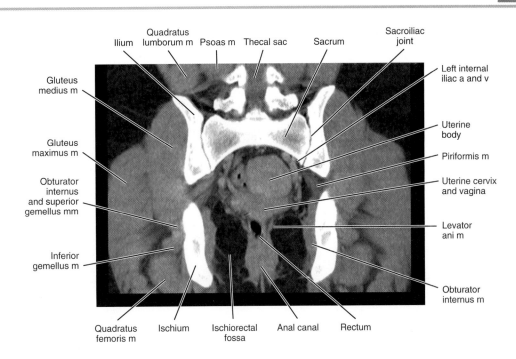

Ilium Quadratus lumborum m Psoas m Thecal sac Sacrum Sacroiliac joint

Gluteus medius m

Gluteus maximus m

Obturator internus and superior gemellus mm

Inferior gemellus m

Left internal iliac a and v

Uterine body

Piriformis m

Uterine cervix and vagina

Levator ani m

Obturator internus m

Quadratus femoris m Ischium Ischiorectal fossa Anal canal Rectum

Figure 23.3.12

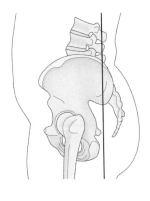

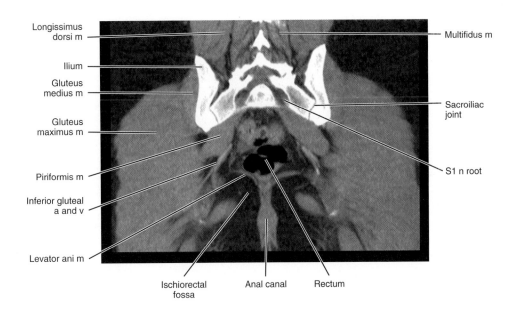

Longissimus dorsi m

Ilium

Gluteus medius m

Gluteus maximus m

Piriformis m

Inferior gluteal a and v

Levator ani m

Multifidus m

Sacroiliac joint

S1 n root

Ischiorectal fossa Anal canal Rectum

Chapter 24

MRI of the Male Pelvis

AXIAL

Figure 24.1.1

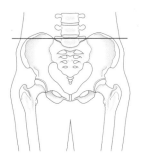

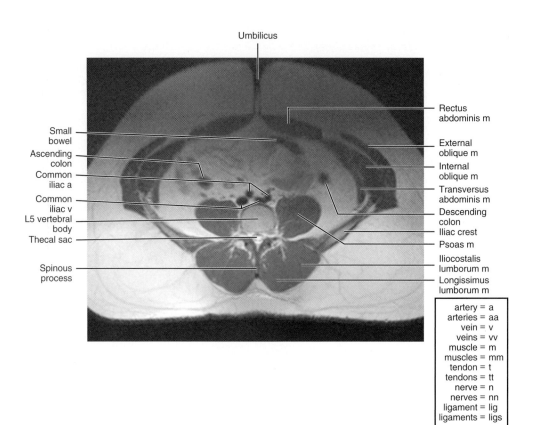

Umbilicus

Rectus abdominis m

External oblique m

Internal oblique m

Transversus abdominis m

Descending colon

Iliac crest

Psoas m

Iliocostalis lumborum m

Longissimus lumborum m

Small bowel

Ascending colon

Common iliac a

Common iliac v

L5 vertebral body

Thecal sac

Spinous process

artery = a
arteries = aa
vein = v
veins = vv
muscle = m
muscles = mm
tendon = t
tendons = tt
nerve = n
nerves = nn
ligament = lig
ligaments = ligs

Figure 24.1.2

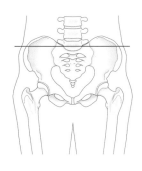

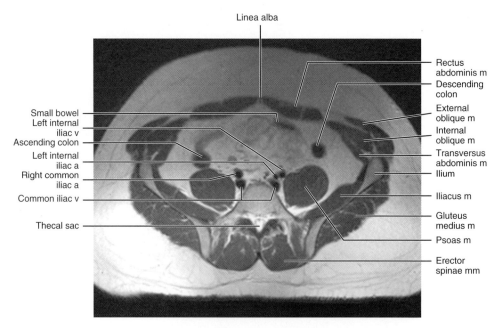

Linea alba

Rectus abdominis m

Descending colon

External oblique m

Internal oblique m

Transversus abdominis m

Ilium

Iliacus m

Gluteus medius m

Psoas m

Erector spinae mm

Small bowel

Left internal iliac v

Ascending colon

Left internal iliac a

Right common iliac a

Common iliac v

Thecal sac

Figure 24.1.3

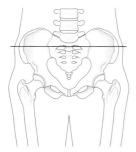

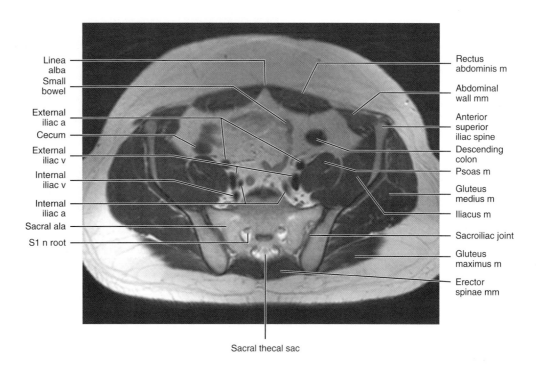

Linea alba
Small bowel
External iliac a
Cecum
External iliac v
Internal iliac v
Internal iliac a
Sacral ala
S1 n root

Rectus abdominis m
Abdominal wall mm
Anterior superior iliac spine
Descending colon
Psoas m
Gluteus medius m
Iliacus m
Sacroiliac joint
Gluteus maximus m
Erector spinae mm

Sacral thecal sac

Figure 24.1.4

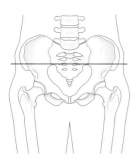

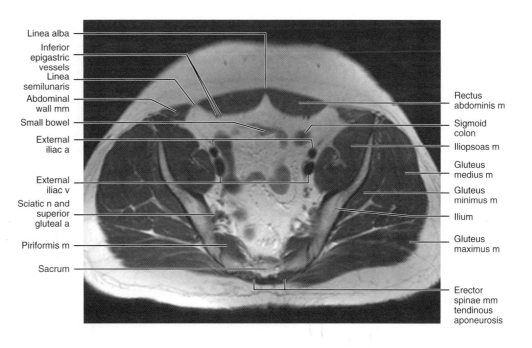

Linea alba
Inferior epigastric vessels
Linea semilunaris
Abdominal wall mm
Small bowel
External iliac a
External iliac v
Sciatic n and superior gluteal a
Piriformis m
Sacrum

Rectus abdominis m
Sigmoid colon
Iliopsoas m
Gluteus medius m
Gluteus minimus m
Ilium
Gluteus maximus m
Erector spinae mm tendinous aponeurosis

Figure 24.1.5

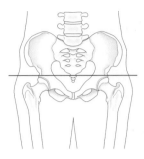

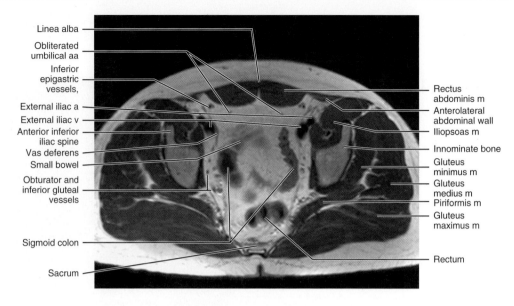

Linea alba

Obliterated umbilical aa

Inferior epigastric vessels,

External iliac a

External iliac v

Anterior inferior iliac spine

Vas deferens

Small bowel

Obturator and inferior gluteal vessels

Sigmoid colon

Sacrum

Rectus abdominis m

Anterolateral abdominal wall

Iliopsoas m

Innominate bone

Gluteus minimus m

Gluteus medius m

Piriformis m

Gluteus maximus m

Rectum

Figure 24.1.6

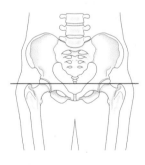

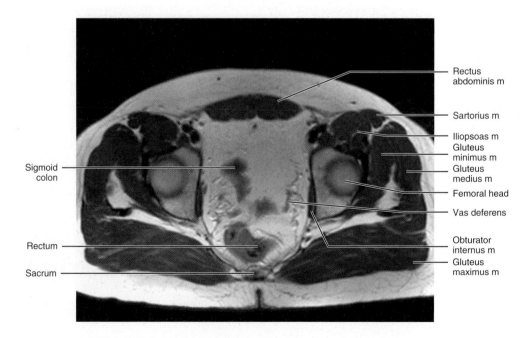

Sigmoid colon

Rectum

Sacrum

Rectus abdominis m

Sartorius m

Iliopsoas m

Gluteus minimus m

Gluteus medius m

Femoral head

Vas deferens

Obturator internus m

Gluteus maximus m

Figure 24.1.7

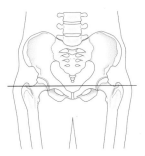

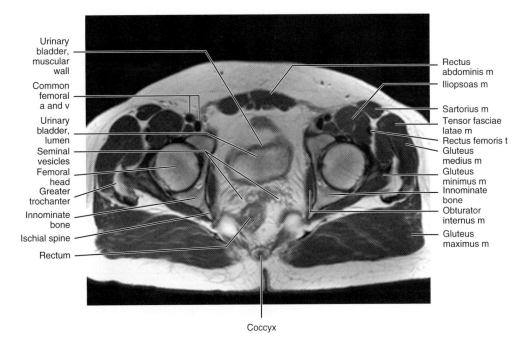

Urinary bladder, muscular wall

Common femoral a and v

Urinary bladder, lumen

Seminal vesicles

Femoral head

Greater trochanter

Innominate bone

Ischial spine

Rectum

Rectus abdominis m

Iliopsoas m

Sartorius m

Tensor fasciae latae m

Rectus femoris t

Gluteus medius m

Gluteus minimus m

Innominate bone

Obturator internus m

Gluteus maximus m

Coccyx

Figure 24.1.8

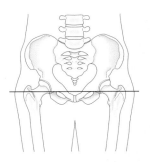

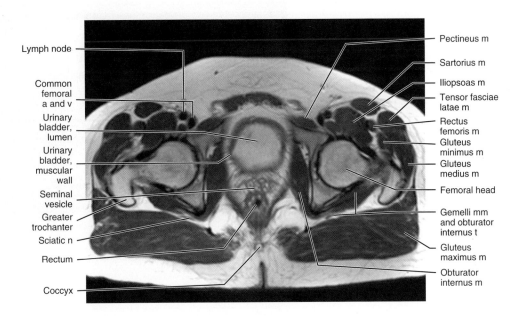

Lymph node

Common femoral a and v

Urinary bladder, lumen

Urinary bladder, muscular wall

Seminal vesicle

Greater trochanter

Sciatic n

Rectum

Coccyx

Pectineus m

Sartorius m

Iliopsoas m

Tensor fasciae latae m

Rectus femoris m

Gluteus minimus m

Gluteus medius m

Femoral head

Gemelli mm and obturator internus t

Gluteus maximus m

Obturator internus m

Figure 24.1.9

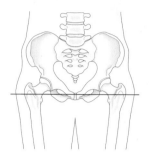

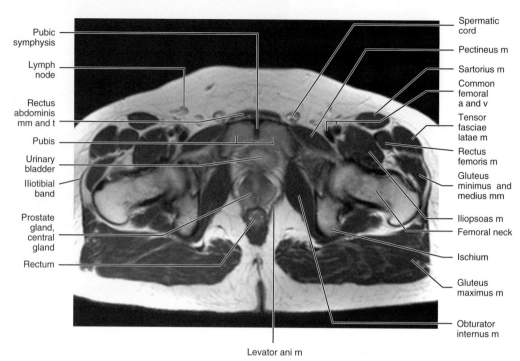

Pubic symphysis

Lymph node

Rectus abdominis mm and t

Pubis

Urinary bladder

Iliotibial band

Prostate gland, central gland

Rectum

Spermatic cord

Pectineus m

Sartorius m

Common femoral a and v

Tensor fasciae latae m

Rectus femoris m

Gluteus minimus and medius mm

Iliopsoas m

Femoral neck

Ischium

Gluteus maximus m

Obturator internus m

Levator ani m

Figure 24.1.10

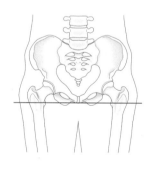

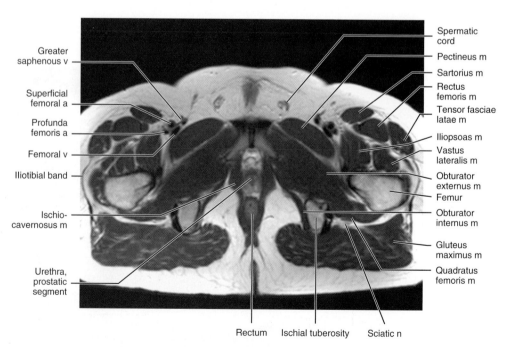

Greater saphenous v

Superficial femoral a

Profunda femoris a

Femoral v

Iliotibial band

Ischio-cavernosus m

Urethra, prostatic segment

Spermatic cord

Pectineus m

Sartorius m

Rectus femoris m

Tensor fasciae latae m

Iliopsoas m

Vastus lateralis m

Obturator externus m

Femur

Obturator internus m

Gluteus maximus m

Quadratus femoris m

Rectum   Ischial tuberosity   Sciatic n

Figure 24.1.11

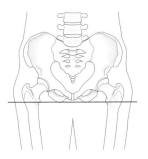

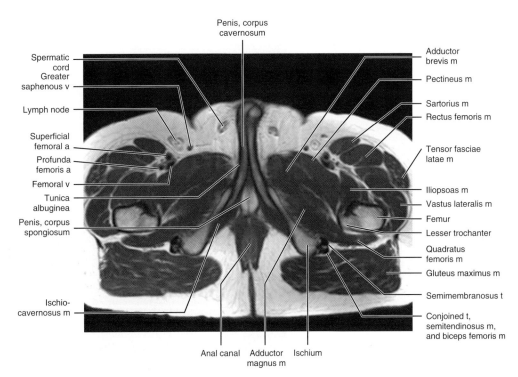

Penis, corpus cavernosum

Spermatic cord
Greater saphenous v

Lymph node

Superficial femoral a

Profunda femoris a

Femoral v

Tunica albuginea

Penis, corpus spongiosum

Ischio-cavernosus m

Adductor brevis m

Pectineus m

Sartorius m
Rectus femoris m

Tensor fasciae latae m

Iliopsoas m
Vastus lateralis m
Femur
Lesser trochanter
Quadratus femoris m
Gluteus maximus m

Semimembranosus t

Conjoined t, semitendinosus m, and biceps femoris m

Anal canal   Adductor magnus m   Ischium

Figure 24.1.12

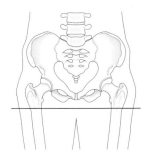

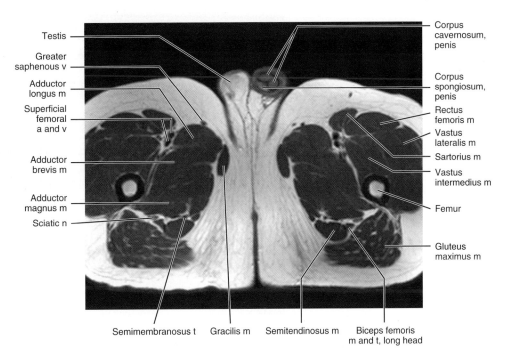

Testis

Greater saphenous v

Adductor longus m

Superficial femoral a and v

Adductor brevis m

Adductor magnus m
Sciatic n

Corpus cavernosum, penis

Corpus spongiosum, penis

Rectus femoris m

Vastus lateralis m

Sartorius m

Vastus intermedius m

Femur

Gluteus maximus m

Semimembranosus t   Gracilis m   Semitendinosus m   Biceps femoris m and t, long head

SAGITTAL

Figure 24.2.1

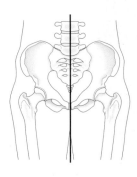

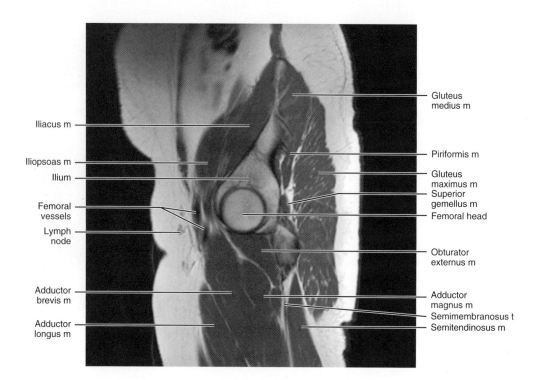

Iliacus m

Iliopsoas m

Ilium

Femoral vessels

Lymph node

Adductor brevis m

Adductor longus m

Gluteus medius m

Piriformis m

Gluteus maximus m

Superior gemellus m

Femoral head

Obturator externus m

Adductor magnus m

Semimembranosus t

Semitendinosus m

Figure 24.2.2

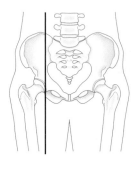

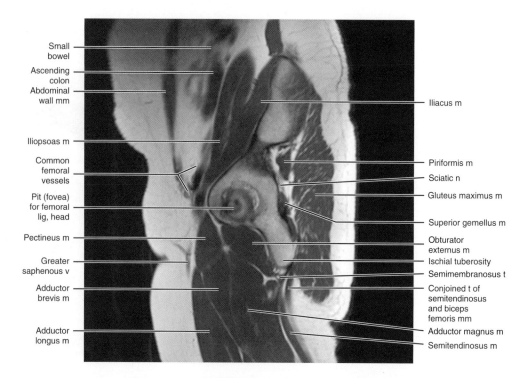

Small bowel

Ascending colon

Abdominal wall mm

Iliopsoas m

Common femoral vessels

Pit (fovea) for femoral lig, head

Pectineus m

Greater saphenous v

Adductor brevis m

Adductor longus m

Iliacus m

Piriformis m

Sciatic n

Gluteus maximus m

Superior gemellus m

Obturator externus m

Ischial tuberosity

Semimembranosus t

Conjoined t of semitendinosus and biceps femoris mm

Adductor magnus m

Semitendinosus m

Figure 24.2.3

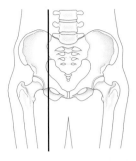

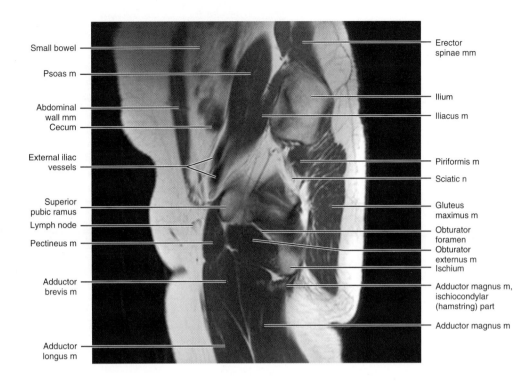

Small bowel

Psoas m

Abdominal wall mm

Cecum

External iliac vessels

Superior pubic ramus

Lymph node

Pectineus m

Adductor brevis m

Adductor longus m

Erector spinae mm

Ilium

Iliacus m

Piriformis m

Sciatic n

Gluteus maximus m

Obturator foramen

Obturator externus m

Ischium

Adductor magnus m, ischiocondylar (hamstring) part

Adductor magnus m

Figure 24.2.4

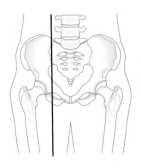

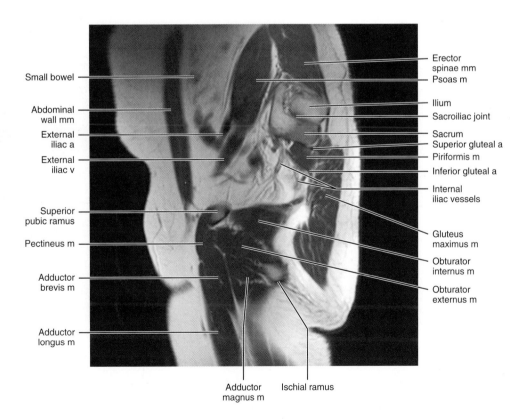

Small bowel

Abdominal wall mm

External iliac a

External iliac v

Superior pubic ramus

Pectineus m

Adductor brevis m

Adductor longus m

Erector spinae mm

Psoas m

Ilium

Sacroiliac joint

Sacrum

Superior gluteal a

Piriformis m

Inferior gluteal a

Internal iliac vessels

Gluteus maximus m

Obturator internus m

Obturator externus m

Adductor magnus m

Ischial ramus

Figure 24.2.5

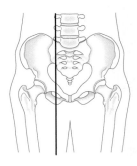

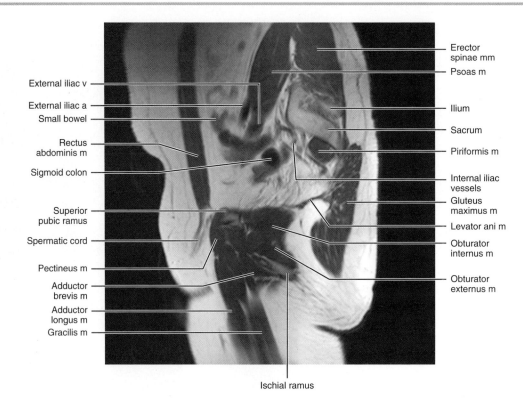

External iliac v

External iliac a

Small bowel

Rectus abdominis m

Sigmoid colon

Superior pubic ramus

Spermatic cord

Pectineus m

Adductor brevis m

Adductor longus m

Gracilis m

Erector spinae mm

Psoas m

Ilium

Sacrum

Piriformis m

Internal iliac vessels

Gluteus maximus m

Levator ani m

Obturator internus m

Obturator externus m

Ischial ramus

Figure 24.2.6

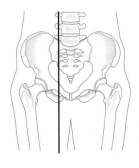

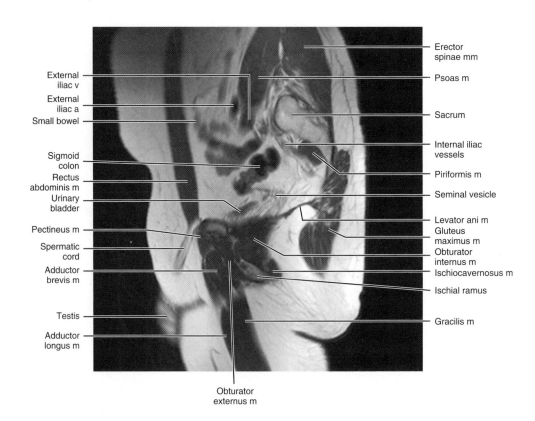

External iliac v

External iliac a

Small bowel

Sigmoid colon

Rectus abdominis m

Urinary bladder

Pectineus m

Spermatic cord

Adductor brevis m

Testis

Adductor longus m

Erector spinae mm

Psoas m

Sacrum

Internal iliac vessels

Piriformis m

Seminal vesicle

Levator ani m

Gluteus maximus m

Obturator internus m

Ischiocavernosus m

Ischial ramus

Gracilis m

Obturator externus m

Figure 24.2.7

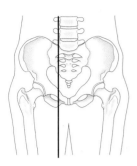

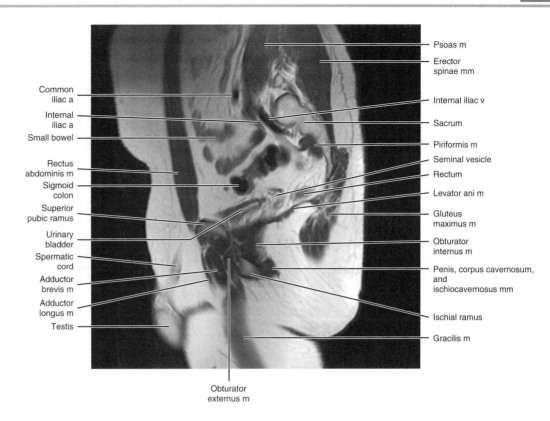

Common iliac a

Internal iliac a

Small bowel

Rectus abdominis m

Sigmoid colon

Superior pubic ramus

Urinary bladder

Spermatic cord

Adductor brevis m

Adductor longus m

Testis

Psoas m

Erector spinae mm

Internal iliac v

Sacrum

Piriformis m

Seminal vesicle

Rectum

Levator ani m

Gluteus maximus m

Obturator internus m

Penis, corpus cavernosum, and ischiocavernosus mm

Ischial ramus

Gracilis m

Obturator externus m

Figure 24.2.8

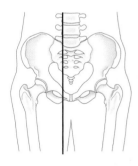

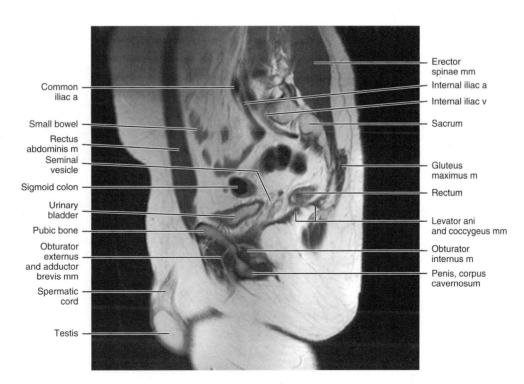

Common iliac a

Small bowel

Rectus abdominis m

Seminal vesicle

Sigmoid colon

Urinary bladder

Pubic bone

Obturator externus and adductor brevis mm

Spermatic cord

Testis

Erector spinae mm

Internal iliac a

Internal iliac v

Sacrum

Gluteus maximus m

Rectum

Levator ani and coccygeus mm

Obturator internus m

Penis, corpus cavernosum

Figure 24.2.9

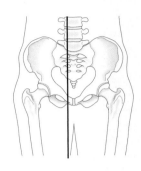

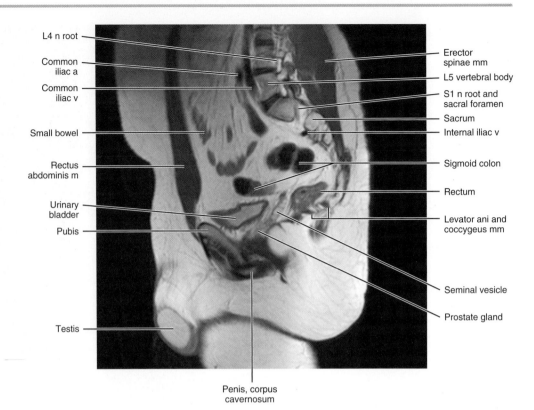

L4 n root

Common iliac a

Common iliac v

Small bowel

Rectus abdominis m

Urinary bladder

Pubis

Testis

Erector spinae mm

L5 vertebral body

S1 n root and sacral foramen

Sacrum

Internal iliac v

Sigmoid colon

Rectum

Levator ani and coccygeus mm

Seminal vesicle

Prostate gland

Penis, corpus cavernosum

Figure 24.2.10

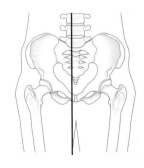

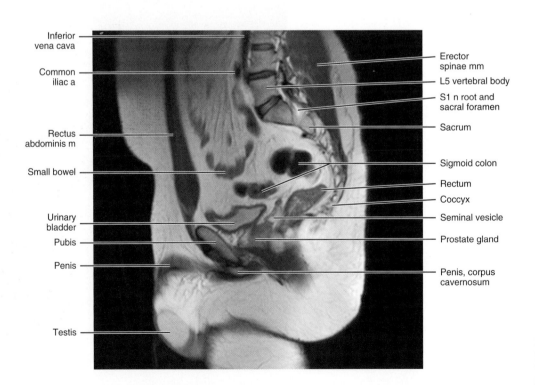

Inferior vena cava

Common iliac a

Rectus abdominis m

Small bowel

Urinary bladder

Pubis

Penis

Testis

Erector spinae mm

L5 vertebral body

S1 n root and sacral foramen

Sacrum

Sigmoid colon

Rectum

Coccyx

Seminal vesicle

Prostate gland

Penis, corpus cavernosum

Figure 24.2.11

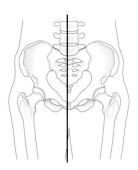

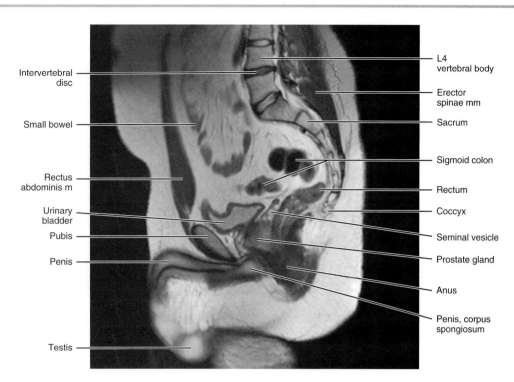

Intervertebral disc

Small bowel

Rectus abdominis m

Urinary bladder

Pubis

Penis

Testis

L4 vertebral body

Erector spinae mm

Sacrum

Sigmoid colon

Rectum

Coccyx

Seminal vesicle

Prostate gland

Anus

Penis, corpus spongiosum

Figure 24.2.12

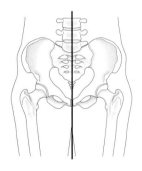

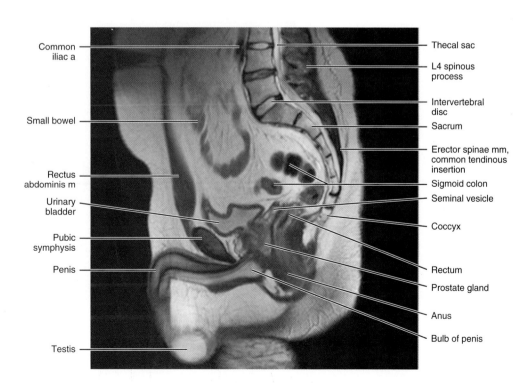

Common iliac a

Small bowel

Rectus abdominis m

Urinary bladder

Pubic symphysis

Penis

Testis

Thecal sac

L4 spinous process

Intervertebral disc

Sacrum

Erector spinae mm, common tendinous insertion

Sigmoid colon

Seminal vesicle

Coccyx

Rectum

Prostate gland

Anus

Bulb of penis

CORONAL

Figure 24.3.1

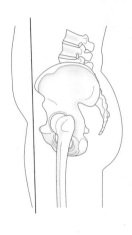

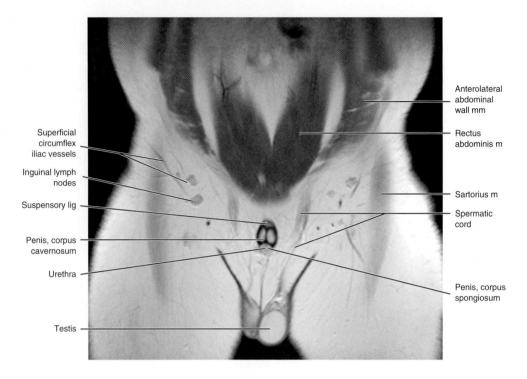

Superficial circumflex iliac vessels

Inguinal lymph nodes

Suspensory lig

Penis, corpus cavernosum

Urethra

Testis

Anterolateral abdominal wall mm

Rectus abdominis m

Sartorius m

Spermatic cord

Penis, corpus spongiosum

Figure 24.3.2

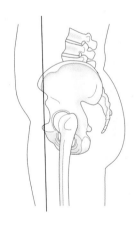

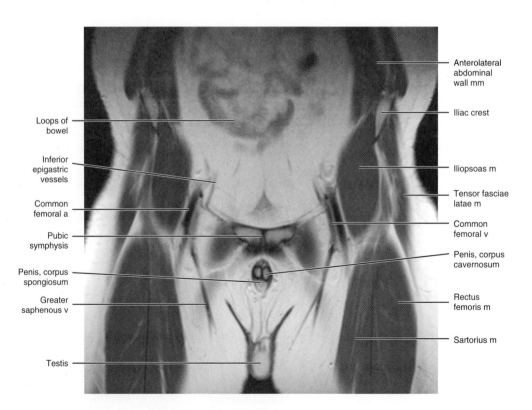

Loops of bowel

Inferior epigastric vessels

Common femoral a

Pubic symphysis

Penis, corpus spongiosum

Greater saphenous v

Testis

Anterolateral abdominal wall mm

Iliac crest

Iliopsoas m

Tensor fasciae latae m

Common femoral v

Penis, corpus cavernosum

Rectus femoris m

Sartorius m

Figure 24.3.3

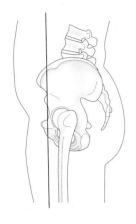

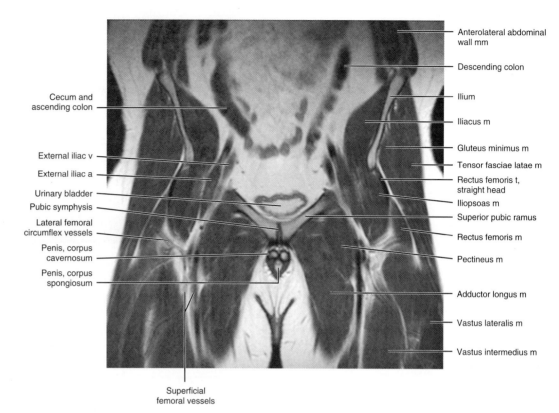

Cecum and ascending colon

External iliac v
External iliac a
Urinary bladder
Pubic symphysis
Lateral femoral circumflex vessels
Penis, corpus cavernosum
Penis, corpus spongiosum

Anterolateral abdominal wall mm
Descending colon
Ilium
Iliacus m
Gluteus minimus m
Tensor fasciae latae m
Rectus femoris t, straight head
Iliopsoas m
Superior pubic ramus
Rectus femoris m
Pectineus m
Adductor longus m
Vastus lateralis m
Vastus intermedius m

Superficial femoral vessels

Figure 24.3.4

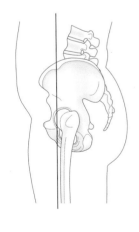

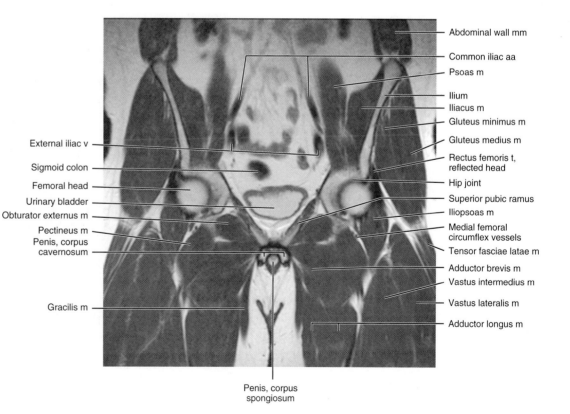

External iliac v
Sigmoid colon
Femoral head
Urinary bladder
Obturator externus m
Pectineus m
Penis, corpus cavernosum

Gracilis m

Abdominal wall mm
Common iliac aa
Psoas m
Ilium
Iliacus m
Gluteus minimus m
Gluteus medius m
Rectus femoris t, reflected head
Hip joint
Superior pubic ramus
Iliopsoas m
Medial femoral circumflex vessels
Tensor fasciae latae m
Adductor brevis m
Vastus intermedius m
Vastus lateralis m
Adductor longus m

Penis, corpus spongiosum

Figure 24.3.5

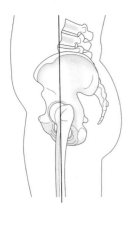

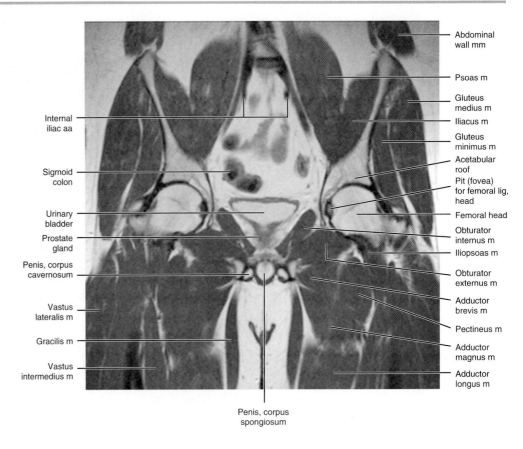

Internal
iliac aa

Sigmoid
colon

Urinary
bladder

Prostate
gland

Penis, corpus
cavernosum

Vastus
lateralis m

Gracilis m

Vastus
intermedius m

Abdominal
wall mm

Psoas m

Gluteus
medius m

Iliacus m

Gluteus
minimus m

Acetabular
roof

Pit (fovea)
for femoral lig,
head

Femoral head

Obturator
internus m

Iliopsoas m

Obturator
externus m

Adductor
brevis m

Pectineus m

Adductor
magnus m

Adductor
longus m

Penis, corpus
spongiosum

Figure 24.3.6

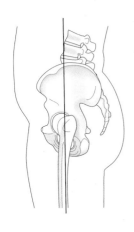

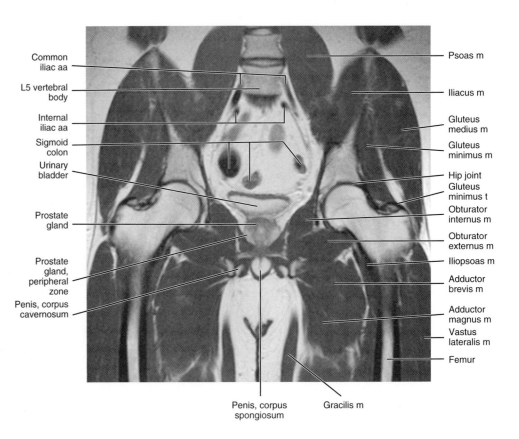

Common
iliac aa

L5 vertebral
body

Internal
iliac aa

Sigmoid
colon

Urinary
bladder

Prostate
gland

Prostate
gland,
peripheral
zone

Penis, corpus
cavernosum

Psoas m

Iliacus m

Gluteus
medius m

Gluteus
minimus m

Hip joint

Gluteus
minimus t

Obturator
internus m

Obturator
externus m

Iliopsoas m

Adductor
brevis m

Adductor
magnus m

Vastus
lateralis m

Femur

Penis, corpus
spongiosum

Gracilis m

Figure 24.3.7

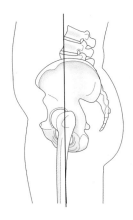

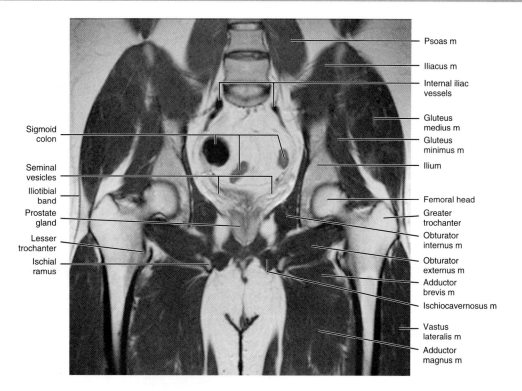

Psoas m

Iliacus m

Internal iliac vessels

Gluteus medius m

Gluteus minimus m

Ilium

Femoral head

Greater trochanter

Obturator internus m

Obturator externus m

Adductor brevis m

Ischiocavernosus m

Vastus lateralis m

Adductor magnus m

Sigmoid colon

Seminal vesicles

Iliotibial band

Prostate gland

Lesser trochanter

Ischial ramus

Figure 24.3.8

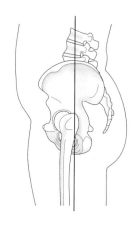

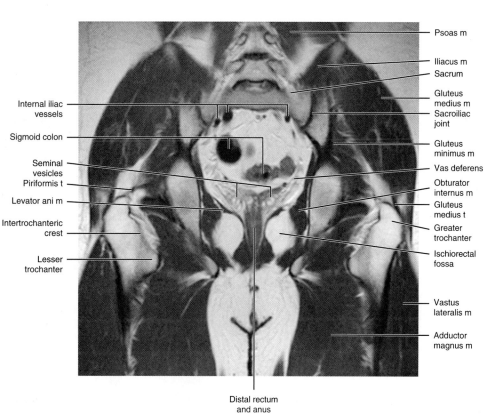

Psoas m

Iliacus m

Sacrum

Gluteus medius m

Sacroiliac joint

Gluteus minimus m

Vas deferens

Obturator internus m

Gluteus medius t

Greater trochanter

Ischiorectal fossa

Vastus lateralis m

Adductor magnus m

Internal iliac vessels

Sigmoid colon

Seminal vesicles

Piriformis t

Levator ani m

Intertrochanteric crest

Lesser trochanter

Distal rectum and anus

Figure 24.3.9

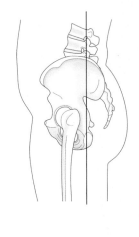

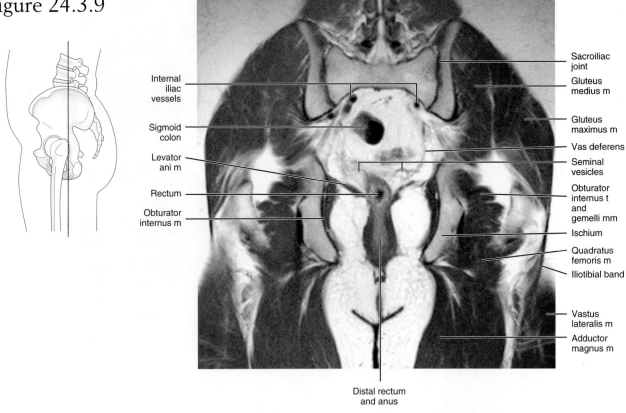

Internal iliac vessels

Sigmoid colon

Levator ani m

Rectum

Obturator internus m

Sacroiliac joint

Gluteus medius m

Gluteus maximus m

Vas deferens

Seminal vesicles

Obturator internus t and gemelli mm

Ischium

Quadratus femoris m

Iliotibial band

Vastus lateralis m

Adductor magnus m

Distal rectum and anus

Figure 24.3.10

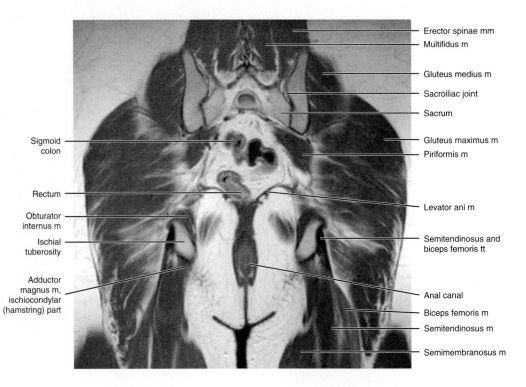

Sigmoid colon

Rectum

Obturator internus m

Ischial tuberosity

Adductor magnus m, ischiocondylar (hamstring) part

Erector spinae mm

Multifidus m

Gluteus medius m

Sacroiliac joint

Sacrum

Gluteus maximus m

Piriformis m

Levator ani m

Semitendinosus and biceps femoris tt

Anal canal

Biceps femoris m

Semitendinosus m

Semimembranosus m

Figure 24.3.11

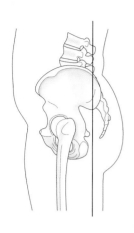

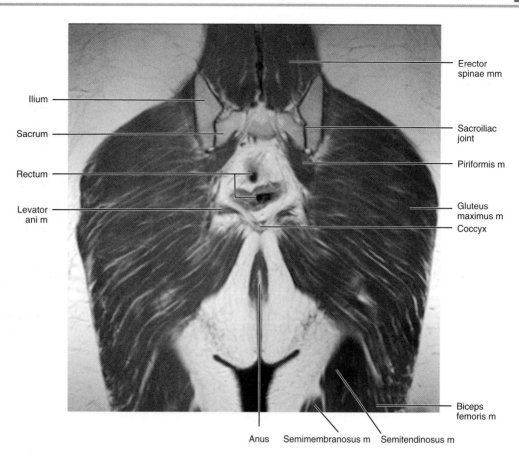

Ilium

Sacrum

Rectum

Levator ani m

Erector spinae mm

Sacroiliac joint

Piriformis m

Gluteus maximus m

Coccyx

Biceps femoris m

Anus   Semimembranosus m   Semitendinosus m

Figure 24.3.12

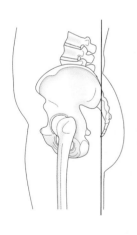

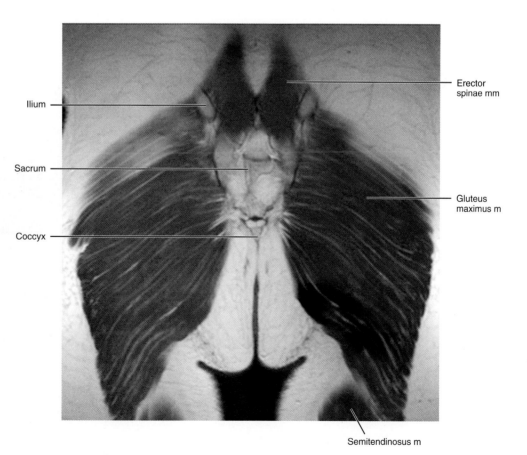

Ilium

Sacrum

Coccyx

Erector spinae mm

Gluteus maximus m

Semitendinosus m

Chapter 25

MRI of the Female Pelvis

AXIAL

Figure 25.1.1

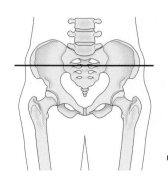

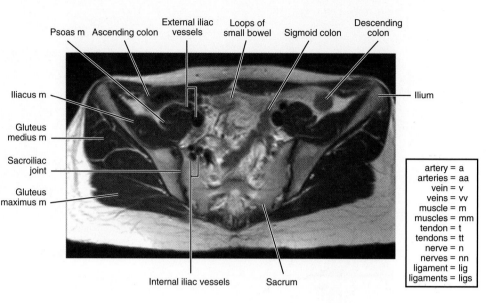

Psoas m   Ascending colon   External iliac vessels   Loops of small bowel   Sigmoid colon   Descending colon

Iliacus m

Gluteus medius m

Sacroiliac joint

Gluteus maximus m

Ilium

Internal iliac vessels   Sacrum

| artery = a |
| arteries = aa |
| vein = v |
| veins = vv |
| muscle = m |
| muscles = mm |
| tendon = t |
| tendons = tt |
| nerve = n |
| nerves = nn |
| ligament = lig |
| ligaments = ligs |

Figure 25.1.2

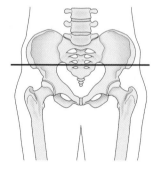

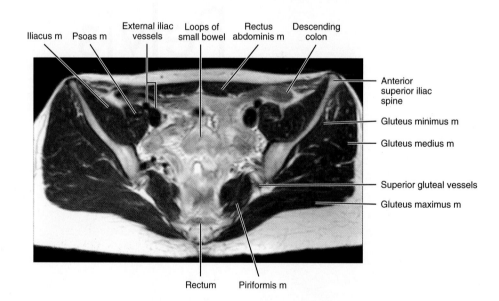

Iliacus m   Psoas m   External iliac vessels   Loops of small bowel   Rectus abdominis m   Descending colon

Anterior superior iliac spine

Gluteus minimus m

Gluteus medius m

Superior gluteal vessels

Gluteus maximus m

Rectum   Piriformis m

Figure 25.1.3

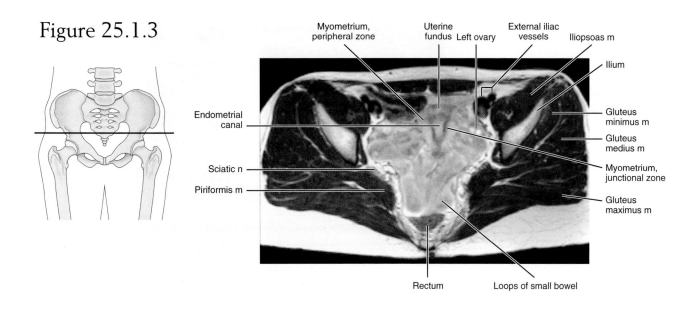

Myometrium, peripheral zone

Uterine fundus

Left ovary

External iliac vessels

Iliopsoas m

Ilium

Endometrial canal

Gluteus minimus m

Gluteus medius m

Sciatic n

Myometrium, junctional zone

Piriformis m

Gluteus maximus m

Rectum

Loops of small bowel

Figure 25.1.4

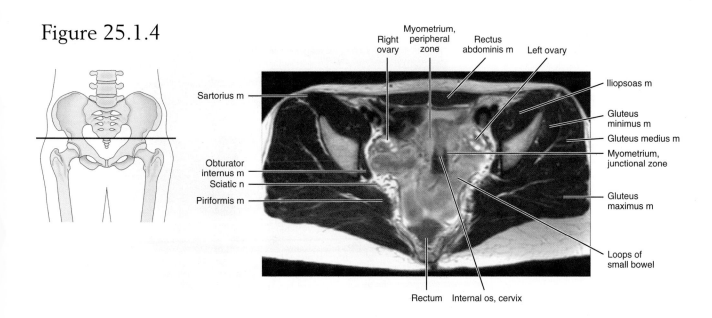

Right ovary

Myometrium, peripheral zone

Rectus abdominis m

Left ovary

Sartorius m

Iliopsoas m

Gluteus minimus m

Gluteus medius m

Obturator internus m

Myometrium, junctional zone

Sciatic n

Piriformis m

Gluteus maximus m

Loops of small bowel

Rectum

Internal os, cervix

Figure 25.1.5

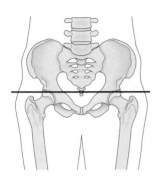

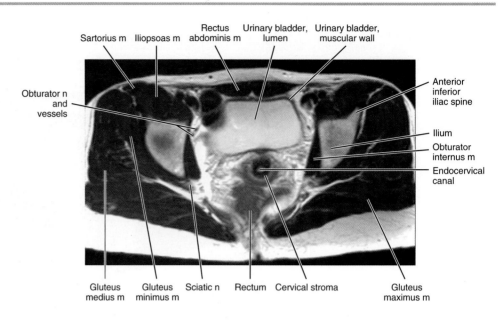

Sartorius m · Iliopsoas m · Rectus abdominis m · Urinary bladder, lumen · Urinary bladder, muscular wall · Anterior inferior iliac spine · Ilium · Obturator internus m · Endocervical canal · Obturator n and vessels · Gluteus medius m · Gluteus minimus m · Sciatic n · Rectum · Cervical stroma · Gluteus maximus m

Figure 25.1.6

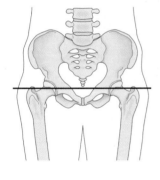

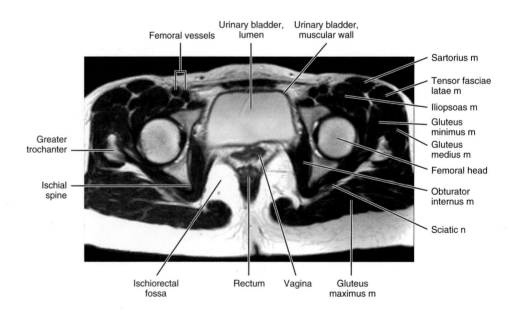

Femoral vessels · Urinary bladder, lumen · Urinary bladder, muscular wall · Sartorius m · Tensor fasciae latae m · Iliopsoas m · Gluteus minimus m · Gluteus medius m · Femoral head · Obturator internus m · Sciatic n · Greater trochanter · Ischial spine · Ischiorectal fossa · Rectum · Vagina · Gluteus maximus m

Figure 25.1.7

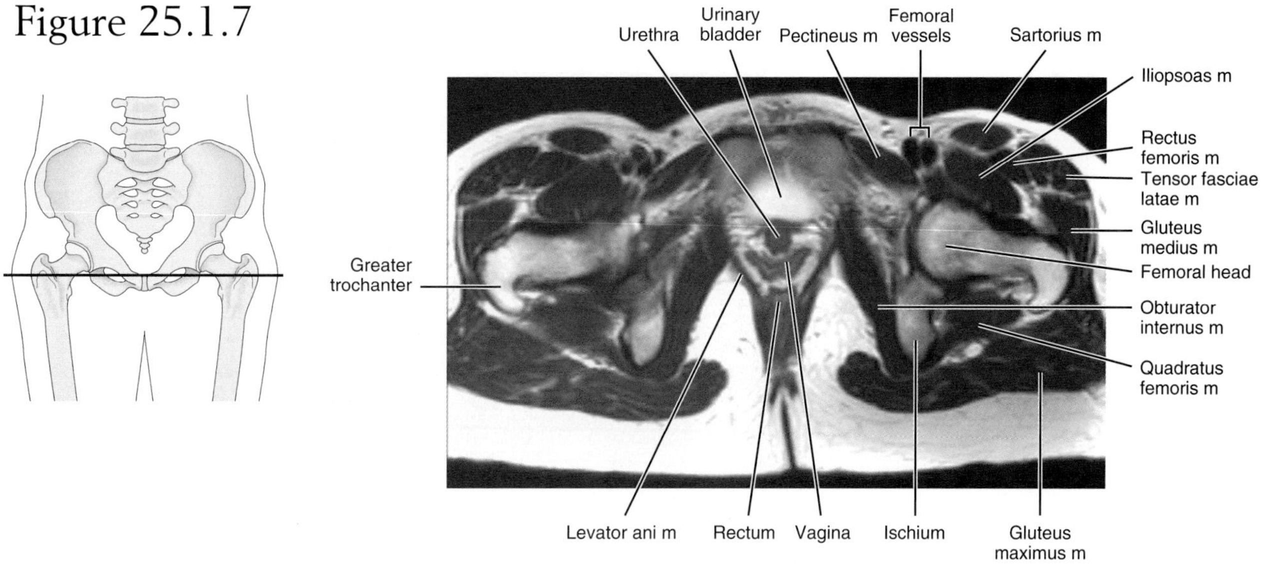

Urethra
Urinary bladder
Pectineus m
Femoral vessels
Sartorius m
Iliopsoas m
Rectus femoris m
Tensor fasciae latae m
Gluteus medius m
Femoral head
Obturator internus m
Quadratus femoris m
Greater trochanter
Levator ani m
Rectum
Vagina
Ischium
Gluteus maximus m

Figure 25.1.8

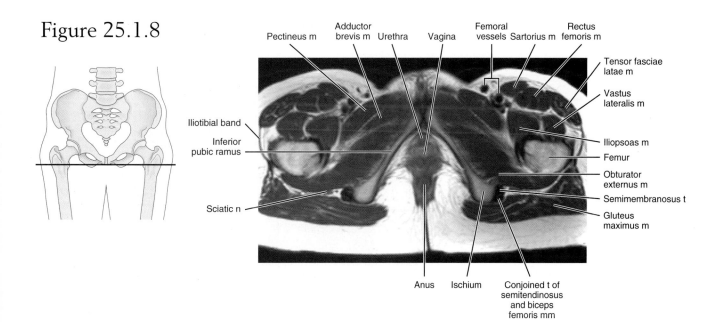

Pectineus m
Adductor brevis m
Urethra
Vagina
Femoral vessels
Sartorius m
Rectus femoris m
Tensor fasciae latae m
Vastus lateralis m
Iliotibial band
Inferior pubic ramus
Iliopsoas m
Femur
Obturator externus m
Semimembranosus t
Gluteus maximus m
Sciatic n
Anus
Ischium
Conjoined t of semitendinosus and biceps femoris mm

SAGITTAL

Figure 25.2.1

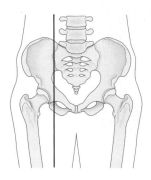

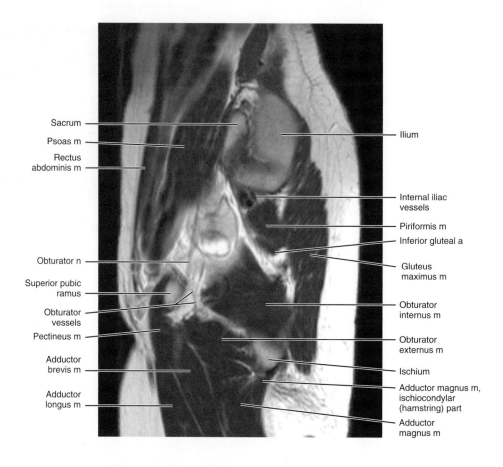

Sacrum

Psoas m

Rectus abdominis m

Ilium

Internal iliac vessels

Piriformis m

Inferior gluteal a

Obturator n

Gluteus maximus m

Superior pubic ramus

Obturator vessels

Obturator internus m

Pectineus m

Obturator externus m

Adductor brevis m

Ischium

Adductor magnus m, ischiocondylar (hamstring) part

Adductor longus m

Adductor magnus m

Figure 25.2.2

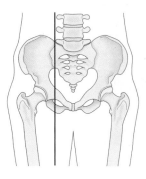

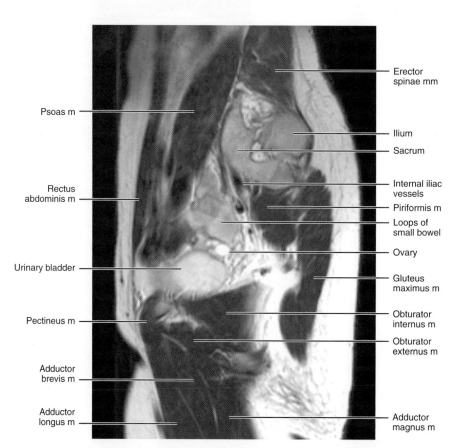

Psoas m

Erector spinae mm

Ilium

Sacrum

Rectus abdominis m

Internal iliac vessels

Piriformis m

Loops of small bowel

Ovary

Urinary bladder

Gluteus maximus m

Pectineus m

Obturator internus m

Obturator externus m

Adductor brevis m

Adductor longus m

Adductor magnus m

Figure 25.2.3

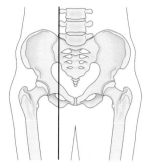

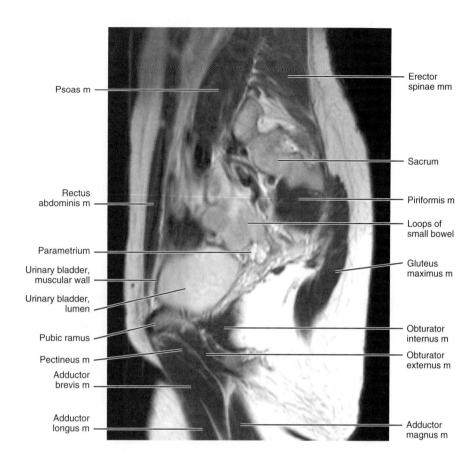

Psoas m

Rectus abdominis m

Parametrium

Urinary bladder, muscular wall

Urinary bladder, lumen

Pubic ramus

Pectineus m

Adductor brevis m

Adductor longus m

Erector spinae mm

Sacrum

Piriformis m

Loops of small bowel

Gluteus maximus m

Obturator internus m

Obturator externus m

Adductor magnus m

Figure 25.2.4

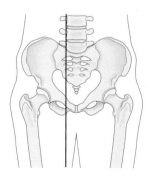

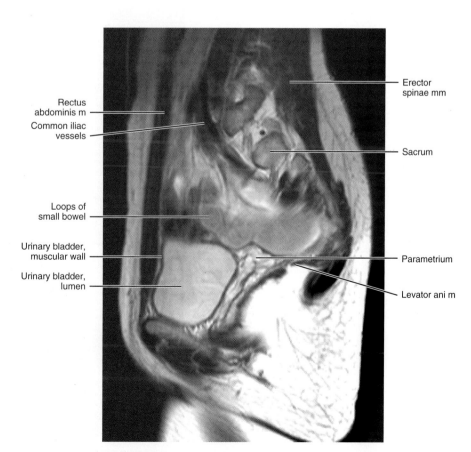

Rectus abdominis m

Common iliac vessels

Loops of small bowel

Urinary bladder, muscular wall

Urinary bladder, lumen

Erector spinae mm

Sacrum

Parametrium

Levator ani m

Figure 25.2.5

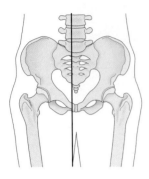

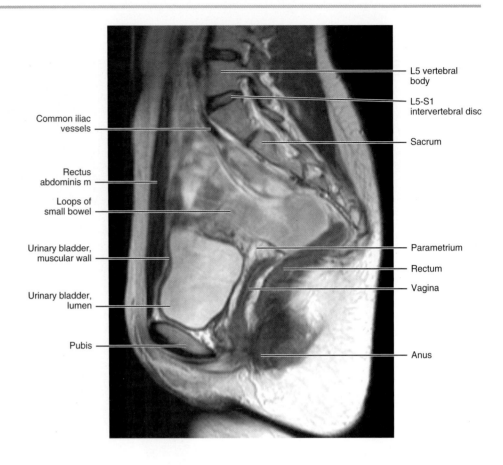

Common iliac vessels

Rectus abdominis m

Loops of small bowel

Urinary bladder, muscular wall

Urinary bladder, lumen

Pubis

L5 vertebral body

L5-S1 intervertebral disc

Sacrum

Parametrium

Rectum

Vagina

Anus

Figure 25.2.6

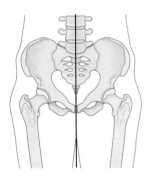

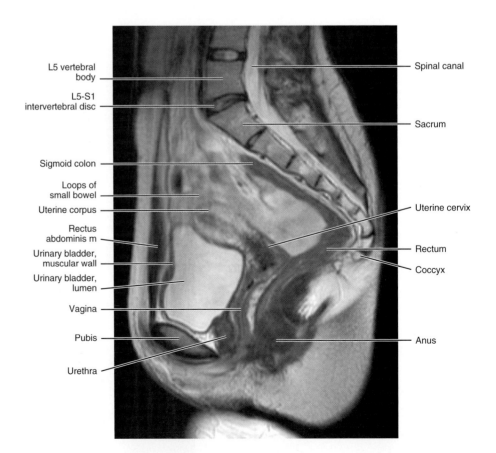

L5 vertebral body

L5-S1 intervertebral disc

Sigmoid colon

Loops of small bowel

Uterine corpus

Rectus abdominis m

Urinary bladder, muscular wall

Urinary bladder, lumen

Vagina

Pubis

Urethra

Spinal canal

Sacrum

Uterine cervix

Rectum

Coccyx

Anus

Figure 25.2.7

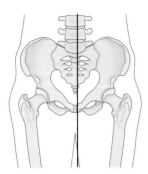

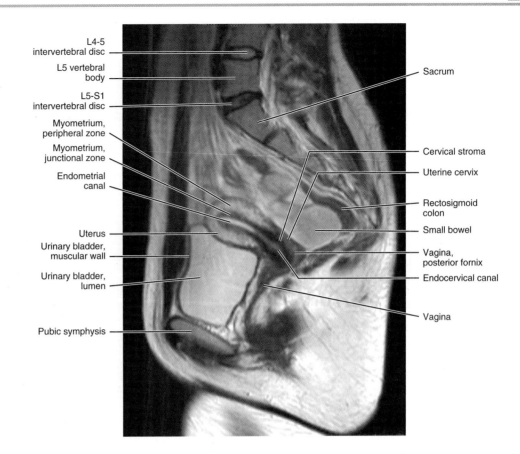

L4-5 intervertebral disc

L5 vertebral body

L5-S1 intervertebral disc

Myometrium, peripheral zone

Myometrium, junctional zone

Endometrial canal

Uterus

Urinary bladder, muscular wall

Urinary bladder, lumen

Pubic symphysis

Sacrum

Cervical stroma

Uterine cervix

Rectosigmoid colon

Small bowel

Vagina, posterior fornix

Endocervical canal

Vagina

CORONAL

Figure 25.3.1

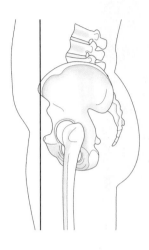

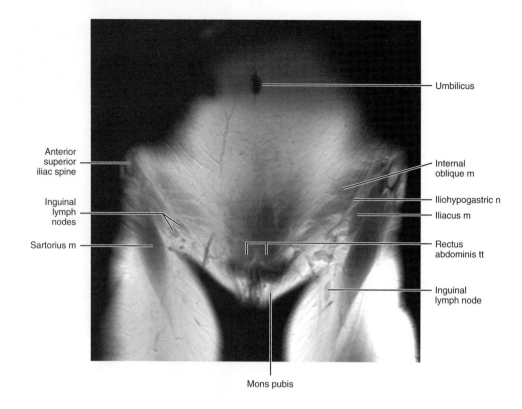

Umbilicus

Anterior superior iliac spine

Internal oblique m

Iliohypogastric n

Iliacus m

Inguinal lymph nodes

Sartorius m

Rectus abdominis tt

Inguinal lymph node

Mons pubis

Figure 25.3.2

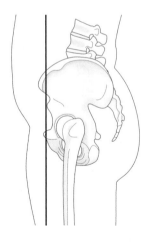

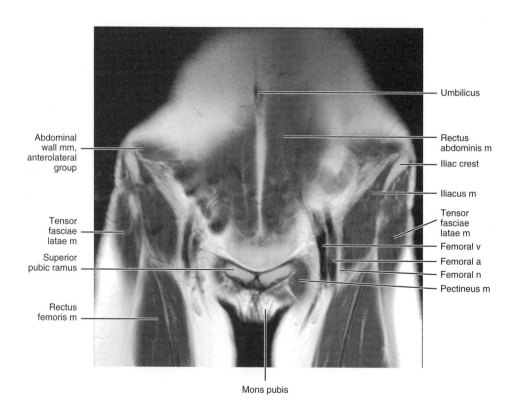

Umbilicus

Abdominal wall mm, anterolateral group

Rectus abdominis m

Iliac crest

Iliacus m

Tensor fasciae latae m

Tensor fasciae latae m

Femoral v

Superior pubic ramus

Femoral a

Femoral n

Pectineus m

Rectus femoris m

Mons pubis

Figure 25.3.3

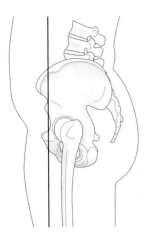

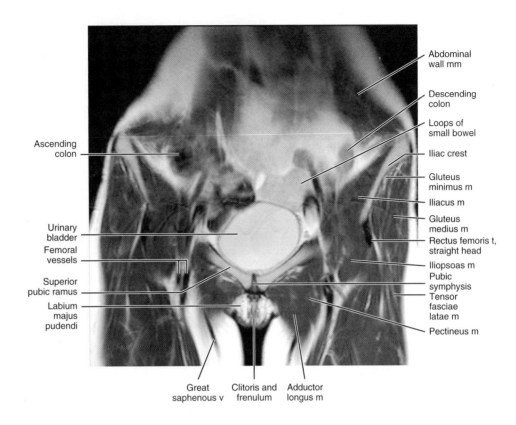

Ascending
colon

Urinary
bladder

Femoral
vessels

Superior
pubic ramus

Labium
majus
pudendi

Abdominal
wall mm

Descending
colon

Loops of
small bowel

Iliac crest

Gluteus
minimus m

Iliacus m

Gluteus
medius m

Rectus femoris t,
straight head

Iliopsoas m

Pubic
symphysis

Tensor
fasciae
latae m

Pectineus m

Great
saphenous v

Clitoris and
frenulum

Adductor
longus m

Figure 25.3.4

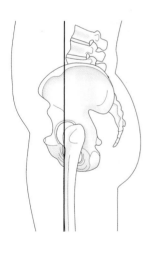

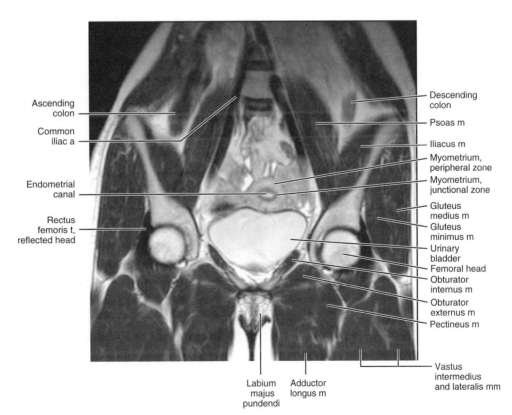

Ascending
colon

Common
iliac a

Endometrial
canal

Rectus
femoris t,
reflected head

Descending
colon

Psoas m

Iliacus m

Myometrium,
peripheral zone

Myometrium,
junctional zone

Gluteus
medius m

Gluteus
minimus m

Urinary
bladder

Femoral head

Obturator
internus m

Obturator
externus m

Pectineus m

Labium
majus
pundendi

Adductor
longus m

Vastus
intermedius
and lateralis mm

Figure 25.3.5

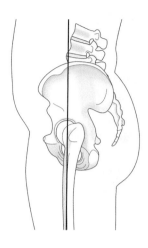

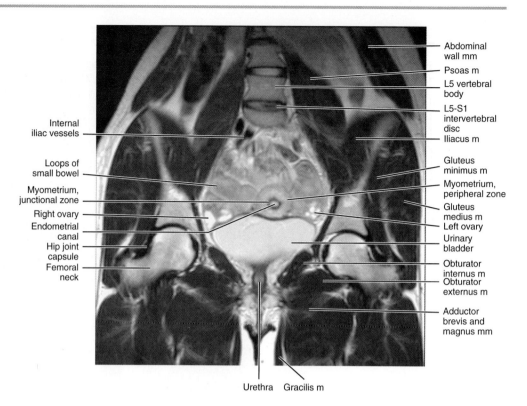

Internal iliac vessels

Loops of small bowel

Myometrium, junctional zone

Right ovary

Endometrial canal

Hip joint capsule

Femoral neck

Abdominal wall mm

Psoas m

L5 vertebral body

L5-S1 intervertebral disc

Iliacus m

Gluteus minimus m

Myometrium, peripheral zone

Gluteus medius m

Left ovary

Urinary bladder

Obturator internus m

Obturator externus m

Adductor brevis and magnus mm

Urethra   Gracilis m

Figure 25.3.6

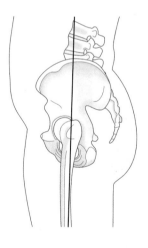

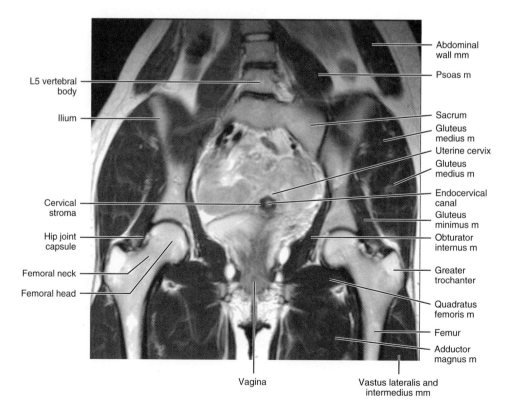

L5 vertebral body

Ilium

Cervical stroma

Hip joint capsule

Femoral neck

Femoral head

Abdominal wall mm

Psoas m

Sacrum

Gluteus medius m

Uterine cervix

Gluteus medius m

Endocervical canal

Gluteus minimus m

Obturator internus m

Greater trochanter

Quadratus femoris m

Femur

Adductor magnus m

Vagina   Vastus lateralis and intermedius mm

Figure 25.3.7

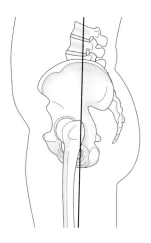

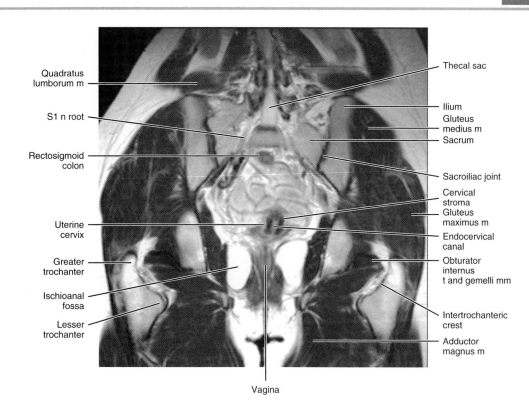

Quadratus
lumborum m

S1 n root

Rectosigmoid
colon

Uterine
cervix

Greater
trochanter

Ischioanal
fossa

Lesser
trochanter

Thecal sac

Ilium

Gluteus
medius m

Sacrum

Sacroiliac joint

Cervical
stroma

Gluteus
maximus m

Endocervical
canal

Obturator
internus
t and gemelli mm

Intertrochanteric
crest

Adductor
magnus m

Vagina

Figure 25.3.8

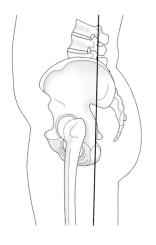

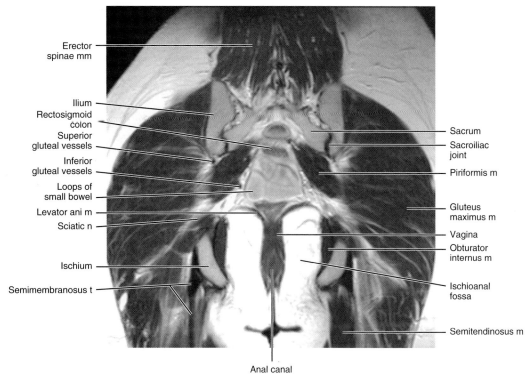

Erector
spinae mm

Ilium

Rectosigmoid
colon

Superior
gluteal vessels

Inferior
gluteal vessels

Loops of
small bowel

Levator ani m

Sciatic n

Ischium

Semimembranosus t

Sacrum

Sacroiliac
joint

Piriformis m

Gluteus
maximus m

Vagina

Obturator
internus m

Ischioanal
fossa

Semitendinosus m

Anal canal

Figure 25.3.9

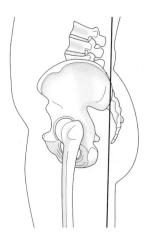

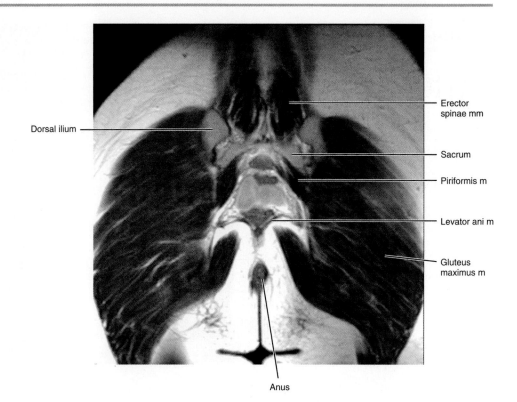

Dorsal ilium

Erector spinae mm

Sacrum

Piriformis m

Levator ani m

Gluteus maximus m

Anus

Index

Note: Page numbers followed by t indicate tables. a. = artery; ABER = abduction external rotation; lig. = ligament; ligs. = ligaments; m. = muscle; n. = nerve; t. = tendon; v. = vein